D1614217

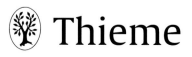

Intervertebral Disk Diseases

Causes, Diagnosis, Treatment, and Prophylaxis

Juergen Kraemer, MD

Professor Emeritus
Formerly Orthopedic University Clinic
St. Josef Hospital
Bochum, Germany
Institute for Spine Research
at the Ruhr University
Bochum, Germany

3rd edition

With contributions by
Monika Hasenbring, Robert Kraemer, Ethan Taub,
Theodoros Theodoridis, Hans-Joachim Wilke

560 illustrations

Thieme
Stuttgart · New York

Library of Congress-in-Publication Data
Krämer, Jürgen, 1939-

  [Bandscheibenbedingte Erkrankungen. English]
  Intervertebral disk diseases : causes, diagnosis, treatment, and prophylaxis / Juergen Kraemer ; with contributions by Monika Hasenbring ... [et al.] ; translated by Ethan Taub ; illustrators, Christiane and Michael von Solodkoff. – 3rd ed.

     p. ; cm.
  Includes bibliographical references and index.
  ISBN 978-3-13-582403-1 (alk. paper)
  1. Intervertebral disk—Diseases. 2. Intervertebral disk—Surgery.
I. Title.
  [DNLM: 1. Intervertebral Disk. 2. Intervertebral Disk Displacement. 3. Magnetic Resonance Imaging. 4. Spinal Diseases. WE 740 K89b 2008a]
  RD771.I6K7313 2008
  617.5'6–dc22

       2008031810

This book is an authorized and revised translation of the German edition published and copyrighted 2006 by Georg Thieme Verlag, Stuttgart, Germany. Title of the German edition: Bandscheibenbedingte Erkrankungen. Ursachen, Diagnose, Behandlung, Vorbeugung, Begutachtung.

Translator: Ethan Taub, MD, Basel, Switzerland

Illustrators: Christiane and Michael von Solodkoff, MD, Neckargemünd, Germany

Important note: Medicine is an ever-changing science undergoing continual development. Research and clinical experience are continually expanding our knowledge, in particular our knowledge of proper treatment and drug therapy. Insofar as this book mentions any dosage or application, readers may rest assured that the authors, editors, and publishers have made every effort to ensure that such references are in accordance with **the state of knowledge at the time of production of the book.**

Nevertheless, this does not involve, imply, or express any guarantee or responsibility on the part of the publishers in respect to any dosage instructions and forms of applications stated in the book. **Every user is requested to examine carefully** the manufacturers' leaflets accompanying each drug and to check, if necessary in consultation with a physician or specialist, whether the dosage schedules mentioned therein or the contraindications stated by the manufacturers differ from the statements made in the present book. Such examination is particularly important with drugs that are either rarely used or have been newly released on the market. Every dosage schedule or every form of application used is entirely at the user's own risk and responsibility. The authors and publishers request every user to report to the publishers any discrepancies or inaccuracies noticed. If errors in this work are found after publication, errata will be posted at www.thieme.com on the product description page.

© 2009 Georg Thieme Verlag KG
Rüdigerstrasse 14, 70469 Stuttgart, Germany
http://www.thieme.de
Thieme New York, 333 Seventh Avenue,
New York, NY 10001, USA
http://www.thieme.com

Cover design: Thieme Publishing Group
Typesetting by primustype Hurler GmbH, Notzingen, Germany

Printed in Germany by Appl aprinta druck, Wemding

ISBN 978-3-13-582403-1   1 2 3 4 5 6

Contributors

Professor Monika Hasenbring, PhD
Department of Medical Psychology
at the Ruhr University
Bochum, Germany

Robert Kraemer, MD
Centro Medico Tecnon
Barcelona, Spain

Ethan Taub, MD
Supervising Physician
Department of Neurosurgery
University Hospital of Basel
Basel, Switzerland

Theodoros Theodoridis, MD
Institute for Spine Research
at the Ruhr University
Bochum, Germany

Professor Hans Joachim Wilke, PhD
Institute for Research in Trauma Surgery
and Biomechanics
University of Ulm
Ulm, Germany

Preface

There have been numerous developments in the diagnosis and treatment of intervertebral disk diseases since the last edition. In many industrialized countries, back problems attract increasing attention; it is now generally understood that they affect a very high proportion of the population and give rise to enormous costs. Low back pain also forms a central topic of the Bone and Joint Decade, which is currently in progress.

This new English edition is the product of a thorough revision. It incorporates the most recent additions to our understanding of spine biomechanics, which were contributed by Professor H. J. Wilke (engineering). The sections on psychology and the treatment of pain were updated by Professor M. Hasenbring (medical psychology).

The clinical diagnosis of disk diseases is now centered on magnetic resonance imaging (MRI). This all-encompassing radiological study has largely displaced myelography, discography, and finally even CT as the diagnostic method of choice for disk diseases. This book contains many striking images of MRI scans, taken from an atlas that I compiled a few years ago together with Professor O. Köster (a radiologist). In my own institution, the last few years have witnessed new developments in both the conservative and the operative treatment of disk diseases. Spinal injection techniques have been improved in collaboration with Dr. T. Theodoridis, while the microsurgical treatment of lumbar disk herniation has been improved in collaboration with Professor J. Herdmann (neurosurgery) and Dr. Robert Kraemer (orthopedic surgeon).

I would like to thank Dr. Ethan Taub for his thorough editing and his additions to our original work. His contribution is of immense value for a better international understanding of intervertebral disk diseases.

My thanks also go to all those who have enabled me to write a monograph on such a wide topic. I also thank Georg Thieme Verlag for the large and attractive format of the book.

Juergen Kraemer

Table of Contents

Introduction

Of all the disorders affecting the intervertebral disks, **degenerative conditions** are by far the most common, to such an extent that conditions of other causes—neoplastic, infectious/inflammatory, and developmental—are of only secondary clinical importance. Degenerative disturbances of the structure and function of the intervertebral disks have attracted a great deal of attention in recent decades, both because of their wide intrinsic variety and because of their widespread effects on other organs. At first, the discovery of the causal relation between disk prolapse and sciatica led physicians interested in the subject to concentrate on the structural, rather than functional, properties of the disks. This almost exclusive focus on **pathoanatomical changes** led to a situation in which functional disturbances of the spine unaccompanied by objectively detectable structural abnormalities were most often dealt with, not by physicians, but by other types of practitioners. It was soon realized that mere removal of the disk prolapse did not solve all of the patient's problems. All too often, there was a remarkable discrepancy between the patient's radiologically defined pathoanatomical condition on the one hand, and the symptoms on the other.

Despite a widely expressed belief to the contrary, structural and functional disturbances of the motion segment do not always appear simultaneously. Morphological abnormalities do not cause symptoms in every patient. Indeed, various types of deformity, such as scoliosis and juvenile kyphosis, are often asymptomatic.

> The main determinant of whether symptoms will arise is the *length of time* over which the structural deformity of the motion segment developed.

Sudden impingement on a nerve root by a fracture or disk prolapse produces very severe symptoms. If a nerve is gradually stretched, however, as in idiopathic scoliosis or spondylolisthesis, the organism is able to adapt so that no neurological symptoms will arise.

Our current **functional–dynamic approach** is based on recent advances in biochemistry and biomechanics. It is possible for the function of the spine as a whole to be impaired by changes in tissue volume and consistency, deep within the intervertebral disk, that cannot be detected with the usual morphological techniques. Each disk, the vertebrae above and below, and the associated spinal ligaments and muscles make up a

functional unit that Junghanns (1951) appropriately named the "motion segment." A disturbance in any component of this unit inevitably affects all of the other components as well. The mechanical stress of movement is distributed among all components of the motion segment, but the intervertebral disk is more vulnerable to disease than the rest, because of the special nature of its metabolism. Symptoms most commonly arise in the lower motion segments of the cervical and lumbar spine, which are sites of transition between relatively fixed and relatively mobile parts of the trunk. Furthermore, the structures delimiting the intervertebral disks at these levels lie in close proximity to the spinal nerve roots and are thus likely to impinge on them if they become pathologically deformed.

Of necessity, therefore, any monograph on intervertebral disks must concern itself largely with pathological states of the lower cervical and lumbar segments. As the title of this book implies, we have consciously chosen to focus the present discussion on **clinical disorders.** Other topics such as embryology, histopathology, electron microscopy, and special surgical techniques are discussed here only as far as their practical importance warrants. The common features of all intervertebral disk disorders have been highlighted to facilitate diagnosis and simplify treatment. One such feature is the positional dependence of the pain, i. e., its tendency to vary with the patient's posture or lying position.

All diagnostic and therapeutic measures must be chosen with care to satisfy four important conditions, as stated by the *MIRACLE* principle: a good intervention is one that has

> **M**inimal
> **I**nvasiveness,
> **R**isks,
> **A**nd
> **C**ost,
> but has a
> **L**asting
> **E**ffect.

The *MIRACLE* principle must be stressed, because, while the available diagnostic and therapeutic techniques are becoming ever more complicated and expensive, most disk diseases still take a relatively benign course. Most of the patients affected are fairly young; thus, no matter

1

what course of therapy is decided on and pursued, it should conclude with the physician's giving the patient a **set of behavioral instructions** for the future. Only a few years ago, the development and progression of intervertebral disk disease still seemed to be inexorable, and we physicians were cast in the role of helpless onlookers. Today, by contrast, a program of **back school,** combined with a rational strategy of rehabilitation and disease prevention, can be used successfully to lessen the frequency and intensity of cervical and lumbar syndromes.

We polled a number of European centers for spinal disorders by questionnaire (Bernsmann 2000) and identified *magnetic resonance imaging (MRI)* as the diagnostic technique for disk disease that was most favored by the respondents, and *physiotherapy* as the most favored treatment, in accordance with the *MIRACLE* principle enunciated above.

2 History and Terminology

■ History

Spinal degenerative changes and intervertebral disk diseases are as old as humanity itself. Skeletal remains from all periods, from the era of early humans to modern times, yield plentiful evidence of damage to the vertebral column by wear and tear. Even though intervertebral disk diseases and the related pains in the shoulders, neck, low back, and lower limb are now quite common and are often held to be "diseases of civilization," it turns out that our remote forebears suffered from them as well. Nor can it be said that the high prevalence of these conditions merely reflects today's longer life expectancy, because they often affect relatively young people.

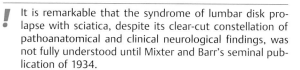

! It is remarkable that the syndrome of lumbar disk prolapse with sciatica, despite its clear-cut constellation of pathoanatomical and clinical neurological findings, was not fully understood until Mixter and Barr's seminal publication of 1934.

Decades before Mixter and Barr, anatomical dissection methods and surgical technique had advanced to the point that their discovery could easily have been anticipated. Indeed, some of the major medical writers of the ancient world and the Middle Ages had already surmised that the cause of sciatica lay in the intervertebral disk (**Table 2.1**).

Table 2.1 History of the medical and scientific understanding of intervertebral disk disease

Author(s)	Year	Event
Hippocrates	460–377 BC	Description of sciatica as "hip pain"; treatment by cauterization with a hot poker
Galen of Pergamon	AD 129–199	Lifestyle as cause of sciatica. Treatment: bloodletting in popliteal fossa, emetics
Andreas Vesalius	1543	Thorough description of the intervertebral disks
Sydenham	1624–1689	Coins the term "lumbago"; treatment by vomiting, purging, and sweating
Cotugno	1736–1822	Precise description of the signs and symptoms of sciatica. Treatment with warm compresses, massage, poultices
Bretschneider	1847	Describes the so-called sciatic pressure points
Valleix	1852	Re-describes the "Valleix" pressure points already described by Bretschneider
Lasègue	1864	Describes sciatica in *Considérations sur la sciatique*
Charcot	1888	Thorough description of the postural abnormality accompanying sciatica
Krause and Oppenheim	1909	Cauda equina compression by disk tissue
Goldthwait	1911	Recognition of intervertebral disk lesions as a cause of sciatica and cauda equina compression
Dandy	1919	Description of pneumoencephalography (and pneumomyelography)
Sicard and Forestier	1922	Injection of lipiodol into the lumbar theca as a positive contrast medium for the localization of spinal tumors
Schmorl	1928	Description of disk herniation into the vertebral body (Schmorl's nodes)
Mixter and Barr	1934	Description of disk herniation as a cause of sciatica; treatment by operative removal of the prolapsed material via hemilaminectomy

2

Table 2.1 (Continued)

Author(s)	Year	Event
Bärtschi-Rochaix	1949	Degenerative changes of the cervical disks as a cause of "cervical migraine"
Junghanns	1951	Coins the term "motion segment," laying the groundwork for the modern biomechanical and biochemical understanding of the disk
L. Smith	1964	Intradiscal chymopapain injection for the treatment of disk protrusions
Oldendorf, Hounsfield, Ambrose	1961, 1973, 1973	Development of compter tomography (CT) for pathoanatomical diagnosis of many conditions, including spinal diseases
Lauterbur, Mansfield	1973	Development of magnetic resonance imaging (MRI)

Pre-Christian Times

Hippocrates (460–437 BC), for example, described a patient with pain in the hip, lower portion of the sacrum, and buttock, radiating into the leg. His treatment consisted, among other things, of baths and warm compresses, both of which are still in use today (Hippocrates 1897).

AD 1–1700

Galen of Pergamon (AD 128–199) held that certain aspects of the patient's lifestyle, such as sexual excess, over-consumption of wine, and idleness, were major contributing causes of sciatica. His treatment consisted in purification of the body, e. g., by bloodletting.

There were no major advances in the understanding of intervertebral disk disease for many centuries thereafter, notwithstanding the first precise description of the intervertebral disk by **Vesalius** in 1543 (see References) and the description of lumbago by **Sydenham** (1624–1689).

1700–1900

It was not until 1764 that **Cotugno** (1736–1822) published the first comprehensive work dealing with sciatica, *De ischiade nervosa commentarius* ("remarks on nervous sciatica"). His observations regarding diagnosis and treatment advanced the understanding of this condition so greatly that it came to be known in medical circles as "malum Cotunii"—Cotugno disease. The decades that followed saw further advances by others whose names are connected with clinical tests that are still in use today. The pressure points along the course of the sciatic nerve that were described by **Valleix** in 1852 are still known by his name, even though they had already been precisely described by **Bretschneider** 5 years earlier. One searches in vain for the sciatic nerve stretch test, the so-called "Lasègue test," in *Considérations sur la sciatique,* Lasègue's magnum opus of

1864; it was first described in writing in 1881 by Lasègue's former student, **Forst** (cited in Finneson 1980).

The markedly abnormal posture of the trunk that accompanies sciatica due to disk prolapse was presumably known to physicians of earlier centuries but was first correctly described in 1888 by **Charcot**, the pioneer neurologist of Paris.

From 1900 Onward

Even though Charcot had already associated sciatica with a problem in the lumbar spine, the crucial observation that intervertebral disk lesions could cause cauda equina compression and sciatica was first made decades later by **Krause and Oppenheim** (1909) and by **Goldthwait** (1911). No further studies on the subject were made right away; it took 20 years for others to become convinced of the correctness of Goldthwait's idea by corroborating it in their own, larger series of patients. The decisive factor was the development of radiological studies involving the intraspinal injection of contrast substances—first air, as used by **Dandy** (1919), and then lipiodol, as used by **Sicard and Forestier** (1922). Regrettably, the pathologist **Schmorl**, who published his systematic study of the spine in 1928, lacked contact with clinicians who treated patients suffering from low back pain and sciatica. Otherwise, he and his co-workers would surely have grasped the clinical importance of their many discoveries. He described protuberances from the surface of the vertebral body (osteophytes), narrowing of the intervertebral disk, destruction of the anulus fibrosus, and displacement of disk tissue into the spongiosa of the vertebral body in what are now called *Schmorl's nodes.*

Finally, the seminal paper on intervertebral disk disease was published in 1934 by **Mixter and Barr,** who clearly described the production of sciatica by lumbar disk herniation and demonstrated the effectiveness of surgical treatment in 58 patients. Further improvements in the diagnosis and treatment of lumbar disk herniation came in the following years and decades.

The improved understanding of the etiology and pathogenesis of lumbar disk syndromes led to comparable advances in the cervical spine. **Bärtschi-Rochaix,** in 1949, described the causation of shoulder–arm syndrome and of pains in the nuchal region and occiput by loosening and displacement of the cervical intervertebral disks.

This recognition of the mechanically induced degenerative changes of the intervertebral disk as the major pathogenetic factor in disk disease was followed, in the ensuing decades, by further study of the biomechanical and biochemical properties of the disk. **Junghanns** (1951) brought about a significant advance by identifying the *motion segment* as the functional unit of the spine.

The introduction and further refinement of magnetic resonance imaging (MRI; Lauterbur and Mansfield 1973) was a major advance in the radiological depiction of intervertebral disk diseases. In recent years, MRI has largely replaced earlier, invasive diagnostic techniques, such as discography and myelography; computer tomography (CT), too, which involves ionizing radiation, is now losing ground to MRI as the imaging study of choice.

More information on current developments in spinal surgery, including minimally invasive techniques, can be found in Krämer (2004) and in Bornstein, Wiesel, and Boden (2001).

■ Terminology

> *!* All diseases that arise directly or indirectly from pathology of the intervertebral disks are designated "intervertebral disk diseases" or "discogenic diseases."

Anatomy and Pathology

The category of discogenic diseases is broadly defined, so that it also includes conditions whose symptoms arise from the intervertebral joints and ligaments, but whose ultimate cause lies in pathological processes of the intervertebral disk. The disk is a biomechanical unit, even though the tissues that constitute it do not have a single embryological origin. At autopsy, a single, disk-shaped structure can easily be dissected free of the vertebral end plates above and below. The intervertebral disk lacks some of the structures that would be needed to classify it as a joint or half-joint (**von Luschka** 1858); it was more correctly called a *synchondrosis* by **Lindemann and Kuhlendahl** (1953).

> *!* The structures linking the articular facets of two adjacent vertebrae are true joints and are called the intervertebral joints.

The term "facet joint" is sometimes used as a synonym for "intervertebral joint." This may be a useful abbreviation but it does not contain any additional information, because, as we have seen, the *only* true joints between two adjacent vertebrae are the intervertebral joints. In the thoracic spine, the joints between a rib and a transverse process are called the costotransverse joints.

> *!* The motion segment is the functional unit of the spine. It consists of two vertebral bodies, the disk between them, and the associated soft tissues.

Protrusion and prolapse

Even though the pathological changes of the intervertebral disk and their relevance to disease states have been studied for less than a century, there have already been several shifts of expert opinion regarding their causation and treatment, resulting in corresponding shifts of terminology.

Before Mixter and Barr (1934) were able to show that sciatica is often caused by a disk lesion and consequent nerve root compression, other authors, including **Steinke** (1918), Clymer (1921), **Adison and Ott**, and **Elsberg** regarded the prolapsed disk tissue as a kind of cartilaginous tumor, which they designated as a ventral extradural "chondroma."

Bradford and Spurling (1950) referred to bulging of an intact intervertebral disk as a *disk protrusion,* which they contrasted with true disk rupture and herniation of the nucleus pulposus. Accordingly, we use the term *protrusion* for posterior bulging of the disk contour while the anulus fibrosus remains intact.

When the anulus fibrosus is perforated and disk tissue penetrates it dorsally or dorsolaterally in the direction of the epidural space, we speak of a disk *prolapse.* Transitional situations are described on p. 153.

The term "herniation" is liable to misinterpretation, as it is already used to describe certain pathological extrusions, e. g., of the peritoneum or the diaphragm, where the anatomical relations are decidedly different. For instance, the contents of an inguinal or diaphragmatic hernia are always surrounded by several layers of tissue (the hernia sac), which is not so in the case of a disk prolapse.

A displacement of disk tissue in the interior of an intervertebral disk without any significant outward bulging of the disk contour is called an internal disk derangement or, in the original French, a *dérangement in-*

2

terne. Fragments of the disk that have lost their continuity with the remainder of the disk are called "sequestrated disk fragments."

Age-dependent attrition and tears of the intervertebral disk are part of the normal aging process and are often called intervertebral chondrosis, after **Schmorl and Junghanns** (1968). This term includes all changes due to intervertebral disk degeneration, not just in cartilage (as one might suppose from the term "chondrosis"), but rather in any part of the disk. **Discosis** would seem to be a more appropriate designation. It gives us the pair discosis/discitis, analogous to arthrosis/arthritis, where the suffix "-osis" denotes a degenerative process.

> **!** The term "discosis" refers to all pathoanatomical, biochemical, and biomechanical changes of the disk resulting from disk degeneration.

The term "regressive changes" can also be used in this context, as the disk is unable to regenerate itself. Disk degeneration (discosis) is not a disease in itself, but it renders the individual susceptible to disease. The same is true of the changes of the vertebral end plates that arise in tandem with the degenerative disk changes. Schmorl coined the term **osteochondrosis** for the combination of wear-and-tear of the intervertebral disk with reactive condensation of the neighboring vertebral end plates.

Radiologically the most impressive change associated with disk degeneration is **spondylosis**, a condition in which smaller or larger, reactive bony spurs (anterior osteophytes) develop at the periphery of the vertebral bodies, at sites where the anterior longitudinal ligament separates itself from the vertebral body. Spondylotic bony spurs are only rarely seen on the *dorsal* side of the border between the vertebral body and the disk, because the *posterior* longitudinal ligament is firmly attached to the anulus fibrosus. If posterior osteophytes do form, the condition is called retrospondylosis.

Spondylosis and osteochondrosis often appear in the list of diagnoses in clinical and radiological reports, but it should be remembered that neither of these conditions is a disease; they are normal, age-related appearances, like gray hair and wrinkled skin. Aging is a physiological process that affects all of the tissues of the body. The unusual feature of the aging process as it affects the human intervertebral disk is that its effects are manifest earlier here than elsewhere, because of the relatively unfavorable nutritional status of the disk tissue and the major mechanical stresses to which it is subject.

> **!** Premature aging is the biologically determined fate of human disk tissue. Spondylosis and osteochondrosis can be found in all older people, regardless of whether or not they have symptoms.

We will retain the term "disk degeneration" alongside the term "discosis," because this term is in common international use, even though "degeneration" seems to connote a pathological process, which is misleading in this context. Degeneration is a purely morphological description without clinical relevance, as structural changes do not imply either disturbed function or a symptomatic patient.

> **!** It is proper to speak of degenerative disk *disease*, i. e., disk disease due to degenerative changes, only when a functional disturbance or pain is present.

Deviations of the spinal axis in the frontal and sagittal planes place the disks under asymmetrical mechanical stress. Degenerative processes run their course more rapidly on the compressed side of the disk (i. e., the side in the concavity of the axial deviation), because this side is less well nourished than the other. Tears and other types of attrition tend to appear on this side first.

> **!** Postural abnormalities predisposing to premature discosis, such as pelvic tilt, thoracic kyphosis, hemivertebra, scoliosis, and so forth, are called prediscotic deformities (in analogy to the prearthrotic deformities of the joints).

Like the term "discosis, " the term "prediscotic deformity" refers to a morphological substrate that *predisposes* to disk disease but should not be considered a disease in itself.

Infection or inflammation is denoted by the suffix "-itis": a disk infection is called **discitis**, while an infection of the vertebral body is called **spondylitis**. Most cases of local infection involve both the disk and the vertebral body and should therefore, strictly, be called **spondylodiscitis**. Nonetheless, in medical usage, bacterial infections of both the disk and the vertebral body are often simply called spondylitis, even though it is the disk infection that produces the more prominent symptoms. The term "spondylodiscitis" is generally used only for rheumatic inflammatory conditions at the interface between the vertebral body and the disk.

Clinical Syndromes

The terms cervical, thoracic, and lumbar syndrome are imprecise and convey no information about the etiology or pathogenesis of the condition so described. They merely imply that the patient has symptoms arising from the corresponding portion of the spine. (According to Leiber and Olbrich 1990, a "syndrome" is a constellation of symptoms that tend to appear together and have a typical history, course, and prognosis.) Nonetheless, the retention of these terms appears justified: first, because they are already established in common medical

Table 2.2 Commonly used terms and synonyms

Term	Synonyms	Remarks
Anulus fibrosus	Fibrous ring	Periphery of disk, composed mainly of fibers
Cartilaginous end plate		Layer of hyaline cartilage covering the vertebral end plate
Cervical myelopathy	CMS (international abbreviation)	Dysfunction of the cervical spinal cord, possibly due to spinal cord compression caused by degenerative changes of the spine
Cervical syndrome	CS (international abbreviation)	Symptoms due to functional disturbances and degenerative changes of the cervical spine
Cervicobrachial syndrome	CBS (international abbreviation), cervical radiculitis, shoulder-arm syndrome, cervical root syndrome, cervicobrachialgia	Cervical syndrome with radiation into the upper limb
Cervicocephalic syndrome	CCS (international abbreviation), cervical migraine, cervical headache	Cervical syndrome with headache, vertigo, and disturbances of hearing, vision, and swallowing
Chemonucleolysis	Discolysis, nucleolysis	Softening or dissolution of disk tissue by intradiscal injection of a chemical substance
Costotransverse joint		Joint between a rib and the associated transverse process
Discectomy	Disk surgery, prolapse surgery, nucleotomy, discotomy	A surgical operation on the disk
Discitis	Disk infection	Isolated infection of the disk
Disk degeneration	Discosis, intervertebral chondrosis, degenerative disk disease	All biomechanical and pathoanatomical changes of the disk resulting from degenerative processes
Facet syndrome	Pseudoradicular syndrome	Pain arising in the intervertebral joints, nonsegmental, with or without radiation into a limb
Facetectomy		Removal of part of an intervertebral joint
Fenestration	Flavectomy	Removal of the ligamentum flavum to open the dorsal aspect of the spinal canal
Foraminotomy		Surgical widening of a narrow intervertebral foramen
Hemilaminectomy		Removal of half of a lamina, from the midline to the intervertebral joint
Interlaminar space	Foramen interarcuale	The dorsal opening of the spinal canal between two laminae, which is spanned by the ligamentum flavum
Internal disk derangement	Dérangement interne	Abnormal displacement of tissue within an intervertebral disk
Intervertebral disk	Disk (for short)	The tissue between two vertebral bodies
Intervertebral disk diseases	Discogenic diseases	All disease states arising directly or indirectly from the disk or disks
Intervertebral foramen	Neural foramen	The lateral opening of the spinal canal between two vertebrae, traversed by the segmental spinal nerve
Intradiscal injection	Disk injection	Direct injection of a medication into the disk
Intrathecal injection	Intrathecal instillation	Direct injection of a medication into the subarachnoid space
Laminectomy		Removal of an entire lamina up to the intervertebral joints on both sides
Laminotomy		Removal of part of a lamina without breaching its continuity across the midline

2

2

Table 2.2 (Continued)

Term	Synonyms	Remarks
Local cervical syndrome	LCS (international abbreviation)	Pain confined to the cervical spine
Low back pain	Local lumbar syndrome	Pain confined to the lumbar region near the midline
Lumbago		Acute form of local lumbar syndrome
Lumbar disk disease	Lumbar spine syndrome, lumbar disk syndrome	Symptoms due to functional disturbances and degenerative changes of the lumbar spine
Lumbar radiculitis		Lumbar syndrome with dermatomal pattern of radiation into the lower limb
Motion segment	Segmentum mobilitatis	Functional unit of the spine
Nucleus pulposus		The center of the intervertebral disk, consisting mainly of matrix substance
Sciatic list	Sciatic scoliosis	Typical abnormal posture of the spine in lumbar root syndrome
Sciatica	Sciatic pain	Lumbar syndrome involving the sciatic nerve (L5, S1, or possibly L4 or S2 roots)
Segmental instability	Intervertebral instability	Loss of stability of the motion segment due to loss of disk turgor
Sequestrated disk fragment	Free fragment	Fragment of disk that has broken away from the remainder of the disk
Spinal fusion	Spondylodesis, stabilization	Ventral or dorsal surgical stabilization of a motion segment
Spinal stenosis	Spinal canal stenosis	Narrowing of the spinal canal
Tight hamstrings		Reflex contraction of the ischiocrural muscles and spinal extensors
Upper lumbar radiculitis	Femoral neuralgia	Lumbar syndrome involving the L2, L3, and (possibly) L4 roots

usage, and, second, because disk diseases are so common, particularly in the cervical and lumbar regions, that symptoms of any other cause in these areas are the exception to the rule.

For effective communication between physicians in hospitals or in the community, we find it useful to characterize the type of disk disease that is present as specifically as possible, and at the earliest possible stage, by giving it a precise name. The three local syndromes mentioned above, in which the patient's complaints are limited to the *spine itself* in the corresponding regions, are the most common, but there are also clinical syndromes with radicular, medullary, or cephalic symptoms. There are already generally accepted terms for the cervical spine, which are given together with their international abbreviations in **Table 2.2.** In the lumbar region, purely local pains are distinguished from pains radiating into the lower limbs. The displaced or expelled tissue consists not only of nucleus pulposus, but indeed of all the components of the intervertebral disk, including the cartilaginous end plate and anulus fibrosus; the disease is therefore called disk prolapse, and the operation is called discectomy.

The term **local lumbar syndrome** comprises all disk-related complaints in the lumbar region that are not ac-

companied by segmental radicular irritative phenomena. This term corresponds quite closely to the usual English term, "low back pain."

Lumbar symptoms can be either acute or chronic. These should not all be lumped together under the term "lumbago, " which properly refers only to the *acute* form of the local lumbar syndrome. "Lumbago" was defined by the Roman lexicographer Sextus Pompeius Festus as *vitium et debilitas lumborum,* "a defective condition and weakness of the loins." In current medical usage, the word refers to acute, severe pain in the lumbar spine, exacerbated by movement, and often associated with an abnormally stooped posture. The German folk term for this condition is *Hexenschuss,* or "witch's shot, " occurring as early as the 16th century. The notion of a malign, supernatural influence clearly has much older, pagan roots: it was already current among the Anglo-Saxons (another Germanic people) half a millennium earlier. An 11th-century manuscript now in the British Museum contains a metrical charm entitled *For a Sudden Stitch,* which reads, in part:

…this the to bote ylfa gescotes,

this the to bote hægtessan gescotes; ic thin wille helpan. ("This to cure you of elf-shot, this to cure you of hag-shot; I will help you.")

If one compares the image of a stooped and staggering patient with acute lumbago with the traditional notion of how a witch is supposed to look, one can easily surmise how the notion of a "hag-shot" might have arisen.

> **!** The patient with lumbago resembles the witch who shot him.

Incidentally, the term "lumbago" is also used in veterinary medicine, but with a different meaning—a prolonged episode of muscle stiffness in the horse, lasting 12–14 hours.

The collective term for radicular signs and symptoms due to lumbar disk disease is "lumbar radiculitis." Not every pain that radiates into the leg is sciatica. There are also upper lumbar root syndromes due to compression of the ventral branches of L2 and L3, which do not join the sciatic nerve.

In addition to the terms "lumbar syndrome" and "lumbar radiculitis, " Anglo-American terminology also includes such expressions as "low back pain" and "leg and back pain, " which are commonly found in medical literature for the lay public.

Simple back pain is mechanically induced, exacerbated by movement, and short-lasting. It usually affects individuals between the ages of 20 and 60.

Complicated back pain has the same general features but lasts longer and is often accompanied by factors predisposing its transition to chronic pain. The patient feels unwell. We find the terms "specific and nonspecific back pain" (Waddell 2004) to be potentially misleading, because the same terms are used in other contexts to distinguish, e. g., tuberculous from nontuberculous disorders (specific and nonspecific spondylitis; Peters 2004).

Pain radiating from the back into the lower limb, be it radicular pain (as in lumbar radiculitis) or pseudoradicular pain (which usually arises in the facets), can also be called **back and leg pain. Alarming spinal syndromes** ("red flags") imply the possibility of serious disease and can arise in any age group.

Summary

Intervertebral disk diseases tend to arise in relatively young individuals and are known to have plagued our shorter-lived prehistoric forebears. The great physicians and scientists of the ancient and medieval periods classified them by the site of the symptoms they produced, e. g., hip pain (Hippocrates), and treated them by the usual methods of the times, such as cautery, bloodletting, and sweating. A better understanding of disk-related syndromes was possible only after the birth of neurology in the 19th century. The real breakthrough in our knowledge of the etiology and pathogenesis of nerve root compression syndromes was made in the early 20th century, when it was finally discovered that intervertebral disk prolapse could cause sciatica and that the condition could be effectively treated by discectomy. Rapid advances in diagnostic techniques soon followed: first myelography, then CT, and then MRI. Many new forms of treatment were developed, too, most of them surgical. It is still too early to evaluate all of these from a historical perspective.

Today's neuroimaging techniques give us a clear view of the pathoanatomical processes affecting the motion segment, but the clinical classification of disk syndromes nonetheless remains a difficult problem. This is reflected in the terminology as well, particularly in such general terms as lumbar syndrome, simple back pain, and pseudoradicular syndrome.

Conclusion

Disk diseases have existed since the dawn of humanity but are only just beginning to be understood. The current, imperfect clinical terminology reflects the difficulties we still face in classifying our patients' symptoms in accordance with the pathoanatomical changes revealed by the ever-improving methods of neuroradiology.

3 Epidemiology

■ Lifetime Prevalence

Disk-related complaints, particularly low back pain, are very common. Almost all of us will suffer at some time during our life from symptoms related to degenerative changes of the intervertebral disks: the pathoanatomical studies of Schmorl (1932), Schmorl and Junghanns (1936), Coventry (1945), Hirsch (1960), and, in our institution, Tiedjen and Müller (2001) have shown that all humans over the age of 30 have degenerative changes in their intervertebral disks. The frequency of spondylosis and osteochondrosis, which represent the final stage of degenerative disk disease, rises steadily with age and approaches 100% by age 80 or 90.

Pathoanatomically identified degenerative changes and radiological signs of disk degeneration are not necessarily accompanied by symptoms. Many individuals with documented degenerative changes are asymptomatic, or else their symptoms are not severe enough to require medical help. These "patients" with degenerative disk disease remain undetected by insurance statistics.

> **!** Controlled studies have revealed that every older person occasionally experiences low back pain. The lifetime prevalence of this symptom is thus 100%.

There is no evidence that the prevalence of back pain has increased over the past 50 years; what has changed is the way that individuals, the medical community and society respond to back pain (Schöne 2004).

■ Point and Annual Prevalence

The point prevalence of back pain is 35%; i. e., 35% of individuals will state that they are experiencing back pain on the day they are questioned, and its annual prevalence is 70% (Raspe and Kohlmann 1993, TNS-Emnid 2004, Kohlmann and Schmidt 2005, Schmidt et al. 2007). Back pain is thus at or near the top of the list in all statistical studies of human ailments ranked by frequency. The first serious illness requiring medical help in adulthood is usually a musculoskeletal illness, most often involving the spine (Ludwig et al. 1999).

Many international surveys of low back pain report a point prevalence of 15–30%, a 1-month prevalence between 19% and 43%, and a lifetime prevalence of about 60–80%. The exact figures in different studies appear to depend mainly on the wording of the question rather than any difference in the individuals studied (Nachemson 2004).

■ Localization and Frequency

The different regions of the spine are affected by intervertebral disk disease to different extents. An epidemiological review of our clinical experience of disk disease revealed that 36% of our cases involved the cervical spine, and 62% the lumbar spine (**Fig. 3.1**).

No exact figures are available regarding the relative frequency of various types of symptom (back pain vs. back and leg pain). Waddell's estimates (2004) accord with those of other published reports (Bogduk 2000, Caspar 2001, Deyo 2004) and are as follows:

3

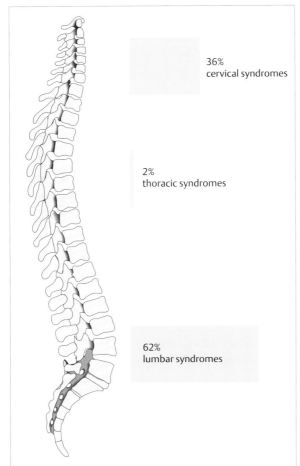

36%
cervical syndromes

2%
thoracic syndromes

62%
lumbar syndromes

Fig. 3.1   The relative frequencies of disk diseases in the three regions of the spine, calculated from a large series of outpatients.

- low back pain, 93%
- back and leg pain, 5%
- alarming spinal symptoms (red flags), 2%.

The high frequency of disk disease is reflected in medical, insurance, and pension statistics and in health policy decisions. Every tenth patient in a general medical practice, and every other patient in an orthopedic practice, is seeking medical help because of disk disease (Orthopädie-Memorandum 2001). Wilweber-Strumpf et al. (2000) questioned patients visiting orthopedic practices and found that half were there because of acute or chronic pain, which was most commonly located in the back (53.4%). The society-wide consequences of disk disease are manifest in the fact that, in Germany, back pain is the single most common cause of days lost from work by persons covered by mandatory health insurance. Statistics reveal that, on the average, back pain puts each insured person out of work for 2–3 days per year (Kohlmann and Schmidt 2005).

Back pain due to intervertebral disk disease is also a leading reason for reimbursement by social security disability insurance. In Germany, in 2002, 30% of the payments of the mandatory social security–medical rehabilitation scheme were for diseases of the spine and back (the single most common cause) and 17% of all new cases of disability reimbursement are due to disk disease (German Back Pain Guidelines 2006).

The available estimates of the overall societal cost of back pain in Germany have fluctuated over the past few years from 16 to 22 billion euros per year ($20–27.5 billion per year) (Hildebrandt et al. 2005). This sum equals approximately 1% of the gross national product.

■ International Figures

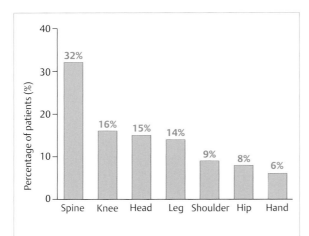

Fig. 3.2   The site of pain in patients complaining of pain, in 16 European countries (European Pain Survey 2003).

These figures on the epidemiology of back and neck pain in Germany are comparable to those in the international literature. The point, annual, and lifetime prevalence of these conditions in other countries are the same as in Germany (Nachemson and Jonsson 2000). The prevalence of pain due to degenerative spinal changes, as determined by German disease statistics, equals the prevalence found in the European Pain Survey of 2003. This survey involved a telephone poll of 46 394 adults in 16 European countries, carried out in the years 2002 and 2003, as well as 48 039 interviews with individuals suffering from chronic pain. All across Europe, the most common site of chronic pain was in the back (**Fig. 3.2**).

Back pain has enormous economic consequences, with total costs exceeding $100 billion per year. Two-thirds of these costs are indirect, due to lost wages and reduced productivity. Fewer than 5% of patients who sustain an episode of low back pain each year account for 75% of the total costs (Katz 2006).

Summary

The German-language and international literature contains precise data on the frequency and distribution of intervertebral disk diseases. The most common symptom is so-called simple low back pain. Disk disease is rarely a very serious problem; it can generally be treated conservatively with simple methods. Nonetheless, this category of disease, because it is so common, still takes an enormous financial toll on our society, not just through the consumption of medical resources, but also by being the most frequent cause of days lost from work and of early retirement.

Conclusion

Disk diseases are very common.

3

4 General Anatomy, Physiology, and Biomechanics

■ Development of the Intervertebral Disk

An understanding the pathoanatomical changes affecting the intervertebral disk in adulthood requires knowledge of its developmental history in utero and in early childhood. Even at these very early stages of development, evidence can often be found indicating that the process of disk degeneration—which affects humans at a relatively young age—has already begun. The more important developmental studies of the normal and abnormal spine are those of Töndury (1947, 1955, 1958, 1968, 1970, 1981) and his colleagues Larcher (1947), Prader (1947), and Ecklin (1960), as well as those of Bell et al. (1990) and Bogduk (2000). These researchers were able to demonstrate, in serial histological sections, the **regression of the notochord** and the development of the vertebral bodies and primordial intervertebral disks (**Figs. 4.1–4.3**).

An axial cord of cells that is at first only one cell thick, called the notochord (from the Greek *notos*, "back") or chorda dorsalis, is found in the embryos of all chordate animals and gives them their name. In lancelets

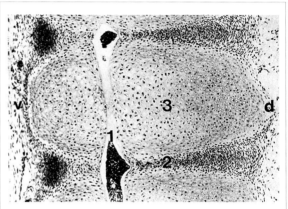

Fig. 4.1 Midline sagittal section of the primitive vertebral column of a 12 mm embryo. The notochord (1) runs craniocaudally through the primordial intervertebral disks (2) and vertebral bodies (3). v = ventral, d = dorsal. (Original photograph courtesy of Prof. Christ, Anatomical Institute, Univ. of Bochum, Germany.).

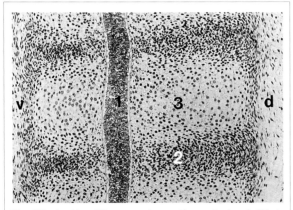

Fig. 4.2 In the 30 mm embryo, the notochord (1) is thickened at the level of the intervertebral disk (2). During the course of further development, the notochord normally disappears entirely from the primordial vertebral bodies (3). d = dorsal. (Original photograph courtesy of Prof. Christ, Anatomical Institute, Univ. of Bochum, Germany.).

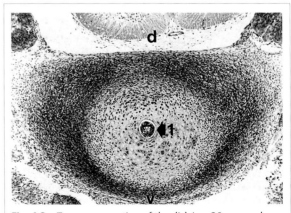

Fig. 4.3 Transverse section of the disk in a 30 mm embryo. The notochord (1) lies at the center. The peripheral, thickened portion of the disk blastema will develop into the anulus fibrosus. v = ventral, d = dorsal. (Original photograph courtesy of Prof. Christ, Anatomical Institute, Univ. of Bochum, Germany.).

4

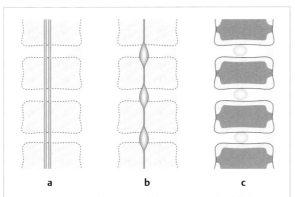

a   b   c

Fig. 4.4 a–c Development of the intervertebral disk.
a 12 mm embryo. Primordial vertebral column with cartilaginous vertebral bodies and intervertebral disks with longitudinally running fibrils in the outer zone; the notochord traverses all segments.
b 50 mm embryo. The notochord has been pressed out of the vertebral bodies, and remnants of it are found only in the intervertebral disks.
c 6-year-old child. Notochord remnants are found only in the central portion of the intervertebral disks. Central ossification of the vertebral bodies. The transitional zone between the vertebral body and the intervertebral disk forms plates of cartilage with cartilaginous margins that later give rise to bony margins (cf. **Fig. 4.5 a–c**).

(Cephalochordata) and tunicates (Urochordata, sea squirts), the notochord remains the only axial skeleton for the entire life of the organism. In vertebrates, the notochord disappears at an early stage of embryonic development and is replaced by the cartilaginous or bony spine. Only a few weeks after conception, the embryo (measuring 12 mm from vertex to sacrum) contains a spinal column with distinct vertebrae and intervertebral disks; these are pierced by the notochord, which is still present along the entire length of the spine (**Fig. 4.1**).

Later in development, the notochord is squeezed out of the primordial vertebral bodies by the growing cartilage cells, so that it ultimately persists only as droplike remnants in the center of the intervertebral disks, marking the location of what will later be the nucleus pulposus. The primordial disk tissue surrounding the notochordal remnant consists of outer and inner zones. The outer zone will later become the **anulus fibrosus.** Even at an early stage of development, it already contains longitudinally running fibers that radiate into the cartilaginous layer of the primordial vertebral body. These are the forerunners of Sharpey's fibers in the transitional zone between disk and vertebra. The outer zone contains many fibers and few cells; it undergoes a smooth transition to the pulpy inner zone around the notochord, which contains fewer structures (**Fig. 4.4**).

The parachordal inner zone and the somewhat eccentrically situated notochordal remnant together give rise to the nucleus pulposus. While the center of the vertebral body gradually ossifies, a cartilaginous plate forms at the interface of the vertebral body and the disk. The cartilaginous margin of this plate will later give rise to the bony margin of the vertebral body.

All of the disk structures destined to play a role in the biomechanical function of the spine are already present at birth.

> **!** The growing intervertebral disk still possesses its own blood supply during embryonic development and infancy.

These blood vessels arise in the vascular network lying just outside the spine, particularly in the intervertebral foramina, and travel directly into the anulus fibrosus, radially penetrating its layers (lamellae) and forming interlamellar capillary networks. There are two types of blood vessels that supply the disk: peripheral and central axial. They never penetrate into the inner layers of the anulus fibrosus or into the nucleus pulposus. Thus, from the very beginning of its development the central portion of the intervertebral disk is nourished exclusively by diffusion.

The vertebral bodies and the intervertebral disks do not reach their final form till early adulthood. The vertebral bodies grow from the proliferative zones of the cartilaginous end plates. The side of the end plate facing the bone marrow bears a typical zone of cartilage growth and degradation that remains present till about age 20.

Areas of ossification appear within the ring of cartilage at the edge of the cartilaginous end plate, joining together at about age 12 to form a bony ring which then fuses with the vertebral body. The lamellae of the anulus fibrosus are anchored to this bony marginal ring by Sharpey's fibers (**Fig. 4.5**).

The anulus fibrosus and the nucleus pulposus increase in size by interstitial appositional growth. Dense lamellar bundles form in the outer layers of the disk and pass between the two vertebral bodies in variably intertwined helical configurations.

The lamellae of the anulus fibrosus are weaker and less densely packed the further they are from the periphery of the disk; thus, even when the disk is fully mature, its center—the nucleus pulposus—consists mostly of structureless matrix. Töndury (1955) and Schaaf et al. (2004) found that the connective tissue cells in the anulus fibrosus, which produce fibers and matrix, receive a blood supply only until about the second year of life. The nourishing vessels regress thereafter, so that the anulus fibrosus is avascular even in a 4-year-old child. The function of this vascular regression is not known. On the contrary, the human intervertebral disk, rich as it is in cells and fibers, might seem to require an abundant blood supply, in view of the continual synthesis and degradation of macromolecules taking place within it. The regression of the blood supply of the intervertebral disk roughly coincides with the assumption of an upright posture at the age of about 1 year. One may suspect a connection between the avascularity of the disk and the mechanical stresses continually placed on it by standing and walking.

The arteries and veins of the vertebrae lie in the empty spaces left by the hard, bony trabecular system and are thus not exposed to axial mechanical stress. In contrast, the pulpy, homogeneous tissue of the interior of the disk physically resembles a fluid. Thus, depending on body position, the intradiscal pressure can be high enough to cause prolonged compression of the intradiscal vessels, leading in turn to an impairment of metabolism in the disk tissue.

> **!** The reduced supply of nutrients to the intervertebral disk adversely affects both the quantity and the quality of the intradiscal connective and supporting tissues.

In the ensuing years, the anulus fibrosus and the nucleus pulposus increase in volume by interstitial appositional growth, but their growth is outstripped by that of the vertebral body. Thus, the **ratio of vertebral height to disk height** gradually increases from 1:1 at birth to 3:1–5:1 by the end of the axial growth phase. Qualitatively, too, the intervertebral disks of adolescents display involutional changes suggesting premature aging, mainly because of a rapid loss of water content.

Changes in the consistency and color of the disk tissue over the first few years of life can easily be seen with the naked eye in fresh autopsy specimens. In neonates and infants, the cut surface of the intervertebral disk appears glassy, gelatinous, and semi-liquid (**Fig. 4.6**). Even in a 2-year-old, for example, one can wipe away the semi-liquid central portion of the disk with a cotton swab, but in the adult disk this is no longer possible.

Even **after the completion of axial growth,** the disk undergoes further regressive changes that alter its appearance. In advanced age, the central disk tissue loses its original, homogeneous, gelatinous character and instead looks dry and fibrous. If the motion segment is immobilized by spondylotic spurs, the connective tissue of the disk may become reorganized, and there may be renewed ingrowth of blood vessels into the disk. Hassler (1969) regularly found granulation tissue and blood vessels inside severely degenerated disks.

> **!** The intervertebral disk continues to change throughout life, from infancy to old age, and is particularly vulnerable to disease in certain phases of life. These are the times at which disk-related symptoms tend to arise.

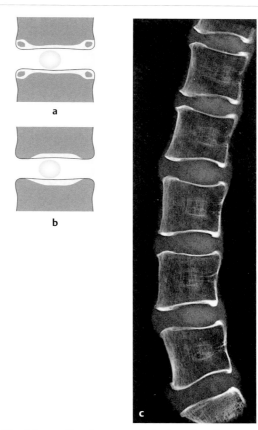

Fig. 4.5 a–c Development of the interface between the vertebral body and the intervertebral disk.
a 12-year-old child. A bony ring, the bony margin, forms within the cartilaginous margin between the ages of 8 and 12.
b Adult. The bony margin fuses with the vertebral body at the age of 14 or 15.
c Lateral radiograph of a midline sagittal section of a 17-year-old boy (saw-cut anatomical preparation).

4

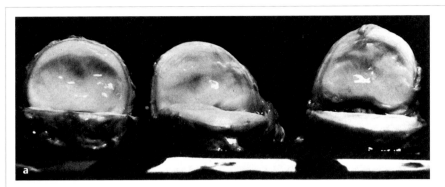

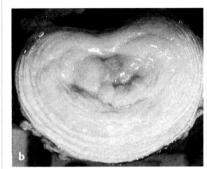

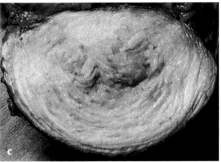

Fig. 4.6 a–c Lumbar intervertebral disks in cross-section.
a 2-year-old boy.
b 15-year-old boy.
c 42-year-old man.

■ Anatomy

The conditions that are known as intervertebral disk disease involve pathological changes not only in the disks themselves, but also in the neighboring tissues, which have closely related functions. In this section, we discuss the normal anatomy in and around the intervertebral disks only in as much detail as necessary for an understanding of pathological changes in these areas. The particular anatomical features of the different regions of the spine will be described in the corresponding chapters.

> ! The motion segment is the building block and functional unit of the spine.

One important component of the motion segment is the intervertebral disk, comprising the nucleus pulposus, the anulus fibrosus, and the cartilaginous end plates (though the end plates belong, embryologically speaking, to the vertebral bodies). Its other components are the lower half of the upper vertebral body and the upper half of the lower vertebral body, the anterior and posterior longitudinal ligaments, the ligamentum flavum (yellow ligament), the intervertebral joints, and all of the other soft tissues found at the level of the motion segment, in the spinal canal, in the intervertebral foramen, and between the spinous and transverse processes.

The human spine generally comprises 25 motion segments, of which the upper two (atlanto-occipital and atlantoaxial) do not possess an intervertebral disk. The **disks** are named according to the neighboring vertebral bodies. There are normally 23 of them: 5 cervical, 11 thoracic, 4 lumbar, and one each at the junctions between the regions of the spine—cervicothoracic, thoracolumbar, and lumbosacral. The lowest disk (L5/S1) is also sometimes called the presacral disk. Individuals with 6 lumbar vertebrae will correspondingly have 5 lumbar disks (**Figs. 4.7, 4.8**). In the adult, the disks account for one-quarter of the length of the spine.

The intervertebral disks increase in height going down the spine. They have a trapezoidal shape in the sagittal plane, corresponding to the normal spinal curvatures. The normal convexity of the cervical and lumbar lordoses is due to the greater height of the anterior portion of the cervical and lumbar disks, but the normal thoracic kyphosis is due to the shapes of the vertebral bodies.

> ! The term "intervertebral disk" refers to all of the non-osseous tissues lying between two adjacent vertebral bodies: the cartilaginous end plates, the anulus fibrosus, and the nucleus pulposus.

The **cartilaginous end plates** constitute the interface between the vertebral bodies and the disks. They are composed of hyaline cartilage. After the longitudinal growth of the spine is complete, the end plates terminate at the inner edge of the bony margin of the vertebral body on all sides. The site where the cartilaginous end plate is anchored to the bony end plate of the vertebral body is called the lamina cribrosa ("sieve-like layer"). This is a calcific layer with fine pores through which the marrow spaces of the vertebral body communicate with the end plate to supply nutrients to the intervertebral disk, mostly by diffusion.

The **fibrous ring (anulus fibrosus) of the intervertebral disk** consists mainly of fibers that are interwoven with each other as they take a helically winding path from one vertebral body to the next. Its peripheral zone contains the tough Sharpey's fibers, which are tightly anchored to the bony margins of the vertebral body. The lamellae of the anulus fibrosus are tougher and more numerous ventrally and laterally than dorsally and dorsolaterally; at the latter sites, the anulus fibrosus is thin, composed of only a few, relatively thin lamellae. The transition between the anulus fibrosus and the nucleus pulposus is gradual, without any sharply defined border between the two structures.

The **nucleus pulposus** is built up around the notochordal remnant and therefore does not lie in the exact center of the intervertebral disk, but somewhat more posteriorly. While the spine is still growing longitudinally, the nucleus pulposus contains not just the bubble-like cells of the notochordal remnant, but also the so-called notochordal reticulum, composed of reticulated strands of nuclei that look like notochord cell nuclei, yet lie directly next to one another. The interstices of the reticulum are filled with a slippery fluid matrix. A widely branching cavity is thus generated, which is at first filled with fluid resembling synovial fluid, and later with pulpy tissue that wells up as soon as the disk is cut open (**Figs. 4.9, 4.10**).

In advanced age, the tissue of the nucleus pulposus is easier to push apart, and it contains cavities. It is thus easier to inject 1–2 mL of fluid into the disk of an elderly person than into that of a young adult, whose disk tissue is still highly coherent.

When the intervertebral disk of a young adult is incised, the pulpy tissue of the interior of the disk immediately wells up out of the plane of the cut surface. The reason for this is that, once the nucleus is freed of the constraining framework of the anulus fibrosus and the vertebral bodies above and below, its internal pressure, i. e., its tissue turgor, leads it to assume a more spherical shape.

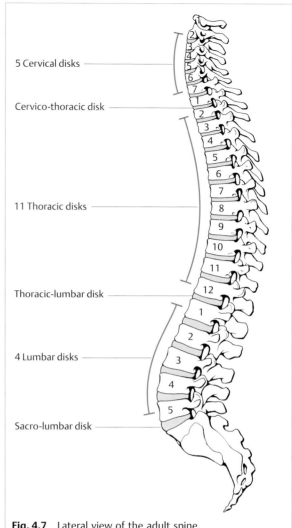

5 Cervical disks

Cervico-thoracic disk

11 Thoracic disks

Thoracic-lumbar disk

4 Lumbar disks

Sacro-lumbar disk

Fig. 4.7   Lateral view of the adult spine.

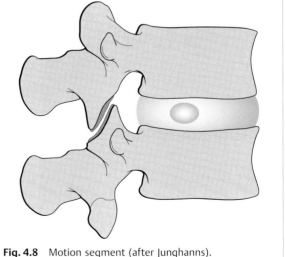

Fig. 4.8   Motion segment (after Junghanns).

4

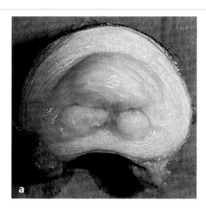

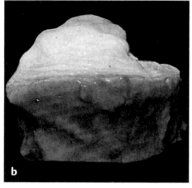

Fig. 4.9 a, b   Lumbar disk of a 17-year-old boy. As soon as the disk is bisected, the nucleus pulposus wells up out of the plane of section.

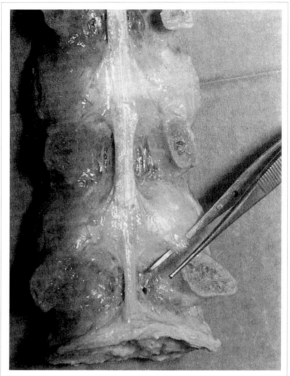

Fig. 4.11   Posterior longitudinal ligament in a dissected specimen of the lumbar spine. The ligament widens at the level of the disk, and some of its fibers course obliquely downward to the root of the lamina. The ligament does not cover the upper lateral portion of the posterior aspect of the disk.

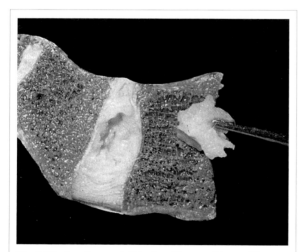

Fig. 4.10   Lumbosacral disk of an 18-year-old man. The mobile tissue in the center of the disk is easily extracted with forceps.

Ligaments

The *anterior longitudinal ligament* is a broad ligamentous band that covers the anterior surfaces of the vertebral bodies and of the anuli fibrosi of the intervertebral disks. It can easily be dissected free of the underlying anular tissue.

The *posterior longitudinal ligament*, on the other hand, is tightly bound to the underlying anulus fibrosus and is more difficult to separate from it. It is broader cranially than caudally; at the lumbar vertebral level, it is no more than a narrow strip (**Fig. 4.11**). Our anatomical studies (Stahl 1977) have revealed that, despite what many anatomy texts say, the posterior longitudinal ligament does *not* entirely cover the posterior aspect of the lumbar disks. Their superolateral portion remains uncovered, and it is presumably no coincidence that disk prolapses are most common at this site. The lateral fibers of the posterior longitudinal ligament run obliquely downward at the level of the disk to terminate on the periosteum of the root of the lamina. Tension on these fibers, from a disk protrusion or other cause, can give rise to periosteal pain.

■ Fine Structure and Biochemistry

Apart from the sparse remnants of the embryonic noto-chord, the human intervertebral disk contains only tissue components that are found in supportive and connective tissues throughout the body. The disk is clearly distinct from the structures around it, and its components are arranged in the intervertebral space in such a way that the mechanical properties of each are ideally suited to the stress occurring locally. Thus, the disk can be thought of as **an organ composed of connective tissue.** Its histologically and biochemically distinct components occupy different spatial positions to fulfill their respective biomechanical roles.

! The anulus fibrosus consists mainly of fibers, the nucleus pulposus of matrix, and the cartilaginous end plates of hyaline cartilage.

These tissues are generated by connective tissue cells, which themselves make up between 20% and 30% of the overall tissue volume. The disk contains fibroblasts, cartilage cells, and a few notochord cells. These connective tissue cells produce matrix and intra- and extracellular fibers. To synthesize extracellular macromolecules, the cells need low-molecular-weight metabolic substrates, including amino acids, salts, glucose, and water. The cell density within the disk is a function of the local nutrient supply; the center of the disk thus contains fewer cells (Stairmand et al. 1991, Ito et al. 2001, Kluba et al. 2005).

! The water content of the nucleus pulposus decreases from 90% in the first year of life to 74% in the eighth decade.

Our studies have shown that the water content varies in different parts of the anulus fibrosus (Kolditz et al. 1985, Krämer et al. 1985). The water is mainly present, not in free form, but rather as a structural component of macromolecules. It is reversibly bound to the free ionized groups on macromolecules; it can be exchanged for the hydrophilic groups of certain substances and thereby move into the interstitial fluid. The water content of the disks can be determined quantitatively by MRI (Panagiotacopoulos et al. 1987, Silcox 1995, Rajasekaran 2004). Our radiologists quantitatively measured the change in water content of the disks from morning to evening, as manifested by changing echo times (Beyer et al. 1986).

In addition to *interstitial fluid,* the disk tissue contains **minerals,** enzymes, organic matrix, and a small amount of fat. It does not normally contain a separate mineral phase; crystals of apatitic calcium phosphates are present only in elderly individuals. McCarty (1964) found brushite and calcium phosphate crystals in human disk tissue. Inorganic ions such as sodium, potassium, and calcium are partly structurally bound,

partly dissolved in the extracellular fluid. Calcium ions are bound to acidic mucopolysaccharides in the matrix, where their concentration may be up to 35 times as high as in the extracellular fluid. The disk is thus rightly called a calcium-trapping organ. Mineralization occurs in tandem with a rise in phosphorus concentration and, often, a gradual precipitation of crystals. The high calcium content of the cartilaginous portion of the disk is accounted for by intracellular calcium. Sodium is partly bound to the matrix; all other ions are found in the interstitial fluid.

The organic **matrix** content of the disk increases from periphery to center, i. e., from the anulus fibrosus to the nucleus pulposus. The matrix contains mainly glycoproteins and high-molecular-weight polysaccharides. The glycoproteins consist of protein and carbohydrate; being mucoprotein secretions, they are viscous and highly hydrophilic. The high-molecular-weight polysaccharides of the matrix are mainly acidic mucopolysaccharides, such as hyaluronic acid, chondroitin sulfate, keratan sulfate, and heparin. These molecules form a highly polymerized, three-dimensional grid that lends viscosity to the matrix.

! By virtue of their high effective hydrodynamic volume, the macromolecules bind a large fraction of the fluid content of the intervertebral disk.

The mucopolysaccharides lend the matrix its elasticity and viscosity through their ability to bind large amounts of water. Mucopolysaccharides and other macromolecules are synthesized partly intracellularly, partly extracellularly. Amino sugars and other building blocks of the acidic mucopolysaccharides are formed intracellularly as intermediate products of glucose metabolism. The cartilage cells are the most important sites of metabolic activity within the disk. They synthesize their own organic matrix, which consists of collagen and a mucopolysaccharide–protein complex. Macromolecule complexes are degraded through the activity of a vitamin-A-dependent cytoplasmic acid protease of the cartilage cells, which is inhibited by cortisone.

The biosynthesis of macromolecule groups in the intervertebral disk is an ongoing cellular activity rather than a one-off event. The extracellular structures break down after a period of time and must constantly be regenerated. Normally, an equilibrium is maintained between macromolecule synthesis and depolymerization. Acidic mucopolysaccharides, for example, are turned over quite rapidly: the biological half-life of chondroitin sulfate is 7–16 days, that of hyaluronic acid 2–4 days (Boström 1958, Davidson and Small 1963, Schiller et al. 1956, Ito et al. 2001).

4

> The biosynthesis and degradation of the extracellular structural elements of the intervertebral disk is possible only through a regular exchange of biochemical substances. Poorly nourished disk cells produce macromolecules of lesser quality and quantity.

The *collagen* content of the matrix accounts for 44–51 % of the dry weight of the disk. **Fibrocartilage** is mainly composed of the amino acids glycine (30%), proline (12%), and hydroxyproline (12–14%), and has a highly organized macromolecular structure. Collagen fibers are located mainly in the anulus fibrosus in the form of densely woven fiber bundles. Light-and electron-microscopic studies have revealed that this tissue becomes denser toward the periphery of the disk (Dahmen 1966, Takeda 1975, Buckwalter 1976, Buckwalter et al. 1985, Urban 2001). In the outermost portion of the human intervertebral disk the fibers are very tightly bundled; between them there are other obliquely running fibers, forming a mesh. The bundled fibers are more or less parallel and are densely arranged in an irregular onion-skin pattern. The cells that produce them lie between the collagen fibrils and are biconvex in shape. The collagen fibers are held together by mucopolysaccharides; the macromolecular superstructure formed by their interlocking molecules is mechanically anchored in the three-dimensional network of the collagen fibers. Such systems hinder molecular diffusion and thus constitute a low-permeability barrier to extracellular transport (Buddecke 1970). Our diffusion studies with different dyestuffs showed that only those with molecular mass less than 400 Da can pass through the wall of the intervertebral disk (Krämer 1973).

> The outermost layer of the disk functions as a selectively permeable membrane.

The initial phase of *collagen fiber synthesis* also takes place within cells. The disk cells produce the soluble collagen precursor molecule known as tropocollagen (Steven et al. 1969). Tropocollagen leaves the cells, then undergoes polymerization in the extracellular space to form insoluble collagen fibers (Eyring 1969, Urban et al. 2004). Like the mucopolysaccharides , collagen macromolecules are involved in a continual cycle of synthesis and degradation. The collagen within fibrils has a biological half-life of 30–60 days. Collagen turnover is slower in older individuals. Collagen is degraded through the action of collagenases.

Enzymes are synthesized in the lysosomes of the disk cells (Pearson 1972, Urban 2001) and act as biocatalysts to accelerate metabolic processes. They play important roles in both the synthesis and the degradation of many compounds.

> The levels of enzymatic activity and the short biological half-lives of certain major macromolecules reveal that metabolic processes within the intervertebral disk are continually active. They are subject to the influence of many different mechanical and biochemical factors, both from within the disk and from outside.

■ Biomechanics

The Disk as an Osmotic System

> The interior of the disk, the cartilaginous end plates, the anulus fibrosus, the paravertebral tissues, and the spongiosa of the neighboring vertebral bodies constitute an osmotic system for the exchange of molecules and fluid.

Electrochemical measurements can be used as a nondestructive and relatively inexpensive method for real-time measurements of changes in invertebral disk hydration in response to mechanical loading in vitro. The method also allows investigation of the effect of fluid expression or imbibition on the transport of electrochemically active solutes such as oxygen into the disk (Grünhagen 2006).

The tissue layers at the periphery of the intervertebral disk serve as a **semipermeable membrane** *whose perme*ability to fluids and dissolved molecules varies according to location. Studies have shown that glucose diffuses mainly through the end plates, while sulfate ions diffuse mainly through the anulus fibrosus (Maroudas 1975, Urban et al. 1976, Holm 1980, Urban and McMullin 1988, Roberts et al. 1989, Urban 2001, Adams and Bogduk 2004, Neidlinger-Wilke 2004).

The extracellular matrix of the intervertebral disk structures contains many molecules also found in cartilage. The extremely polyanionic proteoglycans play a central role, particularly in the nucleus, by creating an osmotic environment leading to retention of water and ensuing resistance to deformation—important for the resilience of the tissue (Feng 2006.)

The interlocking of individual molecules in the outer layers of the anulus fibrosus and the cartilaginous end plates turns the three-dimensional fiber network into a submicroscopic mesh that admits only small molecules, including water and low-molecular-weight metabolic substrates and waste products. A *permeability barrier* thus separates two tissue compartments with very different biological and mechanical properties: the interior of the disk on one side, and the paravertebral tissues and spongiosa of the vertebral body on the other. One major difference between these compartments is the **mechanical (hydrostatic) pressure** to which they are subject. The marrow of the vertebral body, which fills the cavity created by the bony trabecular system, and the soft tissues adjacent to the disk are subject to normal tissue pressures of only a few millimeters of mercury. The intradiscal pressure, on the other hand, may rise to 1 MPa (1×10^6 N/m^2) or more (**Fig. 4.12**), depending on posture and whatever additional weight the individual may be bearing at the moment. If this mechanical pressure gradient were not opposed by other forces promoting the entry of fluid into the disk, the disk would soon dry out, as all of the fluid would be squeezed out of it. Osmotic forces are the most important forces involved in this process. Diurnal hyperosmotic stimulation of a whole-organ disk/end plate culture partially inhibited a degenerative matrix gene expression profile and counteracts cellular metabolic hypo-activity (Haschtmann 2006).

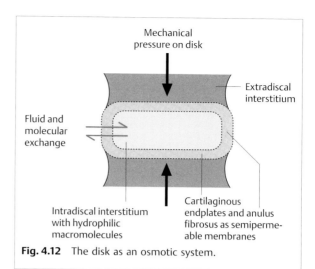

Fig. 4.12 The disk as an osmotic system.

> **!** The macromolecules in the interior of the disk—especially the mucopolysaccharides—are very strongly hydrophilic and are thus able to take up and retain fluid even in the face of an opposing hydrostatic pressure gradient.

The opposing pressure with which concentrated solutions attract water or other solvents across a semipermeable membrane is known as *osmotic pressure.* Osmotic fluid movement is in the opposite direction to the hydrostatic pressure gradient and continues until an *equilibrium* is established between these two kinds of pressure. *Colloid osmotic pressure* is the osmotic pressure due to high-molecular-weight compounds in solution.

Turgor pressure is another important type of pressure in biological tissues, and in the intervertebral disk in particular: it is the mechanical pressure exerted against resistance by a body that is capable of expanding by absorbing water. The expansile pressure of the disk can be measured experimentally. A disk that is compressed and suddenly released will re-expand at once. Both the speed of this expansion and the pressure it exerts are functions of the elasticity of the disk and its ability to absorb water. The disks of younger individuals re-expand more rapidly and more forcefully. Colloid osmotic pressure and turgor pressure, taken together, constitute the **oncotic pressure** of the tissue.

> **!** The interior of the disk, unlike the tissues around it, is subject both to a high hydrostatic pressure and to a high oncotic pressure. These two types of pressure promote the movement of fluid in opposite directions—out of and into the disk, respectively.

The concentration and pressure gradients across the outer layers of the disk are in a reciprocal relation that can be depicted as follows:

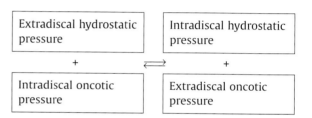

The mechanical pressure outside the disk and the absorptive pressure within it are on one side of this relation, the mechanical pressure within the disk and the absorptive pressure outside it on the other. If either side predominates, fluids and molecules will shift into or out of the disk.

> **!** The reciprocal relation of hydrostatic and oncotic pressure has important implications for the supply of nutrients to the disk and for the function of the motion segment.

The osmotic system of the disk can be influenced by both mechanical and biochemical factors. Short-term changes affecting this system arise mainly on the mechanical side, through increases or decreases of the intradiscal hydrostatic pressure (usually referred to in abbreviated fashion as the *intradiscal pressure,* even though this is, strictly speaking, ambiguous). Large pressure fluctuations within the disk are caused by changes in body position. No other organ is subject to persistently high mechanical pressures of comparable magnitude.

Our diffusion experiments with chemical dyes and radioactive labels have shown that an increase of intradiscal pressure to more than 80 kPa favors outflow of fluid from the disk, and a decrease to less than 80 kPa

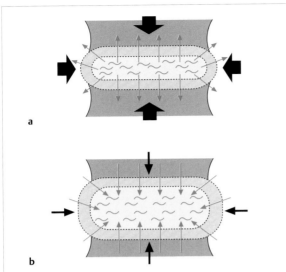

Fig. 4.13 a, b   Changes in intradiscal pressure.
a Increase in intradiscal pressure: when the pressure rises above 80 kPa, fluid and metabolic waste products are pressed out of the disk. The disk loses height and volume. The concentration of macromolecules within the disk increases, so that the intradiscal osmotic pressure rises.
b Decrease in intradiscal pressure: when the pressure falls below 80 kPa, the disk absorbs fluid and metabolic substrates. It increases in height and volume. The concentration of macromolecules within the disk decreases, so that the intradiscal osmotic pressure falls.

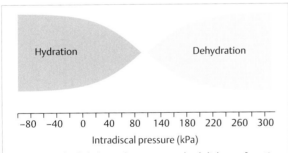

Fig. 4.14   Fluid shifts in the intervertebral disk as a function of its state of hydration.

favors inflow of fluid into it. Fluid flow reverses direction at a hydrostatic pressure between 70 and 80 kPa (see **Fig. 4.13**). Studies of the fluid and electrolyte content of disk tissue before and after compression have confirmed that the processes just described do, in fact, take place. The relative increase of electrolyte content through the loss of water under mechanical stress creates an osmotic pressure gradient that opposes any further water loss (Kolditz et al. 1985).

> ! The amount of fluid influx or efflux across the border of the intervertebral disk is proportional to the difference between the oncotic and hydrostatic pressure gradients.

Heavy mechanical stresses, such as sitting, lifting, and carrying, promote the outflow of fluid from the disk, while a release of mechanical stress, i. e., spinal traction, possibly leading to transiently lower than resting pressure in the disk, promotes fluid inflow into it (see **Fig. 4.14**).

Under physiological conditions, a limit is set to pressure-dependent fluid shifts in the intervertebral disk by the fact that any incoming water dilutes the macromolecules inside the disk and thus lowers the intradiscal oncotic pressure. On the other hand, when the disk is put under high mechanical stress, water can only be squeezed out of it up to a certain point, as water loss concentrates the macromolecules in the disk till the oncotic pressure gradient rises to exactly oppose the hydrostatic pressure gradient. Asymmetrical mechanical stresses on the disk cause water and dissolved molecules to move within the disk from the side of higher pressure to the side of lower pressure. Experimental study has confirmed that the part of the disk that is under greater pressure contains less water (Krämer et al. 1985).

Pressure-dependent fluid shifts within the disk were also observed by Shirazi (1992) in a finite-element simulation model and in the experimental studies of Adams and Hutton (1984) and Monat et al. (1993). These investigators found, as we did, that the ventral portion of the disk contains more water during standing, i. e., lordosis, while its dorsal portion contains more water during sitting, i. e., kyphosis. Further studies on pressure-dependent fluid shifts within the disk have been carried out by Fajman (1998), Malko and Hutton (2000), Williams et al. (2001), Riley et al. (2004), Veen (2004), Hutton (1996, 1999), Urban (2001), Pope (2002), Holm (2004), Urban et al. (2004), Rajasekaran et al (2004), Wang et al. (2007a/b), Masuoka et al (2007), Huang et al (2007), and Iatridis et al (2007).

Measurements of intradiscal pressure reveal that any lateral or anteroposterior bending movement of the trunk changes the overall mechanical stress on the intervertebral disks. Bodily movement thus causes fluid to move into and out of the disks, as well as to shift within the disks themselves. The innermost cells respond to low-to-moderate magnitudes of static compression, osmotic pressure, or hydrostatic pressure with increases in anabolic cell responses. Higher magnitudes of loading may give rise to catabolic responses marked by elevated protease gene or protein expression or activity (Setton and Chen 2006).

> ! Pressure-dependent fluid exchange in the human intervertebral disk is a pumping mechanism that moves water and low-molecular-weight solutes back and forth across the borders of the disk. This mechanism aids both the supply of nutrient substrates to the disk and the removal of waste products from it.

Any change in spinal posture that changes the intradiscal pressure will either accelerate or slow the movement of fluid into or out of the disk, and perhaps reverse its direction. The effective increase in aggrecan concentration which results from fluid expression during the diurnal loading cycle stimulates matrix production and is an important regulator of matrix composition (Boubriak 2006).

> **!** Regular alternation between vertical and horizontal postures improves transport into and out of the disk. Unchanging posture brings pressure-dependent fluid shifting to a halt.

Constancy of posture is especially disadvantageous to the exchange of fluids and molecules in the intervertebral disk when the posture that is maintained is associated with a very high intradiscal pressure.

Changes of Intervertebral Disk Height

Pressure-dependent fluid shifts in the intervertebral disks cause measurable changes in disk height and volume. These changes have major implications for the causation of disk-related complaints, as well as for their treatment. Changes in disk height can be measured directly in radiographs, and indirectly as reflected in changes in **body height.**

Normal fluctuations of body height over the course of the day were described by De Puky (1936), Heiss (1954), Tynell and Troup (1985), Wing et al. (1992), and Brinkmann (2004). Radiologically measurable increases in disk height after traction have been described by many groups (Krusen and McFarlane 1943, De Sèze and Levernieux 1952, Fraser 1954, Crisp 1955, Judovich 1955, Lawson and Godfrey 1958, Lehmann 1958, Cyriax 1959, Worden and Humphrey 1964, Mathews 1968, Colachis 1969, Krämer 1973, Eklund and Corlett 1984, Krag et al. 1985, Ledsome 1996).

In accordance with the pressure-dependent fluid shifts described above, increased compressive stress on the disks, e.g., in the standing or sitting positions, causes a decrease in disk height, while a reduction of compressive stress on the disks, e. g., by lying or spinal traction, causes an increase in disk height. The summation of these changes across all of the intervertebral disks results in a significant change of body height. Humans are normally shorter in the evening than in the morning.

Measurements of body height are subject to error through changes in posture and, in particular, deliberate alterations of the normal curvatures of the spine: one can make oneself taller or shorter at will. Involuntary changes of height result from altered curvature due to changes in the tone of the trunk muscles. Measurements of height must, therefore, be carried out according to a

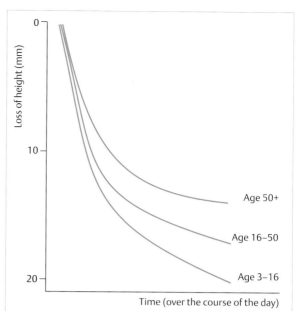

Fig. 4.15 Loss of body height through shortening of the intervertebral disks over the course of the day, in different age groups.

protocol that takes account of the normal curvatures. We generated daily height profiles by measuring height with a special type of grid that enabled us to hold the normal curvatures constant (Gritz 1975). The absolute loss of body height over the course of the day was found to have a mean value of 17.6 mm, equivalent to 1.13 % of body height. The difference in height from morning to evening lessens with advancing age (**Fig. 4.15**). The normal daily height profile can be altered by additional mechanical stress or by a temporary reduction of stress. Stress reduction by horizontal positioning at midday for as little as 1 h causes a mean increase in height of 4.5 mm, or 0.2 % (**Fig. 4.16**).

According to the relation discussed on page 23, the **fluid shifts** in the intervertebral disk are a function of the pressure gradient and depend on the initial conditions (oncotic pressure) and on the fluid filling state of the disk.

> **!** A disk that is tautly filled after prolonged maintenance of a horizontal position loses more height, when placed under stress, than one that has already had most of the fluid pressed out of it.

Conversely, a disk that has been dehydrated by compression fills more rapidly when the mechanical stress is removed than one that is already nearly saturated. Changing concentrations of the various types of macromolecules in the intervertebral disk, which are hydrophilic to varying degrees, keep the disk from being fully compressed even under the substantial mechanical

4

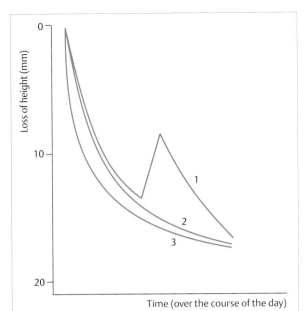

Fig. 4.16 Daily body height profile under conditions of increased and reduced stress in a group of subjects aged 16–50. 1, with 1 h of horizontal positioning at midday; 2, with normal daily stresses; 3, with an additional 10 kg of stress for 1 h in the morning.

A similar re-equilibration phenomenon can be observed in height measurements of astronauts before, during, and after a period of weightlessness. The astronauts were already more than 4 cm taller after only a few days of weightlessness, and maintained a constant height thereafter for the remainder of their trip. After their return to Earth, their spines rapidly became shorter again; there was even a transient "undershoot" (**Fig. 4.17**) (Thornton et al. 1979).

Traction and the Intervertebral Disk

Traction of the spine is an amplified form of mechanical stress reduction. Depending on the weights used at the upper and lower ends of the spine, the intradiscal pressure can even become negative. As the fluid uptake is proportional to the difference between the hydrostatic and oncotic pressure gradients, one expects traction to cause an accelerated increase in disk height and volume. This has been confirmed by measurement in a number of studies (De Sèze and Levernieux 1952, Fraser 1954, Lawson and Godfrey 1958).

After 10 min of traction with a traction bandage, the length of the lumbar spine between T12 and L4 increased by a mean of 4.8 mm, i. e., 1.2 mm per disk. As predicted, the increase in length was greater in younger subjects (Krämer 1973).

> **!** Spinal traction effects a rapid increase in disk height and volume by an amount that would otherwise require 8–9 h of horizontal positioning.

Prolonged traction carries the risk of an excessive increase of disk volume, possibly causing symptoms.

stress of prolonged standing. They likewise limit swelling of the disk under reduced stress, e. g., in a zero-gravity environment. Accordingly, the loss of height under stress is not a linear function of time, but rather an asymptotic approach to a final value. Two-thirds of the loss in height takes place in the first 3 h of the morning. The heavier the individual, the more rapid the loss in height. The exponential shape of the curves shown in **Fig. 4.16** is typical of biological phenomena involving re-equilibration at a new set point.

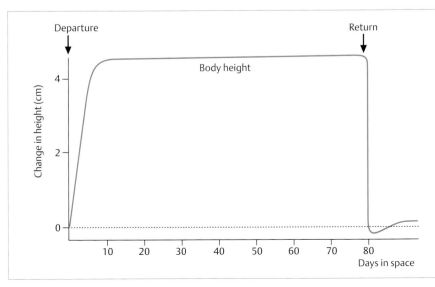

Fig. 4.17 Changes in body height of the Skylab 4 astronauts during and after 80 days of weightlessness in space (from Thornton et al. 1979).

> Conversely, additional, nonphysiological stresses on the spine, e. g., the carrying of heavy loads, cause the disks to dry out to a more than normal degree. The disks lose volume and height, and the (static) stress on the intervertebral joints is increased.

This, too, is a situation that can give rise to symptoms.

Vibration and the Intervertebral Disk

There have been many biomechanical studies of the effect of vibration on the intervertebral disks (Kazarian 1975, Panjabi et al. 1986, Brinckmann and Pope 1990, Holm 1990, Ishihara et al. 1992, Pope and Hansson 1992). Klingenstierna and Pope (1987) showed that vibration caused a loss of disk height that reversed fully within 2 h after the vibration ceased. Epidemiological studies have revealed that low back pain is more common in individuals exposed to large amounts of vibration, e. g., helicopter pilots (Gentlach 1978), truck drivers (Frymorer and Pope 1980), and tractor drivers (Wilder et al. 1982). Whole-body vibrations have this effect only on individuals who are seated in tightly sprung vehicles.

According to Coermann and Okada (1964), energy transfer to the human body is mainly determined by mass only at frequencies lower than 1.5 Hz; at higher frequencies, resonance phenomena come into play. The intrinsic resonant frequency of the spine has been estimated to lie in the range 3.5–8 Hz (Panjabi et al. 1986).

A well-known principle in both engineering and biomechanics states that vibrating a structure at or near its resonant frequency puts it under especially high stress.

> Vibrations at or near the spine's intrinsic resonance frequency cause abnormal pressure-dependent fluid shifts in the intervertebral disk.

The combination of certain postures of the spine with vibrations in the resonance range leads to increased energy consumption, probably because of the 2.5-fold increase in axial stress that experimental studies have shown to arise with vibrations in this range. More energy is consumed because of an increase in muscle activity (i. e., muscle contraction), which can lead to premature muscle fatigue.

We have found that the occurrence of back pain in people who are exposed to various types at vibration at work is more strongly associated with their manner of sitting and postural constancy than with the vibration itself (Kruse and Rezai 1980).

Mechanical Functions of the Intervertebral Disks

The human spine must respond to both static and dynamic forces. The presence of elastic disk tissue between each pair of adjacent incompressible vertebral bodies renders the spine mobile in all directions. The spatial configurations of the intervertebral joints determine the maximum **range of movement** in each direction. The disk, a deformable structure, participates in these movements and makes them possible as far as its finite compressibility and extensibility permit. The relative movement of two adjacent vertebral bodies occurs at the intervertebral joints and is cushioned by the intervertebral disk. The intervertebral joints function mainly as sites of rotation and sliding, rather than as bearers of static weight. The spatial configuration of these joints varies in the different regions of the spine; the correspondingly different pivoting characteristics and possibilities of movement of each region are discussed in the relevant chapters of this book.

The range of movement of a spinal segment is also a function of the initial conditions, i. e., of its state at rest, whether normal or abnormal. Stress-dependent loss of disk height, for example, can alter segmental mobility.

> Extension of the trunk, with hyperlordosis of the cervical and lumbar spine, will compress the nerve root in the intervertebral foramen to a greater extent in the evening, when the disk is shortened by compression, than in the morning, when it is still at its normal height.

Under physiological conditions, the remaining components of the motion segment adapt themselves to the changing height and range of movement of the intervertebral disk. Slowly evolving structural and functional abnormalities, such as scoliosis, are also generally well tolerated because of adaptation. Symptoms tend to arise mainly in response to rapid changes.

The disks not only serve to facilitate movement, but also have important **static functions.** With their very high intrinsic elasticity, they play the role of shock absorbers whenever the spine is subjected to axial stress. The nucleus pulposus acts like a fluid-filled bag, distributing the axial pressure evenly on to the cartilaginous end plates and the anulus fibrosus. The fibers of the anulus fibrosus resist excessive stretching in any direction. A symmetrical axial stress presses the nucleus pulposus from the center of the disk outward, in all directions, against the elastic fibers of the anulus fibrosus; as soon as the stress is released, the nucleus pulposus can return to the center.

Our quantitative studies of the lumbar spine with mercury strain gauges showed that the longitudinal ligaments cannot be excessively stretched under normal conditions, but are put under increased stress by inter-

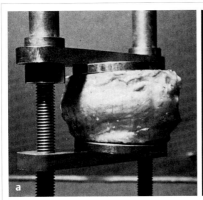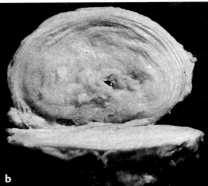

Fig. 4.18 a, b The response of the intervertebral disk to asymmetrical compression.
a Asymmetrical compression of a lumbar disk specimen with 150 kPa of pressure.
b The same disk specimen sliced open immediately after asymmetrical compression. The mobile central disk tissue has moved to the less markedly compressed side and is held in check there by the anulus fibrosus. The onion skin–like lamellae of the anulus fibrosus protrude somewhat on this side.

vertebral disk degeneration. The center of rotation of the motion segment moves backward during reclination (extension) and comes to lie behind the posterior longitudinal ligament. When the mechanical stress on the intervertebral disk is asymmetrical, the mobile central portion of the disk (nucleus pulposus) moves toward the side under less stress, i. e., dorsally in forward bending, ventrally in backward bending, and to the opposite side in lateral bending (**Fig. 4.18**).

In an experimental setting, we implanted a metal bolt firmly into the nucleus pulposus in order to follow intradiscal mass shifts radiologically during asymmetrical loading (Stahl 1977, Vogel 1977). The most pronounced shifting occurred in the first 3 min, at a speed of 0.6 mm/min. If the asymmetrical compression was maintained, shifting of the nucleus pulposus toward the side under less stress continued for several hours, albeit at a lower speed. Krag et al. (1987), Schnebel et al. (1988), David et al. (2001), Pope (2003) and Torio et al (2006) also showed, both experimentally and in computer simulations, that the nucleus pulposus always moves to the side under less stress. Positional MRI clearly demonstrated that nucleus pulposus translated posteriorly as lumbar flexion, and translated anteriorly as lumbar extension in the sitting position (Torio 2006). Thus, when a posture placing an asymmetrical load on the intervertebral disk is held for a long period of time, the nucleus pulposus becomes increasingly "decentralized." This is a very important factor in the development of disk-related symptoms and a highly relevant consideration in their prevention.

If the asymmetrical stress is suddenly released, the viscous tissue of the nucleus pulposus (**Fig. 4.18 b**) initially remains in its altered position, then starts to move back toward the center—at first very slowly, then slightly faster. The ability of the central, mobile disk

tissue to shift in response to asymmetrical loading of the intervertebral disk diminishes with age. The heavier the asymmetrical load and the longer it is applied, the more the nucleus pulposus tends to remain in its decentralized position. Its movement back toward its initial position can be made more rapid by symmetrical compression or traction.

> **!** The physiological ability of the nucleus pulposus to change its position and the elasticity of the anulus fibrosus make the disk a highly elastic and adaptable biomechanical system that can cope with the major static and dynamic stresses placed on the human spine, as long as its tissue turgor is normal and the spine is not bent beyond its normal range of motion.

This system is stable enough to withstand even very strong or violent stresses. Maximal bending, compression, or twisting of the spine, either in the experimental situation or in accidents, usually causes a vertebral body fracture rather than a disk injury, provided that the disks are intact to begin with. In the chain of vertebral bodies and disks that makes up the spinal column, the disk with its ligamentous supporting structures is the stronger type of link, withstanding greater stress and heavier traumatic forces than the vertebral body. On the other hand, once the anulus fibrosus loses its intrinsic elasticity because of tears and attrition, and the nucleus pulposus tissue at the center of the disk becomes more mobile than normal, the disk becomes vulnerable to stress and injury.

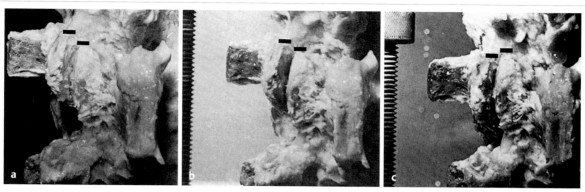

Fig. 4.19 a–c   Posterior views of a lumbar motion segment: **a** before compression; **b** after 12 h of compression; **c** after 24 h of compression. The facets of the intervertebral joint have shifted with respect to each other, in telescopic fashion.

■ The Disk and the Intervertebral Joints

The intervertebral joints play an important role in the function of the motion segment and in the pathogenesis of symptoms indirectly related to the intervertebral disk. Changes of disk height and volume always alter the position of the intervertebral joints. These are genuine joints with hyaline cartilage surfaces, a synovial lining, synovial fluid, and a joint capsule.

The literature to date contains varying information on the potential role(s) of the intervertebral joints as a source of **pain in the spine.** Lange (1936) described changes in the positions of the articular facets as a possible source of low back pain. Further studies on this topic have been carried out by Töndury (1947), Emminger (1955), Güntz (1958), Keller (1959), Zukschwerdt et al. (1960), Brügger (1971), Eisenstein and Perry (1985), Bogduk (2000), Panjabi (2004), and Cavanaugh et al. (2006). Emminger (1955) described synovial folds that project, meniscus-like, into the joint cleft and are said to become entrapped there under certain conditions. The evidence for the existence of this phenomenon, and for the histological nature of the entrapped material (if any), still remains inadequate. Another controversial point is the assertion of many authors that the intervertebral joints can sometimes become "blocked" and can then be freed by special types of "manipulation."

Our biomechanical studies of the motion segment have revealed changes, not only of the disks, but also of the joint facets and capsules (Krämer 1973, Kaschner 1976, Hedtmann et al. 1989). The intervertebral joints are mortise hinge joints that allow movement only in certain directions, depending on their position. Like the joints of the limbs, they are surrounded by a capsule made of elastic fibers. Recesses of variable size are found at the upper and lower edges of the joint.

Axial compression of the spine with symmetrical loss of disk height causes the articular surfaces to telescope into each other in the craniocaudal direction (**Fig. 4.19**). The articular surfaces move in a similar telescopic fashion on flexion and extension of the spine. The differing orientations of the joints at different spinal levels account for the fact that movement of the upper spine is mainly in the frontal plane, whereas that of the lumbar spine is mainly in the sagittal plane. The sagittal orientation of the lumbar intervertebral joints also permits a certain amount of relative movement of two adjacent vertebrae in the dorsoventral direction, even when the articular processes are intact (dorsal dislocation, pseudospondylolisthesis). At cervical and thoracic levels, the more frontal orientation of the joints prevents this type of movement.

We studied the behavior of the lumbar joint capsules in different types of movement by arthrography and by casting the joints with synthetic materials (Kaschner 1976). Dissection of the joints never revealed any menisci or any interposed meniscus-like material. Heavy tension on the joint capsule was found to be produced mainly by loading with an increased lumbar lordosis (i. e., extension = reclination). This type of movement also lowers the volume of the joint, as the joint surfaces are pressed more closely together in extension (Hille and Schulitz 1983, Lorenz 1983, Dunlop et al. 1984, Thols 1986, Rauschning 1987, Bogduk 2004). We used mercury strain gauges to study the extensile behavior of the intervertebral joint capsules. The increased capsular tension caused by slackening and loss of height of the intervertebral disk can be relieved by mild flexion. Mild forward bending with decompression of the disk reduces the tension on the capsules to the greatest

4

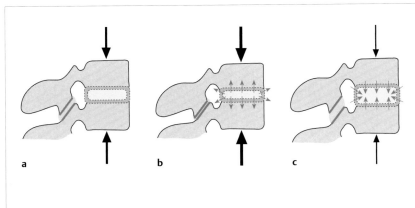

Fig. 4.20 a–c   Loss of height of the intervertebral disk and of the intervertebral joints.
a Initial height in neutral position.
b Increased axial stress causes fluid outflow, loss of disk height, and increased pressure on the intervertebral joints.
c Prolonged reduction of axial stress leads to inflow of fluid to the disk, with a resulting increase in disk height; the intervertebral joint capsule is stretched (put under tension).

possible extent and makes the joint cavities larger, simultaneously reducing the pressure on the articular surfaces. A flexion orthosis (brace) has the same effect (Thols 1986). Our experimental studies on the shifting of the center of rotation of the motion segment after discectomy (Steffen et al. 1991) yielded further support for the usefulness of flexion therapy.

These experiments, together with our earlier studies of the intervertebral joints, reveal that *the disk and the intervertebral joints constitute a functional unit that can react elastically even under strong mechanical stress.* The elasticity of the disk is the main reason why the system always returns to its initial state after symmetrical or asymmetrical compression, extension, or torsion. The intervertebral joint, as long as its capsule is intact, does not become dislocated or locked, even when the disk height is markedly reduced (by discectomy) or when the vertebral bodies are rotated or distracted. Very strong mechanical stress tends to fracture a vertebra rather than cause an intervertebral disk or joint lesion.

Symptoms tend to arise from the intervertebral joints only when the joint capsules are under abnormally high tension or the joint surfaces are subjected to abnormally high pressures.

> **!** The initial conditions predisposing to excessive mechanical strain of the intervertebral joints are almost always due to slackening, volume changes, or irreversible collapse of the intervertebral disk.

When a traumatic or degenerative **slackening of the intervertebral disk** interferes with the normal motion-resisting or shock-absorbing function of the disk tissue, the movements induced by contraction of the powerful muscles of the trunk are relayed to the intervertebral joints in undamped and uncontrolled fashion. Typical intervertebral joint pain ensues (p. 195). If the disk slackening and joint overstrain persist, spondylarthrosis develops. The interaction of changes in facet joints and disk in the three-joint compex (Kirkaldy-Willis, 1988)

leads to enlargement of the articular processes with following spinal stenosis.

Major changes in the **volume of the intervertebral disks** over relatively short periods of time can also cause joint pain. Persistent axial compression of the spine causes a marked loss of disk height. If the intradiscal oncotic pressure is low, the volume of the disk can drop relatively rapidly, with the result that greater pressure is transmitted to the intervertebral joints (**Fig. 4.20 b**). Conversely, prolonged reduction of axial compression, and/or traction, of the spine in the presence of high intradiscal oncotic pressure leads to increased fluid uptake into the disks and an increase of disk height. The intervertebral joint capsules are overstretched (**Fig. 4.20 c**). The capsular stretching and joint compression that are due to fluctuations in intervertebral disk volume can be aggravated by certain movements of the spine, e. g., hyperextension (hyperlordosis).

When the disk has lost several millimeters in height through irreversible collapse, e. g., due to degenerative changes, after discectomy, or after percutaneous chemonucleolysis, the intervertebral joints have a different initial position. In this situation, even movements within the physiological range of motion might produce symptoms by stretching the joint capsules beyond their usual final position, or by putting abnormally high pressure on the joint surfaces (**Fig. 4.21**).

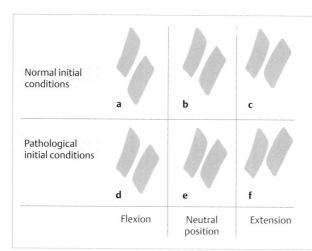

Normal initial
conditions

a   b   c

Pathological
initial conditions

d   e   f

Flexion   Neutral
position   Extension

Fig. 4.21 a–f Configuration of the intervertebral joint in flexion and extension under normal **(a–c)** and pathological **(d–f)** initial conditions. The abnormal configuration of the pathological joint in neutral position **(e)** is easily normalized with mild flexion (reduction of the lumbar lordosis). Extension is synonymous with reclination, backward bending, and increasing the lumbar lordosis.

■ Therapeutic Approaches

Our studies of the intervertebral joint capsules and ligaments (Hedtmann, Fischer and Krämer 1989, Hedtmann et al. 1989) have conclusively shown that the painful capsular and ligamentous overstretching caused by disk slackening and collapse can be reversed by mild flexion, i. e., reduction of the lumbar lordosis (**Fig. 4.22**). These studies provide the theoretical underpinning of the flexion therapy that we recommend, including step positioning, cube gymnastics, and a flexion orthosis.

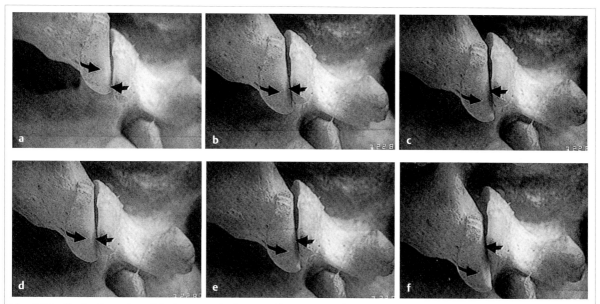

Fig. 4.22 a–f Configuration of the intervertebral joints in flexion, neutral position, and extension (i. e., with a reduced, neutral, or increased lumbar lordosis) in a normal lumbar motion segment (upper row) and in a lumbar motion segment that has been loosened with physiotherapy (lower row).
a Flexion, normal segment. The facet surfaces glide apart; physiological joint capsule tension.
b Neutral position, normal segment. The facet surfaces are precisely opposed to one another; reduced joint capsule tension.
c Extension, normal segment. The facet surfaces are telescoped into each other; physiological joint capsule tension.
d Flexion, loosened segment. The joint resembles the untreated joint in neutral position (**b**), with normal joint capsule tension.
e Neutral position, loosened segment. The joint resembles the untreated joint in extension (**c**).
f Extension, loosened segment. The facet surfaces are telescoped into each other more than in extension of the untreated joint (**c**); pathological joint capsule tension.

We have seen that the configuration and range of motion of the intervertebral joints are altered by processes primarily involving the intervertebral disk. It is also the case that an intervention at the level of the joints can effect a certain degree of stabilization of the entire motion segment. This can be accomplished, for example, with spondylodesis at the joints and application of bone chips to the laminae and transverse processes. Such techniques are more effective when something is simultaneously done to reduce the lumbar lordosis, e.g., a distraction spondylodesis, with or without instrumentation.

The effects that changes in the intervertebral disks exert on the intervertebral joints, and vice versa, vary from one region of the spine to another (cervical, thoracic, and lumbar), depending on the range of motion permitted by the particular configuration of the articular facets in each region. Further details are provided in the chapters on the individual regions of the spine.

Summary

The human spine undergoes normal development in utero and in the first 2 years of life, like other organs of the body. The microscopic and macroscopic structural elements of the motion segment are well adapted to the horizontal stresses associated with crawling on four limbs. On the other hand, the continual vertical stress placed on the intervertebral disks by the upright posture is nonphysiological for the cells and connective tissue structures of the nucleus pulposus and anulus fibrosus. Paucity of movement also harms the nutritive state of the intervertebral tissues.

The intervertebral disk is avascular in adults and obtains nutrients by diffusion through an osmotic system. The existence of pressure-dependent fluid shifts within the disk has also been confirmed by recent studies. A regular alternation of mechanical stress and relaxation aids intradiscal metabolism, but a constantly maintained posture—particularly one in which the spine is under stress—impairs it.

All changes in the anterior portion of the motion segment affect the intervertebral joints as well. The destiny of the joints is bound to that of the disk. Persistent loss of disk height puts the intervertebral joints under nonphysiological amounts of stress, which may cause arthrosis or spinal canal stenosis.

Conclusion

The anatomy and biomechanics of the spine seem to have been designed for quadrupeds, as it is not fully up to the tasks placed on it by humans.

5 Nondegenerative Disk Diseases

5

■ Developmental Disturbances

Notochord Remnants

The regression of the embryonic notochord can be inhibited at any stage of development, giving rise to a wide variety of structural anomalies of the motion segments. A notochord that persists almost in its entirety appears as a cylinder of soft tissue that passes through the entire length of the vertebral body and widens out in the disk space as a fusiform, intervertebral notochordal swelling. This exceedingly rare anomaly has been described to date only by Schmorl (1932) and Schmorl and Junghanns (1968). A lesser degree of persistence of notochordal tissue produces concave indentations in the dorsal third of the upper and lower end plates, with abnormal thinning of the cortical bone. These are sites where the notochordal canal, which previously traversed the vertebral body, has not closed normally. The overlying cartilaginous end plates, too, are always somewhat thinner than usual. At these sites, disk material may protrude into the spongiosa of the vertebral body, forming so-called Schmorl's nodes (Schmorl 1932), which are relatively common and are often found incidentally on spinal radiographs. Schmorl's nodes are an asymptomatic, clinically insignificant finding that should not be mistaken for spondylitis or vertebral body fractures. Characteristic features of notochord remnants are their location in the posterior third of the upper and lower end plates of the vertebral body and their presence in multiple motion segments (**Fig. 5.1**).

Developmental Disturbances of the Vertebral Bodies and Intervertebral Disks in Childhood

Persistence of notochord remnants should not be confused with impaired ossification of cartilage at the interface of the vertebral body and intervertebral disk. The latter condition is due to a developmental disturbance during childhood affecting both the vertebral bodies and the intervertebral disks and is mainly seen in their *anterior* portions. Its cause is not fully understood.

> The high oncotic and hydrostatic pressure of intervertebral disk tissue in children and adolescents can cause it to burst through the cartilaginous and bony end plates at sites of least resistance. The disk tissue destroys growth zones and protrudes into the spongiosa of the vertebral body.

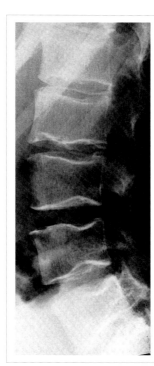

Fig. 5.1 Lateral plain radiograph of the lumbar spine in an asymptomatic 20-year-old man. Notochordal regression anomaly with arch-like impressions in the posterior third of the upper and lower end plates.

Apart from notochord remnants, a number of other possible causes have been suggested for local weakening of the resistance of the cartilaginous and bony end plates to the enormous expansile pressure of the disk. These include vascular channels (Böhmig 1930), local defects of ossification (Schmorl 1932), and local fiber degeneration (Aufdermaur 1968). Mau (1974) considered changes of this type to be compatible with those of enchondral dysostosis.

The severity of the deformity caused by protrusion of the intervertebral disks into the vertebral bodies depends on the size of the protrusions and the stage of development at which they arise. Each region of the spine is affected in its own characteristic way, because the different regions are exposed to different mechanical stresses.

Involvement of the thoracic spine produces the characteristic picture of adolescent kyphosis (Scheuermann disease). The growth of the vertebral bodies is impaired, so that they remain of lesser height ventrally than dorsally; *Schmorl's cartilaginous nodes* are seen, and the contours or the upper and lower end plates are irregular. At the same time, the anterior portions of the intervertebral disks are narrowed.

! The abnormal development of the intervertebral disks in Scheuermann disease is a secondary manifestation. It is caused by increased pressure on the disk tissue lying in the anterior portion of the disk space, i. e., in the inner aspect of the kyphosis.

As mentioned on page 24 above, an asymmetrical stress on the intervertebral disk causes shifting of fluid and molecules within the disk. In Scheuermann disease, water and dissolved metabolic substrates move from the anterior portion of the disk (on the concave side of the kyphosis) to its posterior portion (on the convex side). With persistent asymmetrical compression, the cells of the anterior portion of the disk receive an inadequate supply of the substrates needed for the generation of disk tissue. As a result, the interstitial, appositional growth of the disk is deficient in this area. Thus, in Scheuermann disease, just as in structural scoliosis, the abnormally shaped intervertebral disks account for a large proportion of the fixed axial deviation of the spine in the sagittal plane.

In the thoracic region, the anterior portions of the intervertebral disks are continually under high mechanical stress and therefore begin to manifest degenerative changes relatively early. The disks age rapidly; they prematurely become partially immobilized in an abnormal posture while the normally loose disk tissue is replaced with fibrous tissue. Particularly in the early stage of adolescent kyphosis, when the spine is still adequately mobile, the goal of treatment should be to optimize the metabolic functioning of disk tissue through a regular alternation of mechanical stress (compression) and relaxation.

In the thoracolumbar junction and the lumbar spine, the developmental structural anomalies occurring at the interfaces of the disks and vertebral bodies differ from those seen in the thoracic spine, because these different regions are subject to different mechanical stresses. The lumbar changes are often referred to as the "lumbar type of Scheuermann disease," though Scheuermann himself, in 1921, described only changes of the mid- and lower thoracic spine.

Disk herniations into the spongiosa of the vertebral body tend to be larger in the lumbar than in the thoracic spine and to impair the growth of the motion segment in such a way as to cause a considerable degree of deformity. Peripheral portions of the vertebral body may become separated from its main portion by disk tissue, and deep invaginations into the vertebral body may arise (**Fig. 5.2**).

The radiological diagnosis is usually readily apparent from the simultaneous involvement of multiple segments and the reactive growth that is seen in the adjacent vertebral bodies, often in the form of bony protrusions toward the disk space corresponding to invaginations in the opposite end plate (**Fig. 5.3**).

This type of developmental disturbance has both endogenous and exogenous causes. The cartilaginous end plates of the vertebral bodies contain circumscribed areas of diminished resistance while still in their primordial stage. The very high expansile pressure of the disk tissue, in combination with hydrostatic pressure, damages the growth zone of the vertebral body. Defects arise and are then filled by the expanding disk tissue.

The release of mechanical stress in the axial direction at this site in the disk results in greater than normal bone growth in the ossification layer of the next vertebral body. Its bony end plate therefore develops a bump, or protrusion, pointing in the direction of the disk space. These changes can only arise during development. The importance of mechanical stress on the disk as a cause of these juvenile developmental anomalies is also implied by the fact that they arise in the same regions of the spine that most often sustain compression fractures in accidents involving sudden axial stress.

Though the radiological findings may be quite impressive, one must take care not to ascribe undue importance to them or to cause needless anxiety by communicating them to the patient. The observed deformities often contrast markedly with the patient's complaints of pain, which are usually localized to other areas of the spine and are most commonly due to the ordinary disk-related disturbances of the lumbar and lower cervical motion segments. In fact, symptoms arising from the deformed disk segments are notably rare. The disk tissue has little tendency to become displaced, because it is anchored to its surroundings by the cartilaginous nodules within the bony spongiosa and by the protrusions of the end plates into the disks.

! The affected intervertebral disk is narrowed and the motion segment to which it belongs is biomechanically inactive.

Although juvenile developmental anomalies of this type generally produce no symptoms in the segments directly affected, they do impair the biomechanical quality of the *neighboring* intervertebral disks and related structures. Even while the spine is still in its developing phase, these structures cannot withstand the expansile pressure of the disk tissue. It is thus not surprising that disk-related complaints are more common in individuals with this kind of anomaly, as reported decades ago by Alajouanine and Thurel (1949), Kuhlendahl (1953), Hanraets (1959), Brocher (1973), and Idelberger (1984). Mau (1974) found that evidence of dysostotic weakness of the metaphyses was more common in patients with disk herniation than in normal controls. The multisegmentally distributed juvenile developmental anomalies usually cause deviations of the spinal axes in the sagittal and frontal planes; therefore, as a secondary effect, the disks in the adjoining areas of the spine are subject to abnormal and excessive mechanical stress. This is why affected individuals are more than usually subject to intervertebral disk disease.

Congenital Anomalies

The juvenile developmental anomalies discussed above arise during the growth phase, partly under the influence of gravity. In contrast, certain other anomalies of the intervertebral disk are already present at birth. The disk between two vertebrae may be congenitally absent – a "block vertebra." Incomplete block vertebrae with a markedly attenuated, hypoplastic disk sometimes present difficulties in differential diagnosis; in particular, spondylitis must be ruled out. The diagnosis of a congenital anomaly is supported by the lack of clinical evidence of inflammation; by the concave anterior border of the block vertebra, whose overall size is abnormal compared to the neighboring ones; and by the sharp demarcation of the disk remnants from the vertebral bodies. Congenital anomalies of the disks are not usually accompanied by any areas of bony sclerosis or bony defects in the vicinity of the end plates, but the laminae and spinous processes are often fused. The motion segments corresponding to the block vertebrae do not give rise to any symptoms, even when their neural foramina are markedly narrowed or occluded with bone. This painless block state is analogous to the desired result of spinal fusion procedures. The congenital fusion of two adjacent vertebrae can, however, produce painful functional disturbances of the motion segments above and below, which are subject to increased mechanical stress. This is particularly true when the vertebrae are fused in an abnormal position.

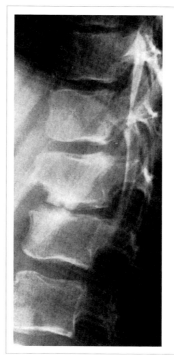

Fig. 5.2 Juvenile developmental disorder of the lumbar spine in a 12-year-old boy, with deformation of an intervertebral disk and of the adjacent vertebral body end plates. The clinical presentation was consistent with paravertebral muscular insufficiency.

5

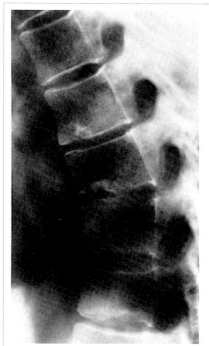

Fig. 5.3 Juvenile developmental disorder of the lumbar intervertebral disks and vertebrae in an active, asymptomatic female athlete, aged 25.

Partial anterior block formation over multiple segments is not a congenital anomaly but, rather, a result of Scheuermann disease or of severe senile kyphosis of the thoracic spine.

■ Inflammatory and Infectious Disorders

Bacterial Infection of the Intervertebral Disk

Bacterial infection is a relatively rare but nonetheless important cause of intervertebral disk disease. It is easily overlooked, particularly in its early stages, because degenerative diseases are much more common.

Bacterial infection of the disk can be caused by specific pathogens (e. g., the tubercle bacillus) or by nonspecific ones (staphylococci, streptococci, *E. coli,* and others). Nonspecific infections arise most commonly in the lumbar motion segments. Infection with Gram-negative organisms (*E. coli, Bacillus proteus*) has recently become more common. Isolated discitis without primary involvement of the vertebral body is caused by direct entry of the pathogenic organism into the disk, usually as a complication of a medical procedure such as discotomy or disk puncture. Hematogenous discitis is theoretically possible only when there are blood vessels within the intervertebral disk, i. e., only in infants and in old people with advanced degenerative disk disease.

Schmorl (1932) found very few cases of primary hematogenous disk infection in his extensive clinical series. In one such case, for example, an abscess developed in the nucleus pulposus of a vascularized second lumbar disk in a patient with tonsillitis complicated by bacterial sepsis.

Most of the "primary disk infections" in adults that have been reported in the literature are, in fact, more likely to have been secondary to vertebral body infection in the vicinity of the end plates (a condition that often cannot be seen on plain radiographs and can only be diagnosed by tomography). Bacterial infection of the disk itself is radiographically characterized by narrowing of the disk space and by subchondral end plate de-

fects with a surrounding sclerotic zone. Unlike Schmorl's nodes, the sclerotic zones around foci of infection are not sharply demarcated; rather, they extend far into the vertebral spongiosa, without any clear border. The vertebral body end plates above and below the infected disk also appear to be unfocused, with blurred contours. Bacterial infection of the disk can spread cranially and caudally beneath the anterior longitudinal ligament and give rise to an extensive, spindle-shaped abscess. Disks at neighboring levels can also be secondarily infected in this way. Paravertebral abscesses in the lumbar region can spread along the psoas sheath, causing a widening of the psoas shadow in a plain radiograph.

Disk infection is difficult to diagnose in its early stages because plain radiographs often show no change beyond a mild narrowing of the disk space. Scintigraphy may reveal increased local activity, but the main diagnostic criteria are clinical: a history of recent infection elsewhere in the body (tonsillitis/pharyngitis, furuncle, abscess), fever, and localized back pain on manual pressure or shaking of the spine. Laboratory testing, CT, and plain tomograms confirm the diagnosis. Later on in the course of disk infection, one may see bony bridges traversing the disk space, a characteristic finding. The radiological distinction between specific and nonspecific intervertebral disk infections is usually only one of degree. Nonspecific infection more commonly takes a fulminant course and shows a more marked bony reaction, with the formation of wide bony bridges and sclerotic areas (**Fig. 5.4**).

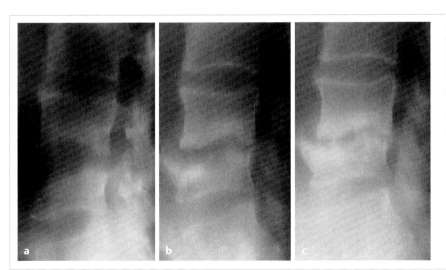

Fig. 5.4 a–c Nonspecific spondylitis at L4/L5 in a 62-year-old man. At first, there is spondylodiscitis with loss of vertebral body bone opacity (**a**); within a few months, the bone consolidates and develops large spondylotic processes (**b**, **c**).

Rheumatic Inflammation of the Intervertebral Disk

Nonbacterial discitis occurs in rheumatic inflammatory diseases, particularly in ankylosing spondylitis and rheumatoid arthritis (Behrens 2005, Rehart and Henninger 2005, Schröder 2005). Dihlmann (1987) found evidence of spondylodiscitis in tomographic images of the lumbar spine in 18% of a series of patients with florid ankylosing spondylitis. Unlike bacterial spondylitis, rheumatic inflammation of the disk and adjoining areas of the vertebral body is characterized from the beginning by a broad zone of opacification in the spongiosa surrounding the defect, which may appear in multiple segments at once. Spondylodiscitis often arises in segments in which there are no syndesmophytes. In rheumatoid arthritis, plain radiographs reveal both narrowing of the intervertebral disks (discitis) and erosion of the vertebral body end plates, with reactive sclerosis (spondylitis). As the disease progresses, block vertebrae may form. The cervical disks are most often affected. The inflammatory granulomatous process begins at the uncovertebral joints. Unlike bacterial infection, nonbacterial rheumatic inflammation of the intervertebral disk causes no particular clinical symptoms, nor does it require any specific treatment.

■ Tumors

Even though the intervertebral disks contain connective and supportive tissue cells that are constantly being renewed, no primary tumors of the disks have ever been described to date. Schmorl (1932) and Schmorl and Junghanns (1968) did not find a single case in their extensive clinical series. Disk prolapses and protrusions were, at one time, wrongly held to be cartilaginous tumors that had supposedly arisen in the disks.

Metastases to the vertebral bodies are relatively common, and any tumor tissue found in an intervertebral disk is the result of extension from neighboring vertebral bodies. The tumor tissue spreads into the disk along pre-existing fissures, deposits of fibrous tissue, blood vessels, or bony spicules. Tumors of the abdominal cavity or mediastinum can also impinge on or infiltrate an intervertebral disk. In general, however, the disk remains intact for a remarkably long time, despite the presence of tumor tissue in its immediate vicinity; thus, the finding of a well-preserved disk next to a destroyed vertebral body can be taken as evidence of neoplasia. Inflammation always affects the disk as well as the vertebral body.

■ Involvement of the Intervertebral Disks in Systemic Illness

Possible Reactions

Because it is not directly linked to the circulation, intervertebral disk tissue participates only after a delay, if at all, in the body's general response to systemic illness. Even a few hours after death (the extreme case of a systemic disturbance!), the physiological tissue turgor, diffusion-related processes, and volume fluctuations of the intervertebral disks can still be demonstrated in vitro. Our own studies have shown the disk tissue to be relatively insensitive to external influences such as hypoxia, temperature fluctuations, and pH changes. Systemic sepsis in infancy could, in theory, lead to hematogenous discitis, but this is very rarely seen in practice. Other severe systemic disturbances, such as coma, acidosis, alkalosis, nutritional deficiencies, and metabolic abnormalities, produce no visible change in the disk tissue. The only systemic conditions that regularly affect the intervertebral disks are the generalized diseases of connective tissue, as well as all pathological conditions causing changes in the tissues adjacent to the disks, most commonly the vertebral bodies.

Achondroplasia

In this autosomal dominant genetic disorder, the proliferation of cartilage cells in growth zones is inadequate. The individual's longitudinal growth (height) is deficient, and the spine grows abnormally. In affected neonates, the centers of ossification of the vertebral bodies are flat wafers with an irregular, zigzag anterior edge. In adult achondroplasts the vertebral bodies are of abnormally reduced height; they protrude backward, narrowing the spinal canal from its anterior aspect. Meanwhile, the canal is narrowed from its posterior aspect, too, because of premature union of the vertebral arches (laminae) in the midline. Accordingly, the studies of the spine in achondroplasia by Donath and Vogt (1927), Bergström (1971), and Nelson (1972) all revealed

5

5

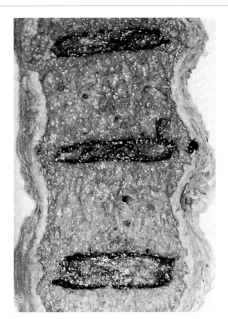

Fig. 5.5 Ochronosis in a 24-year-old man, with dark discoloration of the intervertebral disk tissue (specimen courtesy of the Pathological Institute, University of Düsseldorf).

narrowing of the vertebral canal, reduction of the interpedicular distance, and shortening of the vertebral arches. This disorder is a paradigmatic example of a genetically based spinal canal stenosis. It therefore seems unnecessary to postulate an additional, genetically based abnormality of the intervertebral disks to account for the greater frequency and intensity of disk-related complaints among achondroplasts, but this supposition is nevertheless commonly made. The literature contains a number of observations of disk prolapse in achondroplasts leading to cauda equina syndrome and paraplegia (Vogel and Osborne 1949, Schreiber and Rosenthal 1952, Kuhlendahl and Hensell 1953). Kuhlendahl and Hensell (1953) considered achondroplasia to be a systemic disorder that renders the lumbar spine more than normally susceptible to disk prolapse induced by mechanical stress. Today, more than 50 years later, basic histological and biochemical studies on the nature of the disk tissue in achondroplasia are still lacking.

The studies of Verbiest (1954) revealed that marked narrowing of the spinal canal can cause nerve root compression syndromes. Thus, in achondroplasts, even relatively small disk protrusions or vertebral body displacements can produce severe neurologic deficits.

> ❗ The increased frequency and intensity of disk-related complaints in achondroplasts seem to be due to a combination of two factors: poor quality of the disks themselves, and spinal canal stenosis.

Ochronosis (Alkaptonuria)

Ochronosis is another systemic disease affecting the intervertebral disks, among other organs. In this rare inherited metabolic disorder, the enzymatic cleavage of certain amino acids, including tyrosine and phenylalanine, is impaired. Their degradation proceeds no further than the homogentisic acid stage, and this substance is deposited in bradytrophic tissues, including the intervertebral disks.

The renal excretion of homogentisic acid in ochronosis gives the urine its characteristic dark color. The disks, too, are darker than normal (**Fig. 5.5**). Signs of attrition appear prematurely in all portions of the disk, producing the appearance of extensive osteochondrosis, particularly at the lumbar and lower cervical levels, where the disks are subject to the greatest mechanical stress. Meanwhile, the large joints of the lower limbs (hip, knee, ankle) display marked, symmetrical arthrotic changes. Plain radiographs sometimes reveal a sickle-shaped collection of gas in the anterior portion of one or more disks (a vacuum phenomenon). Fissures and calcifications can also arise. Ochronosis should be suspected in any young patient presenting with generalized osteoarthrosis deformans, including disks with premature evidence of wear and tear, i. e., prematurely severe osteochondrosis. The presence of homogentisic acid in the urine confirms the diagnosis.

Descriptions of intervertebral disk involvement in ochronosis in the literature have so far been confined to case reports (Cervenansky et al. 1959, Feild et al. 1963, McCollum 1965, Emel et al. 2000). In all of these reported cases, the patients suffered from back pain, and some of them also had pain radiating into the legs. The small number of patients does not permit any inference of a causal connection between ochronosis and disk-related complaints.

Loss of Bone Density in the Vertebral Bodies

When the expansile pressure (tissue turgor) of the intervertebral disk tissue exceeds the resistance of the vertebral body, the height of the disk increases at the expense of the height of the vertebral body. Because the expansile pressure of the disk is greatest in the area of the nucleus pulposus, the result is a characteristic biconcave deformity of the end plates in the dorsal portion of the vertebral body. This deformity diminishes the hydrostatic mechanical pressure in the midportion of the disk, which therefore takes up more fluid, in accordance with the relation discussed on page 23. Cystic extensions of the anulus fibrosus cavity may develop; they can be seen on radiographs as hypodense areas in the intervertebral space. Histological examination reveals cartilage cells that have become inflated by the uptake of water.

Osteoporosis is among the spinal disorders that commonly cause secondary changes in the intervertebral disks. In osteoporosis, the rate of bone generation is reduced, while bone degradation continues normally. Thus, the strength of both cortical and cancellous bone is impaired. The bony trabeculae are thinned, and some of them disappear, so that the marrow spaces enlarge. The pathologically diminished mechanical resistance of bone enables the intervertebral disks to protrude into the vertebral bodies—not in localized fashion, as in Schmorl's nodes, but rather as smooth, broad-based impressions into the end plates (**Fig. 5.6**). The disks increase in volume because of their intrinsic expansile pressure, while the vertebral bodies become smaller. Disintegration of the vertebral body is most pronounced where the bone is under the greatest pressure from the neighboring disk. In the thoracic spine, the pressure is greatest anteriorly and the vertebral bodies become wedge-shaped. At the thoracolumbar junction and in the lumbar spine, the pressure is mainly axial (in the center of the vertebral body), and a biconcave vertebral deformity results. The impressions into the two surfaces of a single vertebral body may be so marked that they nearly meet in the middle, with the two disks almost touching each other ("fish vertebra").

Softened vertebral bone deforms in response to pressure from a neighboring intervertebral disk only if the turgor (expansile pressure) of the nucleus pulposus is preserved. This explains why fish vertebrae are seen only in osteoporosis that begins at an early age.

Other bone diseases, too, can weaken vertebral bone so that the disks produce broad-based impressions in the vertebral body end plates. The process of vertebral body disintegration and compensatory disk expansion is, in principle, the same no matter what the cause. The precise etiologic diagnosis can only be established from other kinds of evidence, such as the localization, extent, and progression of such changes, as well as other clinical parameters. Normal or enlarged disks and neighboring disintegrated vertebrae, in an adult patient, are seen not only in osteoporosis, but also in metastatic cancer, plasmacytoma, osteomalacia, osteitis fibrosa cystica (von Recklinghausen disease of bone, i. e., the bone changes associated with advanced hyperparathyroidism), and fractures. On the other hand, involvement of the disk, as well as the vertebral body, by the pathological process suggests an infectious disease rather than one of these conditions.

Weakening of vertebral bone with secondary changes of the intervertebral disks can also occur in childhood. **Osteogenesis imperfecta** is a prominent cause. In this hereditary disease, inadequate matrix synthesis in all mesenchymally derived tissues leads to pathological softening and fragility of bone. Further hallmarks of the disease include blue sclerae and oto-

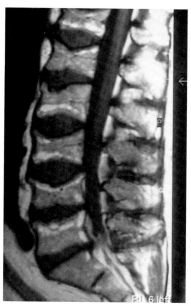

Fig. 5.6   Balloon-like expansion of the lumbar intervertebral disks in early-onset osteoporosis, with arch-like impressions of the upper and lower vertebral body end plates.

sclerosis. The congenital variant (osteogenesis imperfecta congenita) usually leads to death in infancy or early childhood, but there is also a form with later onset, in which the vertebrae and intervertebral disks develop typical changes. Thoracic "wedge vertebrae" and lumbar "fish vertebrae" arise in adolescence, resembling the findings in elderly people with osteoporosis. In extreme cases, the disks are very tall, and the vertebral bodies are flattened. Asymmetrical vertebral body degeneration leads to scoliosis and increased kyphosis. In some of the families of people with osteogenesis imperfecta, there seem to be a greater than average number of otherwise normal individuals with presenile osteoporosis, which Idelberger (1984) considers a *forme fruste* of the disease.

Generalized softening of the vertebral bodies and secondary disk changes can also occur as an acquired disorder during childhood. In **rickets**, the disks in the kyphotic segments are subject to considerably increased stress and therefore tend to display early signs of attrition. Fish vertebrae and flat vertebrae are rare in rickets, however, as it is more common for the disease to affect predominantly the rapidly growing long bones of the limbs.

5

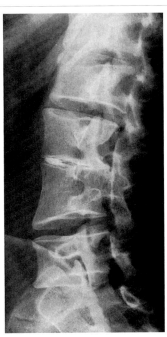

Fig. 5.7 Disk calcification and partial block vertebra in a 20-year-old man (asymptomatic).

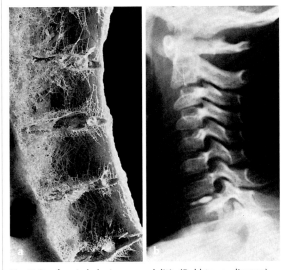

Fig. 5.8 a, b   Ankylosing spondylitis (Bekhterev disease).
a Calcification of the intervertebral disks and severe osteoporosis of the vertebral bodies (specimen courtesy of the Pathological Institute, University of Düsseldorf).
b Central calcification of the C7–T1 disk in a 4-year-old boy (incidental finding).

Disk Calcification and Ossification

Calcification arises in bradytrophic tissues through the crystallization of calcium salts. In the intervertebral disk, calcification may occur in either the nucleus pulposus or the anulus fibrosus. If the nucleus pulposus is calcified, then its dimensions can be measured from plain radiographs (which is not otherwise the case). Such calcifications were demonstrated radiographically as early as 1930 by Calvé and Galland. Schmorl (1932) reported a few cases of intervertebral disk calcification among his extensive collection of vertebral column specimens; the deposits were either of calcium carbonate or of calcium phosphate. People with gout can also have urate crystals in their intervertebral disks. Tomographic images reveal finely grained deposits in the interstices of the nucleus pulposus, or spotty calcifications in the anulus fibrosus (Schmorl and Junghanns 1968).

Intervertebral disk calcification occurs in inactivated motion segments (**Fig. 5.7**) and as a degenerative phenomenon in elderly people. It is a relatively rare finding, usually affecting only one or a few disks; it has not been shown to bear any particular relationship to systemic metabolic disturbances.

Calcific radiodensities in the intervertebral disk can also correspond to sites of true bone formation, i. e., ossification. Ossification can only occur after vascularization of the disk and ingrowth of vascular connective tissue, which are, in turn, most commonly the result of a prior inflammatory process or injury. Bone-forming cells migrate into the disk along with the connective tissue. Even the entire disk may be replaced with cancellous bone, as is often seen, for example, in ankylosing spondylitis (Bekhterev disease, **Fig. 5.8**).

The literature also contains many reports of disk calcifications in children and adolescents (Baron 1924, Buse 1963, Schmorl and Junghanns 1968, Coventry 1970, Wong et al. 1972, Blomquist et al. 1979, Brocher and Willert 1980, Crock 1983, Ventura et al. 1995, Li Yang et al. 2004). Bär and Fischer (1973) reported intervertebral disk calcification in a 10-year-old boy after a sports accident. The causes of calcification in such cases are unknown; hypothetical etiologies include an inflammatory (rheumatic) process, a bacterial infection, and trauma (Eyring 1969). Disk calcifications in young patients have the potential to regress, similarly to the para-articular calcifications of humeroscapular periarthropathy.

> **!** Calcification and ossification of the intervertebral disk are of no clinical significance. Their course and prognosis are benign.

Partial or total immobilization of a motion segment through calcification corresponds to the end stage of healing that we actually strive to obtain when we undertake spinal fusion procedures or intradiscal injections.

Summary

Nondegenerative disk diseases play a much less prominent role in clinical practice than degenerative disk diseases. This statement applies not only to the hereditary, congenital disorders discussed in this chapter, but also to acquired disorders (with the sole exception of discitis). Notochord remnants, developmental anomalies, and congenital malformations often produce very impressive radiological abnormalities while having little or no clinical relevance. The normally avascular intervertebral disks are only indirectly affected by infectious and neoplastic processes. Hematogenous infections and metastases attack the vertebral bodies first, then penetrate the disks by direct extension.

Systemic illnesses, such as diabetes, nutritional disorders, and cardiovascular disease, have no direct effect on disk tissue. The characteristic intradiscal deposits of alkaptonuria (ochronosis) are as harmless as the intradiscal calcifications, of various causes, that have been described mainly in children and adolescents. Balloon-like expansion of the intervertebral disks, as seen in osteoporosis, is due to weakening of the mechanical resistance of the vertebral body end plates and indicates that the turgor pressure of the disks is well preserved.

Conclusion

Genetically based anomalies of the intervertebral disks, intradiscal calcifications, and the changes of disk shape that are seen in osteoporosis are all innocuous findings.

5

6 Discosis

Definition

! The term "discosis" encompasses all biomechanical and pathoanatomical changes in the intervertebral disk that are associated with disk degeneration.

Synonyms: Disk degeneration, degenerative disk disease, chondrosis intervertebralis.

Classification

There are three stages of discosis (**Fig. 6.1**):
- the first, or early, stage, in adolescence and young adulthood
- the second stage, in middle age
- and the third stage, in old age.

The **first stage of discosis** begins with regression of the intradiscal vessels between the ages of 2 and 4 years.

From this time onward, the disk tissue receives nutrients only by diffusion. In childhood, the disk continues to function adequately as an osmotic system, so that its fibroblasts and chondrocytes are assured a sufficient supply of nutrients. The lower body weight of children and, above all, their relatively high degree of physical activity create favorable biomechanical conditions for the nourishment of the fiber-producing cells of

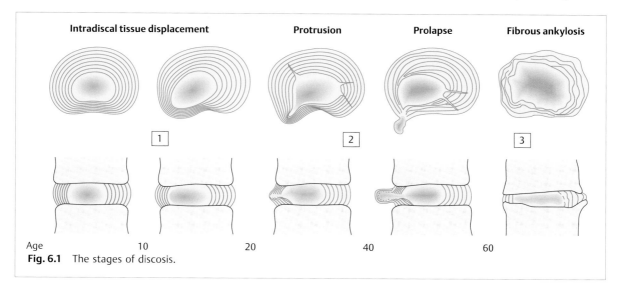

Fig. 6.1 The stages of discosis.

6

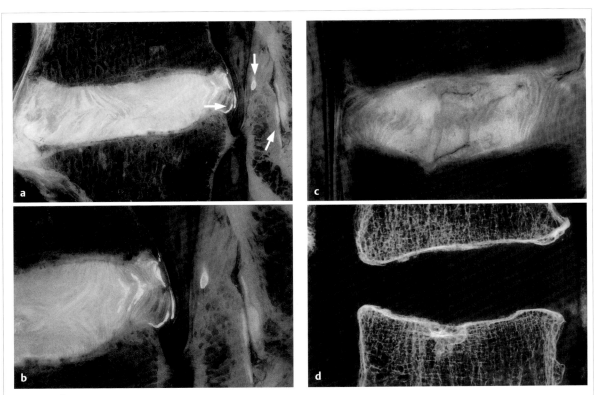

Fig. 6.2 a–d

a, b Sagittal section of the L4–L5 motion segment (anatomical preparation). Disseminated calcifications in the dorsal lamellae of the anulus fibrosus and the posterior longitudinal ligament. Isolated focus in the ligamentum flavum (arrow). Note the facet joint space (arrow). "Geographical" pattern of the disk in both the nucleus pulposus and the anulus fibrosus. The disk protrusion extends beyond the posterior edge of the vertebral body. Fissures in the anulus fibrosus: discosis, stage 2.

c, d L3–L4 motion segment, with a fissure in the anulus fibrosus extending into the upper cartilaginous end plate of L4, with displacement of disk tissue into the vertebral body. Geographical disk structure and fissures, corresponding to stage 2 discosis (from Ludwig, Tiedjen, and Kramer 2004).

the intervertebral disk. As body weight increases, so does the axial load on the disk, particularly in the lower lumbar segments. Furthermore, as children grow into adolescents and adults, their level of physical activity decreases as they become relatively sedentary, first at school and then at work. The fibrous lamellae of the disk, which are no longer adequately nourished and thus no longer able to withstand the strong outward pressure of the central, mobile disk tissue, begin to protrude outward. The earliest disk-related complaints may arise at any time between age 12 and age 20, when intradiscal shifting of disk material suddenly causes stretching or bulging of the posterior longitudinal ligament. In adolescents, this produces the clinical picture of iliolumbar extension stiffness (see Chapter 11).

The **second stage of discosis** affects adults aged 20–60. The poorly nourished fibroblasts and chondrocytes produce poorer-quality fibers that are no longer able to withstand the expansile pressure of the central, mobile portion of the disk, which, at this time of life, is still intact. The anulus fibrosus develops both radial and circular tears, into which the tissue of the nucleus pulposus protrudes. Entire sequestra composed of tissue from the anulus fibrosus and the cartilaginous end plates can form and then, under asymmetrical axial loading, follow the path of least resistance outward, sometimes beyond the boundary of the intervertebral disk. Disk protrusions and prolapses are the result. As long as the external layers of the anulus fibrosus are intact, it is still possible for the displaced tissue to return to its original position. In a disk prolapse, however, the displaced tissue penetrates the anulus fibrosus and can no longer go back inside the disk. Dorsally or dorsolaterally pointing disk prolapses come into contact with the posterior longitudinal ligament, which derives its sensory nerve supply from the meningeal branch of the spinal nerve. The resulting symptoms consist of locally circumscribed lumbago, chronic discogenic low back pain, and/or root compression syndrome (**Fig. 6.2**).

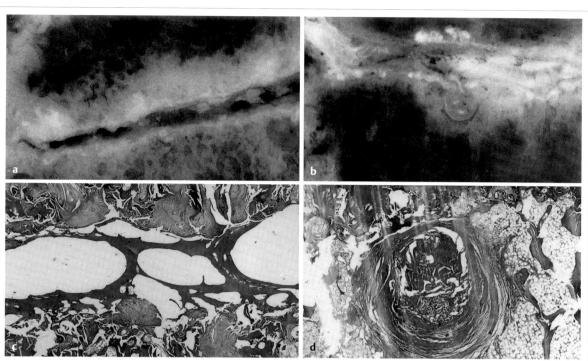

Fig. 6.3 a–d Comparative gross and microscopic findings of advanced discosis (stage 3) (from Ludwig, Tiedjen, and Kramer 2004).
a L5/S1 intervertebral space, with subtotal destruction of the disk, loss of height, and focal zones of contact between the upper and lower end plates (magnification 4×).
b Histological section of the central part of the intervertebral space, with fibrous connective tissue deposits between the trabeculae of the bone marrow space. The intervertebral space contains a number of bony trabeculae. Same specimen as **a** (magnification 63×, H & E stain).

c Macroscopic photograph of disk tissue entering the vertebral body end plate at L4/5. Marked loss of disk height and end plate sclerosis. Consolidated Schmorl's node under the inferior vertebral body end plate.
d The histological section corresponding to **c**. Concentric, fibrous lamellae of connective tissue surround the displaced tissue. Fat is seen in the neighboring marrow space (magnification 63×, H & E stain).

Pathoanatomical changes within the disk tissue, including fiber disruption, tissue loss due to prolapse, and dehydration, produce a further manifestation of the second stage of discosis: **segmental instability.** Slackening of the initially tautly elastic disk tissue loosens the mechanical link between adjacent vertebrae, enabling movements of nonphysiological amplitude and direction. This kind of instability may not be directly visible. It can often be detected only with the aid of functional images, e. g., lateral radiographs on forward and backward bending. Degenerative instability also causes slippage (olisthesis) of the vertebrae relative to one another, either ventrally or dorsally (retrolisthesis). Symptoms are produced by impingement on the neural elements in the vertebral canal or the intervertebral foramen. Most therapeutic procedures are undertaken in the second stage of discosis, because it is in this stage that disk displacement and slackening most commonly produce intense local and radicular manifestations.

In the **third stage,** the displacement of central, mobile disk tissue (loosening, protrusion, prolapse) ceases to progress. After age 60, the disk tissue loses water and becomes fibrotic and firm, and therefore less liable to dorsal displacement. Calcification of the ligaments that span the intervertebral space as part of the spondylotic process contributes further to the fixation of the motion segment (**Figs. 6.3, 6.4**). The pathoanatomical changes may appear quite impressive at this stage, but, as their net effect is partial stabilization, the patient is usually spared severe symptoms. This is the so-called "**comfortable rigidity of the aging spine.**" The age distribution curves for disk diseases show that protrusions and prolapses do, indeed, occur in old age, but with a different pattern than in middle age, mainly affecting the upper lumbar segments and producing extradiscal sequestra that are projected craniolaterally. Spondylogenic symptoms after age 60 tend to be caused not by disk pathology per se, but by secondary degenerative changes in the dorsal part of the motion segment. The

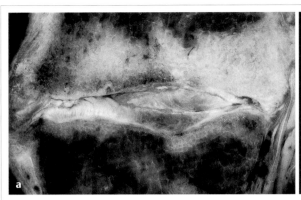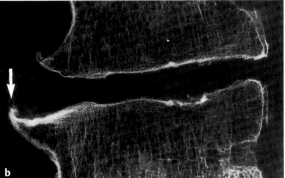

Fig. 6.4 a, b   Advanced discosis (stage 3) with ventral osteophyte formation and condensation of the adjacent bone marrow space (arrow) (from Ludwig, Tiedjen, and Kramer 2004).

most common problems are spondylarthrosis and degenerative spinal canal stenosis, with chronic radicular irritation syndrome due to lateral bony compression of the nerve roots, manifested as spinal claudication.

Etiology

The spine of a quadruped consists, in principle, of a horizontal chain of identical segments supported at two points. The vertical human spine is subject to much greater gravitational stresses.

> **!** We humans owe disk disease mainly to our upright posture.

Schmorl's nodes, i. e., circumscribed protrusions of disk tissue into the vertebral end plates, are not found in quadrupeds. The vertebral columns of certain flightless birds, whose bipedal stance places gravitational stress on the spine much as it does in humans, display abnormalities of a comparable type (Klapp 1958). Exner (1954) described severe forms of spondylosis deformans in anthropoid apes with upright posture. Yamada (1962), Wassilev and Dimova (1970), and Cassidy et al. (1988) forced mice to walk upright by amputating their forelegs. One year later, the anulus fibrosus and cartilaginous end plates displayed structural changes attributable to vertical stress. Similar observations in animals were made by Palmer and Lotz (1993), Edwards et al. (1998), and Unglaub et al. (2003).

> **!** Though genetic differences between individuals are important, the main cause of generalized disk degeneration in humans is the **premature aging of bradytrophic tissue** induced by static mechanical forces.

The human intervertebral disk does not begin as bradytrophic tissue. In infancy, when the disk is not under any particular mechanical stress, intense metabolic ex-

change takes place across the intradiscal vessels. Twisting and bending of the trunk, as the infant crawls, further aid fluid exchange across the boundaries of the disk.

The assumption of an upright posture fundamentally alters the biomechanical situation of the disk. The intravertebral vessels are protected by the bony trabecular system, but the vertical compressive pressure on the disk (the sum of the weight of the body above the disk and the muscle tone across it) is transmitted directly to the blood vessel walls within the pulpy, homogeneous disk tissue. Because the arteriolar and venous pressure is lower than the hydrostatic pressure, the blood is pressed out of these vessels, which collapse, suffer pressure atrophy, and finally disappear. The nutrient supply of the fibroblasts and cartilage cells diminishes in a relatively short time because they are isolated from the bloodstream. Metabolic exchange can now take place only across long distances within the disk tissue, through transport mechanisms that are less effective than the previous normal vascularization.

Insufficient nutrient supply is associate with a lowered oxygen/glucose concentrations and acidic pH, and adversely affects the ability of disk cells to synthesize and maintain the disk matrix leading to disk degeneration (Mokhbi-Soukane 2006).

> **!** The disk is the largest contiguous structure in the body that lacks its own blood supply.

The developing disk, accustomed to adequate perfusion, low mechanical stress, and much movement, is suddenly subjected to new, unfavorable conditions when the infant begins to stand and walk. The inadequate capacity of the cells within the human disk to adapt to the new situation leads to a qualitative degeneration of its connective and supportive tissue, with early signs of wear and tear. This explains why degenerative disk disease sometimes occurs in childhood. Töndury (1968) found microscopic signs of degeneration in the disks of

4-year-old children. The anatomical and clinical data imply that discopathy in all three major regions of the spine can occur at puberty or earlier (Idelberger 1959). The youngest patient undergoing surgery for disk prolapse in the series of Daschner et al. (1971) was 13 years old; in three other series, the youngest patients were 10, 16, and 9 years old (Ford 1960, Mittelmeier 1970, Seyfarth 1970). Of the 2755 patients operated on for discogenic neural compression by the Düsseldorf University Neurosurgical Clinic (Barghoorn 1975), 36 were 18 years old or less; these patients mainly suffered from massive monoradicular sciatica. There are many other reports of disk prolapse in childhood (Key 1950, King 1959, O'Connell 1960, Epstein and Lavine 1964, DaSilva et al. 1977, Parsch and Eulenburg 1983, Bradbury 1996, Ishihara 1997, Panayiotis 1998, Balagué 2001, Schlenzka 2001, Arendt 2002, Kjaer 2005).

! Beyond age 30, it is rare to find a human spine that shows no sign of degenerative changes in the disks.

In most individuals, the active and passive transport mechanisms across the boundaries of the disk cannot sustain, over the decades, a constant, adequate supply of nutrients to its cells.

! A sedentary lifestyle with prolonged maintenance of unfavorable postures impairs movement-dependent fluid shifts across the boundaries of the disk.

Trauma and transient overloading impair the nutrient supply of the disk cells much less than a prolonged absence of movement.

In addition to the verticality of the spine and invariance of posture, **genetic factors** also contribute to the early appearance of regressive changes in the intervertebral disks. An endogenous component is postulated by many authors (Hanraets 1959, Armstrong 1965, Schmorl and Junghanns 1968, Wilson 1968, Braun 1969, Brocher 1973, Töndury 1981, Idelberger 1984, Simmons 1996, Matsui 1998, Kawaguchi 2002, Battié 2004, Bernadino 2004, Lattermann 2004). According to Idelberger (1952), some individuals have a constitutional predisposition to premature disk fatigue. Hanraets (1959) and Wilson (1968) showed familial clustering of disk disease. According to Wilson (1968) and Beard and Stevens (1985), the quality and configuration of the collagen fibers in the anulus fibrosus are influenced by genetic factors. Battié and Videmann (2004) found that near relatives of patients with disk prolapses are more likely to have spine-related complaints than near relatives of normal control individuals. Hestbaek et al. (2006) in their twin study demonstrated a correlation between low back pain in childhood/adolescence and low back pain in adulthood.

The existence of an inherited predisposition to disk disease thus cannot be rejected out of hand, but there is no apparent connection to any particular habitus, as is the case for some other diseases (diabetes mellitus, peptic ulcer disease). Our own studies in a large set of patients have unequivocally shown that disk lesions are equally common in individuals of athletic, leptosomal, pyknic, or dysplastic build (Krämer 1978).

Videman et al. (2006) identified new genes associated with signs of disk degeneration and presents evidence of a multigenic etiology.

■ Pathogenesis

The worsened metabolic situation beginning in childhood alters not only the chemical composition, but also the anatomical structure of the intervertebral disk. Because of their inadequate supply of energy and nutrients, the fibroblasts form fibers and matrix of deficient quality, and finally disintegrate. Many histological studies of disk material from unselected autopsy cases have shown this to be the case. The degenerative process begins in the disk (Eubanks 2006).

Overview of the literature. Basic studies have been undertaken by Hirsch and Schajowitz (1952–1953), Hirsch et al. (1953, 1963), Hirsch and Nachemson (1954), Hirsch (1960, 1966), Hirsch and Bobechenko (1965), Feng (2000), Roughley (2004), Battié and Videmann (2004), An et al. (2004), Crock (2004), Hansson (2004), Naturajan et al. (2004), Haefeli et al. (2005), Roh et al (2005), An and Masuda (2006), Brisby (2006),

Guehring et al. (2006), Natarajan (2006), Setton (2006), and Unglaub et al. (2006). Growth factors, such as bFGF and TGF-β1, macrophages, and mast cells may play a key role in the repair of the injured anulus fibrosus and subsequent disk degeneration (Peng 2006).

Kuhlendahl and Richter (1952) found fatty deposits in the disk matrix of adolescents as well as occasional fat droplets in the cells of the anulus fibrosus. Among young adults (aged 25–40), they found further regressive structural changes including incipient dehydration, sharper contours of the fibrous lamellae, and blurring of the border between the anulus fibrosus and the nucleus pulposus. Histological studies regularly show degenerative changes in all structural components of the intervertebral disk beginning in the third decade of life, with cell degeneration, cell loss, fiber degeneration, and loosening of the matrix (Püschel 1930, Schaffer and von Möllendorf 1930, Erlacher 1949, Coventry et al. 1954,

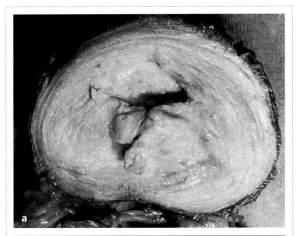

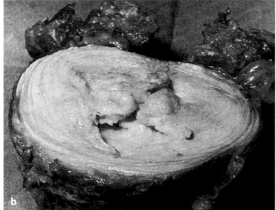

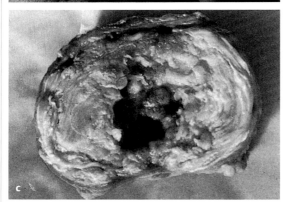

Fig. 6.5 a–c Cavitary system of the third lumbar disk of a 42-year-old man with stage 2 discosis (**a**, **b**), and of a 66-year-old man with stage 3 disease (**c**).

brils of altered density and transverse striation (Dahmen 1966). Further extensive descriptions of histological changes in the intervertebral disk can be found in many publications (Friberg and Hirsch 1950, Lindemann and Kuhlendahl 1953, Güntz 1958, Schmorl and Junghanns 1968, Töndury 1981, Rothman and Simeone 1982, Wiesel and Rothman 1982, Genant 1984, Kirkaldy-Willis 1984, Roberts 1985, Rauschning 1986, Bell et al. 1990, Bernick et al. 1991, An 2004, Crock 2004, Hanson 2004, Bantrizos et al. 2005, Gruber et al. 2007, Waris et al. 2007, Zhang et al. 2008). Studies are under way to describe matrix constituents as targets in matrix breakdown (Feng 2006). The etiology of symptom manifestation in lumbar and cervical spine degeneration is multifactorial and includes cellular, biochemical, and biomechanical causes (Roh 2005).

Biology offers several strategies for restoring the degenerating disk, including the use of recombinant or natural proteins that increase matrix accumulation and assembly, enhance the number of disk cells, or in other ways lead to restoration of the native healthy disk. Recombinant bone morphogenetic protein-7 (osteogenic protein-1) shows promise in this regard. Other growth factors, as well as cytokine antagonists such as the interleukin-1 receptor antagonist, are also good candidates (Evans 2006).

As disk degeneration progresses, concentric and radial fissures develop in the disk. The cavitary system of the nucleus pulposus enlarges and connects to the fissures of the anulus fibrosus (**Fig. 6.5**).

The cavitary system and fissures can also be demonstrated by discography. An intradiscal cavity can be punctured transcutaneously and filled with contrast material or medication. The more severely the disk is degenerated, the greater the amount of fluid that can be injected into it at low pressure (Panjabi et al. 1988). In younger patients, this amount is of the order of 1–2 mL. In older patients, a lumbar disk may admit as much as 5 mL of injected fluid within its confines, without any damage to the borders of the disk or spillage of fluid outside it.

Collections of gas in the cavitary system of the disk are seen in plain radiographs as the so-called "vacuum phenomenon" (**Fig. 6.6**) (Knutsson 1944, Hoeffken 1951, Raines 1953, Armstrong 1965, Schmorl and Junghanns 1968, Genant 1984). The cause of this phenomenon and the composition of the gas are currently unknown.

Yellow and brown discoloration of disk fibers has also been described as a sign of disk degeneration. Güntz (1958), in a systematic study, found that such discoloration occurs only when fissures and tears in the disk tissue extend through gaps in the cartilaginous end plate into the vertebral body and make contact with the vascular structures originating in the bone marrow.

Harris and Macnab 1954, Lang 1962, Dahmen 1966, Rothman and Simeone 1982, Miller et al. 1988). Harris and Macnab (1954) studied the histology of adult nucleus pulposus tissue and found only pyknotic, clumped, degenerate, or shadow cell nuclei. Electron microscopy of adult disk tissue revealed irregular, disorganized fi-

Schmorl and Junghanns (1968) used the term "chondrosis intervertebralis" for wear and tear of the intervertebral disk.

> **!** The term "discosis" is apt, because the degenerative process affects not only cartilage, but all of the other portions of the intervertebral disk as well.

These processes are confined to the disk at first and thus cannot be seen in plain radiographs, except perhaps as narrowing of the disk space or posture-related deviations of the spinal axis. The loss of height of the disks increases the compressive stress on the intervertebral joints and causes narrowing of the intervertebral foramina. The disk tissue, being avascular, cannot repair itself; when disk degeneration is long-standing, certain regenerative changes occur, proceeding from the neighboring vertebral body. As these changes involve both the bone and the cartilage, Schmorl (1932) designated them as **osteochondrosis**. The neighboring vertebral body end plates show sclerotic condensations with irregular contours. In osteochondrosis, unlike spondylitis, the sclerotic zone involves only the portion of the vertebral body that is adjacent to the end plate. As in arthrosis, subchondral cysts are sometimes seen.

Erosive osteochondrosis is a rapidly progressive form of osteochondrosis, often with more severe symptoms, sometimes raising the suspicion of spondylodiscitis, from which it must be differentiated. The key diagnostic criterion for erosive osteochondrosis is preservation of the sclerotic upper and lower end plates in tomographic plain radiographs and CT. The available literature on this condition is sparse (Courtois 1980, Herbsthofer et al. 1996).

Osteochondrosis of the intervertebral disks is found most commonly, and with the greatest severity, in the lower motion segments of the cervical and lumbar regions, because the mechanical stress is greatest at these sites. Generalized disk attrition and loss of turgor pressure slacken the disks and thereby place excessive tension on the ligaments spanning the disk space, particularly the anterior longitudinal ligament. This ligament has no attachment to the disk itself; it is attached to the vertebral bodies on either side of it by Sharpey's fibers on the far side of the bony margin. A bony reaction begins at this site, then progresses along the course of the ligament. **Spondylotic marginal osteophytes** (**Fig. 6.7**) typically have a horizontal take-off from the vertebral body and then a more vertical course. They arise only in the vicinity of the anterior longitudinal ligament on the anterolateral surface of the vertebral body. Small dorsal osteophytes are sometimes seen as well, as in **Fig. 6.8**. The process of neo-ossification involves a steadily expanding region, and osteophyte formation may be so extensive as to constitute *spondylosis hyperostotica* (**Fig. 6.9**). Despite the marked anatomical changes, there are no symptoms. Processes taking place within the disk itself are of greater clinical significance.

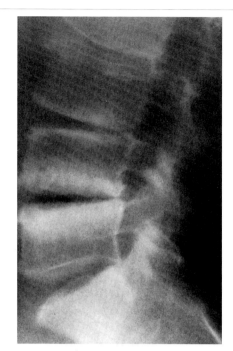

Fig. 6.6 Vacuum phenomenon with gas formation in the ventral portion of the cavitary system of the L4/5 disk in a 68-year-old woman with advanced spondylosis and osteochondrosis (stage 3 discosis). Clinical findings: chronic, recurrent low back pain.

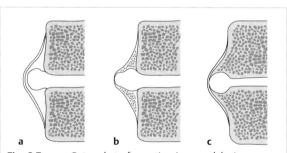

Fig. 6.7 a–c Osteophyte formation in spondylosis.

In advanced degeneration, pieces of the anulus fibrosus may break off, forming so-called disk sequestra. Radial fissures enable **intradiscal mass movements** (as long as the turgor of the nucleus pulposus is preserved). Portions of the nucleus pulposus, as well as anulus fibrosus sequestra, take the path of least resistance along the fissures, and can bulge outward, forming a disk prolapse. The prolapsed material rarely consists only of nucleus pulposus tissue and usually contains parts of the anulus fibrosus and the cartilaginous end plates as well. The expression "disk prolapse" is, therefore, more accurate than "nucleus pulposus prolapse." Radial fissures first appear at precisely the time of life when lumbago and sciatica are most commonly present.

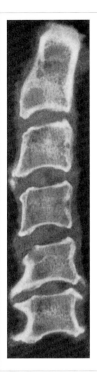

Fig. 6.8 Midline sagittal section of the dissected cervical spine of a 65-year-old man. The spondylotic osteophytes are more pronounced ventrally than dorsally.

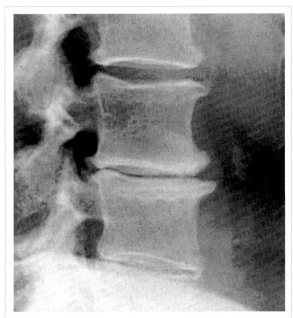

Fig. 6.9 Advanced osteochondrosis and spondylosis with osteophyte development both ventrally and dorsally (stage 3 discosis).

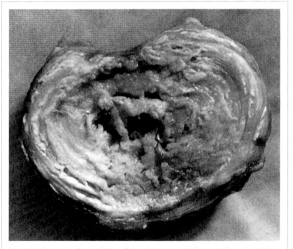

Fig. 6.10 Lumbar disk of an 80-year-old man (stage 3 discosis).

Breaks and tears in the cartilaginous end plates enable the blood vessels and connective tissue of the vertebral body spongiosa to grow into the intervertebral disk (**Fig. 6.10**). If disk remnants are present, the blood vessels grow into them like roots into soil, displacing the disk tissue and replacing it with loose, cell-rich and highly vascularized scar tissue (Töndury 1958). Tough, dried-out disk fibers and spondylotic osteophytes prop up the disk space sufficiently to shield the invading blood vessels from external compressive forces. The re-

sulting fibrous and sometimes bony **ankylosis** leads to the functional inactivation of the motion segment. Though the intervertebral foramen may be markedly narrowed, the loss of disk height and fixation of the motion segment usually cause no pain at all: this process takes decades to run its course, and the remaining components of the motion segment (nerve roots, vessels) have enough time to adapt. Investigators studying intervertebral disk degeneration should bear in mind that there is no correlation between disk degeneration and pain (An and Masuda 2006). Progressive wear and tear of the intervertebral disk is generally considered a "degenerative" process, i. e., as Schmorl and Junghanns (1968) stated, an age-related and thus more or less normal decline of tissue quality, which is the inevitable fate of disk tissue. Töndury (1981) introduced the concept of the life cycle of the intervertebral disk.

> Intervertebral disk degeneration (discosis) is a normal biological regulatory process rather than a disease, but it is nonetheless a major cause of functional disturbances at certain times of life.

The progressive restriction of spinal mobility due to disk degeneration is taken in their stride by most individuals without producing any symptoms whatsoever.

> In general, disk degeneration attains clinical significance only when tears, attrition, and tissue displacement impinge on the immediately adjacent nerves and blood vessels, particularly in the lower motion segments of the cervical and lumbar spine.

■ Biochemical Changes of Aging

The age-related structural changes of the intervertebral disk are accompanied by a decrease in water content and a change of chemical composition. All of these changes affect the biomechanics of the motion segment.

! Low water content is a characteristic sign of aging of the
● intervertebral disk.

Water makes up 88% of the neonatal disk, but the **water content** declines to 83% at age 12 and to 70% at age 72 (Keyes and Compère 1932). In early childhood, the nucleus pulposus contains more water than the anulus fibrosus, but this difference decreases over the years, as shown both in our own studies (Krämer et al. 1985) and by Beard and Stevens (1985). MRI reveals low water content as low signal intensity, i.e., dehydrated disks appear darker than well-hydrated ones (Krämer and Köster 2001). Fluid loss further impairs the nutritive status of the disk, because water is not just a structural component of the intradiscal macromolecules but also serves as a medium of transport for the substrates and waste products of cellular metabolism (**Fig. 6.11**).

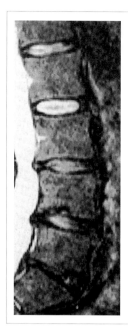

Fig. 6.11 MRI of the lumbar spine (T2-weighted image): the water content of the lower three lumbar vertebrae (dark) is less than that of the upper two (bright), because of disk degeneration.

6

Mineral content. The organic **matrix** of the disk also changes in characteristic ways with age. The calcium content of disk tissue doubles over the course of life, while its potassium content gradually declines because of cell loss. Its magnesium content declines at first till about age 17, then slowly rises again. Its sulfur content declines steadily, but its nitrogen content rises. Changes in **collagen** and **mucopolysaccharides** have important implications for metabolic exchange and biomechanics. Noncollagenous proteins increase, in parallel with the rising nitrogen content. The collagen content of the disk rises till about age 20, then remains nearly constant. The total mucopolysaccharides and proteoglycans change both qualitatively and quantitatively with age (Zöllner et al. 1999, Hutton et al. 2000, Taylor et al. 2000, Weiler et al. 2002, Roberts and Caterson 2004).

! Another characteristic sign of disk aging is the reduction
● of mucopolysaccharide content.

Moreover, the molecular weight of the mucopolysaccharides declines. The hydrating ability of the disk, i.e., its ability to retain fluid even under high pressure, is mainly a function of the number and size of the mucopolysaccharide molecules it contains. The intradiscal osmotic pressure therefore declines with age, and the disk dries out.

■ Biomechanical Basis of Disk Tissue Displacement

The enzymatic depolymerization of macromolecules in the disk gives rise to ionized intermediate products of catabolism whose increased concentration temporarily elevates the **intradiscal oncotic pressure.** By measuring the turgor pressure of the intervertebral disks in individuals of different ages, we have found that disk reexpansion after compression occurs not only with greater force, but also more rapidly, in young and middle-aged individuals than in elderly people. The turgor pressure curves show remarkably high values in individuals aged 30–50. After age 50, however, the turgor pressure of the disk markedly declines (Krämer 1973) (**Fig. 6.12**).

After the age of 30, the central, mobile disk tissue, whose high turgor pressure enables it to expand after compression, is enclosed within an anulus fibrosus whose mechanical resistance has already begun to decline. Even in young adults the anulus is regularly found to contain disorganized fibers and small tears; from age 30–35 onward, full-thickness tears become increasingly common. Microscopic examination of the disk at this age usually reveals a certain amount of matrix expansion and progressive homogenization of the nucleus pulposus, along with evidence of nuclear degeneration in the anulus fibrosus and microscopic tears in its lamellae. These changes impair the solidity of disk tissue.

6

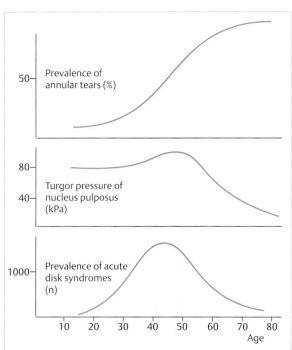

Fig. 6.12 The biomechanical basis of disk prolapse in middle age: high turgor pressure of disk tissue, increased number of tears in the anulus fibrosus.

Table 6.1 Precipitating factors for the pathological displacement of disk tissue

- Elevated mechanical stress on the disk
- Elevated turgor pressure of disk tissue
- Loosening of disk tissue with demarcation of sequestra
- Compressive and shearing forces

> **!** The biomechanical condition underlying disk tissue displacement is present during youth and middle age, causing intradiscal tissue displacement, protrusions, and prolapses.

The increased presence of ionized molecules in the disk leads to the temporary uptake of increased amounts of fluid. This marked volume increase places the anulus fibrosus under high tension even at rest. The disk as a whole therefore becomes relatively stiff and inelastic. The compression experiments of Virgin (1951) and the pressure and strain diagrams of Hartmann (1970) revealed that the overstretched anulus fibrosus fibers, if placed under yet more stress, can cross over into the "border zone" in which they begin to separate and to tear. When the anulus is in this condition, any additional

stress leaves behind an additional amount of irreversible deformation; the fibers fail to return to their original position even after a long time (hysteresis). Thus, after a marked increase in volume, sudden stresses affect the disk almost as if it were made of glass: the anulus fibers—mainly the peripheral ones—may be torn (Gordon et al. 1991).

Although the radial and full-thickness tears of the anulus fibrosus continue to progress with age, as has been unequivocally shown by all histological studies of disk aging, the frequency and intensity of protrusion- and prolapse-related complaints nonetheless decline. The reason for this is that the turgor pressure of the nucleus pulposus decreases, and with it the tendency for the disk tissue to become displaced. The cause of this process of macromolecular depolymerization and the resulting intradiscal pressure elevation remains unknown, as does its precise time course. Naylor (1983) considered the depolymerization to be due to an increased amount of hyaluronidase. Our therapeutic efforts involve, among other things, the instillation of certain substances to accelerate the process of depolymerization (chemonucleolysis), to slow it (hyaluronidase inhibitors), or to neutralize its ionized intermediate products (reduction of turgor pressure).

Aside from the simultaneous presence of high turgor pressure and lessened mechanical resistance of the anulus fibrosus, a number of other biomechanical factors promote disk prolapse. One of these factors is loosening of tissue within the disk itself, resulting in the formation of a relatively large sequestrum that can lose all connection to the surrounding tissue when the intradiscal pressure is raised and compressive and/or shearing forces are applied. The sequestrum then follows the path of least resistance: it moves, for example, toward the convex side of the disk if the disk is asymmetrically compressed. When this displacement (**Table 6.1**) exceeds the physiological limit, the result is a protrusion or prolapse. Often, particularly in medicolegal reports, one reads statements to the effect that a disk prolapse has been caused solely by severe mechanical stress, involving compressive and/or shearing forces. Such events cannot occur, however, unless proceeded by the intradiscal changes listed in **Table 6.1**. It follows that mechanical stress—the "additional impulse," as it was called by Schmorl and Junghanns (1968)—should properly be considered a *precipitating factor* for disk herniation, rather than its sole underlying cause. Understanding the relationship between mechanics and cell metabolism is a priority not only for distinguishing healthy loading from damaging loading but also for providing a baseline understanding required for tissue engineering and gene therapy (Iatridis 2006).

■ Effects on the Osmotic System

Further enzymatic degradation of the intradiscal macro-molecules produces smaller catabolic products, with molecular mass less than 400 Da, which can pass through the semipermeable boundaries of the inter-vertebral disk. If these molecules are not replaced by others newly synthesized within the disk, the intradiscal oncotic pressure will steadily decline. In accordance with the relation shown on page 23, the decline in the oncotic pressure of the disk is accompanied by a decrease in its **water content** and in its absorptive capacity for water. The disk loses volume and height, with a resulting reduction in the tension on the anulus fibrosus fibers at rest. Slackening of these fibers has the further result that movements under mechanical stress are transmitted to the anulus fibrosus less evenly and with less attenuation (damping), so that the fibers now suffer a greater degree of wear and tear than before. The most vulnerable fibers are now the so-called spanning fibers that bind the lamellae to each other and normally prevent large displacements of tissue.

The inelastic disk, vulnerable to tearing, can no longer perform its function in the motion segment as a shock absorber and quasi-joint.

> **!** Slackening of the disk places increased and abnormal functional demands on the remaining components of the motion segment, particularly the intervertebral joints and the ligaments. This, in turn, sets the stage for the development of further symptoms that are the indirect result of disk degeneration.

When the oncotic pressure within the disk is low, relatively mild mechanical stress (relatively low intradiscal hydrostatic pressure) causes a loss of fluid from the disk. The daily fluctuations in body height, due mainly to fluctuations in disk volume, become less pronounced. Adolescents lose 2% of their height from morning to evening, older adults only 0.2%. A further cause of disk dehydration in old age is tearing of the anulus fibrosus, discussed above. These fissures in the boundary of the disk abolish its function as a semipermeable membrane, so that water, solutes, or even macromolecules can leave the disk even when the hydrostatic pressure gradient is relatively small. The osmotic equilibrium at the boundary of the disk is disrupted. The same effect is present in the aftermath of disk injury, including surgical procedures (discotomy).

Progressive dehydration makes the disk tissue even more brittle and susceptible to tearing. In the relatively dry tissue, dissolved nutrients and metabolic waste products cannot diffuse as quickly as before, and a vicious circle finally results in near-total drying out and attenuation of the disk. The loss of fluid and disk mass is reflected in a marked loss of disk height. These degenerative changes first appear in the cervical and lower lumber segments, though they sooner or later affect all of the disks in the spine.

■ Instability of the Motion Segment

Definition

Instability is the lack of stability. In the musculoskeletal system, instability takes the form of a loss of stiffness, e. g., at the symphysis pubis, the sacroiliac joints of the pelvic ring, the elements of the shoulder girdle, or the motion segments of the spine. The disk is the key element of the motion segment that is responsible for stability. If the stiffness of the disk is impaired by degeneration, injury, or discotomy, **discogenic instability** is said to be present. This condition eventually leads to overuse and degeneration of the intervertebral joints, so that, within a few years, typical degenerative changes of the joints (spondylarthrosis) appear, clinically manifest as arthroligamentous low back pain and as spinal canal stenosis due to marginal osteophytes projecting into the spinal canal.

Pathogenesis of Instability

Discogenic instability causes quantitative and qualitative changes of the normal pattern of movement of the motion segment. Krismer et al. (1997) list different definitions of instability and describe it as consisting of the following mechanical abnormalities:
- excessive dorsoventral translational movement
- pathological accompanying movements (coupled motion)
- an enlarged neutral zone
- a pathological center of rotation.

The degenerative loss of disk stiffness is due to structural changes within the disk. In the young disk, the anulus fibers are held taut by the turgor pressure of the nucleus pulposus. When this pressure diminishes, the anulus fibers lose part of their stabilizing function. Krismer et al. (1997) studied the anulus fibers in experiments in which they cut only the fibers running in one particular direction. They found that the anulus fibers limit axial rotation more than the intervertebral joints. Radial, mainly ventrally located anular tears impair the stabilizing function of the anulus. As the anulus progressively degenerates, the intervertebral joints assume a more important role in limiting rotation. It is then only a matter of time before arthrosis of the intervertebral joints develops.

Clinical Significance

Instability, a loss of stiffness, hypermobility, and translational movement with permanent displacement of the vertebral body do not necessarily imply the presence of symptoms. Instability is clinically significant only when it produces pain or limits function. "Clinical instability" therefore seems a more appropriate term. This expression was used by White and Panjabi (1978) to describe the loss of the ability of the spine to move within its normal range, under physiological conditions and in everyday activities, without the appearance of neurological disturbances, major deformities, or intolerable pain. Frymoyer et al. (1979) defined clinical instability as the loss of stiffness of a motion segment to the extent that the application of external force to it is likely to cause a major displacement resulting in a neurological disturbance. Kirkaldy-Willis and Farfan (1982) defined it as a state in which the clinical condition of a patient with back problems worsens upon minimal provocation by movement. In summary, one can say that there exist both
- symptomatic instability and
- asymptomatic instability.

The causes of instability include not only the slackening of the intervertebral disks (discogenic instability) but also changes in the bony components of the motion segment, due, e. g., to fracture, surgical resection of the stabilizing pars interarticularis, or spondylolysis/spondylolisthesis (two conditions of partly genetic origin).

Surgical Indications

Krismer et al. (1997) state that the diagnosis "primary lumbar instability" was created merely to justify the performance of stabilization procedures. This suspicion

is heightened by the fact that there is still no consensus on the proper definition of instability. Functional radiographs obtained on forward and backward bending of the spine, the most important type of imaging study for the diagnosis of instability, very rarely show an anteroposterior displacement of one vertebral body over another with an amplitude greater than the generally accepted cut-off value of 4 mm. Moreover, the intensity of symptoms of degenerative vertebral body slippage is not correlated with the amplitude of the slip.

What is really needed for the proper diagnosis of instability is a technique for the three-dimensional measurement of force–displacement curves in the motion segment (Kayser 2006).

Prognosis and Course of Discogenic Degenerative Instability

Kirkaldy-Willis and Farfan (1982) describe three phases of degenerative instability:
- In the **first phase,** which affects younger individuals, the functional disturbance involving slackening of the disks has, as yet, no radiologically demonstrable correlate. In this phase, intradiscal tissue displacements and disk protrusions may produce acute low back pain or, in some cases, signs of radicular irritation.
- In the **second phase** of instability, during middle age, pain in the back on mechanical stress is accompanied by radiological evidence of instability, including a loss of disk height ("black disks" on MRI) and incipient arthrotic changes of the intervertebral joints. Patients suffer from chronic, recurrent low back pain predominantly arising in the joints and ligaments of the spine.
- The **third phase,** in old age, involves a restabilization of the spine as the joints progressively stiffen. Pain is relatively mild in this phase, though spinal canal stenosis sometimes arises as a result of reactive bony changes in the intervertebral joints.

> **!** Aside from spinal canal stenosis, which is relatively rare, degenerative instability of the motion segments usually takes a benign course. This should always be remembered when a spinal fusion or disk replacement procedure is contemplated.

■ Prediscotic Deformities

Definition

> ! Certain abnormalities of the form and function of the musculoskeletal apparatus accelerate the development of disk degeneration (discosis) in one or more motion segments and are therefore called prediscotic deformities.

The clinically and radiologically evident deformity may lie in the spine itself or elsewhere. Like prearthrotic changes, but even more so, *prediscotic deformities are not pathological in themselves, but merely risk factors for future illness.*

> ! The category of prediscotic deformities includes all abnormalities of the musculoskeletal system that place long-lasting, asymmetrical mechanical stress on one or more intervertebral disks.

Our studies and those of others (MacGibbon and Farfan 1979) have shown that the most common prediscotic deformities leading to the premature appearance of degenerative changes in the lumbar spine are static abnormalities such as scoliosis and hyperlordosis (Strickstrack 1983, Krüger-Sayn 1986, Wansor and Fleischhauer 1986, Nachemson and Jonsson 2000, Herkowitz et al. 2004). Asymmetrical mechanical stress on the disk in childhood impairs interstitial appositional disk growth and thus leads to a deformity of the disk, which is lower on the concave side. Further disturbances arise at the same location after the end of the growth phase. Exner (1954) showed in animal experiments that the more severely compressed portions of the disk degenerate to a greater extent. Lasting asymmetrical loading also impairs metabolic exchange in the part of the disk on the concave side, which bears almost the entire axial load that would otherwise be distributed over the entire disk. The nucleus pulposus and mobile inner portions of the anulus fibrosus become displaced, moving down the pressure gradient to the side bearing the lighter load. The solid components of the anulus fibrosus and the cartilaginous end plates can neither move away from the compressive forces nor transmit them to neighboring structures, as in a fluid. When the curvature of the spine is abnormal, the resting tone in the truncal musculature already suffices to create such a high compressive force in the portion of the disk on the concave side of the deformity that water and low-molecular-weight metabolic substrates can no longer enter it. The metabolism of the cells producing fibers and cartilage in this part of the disk is impaired.

Asymmetrical loading produces typical changes in the disks. On the concave side of scoliosis, the elevated pressure produces premature regressive changes of the anulus fibrosus, which, in turn, make disk displacement more likely. Lasting compression and impairment of the nutrient supply of the fibroblasts lead to premature discosis. The objective findings include a loss of disk height, osteophyte formation, and end plate sclerosis in the affected region of the spine (**Fig. 6.13**).

> ! Disk dehydration and the aging and disintegration of disk tissue occur more rapidly than normal when the disk is continually subjected to increased pressure. In individuals with abnormal curvature of the spine, the end stage of discosis, fibrous ankylosis, is often reached in adolescence.

Thus, at the point of maximum curvature of adolescent kyphosis and scoliosis, one often finds motion segments that have become immobilized with connective tissue.

Disk-related symptoms arise less commonly from the immobilized motion segment(s) than from the neighboring segments that are still at least partially mobile. These segments are under increased biomechanical stress and may therefore suffer tissue damage and displacement.

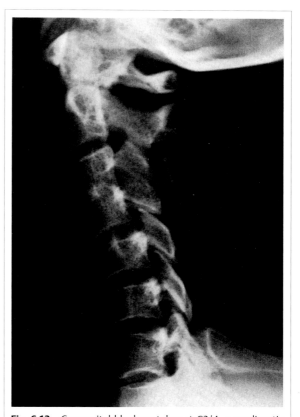

Fig. 6.13 Congenital block vertebra at C3/4, a prediscotic deformity for the neighboring motion segments. This 26-year-old woman had suffered from recurrent neck pain for several years.

Table 6.2 Prediscotic deformities

Cervical spine	Thoracic and lumbar spine
Muscular wry neck	Pathological lordosis (pendulous abdomen, poor posture)
Contracted scar	Scheuermann disease
Block vertebra	Leg length disparity
Vertebral body fracture or infection that has healed in an abnormal position	Spondylolysis/spondylolisthesis
Brachial plexus palsy	Asymmetrical transitional vertebra
Trapezius palsy	Amputation above the knee
	Hypersegmented lumbar spine
	Vertebral body fracture or infection that has healed in an abnormal position

Asymmetrical stress on the intervertebral disk is possible not only in the sagittal plane, but also in the coronal plane. The height of the disk normally differs dorsally and ventrally in the areas of the spine that are physiologically curved. During the growth phase, the disks adapt themselves well to the distance between the upper and lower vertebral body end plates. An increase or decrease in the physiological curvatures after the end of the growth phase puts the anterior or posterior half of the disk under greater mechanical stress, resulting in local premature discosis. A long-lasting forward loading of the trunk—due to pregnancy, poor posture, or obesity, for example—induces *compensatory tilting of the pelvis, exaggeration of the lumbar lordosis,* and therefore continuous mechanical overloading and poor metabolic nourishment of the dorsal half of the lumbar disks. A pendulous abdomen and a stooped posture are, therefore, prediscotic deformities. In general, abnormal lordosis of any cause will always alter the static forces on the lower lumbar region and damage the L5–S1 disk and intervertebral joints. A further common cause is hip arthrosis with flexion contracture.

The most common static deformity of the spine in the sagittal plane is **fixed thoracic kyphosis** in the aftermath of Scheuermann disease. Statistical studies have shown that patients with this deformity suffer from a higher than normal prevalence of lumbar disk disease (Idelberger 1952, Sölderberg and Andrén 1955, Hochheim and Grünbein 1970, Niethard 1982, Nachemson and Jonsson 2000). Aside from an endogenous component (poor quality of the disk cartilage), it is mainly the abnormal static forces that lead to mechanical overloading of the neighboring, nonimmobilized segments of the spine (**Table 6.2**). Severe thoracic kyphosis is usually accompanied by compensatory hyperlordosis of the cervical and lumbar spine. Clinical experience indicates that adolescents with pathological thoracic kyphosis will often develop lumbago and sciatica in their twenties and symptoms of cervical arthrosis 10 or 20 years later.

The lumbar form of juvenile spinal developmental disorder is also a prediscotic deformity, as it is often associated with static abnormalities. The upper portion of the lumbar spine is kyphotic instead of lordotic. Brocher (1973) found a loss of height of the L5–S1 disk in a large percentage of patients with juvenile spinal developmental disorder affecting either the thoracic or the lumbar spine. Compensatory lordosis of the lower lumbar spine heightens the compressive and shearing forces on the L5–S1 disk, causing it to undergo premature attrition, along with its associated intervertebral joints, which become arthrotic.

Abnormalities of the musculoskeletal apparatus also commonly cause deviation of the spine in the *frontal* plane. A long-standing lateral curvature of the spine causes fibrous immobilization of the intervertebral disks and thereby a permanent, curved deformity called **scoliosis**. The most common cause of lateral curvature of the spine is a *lateral pelvic tilt* due to unequal leg length. Though the two legs are never exactly equal in length, a difference in length is only significant if it causes an obvious lateral deviation of the spinal axis. According to Taillard (1964), such a difference is present in 60–75% of all individuals.

Spondylolysis and spondylolisthesis are among the rarer types of prediscotic deformity. The sliding of one vertebral body with respect to another stretches and distorts the intervertebral disk. Continual asymmetrical stress on the intervertebral disk can also be produced by congenital anatomical asymmetries at the lumbosacral junction (**Fig. 6.14**). According to Lange (1986), congenital anomalies at the lumbosacral junction (lumbarization, sacralization) are associated with a rate of disk prolapse that is double or triple the normal rate. In our own studies, we have found that patients with back pain are three times as likely to have an asymmetrical lumbosacral transitional angle as individuals in a control group without back pain (Wansor and Fleischhauer 1986). Further details are given by Aihara and Takahashi (2005).

> **!** Congenital abnormalities at the lumbosacral junction are to be considered prediscotic deformities only when they are asymmetrical and thereby lead to asymmetrical loading of the lumbar motion segments.

A **hypersegmented lumbar spine** is considerably more mobile than normal and therefore requires well-toned paravertebral musculature to hold it in position. Lateral and rotatory deviations (lumbar scoliosis) are more likely to occur if the lumbar spine is hypersegmented. Among individuals with back pain in our series (Wansor and Fleischhauer 1986), the presence of six lumbar

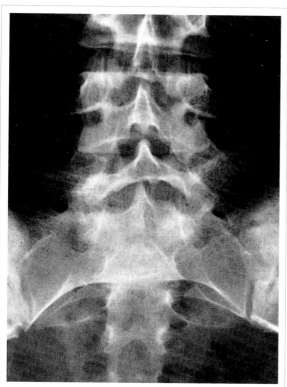

Fig. 6.14 Asymmetrical lumbosacral transitional vertebra, a prediscotic deformity. The disks above the deformity are subject to unevenly distributed mechanical stress. This 19-year-old woman had low back pain and occasional radicular symptoms.

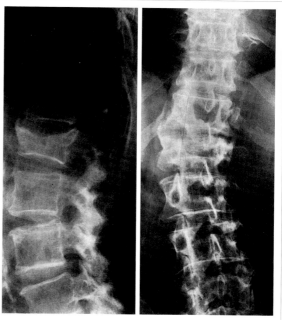

Fig. 6.15 a, b Asymmetrically healed L1 fracture, another type of prediscotic deformity for the lumbar disks below it. The L2/3 intervertebral disk is lower on the concave side. This 58-year-old patient suffered from local and radicular lumbar pain from the time of the accident onward (no one else was involved in the accident, so this was not a medicolegal case with any possibility of financial compensation).

6

vertebrae was twice as common than among individuals in a control group without back pain.

Fewer types of prediscotic deformity affect the cervical spine than the lumbar spine. Cervical **block vertebrae** are relatively common and increase the mechanical stress on the disk immediately below. The same is true after ventral interbody fusion procedures in one or more cervical segments. Prediscotic deformities *outside* the cervical spine include all conditions that cause a **permanently tilted posture of the head and neck,** e. g., muscular wry neck, contracted scars, or the result of amputation of an arm. The scoliotic posture can be compensated for at first, but, in the long term a fixed scoliosis develops.

! In any region of the spine, vertebral body fractures and infections that heal in an abnormal position are prediscotic deformities.

The neighboring disks, though not affected by the primary pathological process, are subjected to asymmetrical mechanical stress and therefore show premature signs of wear and tear. Vertebral body fractures, like fractures of the vertebral arches near the joints, must heal in as near the normal position as possible so that discosis will not develop later (**Fig. 6.15**).

Although prediscotic deformities are not necessarily pathological entities in themselves, but merely predisposing factors to future illness, they should be detected in the course of routine examinations so that their harmful effects can be prevented, as far as possible.

Summary

Just as joint arthrosis involves both pathoanatomical and biomechanical changes, so too does discosis of the intervertebral disks, with the difference that discosis, unlike arthrosis, is a universal accompaniment of human aging. Its cause is the upright human posture, which leads to premature aging and attrition of the bradytrophic disk tissue. The disk tissue is not only continually under mechanical stress, but also receives an inadequate supply of nutrients through the additional harmful effect of the relatively sedentary adult lifestyle.

Degenerative disk changes are not a disease in themselves and are often asymptomatic. In many cases, however, they do produce true disk diseases, which may arise as early as adolescence and reach their highest prevalence and severity in middle age. Among elderly people, the end stage of disk degeneration results in comfortable rigidity of the aging spine.

Many histological, biochemical, and biomechanical studies have revealed the importance of external factors, including occupational stress, in the generation of discosis. Motion segment instability due to degenerative changes is a matter of paticular concern, as it often leads to the consideration of surgical procedures such as spinal fusion or the insertion of a disk prosthesis.

There are both genetic and acquired disturbances of the form and function of the spine and limbs (e. g., differences in leg length) that can be designated as "prediscotic deformities," in the sense that they predispose to the development of discosis and disk diseases.

Disc degeneration is a very complex phenomenon that will require extensive research both biomechanically and biochemically before it can be fully understood (Natarajan 2006).

Conclusion

Discosis affects all humans and is a frequent cause of disk disease in the lower segments of the cervical and lumbar spine.

7 Traumatology

■ Etiologies and Types of Spinal Injury, and the Role of Pre-existing Degenerative Changes

The intervertebral disks, like the other components of the spinal motion segments, are only rarely subject to direct trauma. The spine is an axial organ located in a central position within the body and protected on all sides by soft tissue, so that direct blunt or penetrating trauma rarely affects it. The frequently made diagnosis of "spinal contusion" is probably only rarely correct.

Etiology. Spinal trauma is usually due to an indirect influence such as spraining, bending, or twisting. The segmental construction of the spine, with alternating solid and elastic components, renders it relatively resistant to injury by most types of applied external forces. Spinal trauma is nonetheless commonly encountered in clinical practice, usually as the result of axial compression, e.g., after a fall from a great height, or of sudden bending, with compression on the concave side and distraction on the convex side. There is often a torsional component as well. Trauma of the motion segment can involve the intervertebral disk in a number of different ways, as will be explained.

Types of injury. Trauma of the intervertebral disk can be classified into the following major categories:
- sprains of the motion segment
- disk tears
- vertebral body fractures with disk involvement.

The most commonly traumatized motion segments are those located at the zones of transition between relatively fixed and relatively mobile regions of the spine, i. e., the atlanto-occipital and atlantoaxial segments, the lower segments of the cervical and lumbar regions, and the thoracolumbar junction. An important aspect of disk

trauma and of spinal trauma in general, in all regions of the spine, is that the traumatic deformation and its accompanying pathological features (edema, hematoma) often lies in the immediate vicinity of the spinal cord and its nerve roots, which may be affected by the injury either directly or indirectly. Unlike most injuries elsewhere in the musculoskeletal system, traumatic disturbances of the structure and function of the spine are commonly associated with neurological dysfunction.

The role of pre-existing degenerative changes. The severity of a traumatic disk injury depends not only on the magnitude and direction of the externally applied force, but also on the state of the disk just before it is injured. We have shown experimentally that a healthy intervertebral disk cannot be injured by an externally applied force of practically any kind, unless the vertebral body is fractured first. Similar findings have often been reported in the literature (Göcke 1932, Lob 1951, Ingelmark and Ekholm 1952, Wyss and Ulrich 1953, Hirsch 1954, Güntz 1958, Plaue et al. 1974, Adams and Hutton 1984, Eysel and Fürderer 2004). Motion segments with pre-existing degenerative changes will, however, behave differently. Here, a relatively light loading of the anterior half of the motion segment may suffice to cause posterior displacement of disk tissue beyond the boundary of the disk. Because the *ligaments* between the vertebral bodies are also relatively weak in individuals with disk degeneration, such individuals are also more susceptible to traumatic slippage of the vertebrae. Hinz (1970) showed that, in acceleration–deceleration and bending injuries of the cervical spine, the visible lesions always arise in the segment that was previously most affected by the degenerative process. Thus, identical traumatic forces can produce widely divergent effects in different individuals, depending on their age and on the state of their intervertebral disks. The varying extent of disk degeneration in different individuals, and the vary-

ing magnitude of the causative traumatic forces, often create difficulties of interpretation in the medicolegal assessment of disk trauma.

■ Sprains of the Motion Segment

Etiology and pathogenesis. The mildest type of injury of the motion segment is the sprain, a stretching or distortion of the intervertebral ligamentous connections and joint capsules without any loss of their continuity. Just as in sprains of the limb joints, any violent bending or twisting of the spine beyond its physiological range of motion can overstretch the ligaments and joint capsules of its motion segments, resulting in injury. Such sprains occur most commonly in the cervical region, and "whiplash" (acceleration–deceleration sprain of the cervical spine) is the best-known example. Motion segment sprain due to violent bending and twisting of the spine is less common in other regions because the external stabilization provided by the rib cage and the paravertebral muscles limits extreme excursions of the joints. The frequent diagnosis of "back sprain" is usually incorrectly attached to cases of lumbago that are actually due to intradiscal tissue displacements of degenerative origin.

Clinical features and treatment. When the inter-and paravertebral ligamentous connections and intervertebral joint capsules are briefly overstretched in a spraining injury, small blood vessels are ruptured, resulting in the formation of post-traumatic hematoma and edema, just as in a sprain of a limb joint. The main clinical finding is painful limitation of movement of the affected region of the spine with reflexive spasm of the muscula-

ture. There may also be circumscribed tenderness of the spinous processes of the affected motion segment(s) to percussion and shaking. Plain radiographs show no abnormality except for a possibly abnormal posture (loss of lordosis due to spasm).

> ! The pain and restriction of movement that result from a simple sprain resolve within a few days or weeks as the post-traumatic hematoma and edema are resorbed.

Traumatic functional disturbances in the soft tissues of the spine (sprains) are nearly always reversible, leaving no permanent damage. The healing process can be aided by resting the affected portion of the spine in a soft collar, and anti-inflammatory medications can be used to speed the resolution of edema. Manual therapy is contraindicated, as it can worsen the original sprain.

> ! Simple sprains must be differentiated from traumatically induced intradiscal tissue displacements in disks with pre-existing discosis.

In the latter situation, patients have the typical position-related symptoms, including maintenance of an abnormal posture to reduce strain on the disk, and a positive extension test. The medicolegal assessment of such "post-traumatic" conditions is difficult and always demands careful attention (see Chapter 17).

■ Isolated Traumatic Disk Rupture

The question of whether traumatic disk rupture can occur in the absence of vertebral fracture has been a matter of some controversy in the scientific literature, and even more so in the medicolegal arena. The frequency and severity of isolated traumatic disk rupture are not easy to determine, because this entity cannot be recognized by any telltale clinical or radiological signs. Functional radiographs can demonstrate disk rupture only if the continuity of the disk is entirely disrupted.

Etiology and pathogenesis. Disk rupture can be caused by one of two traumatic processes, compression or distraction. Either of these may be combined with a torsional movement. Combined injuries are common.

Disk rupture through compression by axial loading of the spine always occurs on the basis of pre-existing disk degeneration. We have found, in experimental tests, that axial loading tends to fracture the vertebral body first, rather than rupture the disk. This is confirmed by everyday clinical experience: strains of the spine tend to be located at the thoracolumbar junction, but purported injuries of the intervertebral disks are always located in the segments most commonly affected by disk degeneration, i. e., the lower cervical and lower lumbar segments. In view of the broad, tough ligamentous tissue that is found in a healthy intervertebral disk in an anatomical dissection, it is not surprising that this structure is very hard to damage by compression. Nonetheless, if the integrity of the disk has already been com-

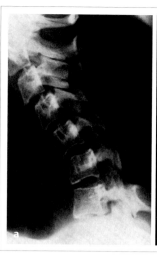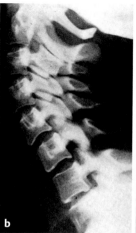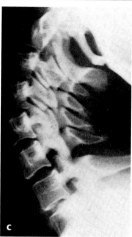

Fig. 7.1 a–c Lateral radiographs of abnormally pronounced dorsal opening (i. e., hyperflexion injury) of the C5/6 intervertebral disk: isolated disk rupture after an acceleration–deceleration injury in a 22-year-old woman.
a In maximum flexion.
b In neutral position (normal).
c In maximum extension.

7

promised by degenerative tears and slackening of the structures enclosing the disk, then axial compression can understandably result in perforation of the disk, with expulsion of a sequestrum.

> **!** In such cases, the traumatic event is merely the precipitating factor for disk rupture, which was already "an accident waiting to happen."

Sudden, strong distraction of the spine would seem to be a plausible cause of isolated disk rupture. Strong forces tending to pull the disk apart can arise, for example, in sudden bending of the spine, on the convex side of the bend. This is the mechanism of disk rupture in hyperflexion and hyperextension trauma, e. g., in acceleration–deceleration injury of the cervical spine and in "jackknife" trauma at the thoracolumbar junction. The intervertebral joints prevent large-amplitude lateral bending of the spine. Any additional torsional movement increases the likelihood of disk rupture.

Primary traumatic disk rupture is a fundamentally different condition from horizontal fissures in the cervical disks or degenerative radial fissures in the disks of the remainder of the spine. Isolated disk rupture is diagnosed by the history of the traumatic event combined with the corresponding radiological image. If the ligaments between the vertebrae are disrupted, functional radiographs will show the affected disk opening more widely than normal (**Fig. 7.1**).

Marked reflexive muscle spasm may render the diagnosis difficult to make, just as in ligamentous injuries of the knee or ankle. The nature of the injury is often not revealed till later, when loss of height of a single disk indicates the site of the problem. Subsequently, osteophytes may grow, often bridging the injured disk in a barrette-like formation. Schmorl and Junghanns (1968) designated post-traumatic bony changes of this type as *spondylosis deformans traumatica*. Osteophytes form

after trauma if the disk has undergone changes similar to those that provoke typical spondylosis deformans, i. e., if the lamellae of the anulus are torn away from the bony margin on either the anterior or the lateral aspect of the vertebral body. (Schmorl 1932 showed that this is a precondition for the formation of osteophytes.) Spondylotic fusion of the disk space after traumatic disk rupture may create a block vertebra. Traumatic spondylosis develops only rarely and therefore is only rarely useful in medicolegal situations as evidence of an isolated disk injury.

Treatment. Healing of the ruptured disk can occur only if the disk is kept in a resting position at all times. Isometric exercises of the trunk, shoulder, and neck muscles can create a "muscular corset" that stabilizes the motion segment from outside.

The adult disk contains no blood vessels and thus cannot regenerate itself. The disk defect is filled exclusively with fibrous tissue that grows after the injured disk is invaded by vessel-bearing granulation tissue. The vessels arise from the paravertebral soft tissue or the vertebral bodies and gain access to the disk through the traumatic tear.

> **!** The motion segment may remain permanently unstable after disk rupture if improper treatment is administered— e. g., manual manipulation—or if the disk fails to heal with a fibrotic scar.

An operative stabilization (fusion) procedure is needed in such cases for the restoration of stability.

■ Vertebral Body Fracture with Injury of the Intervertebral Disk

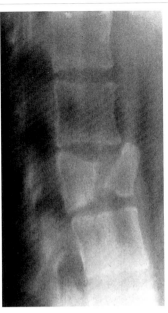

Fig. 7.2 L3 vertebral body fracture in a 23-year-old woman, with involvement of the L2/3 and L3/4 intervertebral disks. Disk tissue has entered the fracture from above and below.

The disk may be injured in combination with either a vertebral body fracture or a laminar fracture. Fractures of the articular processes may be associated with excessive displacement of the vertebral bodies toward one another, and consequent disk rupture. The result may be vertebral subluxation or dislocation, often causing spinal cord compression. Vertebral body fractures in the region of the bony end plates often extend into the cartilaginous end plates as well. The turgor pressure of the nucleus pulposus can then drive some of its disk tissue through the tear in the cartilage and then onward into the vertebral body (**Fig. 7.2**). This process can also be observed experimentally.

An injury to the boundary of the intervertebral disk disrupts the integrity of its osmotic system. Thus, the injured disk not only loses tissue through the penetration of disk tissue into the vertebral body but also loses some of its fluid content. The disk loses height, and the motion segment becomes slack. The bony callus with which the fracture heals and the spondylotic osteophytes that grow along the longitudinal ligaments can span the disk space within a relatively short time, resulting in ankylosis of the motion segment. The end stage often presents problems of radiological interpretation, because the healed state after spinal trauma closely resembles that seen after spinal infection.

Summary

Traumatic injuries of the motion segment, like those of the joints elsewhere in the body, can either leave the bones and soft tissues intact or disrupt their continuity, as in a vertebral body fracture or disk rupture. The severity of the precipitating event, together with the extent of pre-existing discosis (some degree of discosis is always present), will determine whether the injury will be a simple sprain that can heal spontaneously and completely or, for example, a rupture of the anulus fibrosus with disk prolapse. Healthy adults cannot be presumed to have nondiscotic disks. A nondiscotic, intact disk is, in fact, highly resistant to external mechanical shocks, which tend to produce vertebral body fracture rather than disk rupture. In middle age, however, the situation is usually the reverse: the degenerative process has already slackened the disk, and trauma leads to its displacement, rather than to a vertebral body fracture. The fact that discosis is part of normal aging should always be remembered in the medicolegal assessment of acceleration–deceleration injuries of the cervical spine, and whenever the question of a causal relationship between an accident and a disk prolapse is raised.

Any vertebral body fracture that extends to the cartilaginous end plates also involves the neighboring intervertebral disks. The usual long-term sequela is a post-traumatic spontaneous fusion of the motion segment.

Conclusion

The human adult intervertebral disk is vulnerable to injury.

8 Pain: Its Pathogenesis and the Evolution of Chronic Pain

■ Local and Radiating Pain

Local and radiating pain due to intervertebral disk disease are generated by the irritation of different components of the nervous system. The pain may be **referred,** i.e., it may be felt in the distribution of an irritated segmental nerve. Referred pain, by definition, is not felt in the same location as the causative lesion. Brachialgia and sciatica due to nerve root irritation are two common types of referred pain.

Referred pain differs from **organ pain** that is felt at the site of the causative lesion, as in local cervical and lumbar syndromes. There are also certain pain states arising from dysfunction of the sympathetic nervous system, mainly in the area of the body supplied by the cervical nerve roots. The pain in these cases is generally constant, diffusely localized, and accompanied by vasomotor and trophic changes. The sympathetic origin of the pain is reflected in its fluctuation according to the circadian rhythm and other hormonal cycles, as well as its greater frequency in autonomically labile individuals.

Though many symptoms in the back evade precise definition, most disk-related complaints can be attributed in some way to the involvement of particular neural structures in the vicinity of the disks.

■ Nerve Supply of the Spine

Pain-sensitive structures. The human intervertebral disk contains no nerve fibers. Sensory nerve endings have been found to date only in the outermost layers of the anulus fibrosus underlying the posterior longitudinal ligament (Kuhlendahl 1950, Kuhlendahl and Richter 1952, Mulligan 1957, Mendel et al. 1992, Bogduk 2000, Fagan 2003).

These histological findings have their physiological counterpart in the experimental findings of Smith and Wright (1958), who, in the course of disk surgery, attached fine nylon fibers to various structures in the motion segment, as well as to the nerve root. Postoperatively, they were able to duplicate the patient's typical symptoms only by pulling on the posterior portion of the anulus fibrosus, or on the nerve root itself. Kuslich and Ulstrom (1990) stimulated various tissues in the motion segment during lumbar disk operations under local anesthesia and recorded the sensitivity of each to pain. Pain was most easily produced by stimulation of the skin and the compressed nerve root, followed by the anulus fibrosus and the posterior longitudinal ligament. The ligamentous attachments and the joint capsules were less commonly pain-sensitive, while the ligamentum flavum, lumbar fascia, lamina, facet cartilage, and noncompressed nerve roots were completely insensitive to pain.

Puncturing the disk from its anterior aspect, as in cervical discography, is entirely painless. If the disk is in-

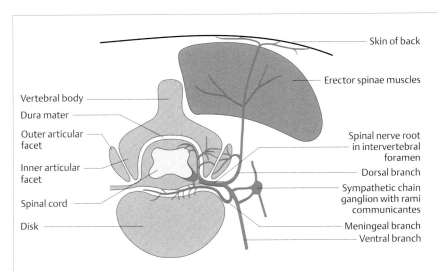

Fig. 8.1 "Autoinnervation" of the structures of the motion segment by the meningeal branch of the spinal nerve. Sensory fibers originate mainly in the intervertebral joint, the posterior longitudinal ligament, and the spinal nerve itself.

Labels in figure:
- Skin of back
- Erector spinae muscles
- Vertebral body
- Dura mater
- Outer articular facet
- Inner articular facet
- Spinal cord
- Disk
- Spinal nerve root in intervertebral foramen
- Dorsal branch
- Sympathetic chain ganglion with rami communicantes
- Meningeal branch
- Ventral branch

tact, no pain or pressure sensations arise when contrast medium or dye is injected into it. On the other hand, if there is a disk protrusion making contact with a nerve root, expansion of the disk may stretch the nerve root, producing pain. This has diagnostic value (see the discussion of the distension test in Chapter 9).

Medial transdural disk puncture at lumbar levels produces no more than a transient, lumbago-like pain at the precise moment that the posterior longitudinal ligament and the dorsal anulus fibrosus are punctured. Just as in disk prolapse surgery under local anesthesia, pressure on the dorsal edge of the disk with a probe induces typical, severe low back pain.

The pain-sensitive structures in the spinal canal—mainly the posterior longitudinal ligament and the dorsal anulus fibrosus, but also the periosteum and intervertebral joint capsules—are supplied by a **special spinal nerve.** In 1850, von Luschka described a branch of the spinal nerve distal to the spinal ganglion, the so-called meningeal branch, which receives sympathetic fibers from the sympathetic chain and then re-enters the spinal canal through the intervertebral foramen (von Luschka 1850). This branch is also called the recurrent branch or the sinuvertebral nerve. Von Luschka's observations were later confirmed by Hovelacque (1925), Roofe (1940), Wiberg (1949), and Bogduk (2000).

The meningeal branch of the spinal nerve branches further after its re-entry into the spinal canal to provide an efferent, afferent, and sympathetic nerve supply to the inner portions of the intervertebral joint capsule, the vertebral periosteum, the posterior longitudinal ligament, and the spinal meninges.

> **!** Mechanically irritable sensory nerve endings are found primarily in the posterior longitudinal ligament, the intervertebral joint capsule, and the spinal nerve itself.

The mixed spinal nerve contains motor, sensory, and sympathetic fibers. As it exits the spinal canal by way of the intervertebral foramen, it splits into a ventral and a dorsal branch. The much larger ventral branch supplies the anterior region of the body, including the limbs, while smaller dorsal branch supplies the skin and muscles of the back. Further branches supply the outer facets of the intervertebral joints and their capsules. The paired dorsal branches, from the occiput to the coccyx, pierce the paravertebral fascia to supply the posterior portions of the corresponding dermatomes. In the thoracic region (T1–T11), the portion of the dermatome supplied by the dorsal branch is relatively narrow, i. e., close to the midline. In the lumbar area, it extends laterally to the outer edge of the erector spinae muscles, and, in the sacral area, it extends to the dorsal foramina. Richter (1977) described entrapment neuropathies of these nerve branches as being responsible for certain painful syndromes, particularly *occipital neuralgia* and *coccygodynia.*

The pattern of nerve supply suggests certain mechanisms for the generation of pain in the motion segment and implies that painful disk syndromes are likely to be complex (**Fig. 8.1**).

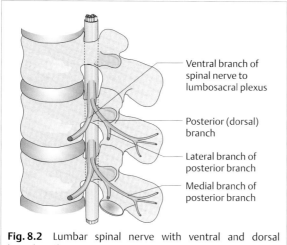

Fig. 8.2 Lumbar spinal nerve with ventral and dorsal branches (from Krämer and Nentwig, after Bogduk 1997).

Ventral branch of
spinal nerve to
lumbosacral plexus

Posterior (dorsal)
branch

Lateral branch of
posterior branch

Medial branch of
posterior branch

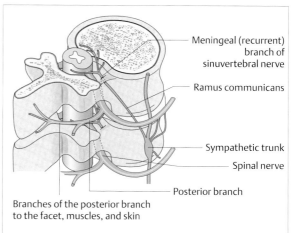

Meningeal (recurrent)
branch of
sinuvertebral nerve

Ramus communicans

Sympathetic trunk

Spinal nerve

Posterior branch

Branches of the posterior branch
to the facet, muscles, and skin

Fig. 8.3 The spinal nerves and their branches (from Krämer and Nentwig, after Bogduk 1997).

■ The Foramino-articular Region

The foramino-articular region of the lower lumbar segments is the site of exit of the spinal nerve from the intervertebral foramen and of its division into terminal branches (see Chapter 11). Its anatomy is, therefore, of special clinical interest, particularly with respect to therapeutic approaches involving local injections.

Figures 8.1–8.3 show the close proximity of the spinal nerves and their branches, their connections to the sympathetic trunk by way of the rami communicantes, and the muscles and joints in this region. The nociceptors of the joint capsules, the posterior longitudinal ligament, and the vertebral periosteum lie directly adjacent to afferent fibers of various nerves. Structural and functional disturbances, mostly caused by the early disk degeneration that is characteristic in humans, lead to reactive changes in the joint capsules. A further consequence (both direct and indirect) is the autonomic response that is induced by irritation of the ramus communicans from the meningeal branch to the sympathetic trunk and mediated by the spinal nociceptive reflex arc. The presence of so many pain-sensitive structures within a compact space suggests the possibility of effective treatment of pain through local injections of anesthetics or anti-inflammatories.

■ Discogenic Pain

Aside from purely mechanical causes of pain, there are other types of stimuli that might irritate the pain-sensitive nerve endings of the motion segment. Just as in other organs (e. g., the teeth or stomach), changes of osmolarity, pH, or chemical composition must be considered as possible causes of motion segment pain.

Nachemson (1969) measured the pH in prolapsed intervertebral disks in vivo with an antimony needle electrode. pH values below 7 were associated with certain inflammatory reactions at the nerve roots that were not seen with pH values in the alkaline range. When the pH was 6.1 or lower, the nerve roots were encased in dense, reactive scar tissue. The chemical composition of the prolapsed disk tissue, independently of its size, can also partially account for the severity of the patient's symptoms. Even in the absence of disk prolapse, nerve structures near the disk (e. g., in the posterior longitudinal ligament) can be irritated by chemical changes taking place within it. Just as in other organs, the poor metabolic condition of the disk sets chemical processes in motion that alter the osmolarity and pH of disk tissue. Nachemson (1969) hypothesized that proteolytic enzymes in connective tissue lysosomes catalyze the release of acidic amino acids from the protein–polysaccharide complexes of the disk matrix, thereby lowering the pH. It may be additionally lowered by an increased concentration of free acidic mucopolysaccharides. Karlsson et al. (1968) and Diamant et al. (1968) reported an inverse relationship between the intraoperatively measured intradiscal pH and lactate levels: when the pH was low the lactate level was high, and vice versa.

The anatomical and biochemical findings of MacCarron et al. (1987), Mooney (1987), and Fagan (2003) suggest that purely discogenic pain—i. e., pain arising in the disk itself—is possible. Thus, if the hydrostatic pressure on a disk is kept high, dissolved acidic metabolites may be pressed out of the disk and excite an inflammatory response in neighboring nerve fibers. If there is a tear in the anulus fibrosus, not much compressive pressure on the disk will be needed for this to take place.

Further studies on discogenic pain have been published by Schwarzer et al. (1995), Nakamura et al. (1996), Coppes et al. (1997), Faustmann (2004), Kniesel (2004), Schaaf et al. (2004), Weisskopf et al. (2004), Peng et al. (2005), and Murata et al (2006a, 2006b).

■ Spinal Deformities without Pain

> ! The severity of pain in the motion segment is correlated less closely with the *size* of the structural abnormality than with the *period of time* over which it arose.

Even very marked deviations of the spinal axis, with torsion, spondylosis, and osteochondrosis, may be asymptomatic if they have developed over many years. The nerve roots, ligaments, and intervertebral joint capsules can apparently adapt adequately to such changes in the long term. On the other hand, even a small dorsal disk protrusion can produce severe pain if it arises suddenly and makes (even minimal) contact with pressure-sensitive neural elements of the posterior longitudinal ligament or the nerve root.

■ Pain Arising from the Posterior Longitudinal Ligament

Pain arising from the posterior longitudinal ligament is dull and poorly localizable. It may be of sudden and very intense onset, as in acute lumbago or acute neckache. It may also develop gradually, as when the dorsal aspect of the intervertebral disk is placed under abnormally high tension for long periods of time by pronounced kyphosis or by an abnormal increase of disk volume. The meningeal branch of the spinal nerve is responsible for intrinsic spinal pain. It is currently unclear whether compression of the spinal dura mater causes pain. Evidence against this possibility comes from the fact that median disk prolapses and spinal tumors sometimes produce little or no pain.

■ Radicular Pain

Mechanical nerve root irritation. Among all structures of the peripheral nervous system, the spinal nerve root is by far the most vulnerable to injury. Compression and stretching are the most common mechanisms. Pain is generated only by pressure on, or pulling of, the meningeal (and thus mesenchymal) tissue that encases the preganglionic segment of the dorsal root. Figure **8.4** shows the segmental distribution of radicular pain by dermatomes.

Radicular pain has the following general features:
- The pain radiates along the dermatome.
- Associated muscle atrophy does not fit the pattern of distribution of any peripheral nerve.
- Any reflex deficit that is seen is attributable to a radicular rather than peripheral nerve lesion.
- There is no accompanying autonomic nerve deficit.

Spinal nerves contain fibers supplying the skin and muscle of the trunk and limbs, as well as the spine itself. Thus, nerve root lesions can produce various combinations of symptoms. The segmental distribution of symptoms is most easily recognizable when the structures innervated by the *ventral* branch of the spinal nerve are prominently involved. The diagnostician should remember, however, that nerve root lesions produce abnormalities not only in the area supplied by the ventral branch on the anterior trunk and limbs, but also in the muscles supplied by the dorsal branch.

Compression of a spinal nerve root produces clearly demarcated segmental sensory and motor disturbances on the trunk and in the limbs. The precise location and severity of the nerve root lesion will determine whether the most prominent symptoms reflect involvement of the ventral or dorsal nerve branch. Dermatomal pain may be of different kinds, depending on the type and severity of nerve root compression; the symptoms may range from isolated, referred pain (band-like pain), without any "objectifiable" signs, to total anesthesia. Smith and Wright (1958) showed that the distance the pain radiates is proportional to the pressure on the nerve root. For example, if a lumbar nerve root is only lightly compressed, sciatica radiates only to the thigh, but stronger compression makes it radiate into the foot.

Cervical and lumbar nerve root compression generally produce no autonomic deficit. Mumenthaler et al. (1998) emphasize the fact that no autonomic efferent fibers to the sympathetic chain exit the spinal cord above T2 or below L2. Thus, the segments most commonly affected by acute and chronic disk disease, C5–C8 and L4–S1, lie well outside the portion of the spinal cord containing the main sympathetic nucleus (the intermediolateral cell column). The absence of accompanying autonomic nerve symptoms, e. g., sweating, in cervical and lumbar radiculopathy is an important diagnostic clue by which these processes can be distinguished from peripheral nerve lesions.

The degree to which a nerve root is compressed by a bulging disk depends both on changes in the volume and consistency of the disk tissue and on position-related changes in the motion segment. Many of the diagnostic and therapeutic measures that are undertaken in patients with disk-related complaints rely on this simple fact.

In previous chapters, we have pointed out that the intervertebral disks of an adolescent or young adult are not mechanically stiff elements, but rather self-contained connective tissue organs whose shape and volume normally fluctuate in response to mechanical stress, relaxation, and asymmetrical compression. The other components of the motion segment, including the nerve fibers, must adapt to these fluctuations. The normally existing space between the posterior border of the disk and the dural sac, with its paired exiting nerve roots, enables movements of the spine, changes of the disk contour, and changes of nerve root length to take place without putting the nerve root under excessive tension or compression. This "reserve space" between the disk and the dura mater contains fat and epidural veins; its width varies among segments. In the intervertebral foramen, too, there is normally enough space between the nerve root and the bony canal in which it is enclosed. The nerve root may be compressed, however, when either of these reserve spaces is narrowed by a disk protrusion or prolapse, or by osteophytes, enlarged vessels, or bony overgrowth (spinal stenosis).

! If an intervertebral disk makes contact with a spinal nerve, the physiological, pressure-dependent fluctuations in the consistency and volume of the disk are transmitted to the nerve. The nerve may not have room to move as freely and may therefore be a source of pain when movement of the spine exceeds a certain range in a given direction.

This explains the highly variable character of disk-related complaints. A nerve root may be compressed not only by disk tissue, but also by bony structures. Though

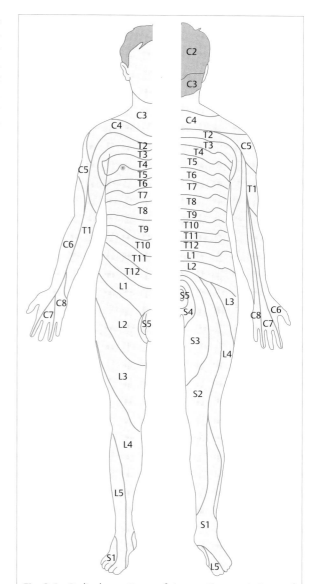

Fig. 8.4 Radicular pattern of innervation: anterior and posterior aspect.

the most common cause is a cervical osteophyte arising from the uncinate process, nerve roots can be compressed in the lumbar spine, too, by arthrotic extensions of the intervertebral joints or spondylotic osteophytes on the posterior surface of the vertebrae. The **pain of osteogenic nerve root compression** typically fails to resolve spontaneously or to respond to conservative treatment. It is usually sharply localized, because the same part of the nerve is always irritated. Surgical treatment is often necessary.

When prolapsed disk tissue enters the epidural space through an anular tear and comes into direct contact with the nerve root, there can also be a **biochemically induced irritation of the nerve root.** Disk tissue normally is not found in the spinal canal, and, when it is deposited there, it excites a foreign-body reaction. Saal and Saal (1989), Olmarker and Rydevik (1993), Willburger et al. (1998), and Olmarker (2004) have experimentally demonstrated the direct toxic effect of disk material on nervous tissue.

> **!** The pain of disk prolapse is caused not just by mechanical trauma, but also by chemical irritation of the nerve root.

Mechanical and chemical irritation produce **grossly visible changes** in the nerve root: initially edema, later atrophy. At surgery, the nerve root is sometimes seen to have a reddish or bluish-purple discoloration. The compressed nerve fibers within the root fire action potentials spontaneously. Compression causes demyelination of nerve root axons and alters their excitability (Wehling 1993, Olmarker 2004, Gupta et al. 2005).

> **!** An already inflamed nerve root is more than normally sensitive to additional mechanical irritation.

The latter statement is routinely confirmed during intervertebral disk surgery whenever the irritated nerve root is lightly touched. Many treatment measures, particularly local injections of novocaine, lidocaine, and cortisone, are intended to lessen the irritability of the nerve root and to desensitize it in a lasting fashion. Therapeutic local anesthesia (TLA) reduces the susceptibility of nerve fibers to mechanical irritation. Even when the disk prolapse (the original source of pain) has been removed and the nerve root is freely mobile once again, the pain and sensory disturbance may persist. There is a fitting analogy here to a half-swallowed fishbone, which leaves a foreign-body sensation in the throat even long after it has been extracted.

■ Intervertebral Joint Pain (Facet Syndrome, Pseudoradicular Syndrome)

Degenerative changes in the intervertebral disk cause not only primary discogenic pain, but also secondary types of pain resulting from the involvement of additional structures, e.g., joint capsule pain and muscle pain.

> **!** The intervertebral joints have many sensory receptors and are an important source of pain in the motion segment.

The joint capsule, synovial membrane, and periosteum of the intervertebral joint facets possess both encapsulated nerve endings (Vater–Pacini corpuscles) and an even greater number of free nerve endings.

The cartilaginous surfaces and partially elastic capsules of the intervertebral joints, like those of all other joints in the body, normally permit movement only in certain directions and with certain amplitudes (excursions). The extremes of possible movement at the intervertebral joint are set by the intervertebral disk. In our own contrast radiographs and compression experiments, we have found that the intervertebral joint normally has an impressively wide range of motion. If the joint excursion suddenly exceeds the physiological range of motion, the joint is sprained. Sprains produce pain by activating the pressure- and stretch-sensitive receptors of the joint capsule.

Loss of disk height, e.g., by discosis, changes the neutral position of the associated intervertebral joints (see p. 29). Movements of the spine that would otherwise be in the normal range may then stretch the joint capsules beyond their physiological limit, causing pain.

The abnormal position of the joint facets also produces excessive, nonphysiological mechanical stress on their cartilaginous surfaces, which suffer erosion. This may result in intervertebral joint arthrosis (spondylarthrosis), which manifests itself as a dull, poorly localizable pain that—unlike primary discogenic pain—fails to improve immediately when the sufferer changes posture to extend the spine. Ghormley (1933) designated pain arising from the intervertebral joint facets as "facet syndrome." This term is now generally used for any type of back or leg pain that does not arise from the nerve root. Mooney and Robertson (1976) showed with arthrographically guided facet injections that pain radiating from the joints into the leg has a particular, nonradicular pattern of distribution. The clinical features of facet syndrome are discussed in greater detail in Chapter 11.

Muscle Pain

The muscles of the shoulder, neck, trunk, hip, and leg can be affected by intervertebral disk disease in two different ways. Irritation of the dorsal branch of the spinal nerve may lead to the continuous firing of motor impulses to the muscle, causing abnormal contraction and/or pain (**Fig. 8.1**). On the other hand, instability of the motion segment due to disk disease may elicit compensatory contraction of the truncal and proximal limb muscles, which may then suffer excessive strain.

Loss of elasticity of the disk fibers and dehydration of the disk matrix are the causes of the most common functional disturbance of the motion segment, i. e., slackening of the intervertebral disk. In its early stage, this disturbance can be compensated for by contraction of the truncal musculature.

> *!* If the functional reserve of the muscles is exceeded, dull back pain is felt, a sign of muscular insufficiency.

The limited ability of the truncal musculature to compensate for disk slackening can cause motion segment dysfunction even in high-performance athletes. The muscles of the back and neck are among the least trainable muscles in the body, even though the nonphysiological demands of today's workplaces often subject them to persistent, severe stress.

> *!* Pain radiating into the truncal and/or proximal limb muscles that is not due to direct irritation of a nerve root is said to constitute a pseudoradicular syndrome.

Pain of this type reflects a disturbed functional relationship between the joints and the muscles that move them (Brügger 1971, Gross 1977, 1984, Mumenthaler and Schliack 1993, Mense 1999, Jerosch 2005). Painful limitation of muscle contraction is usually a sign of joint capsule irritation. Muscle tone is controlled, in part, by receptors in the joint capsules. Prolonged abnormal function causes the muscles to become painful. In the affected musculature, spontaneous pain arises, which can be aggravated by pressure or movement. Thus, for example, irritation of the lower lumbar intervertebral joints induces reflexive pain of the lumbar erector spinae muscles, as well as of the glutei, hamstrings, and calf muscles (**Fig. 8.5**). A muscle that is painful all the way from its origin to its attachment produces pain in a distribution resembling sciatica or brachialgia. Circumscribed areas of tenderness where pressure induces pain in the entire muscle ("trigger points") are a typical indication of pseudoradicular pain. A precisely applied local injection of local anesthetic aids the diagnosis. Pseudoradicular pain may appear either as a harbinger of disk protrusion or as a residual symptom after the surgical or conservative treatment of disk prolapse.

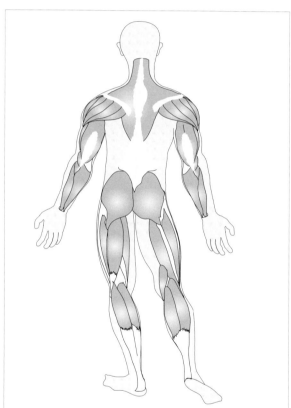

Fig. 8.5 Pseudoradicular pain in the muscles of the shoulder and neck, arising from the cervical intervertebral joints and the shoulder joint, and sciatica-like pseudoradicular pain in the muscles of the hip and lower limb, arising from the lumbar intervertebral and sacroiliac joints.

■ Combined Types of Pain

As we have seen, the various possible sources of pain in the motion segment all lie within a small area, and the nerves bearing the motor, sensory, and autonomic innervation of the motion segment are all interconnected. It is thus not surprising that various combinations of painful symptoms can arise. The term "segment" refers to the part of the body innervated by a particular spinal nerve. The innervated segment has two components: the *dermatome* is the area of skin to which the nerve provides sensory innervation, and the *myotome* is the area of skeletal muscle to which it provides motor innervation. Disturbances affecting either the somatic or the autonomic portion of the ventral branch of a spinal nerve exert certain feedback effects on the spine itself, including the areas innervated by the meningeal and dorsal branches. The various possible components of disk-related complaints are listed in **Table 8.1.** Pain rarely occurs in isolation; patients usually suffer from a mixed combination of symptoms, which continually changes over the course of the illness. Pathophysiologi-

cally, it is assumed that a combination of structural, biochemical, and physiological changes in the peripheral and central nervous system serves as the final common pathway for the "mixed pain" of chronic back pain and sciatica (Baron and Binder 2004). In particular, irritation throughout the motion segment, such as can arise after disk prolapse operations, tends to produce symptoms reflecting the involvement of all nerve branches within the segment.

! A dorsolateral disk prolapse with nerve root compression produces purely radicular pain at first, but, later, combined pain with radicular, pseudoradicular, and tendomyogenic components.

As **Fig. 8.6** shows, reflexive contraction of the erector spinae muscles results in an abnormal displacement of the intervertebral joints, which may painfully overstretch their capsules. Thus, beyond the original radicular pain, the patient also develops pseudoradicular pain

Table 8.1 The components of disk-related pain and their sites of origin

	Site of origin	Pain mechanism	Responsible nerve	
	Posterior longitudinal ligament, dura mater		Meningeal branch	–
Primary discogenic	Spinal nerve	Discogenic	Spinal nerve	Dorsal and ventral dermatome
		Osteogenic	Mainly ventral branch	Motor deficit as well
	Intervertebral joint	Capsular stretch pain	Meningeal and dorsal branches	–
		Arthrosis-related pain		–
Secondary discogenic	Dorsal musculature	Reflex muscle spasm in primary discogenic syndrome	Dorsal branch	Dorsal portion of dermatome
		Inadequate muscular compensation for disk slackening	Dorsal branch	–

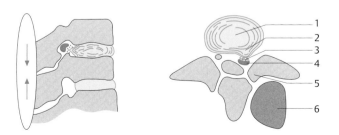

1 Turgor pressure of disk
2 Prolapsed portion of disk
3 Inflamed site of contact of disk prolapse with nerve root
4 Inflammatory swelling of root
5 Pathological displacement of intervertebral joint due to 6
6 Reflexive spasm of erector spinae muscles

Fig. 8.6   The generation of combined types of pain from an originally discogenic disturbance.

and worsened local pain. It is this combined type of pain that must be the target of treatment.

The combined appearance of restricted spinal mobility, muscle spasm, radicular symptoms, and accompanying autonomic signs provides the motivation for the all-encompassing term, "disk syndrome."

> **!** Most pain arising from the muscles or vertebral bodies, and most pseudoradicular symptoms, are quantitative and qualitative variants of the pain of degenerative disk disease.

The choice of treatment is based on the particular component of pain that is most prominent in the individual patient.

Nociception and the Transition from Acute to Chronic Pain

Physiology of Nociception in the Spine

The activation of nociceptors in the motion segment initiates a stereotypic sequence of events that includes the conduction of nociceptive impulses toward the brain, the conscious experience of pain, and the ensuing motor and autonomic reactions to it. Motion segment nociceptors can be activated by mechanical, inflammatory, chemical, or thermal stimuli. The cerebral cortex is responsible for the conscious experience of pain. The spinal cord contains mechanisms controlling the flow of impulses toward the brain and then back to the muscles and the autonomic nervous system.

The flow of nociceptive information that begins with the painful stimulus and eventually results in the conscious experience of pain and in the various responses to it at the spinal level is shown in **Fig. 8.7**. A noxious, i.e., potentially or actually tissue-damaging, stimulus

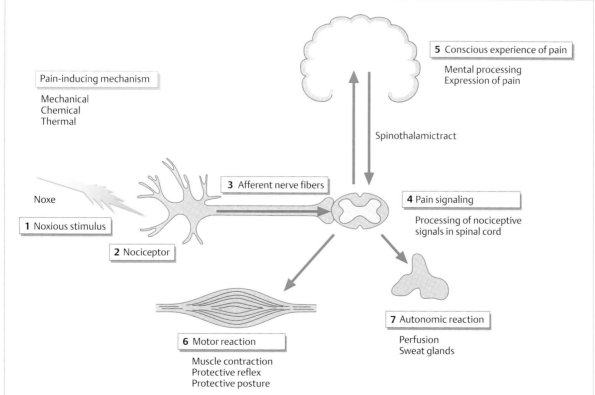

Fig. 8.7 Nociception and pain processing in the bones, muscles, tendons, and joints. The passage of nociceptive impulses from one type of tissue to another (e. g., from afferent nerves to the spinal cord) is shown schematically (from Krämer and Nentwig 1999).

(1) activates nociceptors (2) in the motion segment, which are mainly unmyelinated nerve fibers (pain receptors) that can be brought to fire only by stimuli whose amplitude exceeds the nociceptive threshold. The patient's sensitivity to noxious stimuli in the motion segment is a function both of the density of nociceptors and of their threshold. The sites with the highest density of nociceptors in the motion segment are the joint capsules, the dorsal portion of the anulus fibrosus, and the posterior longitudinal ligament.

Afferent nerve fibers (3) carry the nociceptive impulses into the spinal cord (4), where they cross a synapse onto the nociceptive neurons of the dorsal horn. Within the dorsal horn, the nociceptive impulses induce the release of excitatory neurotransmitters such as L-glutamate and substance P. The flow of nociceptive impulses then proceeds along multiple channels, including the following:

- along the spinothalamic tract to higher centers in the brain (limbic system, thalamus)
- on to segmental neurons that participate in motor and autonomic reflex loops.

The conscious experience of pain (5), along with the mental processing of pain and its conscious expression, is a function of the cerebral cortex. Inhibitory systems are constantly at work in the central nervous system to regulate the individual's sensitivity and responsiveness to pain. Various therapeutic techniques can be used to enhance the activity of these descending and segmental inhibitory systems and thereby relieve pain, including electrical stimulation, opiate medication, afferent stimulation (e.g. acupuncture), mental influences (stress), and physical activity, particularly sports and exercise. **Pain reduction through movement is an important goal of orthopedic pain therapy, particularly with respect to spondylogenic symptoms.**

The motor response (6) to a noxious stimulus involves reflexes that cause the individual to assume a protective posture, e.g., the asymmetrically stooped posture of sciatica. These reflexes are usually mediated by a change in muscle tone. The assumption of a protective posture through the reflexive contraction of some muscle groups and relaxation of others is a defense mechanism for the musculoskeletal system, whose purpose is to limit the effect of noxious stimuli on the nociceptors, i. e., to minimize pain. In torticollis, or in the reflexive posture of sciatica, contact is lessened between the pressure-sensitive nervous structures and the anatomically abnormal structures that compress them. In the orthopedic treatment of acute musculoskeletal pain, it is eminently sensible to let muscle spasm and abnormal postures persist for a few days till the stream of incoming nociceptive impulses is interrupted and the nociceptors are no longer being excited.

The autonomic reaction (7) to a noxious stimulus in the motion segment is part of a spinal reflex arc. Different noxious stimuli have different effects on the autonomic nervous system. The typical effect is a reflexive increase or decrease of local perfusion, one of whose causes is simultaneous muscle contraction (or contracture). The physiological blood-pumping action of the muscles is altered. The autonomic reaction may also include changes in cutaneous temperature or sweating.

Evolution of Chronic Pain

When nociceptors are excited above their threshold by noxious stimuli, the sequence of events described in the last section results in the conscious experience of pain as well as in further pain processing and various types of response to the pain. We are speaking here of **acute pain,** which begins immediately after the delivery of the initiating, tissue-damaging stimulus and warns that further damage may occur unless steps are taken to prevent it. Acute pain signals the need for withdrawal, rest, or "favoring" of the affected part of the body to keep it from being damaged or, if it is already damaged, to enable it to heal.

The transition to chronic pain results when this sequence of events continues to take place, despite the absence of the originally inciting stimulus, through the effect of various exogenous and endogenous factors. Nociceptors, for example, can be so strongly activated by exogenous toxic substances and endogenous inflammatory mediators, such as bradykinin, histamine, prostaglandins, interleukins, and others, that their thresholds become lowered, i. e., they become more sensitive to further stimuli. This is particularly likely to happen when these substances are applied repeatedly. The result is chronic pain that has lost its original warning function. The pain persists even though its original source has healed (or has been removed), and it sends the individual the erroneous message that they must still rest or "favor" the affected body part. The ensuing restriction of physical and social activities further contributes to the evolution of chronic pain.

Acute pain begins when the trauma does, and reaches its peak when tissue damage is at its worst. It decreases over the course of the organic healing process and disappears when this process is completed. Chronic pain, on the other hand, develops in the shadow of the acute pain and then takes on a life of its own even after the originally painful condition has been eliminated.

Temporal Course

There are varying opinions as to how long back pain must be present before it can be called "chronic" (Gershagen and Ljutow 2000, Sandkühler 2001, Zenz and Jurna 2001, Zimmermann 2004, Niesert and Zenz 2005, Kovacs et al. 2005). Suggestions range from 6 weeks to 6 months. Both nociceptive and neuropathic pain can be modulated at higher centers, both at the spinal and the supraspinal levels (central sensitization). The altered magnitude of perceived pain is often referred to as neural plasticity and is considered to play a critical role in the evolution of chronic pain (Brisby 2006).

> **!** Chronic pain is more than just long-lasting pain.

The temporal dimension, however, is only one of the features that distinguish chronic from acute pain. As pain becomes chronic, the pain experience and the so-called "pain behavior" of patients both change. Patients may complain of severe pain even after a very mild mechanical stimulus. They behave differently than in the acute phase—they change physicians frequently, take more and stronger analgesic medication, and are more frequently hospitalized and operated upon. Their identity becomes increasingly defined by the role of a "pain patient" (see also Chapter 13).

Secondary Pain

In spondylogenic pain syndromes, the *primary* pain arising from the motion segment itself (caused mainly by tension on the joint capsules and by nerve root compression) is accompanied by *secondary* pain arising from the musculoskeletal structures outside it, usually as the result of reflexive elevation of muscle tone and postural abnormalities. The shifting of weight to one leg leads to a crooked stance of the trunk and an asymmetrical position of the pelvis, with ensuing chronic pain in the sacroiliac joints and the muscular attachments to the iliac crest and the spinous processes. Secondary pain, like primary pain, may become chronic and lead a life of its own even after the original cause of the pain has been eliminated. This is particularly true of residual uni- or bilateral sacroiliac joint pain in the aftermath of lumbar nerve root irritation.

Chronic spondylogenic pain is characterized not only by its long duration, but also by alteration of the pain experience and of the patient's psychosocial condition.

Painful Syndromes

Chronic spinal pain syndromes usually consist of a combination of nociceptor-mediated and neurogenic pain. The most common examples are the mixed radicular/pseudoradicular syndromes of the cervical and lumbar regions. The patient suffers both from dermatomal neurogenic pain radiating into a limb and (nearly always)

from local pain in the affected motion segment, which arises from nociceptors in the intervertebral joint capsules, the dorsal part of the anulus fibrosus, and the posterior longitudinal ligament. In addition, there is secondary pain originating in other parts of the musculoskeletal system, as a result of elevated muscle tone and of the patient's antalgic postural abnormality. Rational orthopedic pain therapy is based on an analysis of the individual components of the patient's pain, with the following techniques:

- clinical neurological examination, with testing of motor and sensory function, coordination, and reflexes
- manual–medical examination of the individual segments of the spine
- analysis of faulty posture
- analysis of the patient's emotional state.

The orthopedic approach to the treatment of spondylogenic pain is thus multidimensional.

Therapeutic Approaches

The most important orthopedic therapies that are aimed at eliminating the causes of spondylogenic pain are familiar: positioning, orthopedic aids, and manual therapy. In the longer term, patients receive postural and behavioral training (back school—see Chapter 14) as well as physiotherapy and exercise programs. The goal of "causal" pain therapy is to remove the stimuli that excite the nociceptors of the pain-sensitive components of the motion segment, so that the pain process can no longer be initiated (**Fig. 8.8**).

Symptomatic pain therapy, on the other hand, attempts to interrupt the process of nociception *after* it has already been initiated by a noxious stimulus. The pain-related impulses are to be stopped somewhere along their course as they travel from the nociceptors by way of the afferent fibers and spinal cord to the brain, where the conscious experience of pain occurs and the peripheral motor and autonomic responses are coordinated. Different forms of symptomatic pain therapy exert their effects at different points along the pathways of pain conduction, perception, and reaction (Baron and Binder 2004, Junker 2004). Physicians and patients expect symptomatic pain therapy, unlike causal pain therapy, to work immediately. Thus, the most important types include rapid-onset analgesics, local injections, and directly acting physical therapies (e. g., heating and cooling).

8

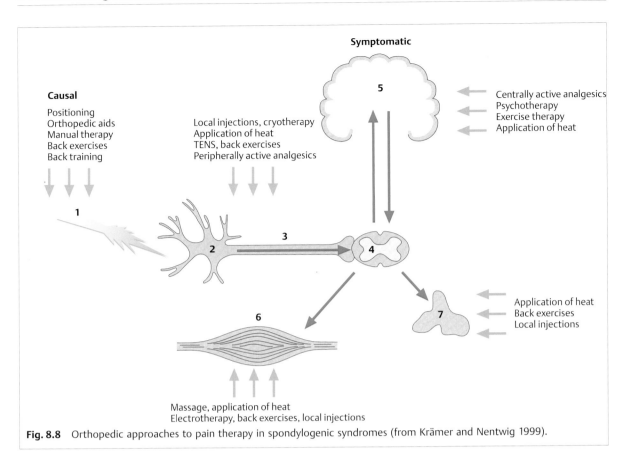

Symptomatic

Causal

Positioning
Orthopedic aids
Manual therapy
Back exercises
Back training

Local injections, cryotherapy
Application of heat
TENS, back exercises
Peripherally active analgesics

Centrally active analgesics
Psychotherapy
Exercise therapy
Application of heat

Application of heat
Back exercises
Local injections

Massage, application of heat
Electrotherapy, back exercises, local injections

Fig. 8.8 Orthopedic approaches to pain therapy in spondylogenic syndromes (from Krämer and Nentwig 1999).

Summary

The high prevalence and diversity of spondylogenic pain syndromes is explained by the presence of highly sensitive nerve endings in various parts of the motion segment. Any of these parts can give rise to pain as the motion segment falls prey to the degenerative changes that so frequently cause premature disturbances of its structure and function. The pain may have its origin in the intervertebral disk, the ligaments, the nerve root, the intervertebral joint capsules, or any combination of these. Deficient expertise and cursory examining techniques often lead to a vague characterization of the pain as "simple low back pain" or a "pseudoradicular syndrome."

A special focal point of the motion segment is the foramino-articular region, in which the spinal nerve and its three branches lie adjacent, on one side, to the inter-

vertebral disk, with its various structural and functional disturbances, and, on the other side, to the intervertebral joint. The foramino-articular region is the usual site of local therapeutic techniques, such as injections. Disk prolapses and joint deformities that change the anatomical relationships in this region often cause severe pain.

Pain is caused not just by mechanical compression of a nerve root by a bulging disk, but also by a chemical irritant effect of disk tissue on the root.

Conclusion

Spondylogenic pain comes in many varieties and tends to become chronic.

8

■ Pharmacological Pain Therapy

Definition

In general, the pharmacotherapy of intervertebral disk diseases is symptomatic and is used as an adjunct to other, nonpharmacological treatments. Analgesic and anti-inflammatory drugs are the mainstay of therapy. There are as yet no drugs that can be used to treat the causes of disk degeneration.

Classification

The medications used to treat disk disease can be classified in various ways:
- analgesics, anti-inflammatories, co-analgesics
- strong vs. mild analgesics (classified according to the WHO scheme)
- opioids vs. nonopioids
- drugs with a greater or lesser risk of side effects.

These medications are given in order to interrupt pain transmission at different points along the pain pathway, which (to repeat) begins with nociception and proceeds via central conduction to the conscious pain experience and the accompanying motor and autonomic reactions. WHO suggests that nonopioid analgesics, such as paracetamol (acetaminophen), should be used first to treat pain because of their relatively mild side effects. If these are not adequately effective, nonsteroidal anti-inflammatory drugs (NSAIDs) can be given; if these, too, fail to bring sufficient relief, opioid analgesics can be given for a short time. Co-analgesics are mainly used in the treatment of chronic pain. The WHO scheme is useful for the treatment of discogenic pain. It involves three stages of medication, to be administered depending on the severity and duration of pain:
- stage 1: nonopioid analgesics
- stage 2: mild opioid analgesics
- stage 3: strong opioid analgesics.

The concomitant administration of an anti-inflammatory (or perhaps a so-called co-analgesic drug, see below) helps keep the opioid dose to a minimum.

Nonopioid Analgesics and Anti-inflammatories

Paracetamol (acetaminophen) has been found to be very useful in the treatment of back pain. It has an analgesic effect similar to that of the NSAIDs, but without any anti-inflammatory effect. Its main advantage over the NSAIDs is the relative rarity of adverse effects. Paracetamol seems to be about as effective as the NSAIDs for the treatment of both acute and chronic pain. Only a few good clinical studies to date have documented these facts, however, and there are no controlled studies of paracetamol vs. placebo (Agency for Health 1994, van Tulder et al. 1997, German Pharmaceutical Commission 2006).

Nonsteroidal Anti-inflammatory Drugs (NSAIDs)

Several placebo-controlled studies have documented the effectiveness of NSAIDs against acute back pain without radicular symptoms, and against chronic back pain (Agency for Health 1994, van Tulder et al. 1997, Koes et al. 1997, German Pharmaceutical Commission 2006). NSAIDs are effective therapy for low back pain. However, patients with acute or chronic low back pain usually require more than one NSAID before being satisfied with their improvement in pain and function (Borenstein 2006). The NSAIDs have not been found to differ significantly from one another in effectiveness. As may be seen from **Table 8.2**, these drugs can have major side effects and interactions with other drugs. Their hepatic and renal side effects are more common in elderly patients. Epidemiological studies of the use of NSAIDs have revealed significant gastrointestinal toxicity (German Pharmaceutical Commission 2006).

Patients requiring NSAID treatment but with an elevated risk of gastrointestinal complications can be treated prophylactically with omeprazole, a proton-pump inhibitor, or misoprostol (German Pharmaceutical Commission 2006). Detailed guidelines for the initiation and maintenance of treatment with analgesics, including NSAIDs, are given in **Table 8.2**. Long-term therapy should be avoided if possible.

Selective COX-2 inhibitors have fewer gastrointestinal side effects than conventional NSAIDs, but some of them have been withdrawn from the market because of an increased incidence of myocardial infarction and thromboembolic events. The remaining available COX-2 inhibitors, celecoxib and parecoxib, are further described in **Table 8.2**.

Opioids

An overview of the more important opioid drugs used in clinical practice is given in **Table 8.3**. There are as yet insufficient data from properly performed studies to support the common assumption that opioids are more effective against back pain than nonopioid analgesics (German Pharmaceutical Commission 2006).

> **!** Nonetheless, there is no doubt about the effectiveness of opioids in disk disease, in view of our understanding of their pharmacological effects, the existing meta-analyses of studies of their use against chronic pain of other kinds, and, not least, the longstanding clinical experiences of physicians and patients alike.

Table 8.2 Overview of clinically important nonopioid medications (from Stehr-Stirngibl in Theodoridis and Krämer 2006)

Generic name	Paracetamol, acetazolamide	Metamizol
Trade name	e. g., Tylenol	e. g., Novalgin
Forms	Tablets, 500 mg Suppositories, 125/250/500/1000 mg Liquid, 1 mL = 200 mg Solution for IV infusion 1000 mg	Solution (drops), 1 mL = 500 mg Tablets, 50 mg Suppositories, 100/300 mg Ampoules 1 g/2.5 g
Single dose	500–1000 mg	500–1000 mg
Maximum daily dose	6000 mg	6000 mg
Dose interval (h)	4–6	6
Adverse effects	Hepatocellular necrosis as an effect of over-dose (antidote: acetylcysteine)	IV: severe hypotension, shock (no bolus injections!), allergic reactions, diaphoresis. Very rare: agranulocytosis.
Contraindications	Hepatic or renal failure	Known allergy to metamizol
Generic name	**Ibuprofen**	**Diclofenac**
Trade name	e. g., Motrin	e. g., Voltaren
Forms	Tablets/capsules, 200/400/600 mg Timed-release tablets, 800 mg Suppositories, 500 mg Dispersable tablets, 600 mg Ampoules (for IM injection)	Tablets/capsules, 25/50 mg Timed-release tablets, 100 mg Resinate capsules, 75 mg Dispersable tablets, 50 mg Suppositories, 12.5/25/50 mg
Single dose	200–800 mg	50–100 mg (children 12.5)
Maximum daily dose	2400 mg	300 mg
Dose interval (h)	8	8
Adverse effects	GI (ulcers), coagulopathy, hepatic and renal dysfunction, allergic reactions	Cf. ibuprofen (more severe GI side effects than ibuprofen); sometimes, severe anaphylactic shock and Lyell syndrome when given parenterally
Contraindications	Steroid medication, known peptic ulcer disease, asthma, pregnancy (acceptable in last trimester for strict indications)	Cf. ibuprofen Allergy to diclofenac
Generic name	**Celecoxib**	**Parecoxib**
Trade name	Celebrex	Dynastat
Forms	Capsules, 100/200 mg	Ampoules (IV/IM), 40 mg/2 mL
Single dose	100–200 mg	40 mg
Maximum daily dose	200 mg	80 mg
Dose interval (h)	12–24	12–24
Adverse effects	Dyspepsia, hypertension, congetive heart failure, edema	Cf. Celebrex
Contraindications	Hepatic or renal failure, asthma, last trimester of pregnancy, nursing	Cf. Celebrex
Generic name	**flupirtin**	**Nefopam**
Trade name	Katadolan, Trancopal Dolo	Ajan
Forms	Capsules, 100 mg Suppositories, 75/100 mg Ampoules, 100 mg	Filmtabs, 30 mg Ampoule, 20 mg
Single dose	100–200 mg	30–90 mg
Maximum daily dose	600 mg	80 mg IV/270 mg po
Dose interval (h)	8	8
Adverse effects	Fatigue, dry mouth, impaired concentration	Tachycardia, hypertension, agitation, dry mouth, impaired concentration, diaphoresis, urinary retention in the elderly
Contraindications	Allergy to flupirtin	Allergy to flupirtin Relative contraindications: old age, epilepsy

8

Table 8.3 Overview of clinically important opioid medications (from Stehr-Stirngibl in Theodoridis and Krämer 2006)

Generic name	tramadol	tilidine, naloxone
Trade name	**e. g., Tramal, Tramal long**	**e. g., Valoron N (retard)**
Potency relative to morphine	1/5–1/10	1/5–1/10
Forms	Drops, 20 = 1 mL	Drops, 20 = 1 mL
	Suppositories, 100 mg	Capsules, 50 mg
	Ampoules, 50/100 mg (1/2 mL)	Timed-release tablets,
	Timed-release tablets, 100/150/200 mg	50/100/150/200 mg
Single dose	50–100 mg	50–100 mg
Single dose (timed release)	50–200 mg	50–200 mg
Maximum daily dose	600 mg	600 mg
Dosing interval (h)	4–6	4–6
Dosing interval for timed-release preparation (h)	8–12	8–12
Special considerations	Frequent nausea/vomiting (timed-release preparations are better tolerated). Inhibits NOR and serotonin reuptake, possibly better for neuropathic pain	Not effective in individuals with severely impaired liver function

Generic name	buprenorphine	
Trade name	**Temgesic, Temgesic forte**	
Potency relative to morphine	20	
Forms	Tablets (sublingual) 0.2/0.4 mg	
Single dose	0.2–0.6 mg	
Maximum daily dose	2.4 mg	
Dosing interval (h)	8–12	
Special considerations	Ceiling effect. Well tolerated, less constipating than morphine. Less tachyphylaxis?	

Generic name	morphine	
Trade name	**MST, MS Contin, etc.**	
Potency relative to morphine	1	
Forms	Morphine solution 0.1–4%	Timed release:
	Suppositories 10/20/30 mg	MST tablets 10/ 30/60/100/200 mg
	Tablets 10/20 mg	MST Continus capsules
	Ampoules (for IV injection) 10/20/100/200 mg	30/50/100/200 mg
		MST retard powder 20/30/60/100/200 mg
Single dose	10 mg	
Single dose (timed release)		30–60 mg
Maximum daily dose	No limit	No limit
Dosing interval (h)	4–6	
Dosing interval for timed-release preparation (h)		8–12
Special considerations	The dose of morphine must be reduced in patients with hepatic or renal failure (accumulation of M6G). Interactions with erythromycin, propofol, and cimetidine may occur, with clinically manifest respiratory depression: titrate naloxone (Note. naloxone effect lasts only about 15 min → continuous monitoring)	

Generic name	hydromorphone	oxycodone
Trade name	**Palladon**	**Oxygesic (timed-release)**
Potency relative to morphine	7	2
Forms	Tablets, 1.25/2.5 mg	Timed-release tablets 10/20/40 mg
	Timed-release tbs 4/8/16/24 mg	
Single dose	1.25/2.5 mg	
Single dose (timed release)	4–8 (16) mg	10–20 mg
Maximum daily dose	No limit	
Dosing interval (h)	As needed (breakthrough pain)	
Dosing interval for timed-release preparation (h)	8–12	8–12
Special considerations	No active metabolites → useful in patients with renal failure. Rarer CNS side effects than morphine, less constipation. Abuse potential?	No active metabolites → useful in patients with renal failure. Little binding to plasma protein → few interactions with protein-bound medications

8

The potential of the opioids to cause adverse effects and drug dependency should always be borne in mind. They can be used in the short term to treat severe, acute back pain that fails to respond to other types of analgesics, or when the other types are poorly tolerated. We have had good results, and no major adverse effects, with the use of oxycodone in acute nerve root compression syndromes (Rubenthaler 2005). Many studies have been published on the outcome of long-term opioid use by patients with chronic pain of nonneoplastic origin (Taub 1982, Maier et al. 2005, Gärtner et al. 2006). The analgesic effect is not lost over time. Most patients continue with this form of treatment and consider themselves adequately treated.

The transdermal route is alternative method for the noninvasive delivery of potent opioids. Among the drugs that are available in patch form, buprenorphine is assigned to WHO stage II–III and fentanyl to stage III (Stehr-Zirngibl 2005). The patch enables continuous delivery of the active substance through the skin at a constant rate (Allan et al. 2005). It takes some time, however, for a therapeutically useful blood level to be reached after the patch is first applied. Thus, acutely arising disk-related pain is more appropriately treated with a timed-release oral opioid preparation.

Muscle Relaxants

Muscle relaxants can be added in the short term if muscle spasm is severe and nonpharmacological measures have brought no relief. These drugs come into the general class of co-analgesics. Though they are very commonly prescribed to treat pain related to disk disease, the available data on their effectiveness in this condition are both sparse and inconsistent. A few studies do indicate that they are more effective than placebo (Pratzel et al. 1996, German Pharmaceutical Commission 2006).

Anticonvulsants

We have found that anticonvulsants can also be useful as co-analgesics in the treatment of pain due to chronic nerve root irritation, whether the cause is discogenic, osseous (spinal stenosis), or postoperative. Carbamazepine was the first such agent used for this indication; the newer agents, gabapentin and pregabalin, have considerably fewer side effects, convenient dosage properties, and a high affinity for their receptors (Stehr-Zirngibl 2005). Their adverse effects include fatigue, dizziness, and orthostatic hypotension.

Summary

The spectrum of symptomatic pharmacological treatment for disk-related symptoms, as reflected in the WHO graded scheme, ranges from simple mild analgesics to opioids. The NSAIDs, which currently retain their popularity among physicians and patients alike, occupy the middle range. They are relatively easy to obtain and can be very effective in adequate doses. Their long-term use, however, carries a high risk of gastrointestinal complications. Thus, for chronic pain, a milder or stronger opioid (depending on the severity of the pain) is generally to be preferred, as these medications are relatively nontoxic. The overall dose of medication can be reduced by multimodal treatment with the simultaneous administration of analgesics, anti-inflammatories, anticonvulsants, and muscle relaxants.

Conclusion

It is worthwhile to treat the pain of disk disease symptomatically with medication. Disc disease being a benign condition, the benefit of pharmacotherapy should be carefully weighed against its potential adverse effects.

9 Cervical Syndrome

■ Definition and Prevalence

> **!** **Definition:** The term "cervical syndrome" refers to all pathological clinical manifestations due to functional disturbances and degenerative changes of the cervical motion segments.

Cervical syndromes are associated with restricted mobility of the cervical spine, increased tension of the shoulder and neck muscles, and (in some cases) radicular signs in the upper limbs, as well as autonomic manifestations. "Cervical syndrome" is a purely clinical term. The painless partial immobilization of the cervical spine that often occurs in old age because of advanced osteochondrosis and spondylosis is not considered a cervical syndrome.

The involutional changes of old age profoundly affect the morphology of the cervical disks, which lie immediately adjacent to important parts of the central nervous system and the vascular system. Clinical manifestations of several different kinds may result, as will be explained below.

Prevalence; age and sex distribution. Symptoms related to changes in the cervical disks are common. Every fifth patient who visits an orthopedist does so because of a cervical disk syndrome. Women are more commonly affected than men, up to age 60 (**Fig. 9.1**). The point prevalence of neck pain (i. e., "neck pain today") in the general population is 30%, and its annual prevalence (i. e., "neck pain within the past year") is 60%. These

figures are only slightly lower than the corresponding ones for back pain (Kohlmann 2001, Borenstein et al. 2004). Similar figures on the prevalence and distribution of cervical spine syndromes were reported by Bovim et al. (1994), Coté et al. (1998), Guez et al. (2002), Borenstein et al. (2004), Fejar et al. (2005), and in the key findings from the Task Force on Neck Pain (Haldeman et al. 2008).

Classification. The cervical syndromes are classified by their cardinal manifestations and duration, and treated accordingly. They are divided into acute and chronic conditions with and without radicular manifestations. The duration of symptoms is correlated with the age of the patient: acute manifestations are more common in younger individuals, while chronic cervical spine conditions are more common in older adults. Traumatic cervical spine syndromes form a class in themselves.

The wide variety of possibilities for the spatial and temporal distribution of pain and other symptoms often makes it impossible to give a more precise and cogent name to a particular instance of a cervical syndrome. The clinical findings are the most important determinant of the treatment to be applied, and the treatment must be continually adapted to the patient's changing symptoms and to their previous response to the treatments already given. "Polypragmasia, " i. e., a multiple-component treatment strategy, is often the best approach.

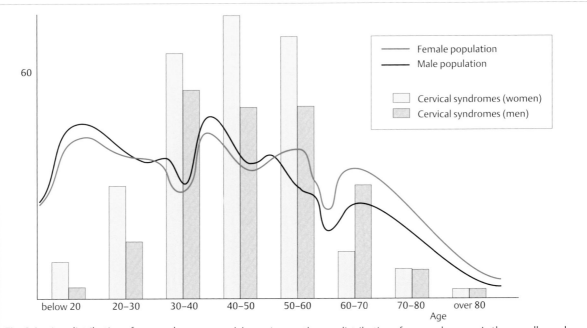

Fig. 9.1   Age distribution of men and women receiving outpatient treatment for cervical syndrome in Düsseldorf and Bochum (North Rhine Westphalia, Germany), compared to the age distribution of men and women in the overall population (population data from the Statistical Yearbook of the State of North Rhine-Westphalia, Germany).

■ Special Anatomy and Physiology of the Cervical Motion Segments

Uncinate Processes

The cervical motion segments differ from those of the rest of the spine in a number of anatomical and biome-

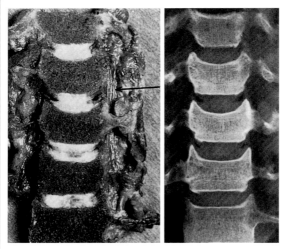

Fig. 9.2 a, b   Coronal section through the mid-cervical spine of a 27-year-old man. The arrow indicates the vertebral artery.
a Anatomical specimen.
b Radiograph.

chanical features that render them more susceptible to early signs of wear and tear, with the consequent development of symptoms. The end plates of vertebral bodies C3–C7 have saddle-like posterior and lateral extensions called the uncinate processes, which in turn give the cervical disks their laterally tapering shape. Furthermore, because of the cervical lordosis, the disks are a third higher ventrally than dorsally. In a frontal anatomical section, the disks look flat and concave upward (**Fig. 9.2**).

The uncinate processes develop during the growth period of the cervical spine and finally assume the shape of shovel-like crests of bone sticking out from the lateral edges of the vertebrae. Because of the uncinate processes, the cervical disks are mainly bordered by bone laterally, unlike the disks elsewhere in the spine. Our studies of cervical spine biomechanics (Stahl 1977) showed that the uncinate processes are located more laterally on the edge of the vertebrae in the upper segments of the cervical spine and more dorsolaterally in the lower segments, with a transition at C6.

Cervical disk degeneration is accompanied by osteophyte formation from the uncinate processes. These osteophytes are often of clinical importance, as they may lie in the immediate vicinity of the cervical nerve roots or the vertebral artery (**Fig. 9.3**). Aufdermaur (1968) showed that osteophytes grow dorsolaterally from the uncinate processes between the ages of 30 and 50. As an individual ages, osteophytes tend to form more laterally, i. e., closer to the vertebral artery.

The transition at C6 regarding the lateral vs. dorsolateral position of osteophytes was mentioned above. In consequence, the formation of large osteophytes is more likely to cause vascular compression in the upper and middle cervical segments and neural compression in the lower cervical segments (Faustmann 2004).

Horizontal Fissures

Von Luschka (1858) was the first to describe horizontal fissures in the cervical disks, which he designated as lateral half-joints. These fissures develop in childhood at the level of the uncinate processes and tend to progress in a medial direction. They are so commonly seen that they are considered a normal finding. Horizontal fissures are a sign, not of degeneration, but rather of adaptation of the cervical spine to allow greater mobility (Töndury 1958, Ecklin 1969, Shark and Parke 1983, Faustmann 2004).

Unlike the degenerative radial fissures of the disks elsewhere in the spine, the horizontal fissures of the cervical disks appear in the midst of entirely normal disk tissue. They begin in the outer lamellae of the anulus fibrosus and gradually narrow as they proceed toward the center of the disk. Often, a meniscus-like wedge of tissue grows into the fissure from the neighboring paravertebral connective tissue. According to Ecklin (1960), an anatomical situation arises that is in all respects comparable to a joint: the fissure possesses an enclosed space with smooth borders, layers of hyaline cartilage on the uncinate process and on the opposite pole (von Luschka's joint facet), a meniscus-like articulation, and, often, tough fibrous bands separating the "joint" from the spinal canal, in the manner of a capsule (Stahl and Huth 1980). In our own anatomical studies, we have found synovium-lined cavities in the uncovertebral region in all decades of life.

> **!** The horizontal fissures increase the mobility of the cervical spine, but they are also a biomechanically vulnerable "site of least resistance" because of their tendency to extend medially and laterally.

Vertebral Artery and Cervical Sympathetic Chain

The uncovertebral region lies in the immediate vicinity of both the vertebral artery and the cervical sympathetic chain. The age-associated changes of the uncovertebral region can impinge on either or both of these structures, producing neurovascular manifesta-

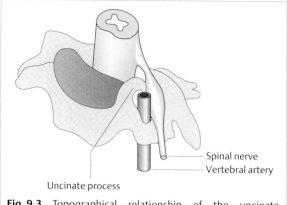

Fig. 9.3 Topographical relationship of the uncinate process, vertebral artery, and spinal nerve.

(labels: Spinal nerve, Vertebral artery, Uncinate process)

tions of various kinds. The cervical sympathetic chain, which communicates with the spinal nerves through the rami communicantes, and its three associated ganglia provide autonomic innervation to the head, neck, and upper limbs. The upper ganglion serves segments C1–C4, and the middle ganglion serves C5–C6; the lower ganglion is fused with the uppermost thoracic ganglion to form the stellate ganglion, which serves C7–T2. The stellate ganglion is the most important relay station among these ganglia, because all of the efferent and nearly all of the afferent sympathetic fibers of the head, neck, upper limb, and upper part of the thorax pass through it. From the sympathetic chain ganglia, the sympathetic fibers travel upward by various routes, including along the sympathetic arterial plexus of the vertebral artery.

The studies of Hovelacque (1925), Werte (1934), Kummer (1984), Kehr and Jung (1985), Bogduk et al. (1988), Lang (1991), Faustmann (2004), and Heller et al. (2005) demonstrate the interconnections of the cervical sympathetic innervation with the cervical spinal nerves and the sympathetic arterial plexus of the vertebral artery. Sympathetic fibers from all three cervical ganglia pass from the sympathetic chain to spinal nerves C4–C8 and partially encircle the vertebral artery.

The vertebral artery originates from the subclavian artery and passes upward through the foramina of the transverse processes of cervical vertebrae C6 through C2. At the level of each intervertebral disk from C5/6 to C2/3, it lies immediately adjacent to the uncinate process. Jung et al. (1974) and Lang (1991) pointed out the relative narrowness of the transverse foramina in relation to the lumen of the vertebral artery. Even head movements within the normal range of motion, in individuals with normal anatomy, can narrow the arterial lumen. The joints of the craniocervical junction create further possibilities for compression of the vertebral artery on movement.

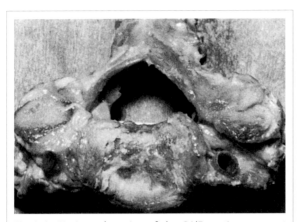

Fig. 9.4 Horizontal section of the C4/5 motion segment of a 23-year-old man. The lumen of the vertebral artery is immediately adjacent to the lateral portion of the unci-nate process and to the soft tissue around the spinal nerve.

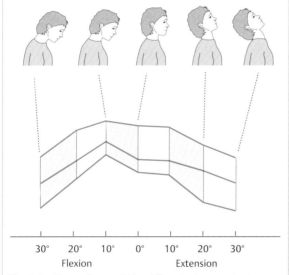

30°	20°	10°	0°	10°	20°	30°
Flexion				Extension		

Fig. 9.5 Dependence of blood flow in the vertebral artery on head posture. Mild inclination (ca. 10°) affords better flow than the neutral position. Any deviation from this opti-mal position is associated with lower blood flow.

! Abnormal positions of the cervical joints, due to trauma or hypermobility of any cause, may narrow the lumen of the vertebral artery at its points of maximum curvature.

Brown and Tissington (1963) found that rotation and re-clination of the head caused marked narrowing of the vertebral artery on the opposite side. The two vertebral arteries constitute a functional unit, i. e., a disturbance of either of the two arteries can be compensated for by the other, because they join superiorly to form the basilar artery. This compensating mechanism is absent, however, if one of the vertebral arteries is nonfunctional to begin with, e. g., because of hypoplasia. The anatomy of the vertebral arteries is variable, and the arteries on the right and left sides may not have the same diameter. A hypoplastic artery on one side may explain the pre-sence of unexpectedly severe symptoms in a patient with relatively mild changes of the uncovertebral joints. Because of the close anatomical relationship of the vertebral artery, sympathetic chain, and intervertebral disks, cervical syndrome can produce vascular and au-tonomic manifestations. The brainstem and inner ear may be affected, as these structures, among others, derive their blood supply from the vertebral artery (**Fig. 9.4**).

Our own studies have demonstrated that blood flow in the vertebral arteries depends on the position of the head (Oppel and Fritz 1986).

! The blood flow in the vertebral arteries is greatest when the cervical spine is in mild flexion.

More pronounced flexion of the cervical spine, the neutral position of the cervical spine, and extension (i. e., reclination of the head) are all associated with a re-duction of blood flow (**Fig. 9.5**). Mild flexion also pro-duces a marked widening of the intervertebral foramina (Grifka et al. 1989, Struckhoff 1994, Tomoaki et al. 2004).

The blood flow in the vertebral artery may be tenu-ous because of arteriosclerosis, anatomical variants, or (most commonly) lateral osteophytes arising from the uncinate processes. If so, any additional factor, such as trauma or an abnormal posture of the cervical spine, may induce vertebrobasilar insufficiency, which can then be compensated for by mild flexion of the neck.

Cervical Nerve Roots and Nerve Root Sleeves

The lower cervical nerve roots and nerve root sleeves are of special clinical significance, particularly with re-spect to cervical spinal nerve analgesia. In this pro-cedure, which is discussed in greater detail toward the end of this chapter, the nerve roots to be treated are flooded with local anesthetic injected via a dorsal ap-proach. The physician doing the procedure must be aware of the topographical anatomic relationship of the bone, specifically the lateral mass of the cervical verte-bra, to the exiting nerve root. As in all other regions of the spine, the proximal segment of a cervical nerve root is bathed in cerebrospinal fluid for a short distance within the so-called nerve root sleeve. If the local anes-thetic is improperly injected into the nerve root sleeve because of faulty technique, it will enter the cervical subarachnoid space and affect the cervical spinal cord, with ensuing respiratory arrest and circulatory collapse.

Standard anatomy textbooks unfortunately tend to depict the central nervous system and the musculo-skeletal tissues surrounding it in separate images, so that the student cannot gain a clear idea of the anatomical relationship of the bones and nerves. Lang (1991) described the apertures of the individual cervical nerve root sleeves receiving the bundled anterior and posterior fascicles of the cervical rootlets. The arachnoid, which typically fuses with the anterior and posterior root a few millimeters proximal to the spinal ganglion, is one component of the inner nerve sheath system. The dura mater of the nerve root sleeves is continuous with the fibrous layer of the perineurium. Frykholm (1951) studied the lower cervical nerve roots and their coverings and found that each root sleeve possesses two openings, one ventral and one dorsal, separated by a dural septum. Each root ostium leads to its own root sleeve, which is a lateral extension of the dural sac (**Fig. 9.6**).

In the anatomy department of our institution, Heinze and Rubenthaler (2004) dissected the spinal nerves of C5–C8 bilaterally, marking their sites of exit from the spinal canal and demonstrating and measuring the nerve root sleeves (**Fig. 9.7**). They studied the relationship of the nerve root sleeves to the encasing bony structures of the intervertebral foramina. The root sleeves were measured with a probe and dissected under 16× magnification to demonstrate the transition to perineurial connective tissue. The root sleeves were then cannulated at their bony site of exit and marked by injection of methylene blue under high pressure. Finally, the intrathecal space was studied radiologically after the injection of contrast medium.

No layer that was separable from the nerve itself could be found lateral to the ganglion, even with sharp dissection. The ganglion lies proximal to the exit of the spinal nerve through the intervertebral foramen. It follows, therefore, that there is a safety zone (extending, in this study, from the outer mark on the root to the deepest point of the root sleeve than can be reached with the probe) in which the direct intrathecal injection of local anesthetic is not possible.

This study also revealed that the C5–C8 nerve roots are thick and lie closely adjacent to one another (**Fig. 9.8**). One must therefore assume that an infiltration of the C7 root for cervical spinal nerve analgesia will also affect the C6 and C8 roots if 5 mL or more of local anesthetic is injected. One can thus treat C8 irritation with an infiltration at C7 in order to minimize the risk of pneumothorax.

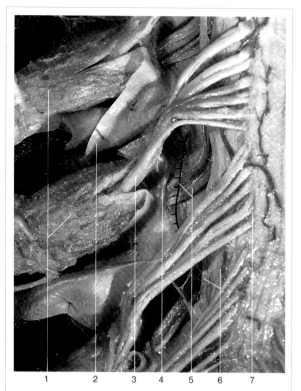

Fig. 9.6 Nerve root sheaths and ostia (opened dorsally) (from Lang 1991).
1 C5 and C6 spinal ganglia.
2 Dura mater (reflected).
3 C6 dorsal root.
4 Dural spur between the ostia for the dorsal and ventral roots.
5 C6 ventral root and millimeter gauge (for scale).
6 Denticulate ligament.
7 Linea radicularis dorsalis (dorsal root entry zone, DREZ).

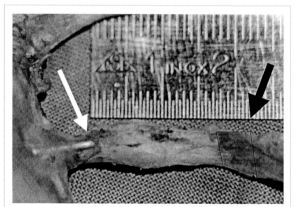

Fig. 9.7 Dissected lower cervical spinal nerve, with mark (black arrow) at the point of its lateral exit from bone. A probe lies in the nerve root sheath (white arrow). The distance from the lateral mark to the tip of the probe is measured with a ruler (from Rubenthaler 2005).

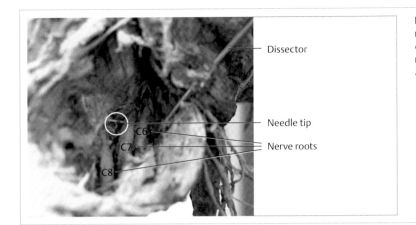

Dissector

Needle tip

Nerve roots

C6

C7

C8

Fig. 9.8 The C5–C8 nerve roots, after removal of the soft tissue covering dorsally. Note the proximity of the roots to each other (from Theodoridis and Krämer 2006).

■ Biomechanics

> ! The cervical spine is the most mobile part of the axial skeleton. The head and neck can be moved in all directions. Much of this mobility is derived from the two uppermost segments, i.e., the segments of the craniocervical junction, which possess no intervertebral disks. The atlanto-occipital joint enables nodding movements, while the atlantoaxial joint primarily subserves rotation.

The remaining segments of the cervical spine all possess intervertebral disks; most of the mobility of the cervical spine is at C4/5–C6/7. The position of the joint facets enables movement in all directions at these levels as well, but forward and backward bending are favored, because the sagittally oriented uncinate processes serve as guides for these movements along their entire range (Jofe et al. 1983, Panjabi et al. 2005). The track-like uncinate processes thus limit rotatory movements of the cervical spine that might place excessive strain on the disks.

Flexion of the cervical spine, like flexion of (e.g.) the knee, is a process of rolling and sliding. The vertebral bodies do not merely tilt, they also slide in the dorsoventral direction, particularly in younger individuals. Radiographs reveal a typical staircase-like arrangement of the posterior edges of the cervical vertebrae. Flexion from the midposition leads to 2–3 mm of anterior displacement of each vertebra with respect to the one immediately below it, and extension leads to 1–2 mm of displacement in the opposite direction (Exner 1954).

Any movement of the cervical spine also alters the width of the intervertebral foramina at each level. Studies of dissected specimens, as well as radiological studies in vivo, have shown that the foramina are wider on the convex side of the laterally inclined cervical spine, and narrower on the opposite (concave) side. Forward bending or kyphosis of the cervical spine widens all of the intervertebral foramina, whereas backward bending or lordosis narrows them. These facts explain the posture that individuals suffering from an acute cervical syndrome typically assume to lessen nerve compression (acute torticollis, wry neck). The position in which the head is held, and the directions in which movement is resisted, are clinical clues pointing to the site of the lesion.

> ! The relatively heavy human head puts the cervical disks under high mechanical stress.

Grob (1968) estimated the stress on the lower cervical disks at 550 kPa with normal head position and muscle tone, and 3900 kPa if muscle tone is absent. Panjabi et al. (2005) carried out biomechanical experiments on the cervical spine that yielded similar results. They also calculated the reduction of stress on the cervical spine that could be obtained with the Glisson kyphotic traction method (stretch test), demonstrating the potential usefulness of this method in the conservative management of cervical syndromes.

The nucleus pulposus of a cervical intervertebral disk changes its position in response to asymmetrical compression of the disk, just as the nucleus pulposus does in other regions of the spine. We studied the question whether the mobile, centrally located tissue of a cervical disk tends to be displaced in the same way as that of a lumbar disk when the disk is asymmetrically compressed. We did so by inserting a small metal bolt into the center of the nucleus pulposus in a dissected cervical motion segment specimen, then following its movements radiographically when the segment was manipulated (Stahl 1977). Asymmetrical compression, as expected, produced displacement of the bolt to the side

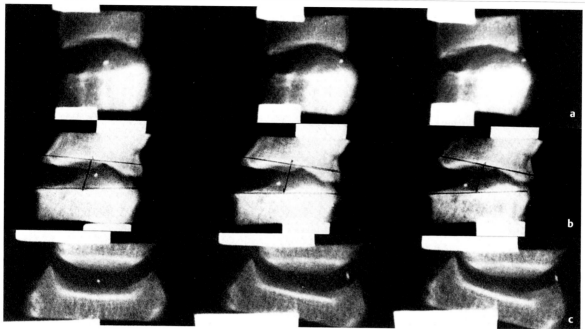

Fig. 9.9 a–c Mobility of central disk tissue (marked with a metal bolt) with asymmetrical compression of the C4/5 intervertebral disk of an 18-year-old man (50–100 kPa of pressure, or 500–1000 N of force).

a Compression of the anterior edge (kyphosis).
b Compression of the posterior edge (lordosis).
c Lateral compression.

that was under less pressure, i. e., dorsally when the stress was greater ventrally (in kyphosis), ventrally when the stress was greater dorsally (in lordosis), and to the convex side on lateral bending (**Fig. 9.9**). The degree of displacement was surprisingly large after no more than a few minutes of asymmetrical compression. If the compression was kept up for some time and then released, displacement of the nucleus pulposus was still evident several hours later. The mobility of the central disk tissue in response to asymmetrical compression is greater in adolescents and young adults than in elderly individuals.

> **!** Any maintained asymmetrical posture of the cervical spine can be expected to cause intradiscal tissue displacement.

Such tissue displacements play a role in the pathogenesis of cervical syndromes.

Special Pathoanatomy and Pathophysiology

Degenerative changes of the lower cervical motion segments begin to appear at an early age, though they are not evident in radiological studies till later on in life. Their main cause is the mechanical stress associated with the larger excursions of movement in these segments, compared to the relatively immobile thoracic spine. The intradiscal pressure is also higher at cervical than at thoracic and lumbar levels, because of the weight of the head. Nor is there, in the cervical spine, any counterpart to the mechanism of reducing the intradiscal pressure in the lumbar spine by raising the intra-abdominal pressure (abdominal pressing, Valsalva maneuver).

Persistent mechanical stress and the wide range of motion of the cervical spine, particularly with regard to rotation, lead to overstretching of the anulus fibrosus, which, in turn, results in anular tears and intradiscal tissue displacement. This situation predisposes to disk protrusion.

> **!** The horizontal fissures are the primary sites of occurrence of pathological changes in the cervical motion segments.

The joint-like construction of the horizontal fissures is biomechanically ideal only for a short time, because

9

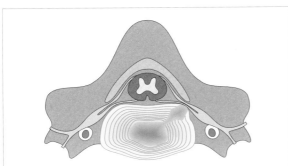

Fig. 9.10 Dorsolateral displacement of central, mobile disk tissue (nucleus pulposus) with compression of a cervical nerve root.

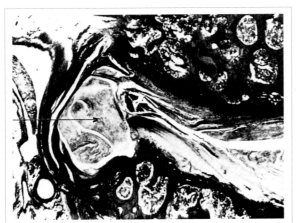

Fig. 9.11 Prolapsed nucleus pulposus tissue (arrow) protruding in mushroom-like fashion under the uncovertebral ligamentous connection. The fissure communicates internally with the anulus pulposus cavity (from Ecklin U. Die Altersveränderungen der Halswirbelsäule. Berlin: Springer; 1960).

of joint capsule. Such protrusions of disk tissue can occur only when the turgor pressure in the disk is normal or elevated, which is the case only in relatively young individuals (**Figs. 9.10, 9.11**). Indeed, Töndury found moderately large cervical disk protrusions only in young people. Elderly individuals had dried-out disk tissue that did not protrude outside the boundaries of the disk even in the presence of full-thickness horizontal tears.

The horizontal fissures can spread so far medially that they actually cut the cervical disk in half. It is then held together only by the joint capsules and the ligaments between the vertebrae. The movement segment is lax and unstable.

> **!** Lateral spread of the horizontal fissures disturbs the osmotic system of the disk.

The boundaries of the intervertebral disk become permeable to larger molecules as well as smaller ones, so that the intradiscal osmotic pressure falls; the disk consequently dries out and loses height. The vertebrae above and below it come closer together, making a greater degree of bony contact at the uncinate processes and the intervertebral joints. The uncinate processes bend laterally and develop **bony appositions.** Reactive thickening of bone occurs on the bony surfaces of the upper vertebra opposite the uncinate processes of the lower one. The uncovertebral region develops a new, supportive function. The uncinate processes and their cartilaginous lining are biomechanically not up to the task, however, and they soon develop arthrosis-like changes as a result.

> **!** The osteophytic reaction of the uncinate processes and the loss of disk height lead to narrowing of the intervertebral foramen.

As **Fig. 9.12** shows, this narrowing is due not only to the bony extensions of the uncinate process that are visible in the radiograph, but also to the radiolucent soft tissue surrounding the bone. Sometimes this soft tissue alone suffices to compress a cervical nerve root and produce clinical symptoms, even in the absence of visible intervertebral foraminal stenosis on an oblique plain radiograph of the cervical spine.

Once the intervertebral foramen is sufficiently narrowed, nerve root irritation and signs of vascular compression can appear. The cervical intervertebral foramina are narrower than the thoracic and lumbar ones and are thus more vulnerable to osteogenic constriction. This constriction is produced by uncovertebral exostoses in combination with the telescoping of the intervertebral joint facets due to osteochondrotic disk collapse, which narrows the upper portion of the intervertebral foramen in particular. Unlike lumbar nerve root irritation, cervical nerve root irritation is usually

these fissures tend to spread both medially and laterally.

Laterally, the outermost fibrous lamellae of the anulus fibrosus remain in place while the disk begins to protrude in the direction of the intervertebral foramen. The fissures also provide a path along which mobile disk material can find its way toward the boundaries of the disk and beyond, though the site of potential egress remains narrow. Töndury (1958) found contained disk protrusions in histological sections of the uncovertebral region even in the cervical spine of children: the overstretched inner fibrous lamellae bulged out through tears in the outer lamellae, without at first overstepping the boundary of the intervertebral disk itself. In adults, Töndury found nucleus pulposus tissue that had nearly found its way out of the disk along the horizontal fissure and was held back merely by the ligamentous bands around the uncovertebral joint, which served as a kind

not caused by direct pressure of the disk on the nerve, but rather by the secondary effects of disk degeneration on the sides of the vertebrae and on the intervertebral joints. The peak age for cervicobrachialgia is accordingly 10 years later than that for sciatica.

All **other degenerative changes,** such as spondylosis, osteochondrosis, and spondylarthrosis, occur in the cervical spine just as they do elsewhere in the spinal column.

> **!** The C5/6 and C6/7 segments are affected earliest and most frequently because they are under the greatest mechanical stress.

Monoradicular nerve root irritation syndromes also affect these motion segments more frequently than others (see **Fig. 9.20**).

> **!** 95–100% of people over age 70 have spondylotic changes of the cervical spine of greater or lesser severity.

Loss of disk height causes a loss of lordosis and a fixed, extended position of the osteochondrotic segments, which is compensated for by hyperlordosis of the segments above and below.

Arthrotic changes of the intervertebral joints (spondylarthrosis) are rarer than was previously thought. As the cervical disks lose height, the uncinate processes come into contact with the vertebral bodies above before the joints can be exposed to any marked elevation of mechanical stress. Intervertebral joint arthrosis is generally more severe in the upper and middle portions of the cervical spine than at C5/6 and C6/7.

Fibrous ankylosis with ingrowth of organized vascular connective tissue finally leads to a comfortable rigidity of the affected cervical motion segments.

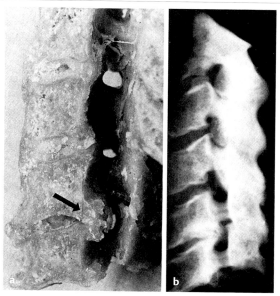

Fig. 9.12 a, b Parasagittal section of the cervical spine of a 65-year-old man: anatomical specimen (**a**) and radiograph (**b**). Note the osteophytic reactions on the uncinate process and on the surface of the vertebral body opposite, with narrowing of the C5/6 intervertebral foramen.

Osteophytes and areas of bony thickening regress once the bony support elicited by slackening of the intervertebral disks is no longer needed. The loss of function resulting from the immobilization of multiple motion segments is well tolerated by older individuals because most of the mobility of the head is provided by the two uppermost (i. e., atlanto-occipital and atlantoaxial) segments.

Summary

The special feature of the **anatomy** of the cervical intervertebral disks is their proximity to important neural and vascular structures. The vertebral artery, the spinal nerve, and the spinal cord are all immediately adjacent to the disk, and these structures may be impinged upon in acceleration–deceleration injuries of the cervical spine, during sporting activities, or during passive movement of the neck in manual therapy. Mild flexion of the neck optimizes (i. e., increases) the distance between the skeletal and neurovascular elements, whereas extension decreases it. This explains the marked positional dependence of disk-related symptoms in the cervical spine.

A special **biomechanical** feature of the human cervical spine is the apparent disproportion between the relatively heavy head and the relatively small cervical disks. This, combined with the wide range of motion of the neck in all directions, results in a high potential for injury. Because of their unfavorable biomechanical situation, the lower cervical motion segments tend to show early signs of wear and tear. Clinical manifestations tend to be produced particularly by such changes occurring in the region of the uncinate process and intervertebral foramen.

Conclusion

The cervical spine moves freely in all directions, bears the relatively large weight of the head, and lies in the immediate vicinity of important neurovascular structures. These features combine to make it one of the more injury-prone areas of the axial skeleton.

■ Clinical Features of Cervical Syndromes

Overview of Symptoms and Their Classification

The **term** "cervical syndrome" refers to any disease state directly or indirectly caused by degenerative changes of the cervical intervertebral disks. Thus, it covers not only conditions with painful limitation of movement of the cervical spine, but also excessive muscle tension in the shoulder and neck, segmental radicular syndromes of the upper limb, cervicogenic headache and dizziness, spinal cord syndromes, cochleovestibular irritative conditions, and various functional disturbances arising in the internal organs. Any systematic classification of such a wide-ranging group of illnesses is necessarily imperfect, regardless of whether it is based on a fundamental subdivision by localization (upper vs. lower) or by disease course (acute vs. chronic).

A strict **separation** of each one of these conditions from all the others is often not possible, because each condition may consist of a large number of different symptoms that change, or vary in severity, over time, and the clinical pictures of different conditions often overlap. We consider a division of cervical syndromes into upper, middle, and lower to be potentially misleading, as it is definitely not the case that all of their symptoms can be attributed, respectively, to pathology in the upper, middle, or lower regions of the cervical spine.

> ! Nearly all cervical syndromes are due to pathology in the *lower* cervical motion segments, no matter which segments manifest the greatest degenerative disturbances of form and function.

A separation of cervical syndromes into acute and chronic is likewise problematic, because the course of disk-related complaints is highly variable.

Our classification is mainly based on the participation of individual spinal nerve roots in the generation of symptoms. In most cases, multiple roots participate, with one root playing the most prominent role.

Patients' Description of Symptoms

The patient's own description of the symptoms is all the more important as a clue for the diagnostician because objective signs are often absent (for which reason medicolegal assessment is often difficult). In our series of patients presenting to private orthopedic practices, we always record the patient's chief complaint in their own words.

The typical pains in the shoulder and neck, combined with stiffness in the cervical spine, tend to arise suddenly and to be precipitated by rotation of the head or by prolonged maintenance of a kyphotic posture for reading, watching television, or working at a desk (**Table 9.1**). Patients often draw a connection between the initial appearance of symptoms and cooling of the shoulder and neck muscles by a draft of air, e. g., in an air-conditioned room or while driving.

> ! A maintained improper posture (generalized cervical kyphosis under mechanical stress), increased muscle tension due to lower temperatures, and muscle tension raising the intradiscal pressure are important pathogenetic mechanisms for cervical syndromes.

The symptoms sometimes appear as soon as the patient wakes up in the morning. They are **position-dependent:** typically, they can be brought on or exacerbated by certain movements and positions of the cervical spine. The patient assumes a protective posture (which takes an extreme form in acute torticollis). Patients often state that they can partially relieve the pain with a movement in the opposite direction or with manual pressure on one side of the head. Patients should be asked specifically about the positional dependence of their symptoms, as this may yield important clues for differential diagnosis.

Worsening of symptoms at night is characteristic of cervical syndromes. The patient is awakened by the pain. Because of the normal diminution of muscle tone and absence of voluntary muscle contraction during sleep, the patient involuntarily assumes positions that induce pain. For example, pronounced lateral bending combined with hyperlordosis narrows the intervertebral foramina on the concave side of the bend. Once the nerves and vessels in the foramen are mechanically irritated, a vicious circle of neurovascular irritation, pain, and muscle contraction is set up. Sleeping prone or propped up on too many pillows can predispose to such situations. The pain is usually combined with a feeling of stiffness. The various kinds of symptom that can arise include *shoulder and neck pain, paresthesiae, occipital pain, tinnitus, syncopal attacks, a feeling of tightness in the chest, and migraine-like phenomena.*

Table 9.1 Typical clinical features of cervical syndrome

- Sudden onset
- Positional dependence
- Pain worse at night

Large anterior spondylotic extensions of the cervical vertebrae may give the patient *dysphagia with a "globus" sensation. Respiratory symptoms* through compression of the trachea and *ocular symptoms* are rarer manifestations.

In addition to the specific symptoms just described, patients also complain of **general accompanying symptoms** such as fatigue, irritability, and impaired concentration. Functional disturbances of the internal organs, including the heart, may also arise. In contrast to the relatively stereotypic complaints of organic heart diseases, spondylogenic pseudo-cardiac symptoms come in a dazzling variety of forms, including palpitations or a stabbing, pulling, rippling or tearing sensation. These symptoms are induced by certain postures of the cervical spine and can be relieved by traction in a Glisson sling.

Most patients presenting with cervical complaints to a physician's office or outpatient clinic seem to have a certain degree of **emotional coloring of symptoms**. We have confirmed this impression in our own outpatient clinic with psychological testing.

> **!** Patients with cervical syndrome have more emotional abnormalities than a comparable group of normal control individuals.

There is no longer any doubt about the purely mechanical and organic cause of cervical syndromes. It therefore seems to be the case that continual, deep pain in the shoulder and neck, present day and night and interfering with sleep, can in the long run disturb the patient's emotional balance. The physician must bear this in mind when dealing with such patients, and especially when prescribing treatment and observing its effects.

Clinical Findings

The clinical findings in patients with cervical syndromes fall into two major categories. In the first category are those findings that generally indicate a disorder of the cervical spine, such as muscle tension in the shoulder and neck, painful restriction of cervical movement, and tenderness to pressure in the entire region of the neck; in the second category are the findings that allow precise segmental localization. These include circumscribed tenderness of a single spinous process to pressure or shaking, restriction of movement of a single motion segment, segmental radicular manifestations, and, lastly, the findings of special tests such as EMG, neurography, myelography, discography, CT, MRI, and the distension test.

The clinical examination begins, as always, with **inspection**. The experienced clinician will immediately notice a certain degree of neck stiffness that is maintained while the patient undresses and dresses. The shoulders are often held high. Above all, the patient takes care not to rotate the head and prefers to turn with the entire trunk. The oblique posture of the head in torticollis (wry neck) is unmistakable and often grotesque. Only by keeping the head in this position can the patient derive some relief of symptoms (as the examiner must remember while testing the range of motion). The cervical spine is not only laterally flexed and rotated, but also bent forward (kyphosed) to a certain degree, as can be seen in a lateral plain radiograph. Our studies have shown that this position decompresses the neurovascular structures in the uncovertebral region to the greatest possible extent.

Palpation reveals tension of the shoulder and neck muscles. Pressure-sensitive local muscle hardening ("myogelosis") is found mainly at the upper edge of the trapezius from the occiput to the acromioclavicular joint, in the scalene region, and in the rhomboid muscles. The spinous and transverse processes are also tender to palpation. The transverse processes of the atlas can be palpated in the mandibulomastoid angle. Tenderness is usually found bilaterally at these preferred sites, but more intensely on the affected side.

Functional testing of the cervical spine in cervical syndromes nearly always reveals a restricted range of motion, though the restriction may be limited to one or a few segments. One should test forward and backward bending (distance of chin from sternum), lateral bending, and rotation. The ranges of motion in each direction should be reported in degrees from the neutral position. The absolute ranges of motion of the cervical spine vary naturally with the length of the neck, the degree of muscularity, and the age of the patient. Thus, pathologically restricted movement is best detected by the difference between the ranges of motion on the two sides and by pain produced at the end of the range of motion in any particular direction.

Testing of segmental mobility is performed with the patient first in the supine position, and then sitting. The edges of the joint facets and transverse processes of each successive segment are fixed by the examiner's hands while the patient carries out rotatory, lateral bending, and flexion–extension movements of the segment above.

Functional testing of the cervical spine should always include a **distension (stretch) test** (also known as the Glisson test). The examiner stands behind the patient, takes hold of the patient's mastoid processes with the palms of the hands, rests the forearms on the patient's shoulders, and pushes the patient's head upward. This maneuver momentarily produces strong axial traction on the cervical spine. If the patient reports temporary relief of shoulder and arm pain, this is of diagnostic sig-

9

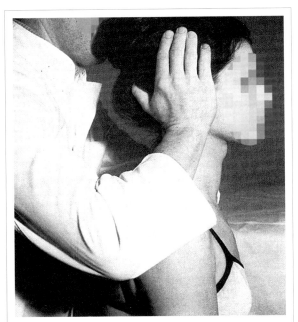

Fig. 9.13 Glisson test of the cervical spine: the examiner holds the patient's mastoid processes in the palms while supporting the forearms on the patient's shoulders and pushing the patient's head upward. This type of grip is also used in manual therapy.

nificance (**Fig. 9.13**) and points to potentially beneficial forms of therapy.

Finally, the clinical examination of a patient with a cervical disk syndrome must always include a **neurological examination.** The single most important piece of localizing information for a cervical radicular irritation syndrome is the patient's description of the pattern of radiation of sensory symptoms. The patient should be asked to outline the band of pain and the area of paresthesia as accurately as possible with one finger. Objective neurological signs such as reflex asymmetry, paresis, muscle hypotonia, atrophy, and hyperesthesia should always be sought as well, though they are relatively rarely seen in cervical disk syndromes.

Radiological Studies

Radiological studies and basic laboratory tests are also a routine part of the evaluation of cervical syndromes. Radiological imaging can effectively rule out tumors (metastases) and infection (spondylitis) as the cause of symptoms. Its usefulness in the precise diagnosis of cervical syndromes and their localization to a particular motion segment is generally overrated, however, and is in fact limited. As already pointed out, cervical spondylosis and osteochondrosis are almost ubiquitous concomitants of aging and are usually of no clinical significance.

The routine radiological evaluation of cervical syndromes consists of anteroposterior and lateral plain radiographs of the entire cervical spine (**Fig. 9.14**). The **anteroposterior view** reveals any deviation of the spinal axis from the vertical in the frontal plane and displays the state of the uncinate processes at middle and lower cervical levels. If the disk has lost height and the uncinate processes make contact with the vertebral body above, they are flattened, so that the end plate is dish-shaped. In advanced spondylarthrosis, joint osteophytes are seen to project from the lateral border of the cervical spine.

The **lateral view** is more important than the anteroposterior view for the exclusion of metastases and infection and for the detection of degenerative disk disease. Disk narrowing, sclerosis of the corresponding upper and lower end plates, and spondylotic projections jutting anteriorly from the lower edge of the cervical vertebrae should not be interpreted as the cause of the present symptoms, but rather as evidence of earlier disk slackening that has, by now, run its natural course.

One should avoid being overly impressed by abnormalities seen in plain radiographs.

> **!** Even massive spondylotic osteophytes, disk collapse, and close approximation of neighboring vertebrae may be associated with only mild symptoms or none at all.

These changes are usually found incidentally. The clinical findings alone are decisive.

> **!** The only radiological finding of direct relevance to an acute cervical disk syndrome is a possible loss of the physiological lordosis due to muscle spasm.

For the lateral radiograph, the patient's head must be in the normal, neutral position, with the neck bent neither forward nor backward. The symptomatic flattening of the lordosis may be limited to one or a few cervical segments. Segmental loss of lordosis, visible as a mild kyphotic kinking of the cervical spine, is caused by reflexive muscle spasm. The patient involuntarily assumes

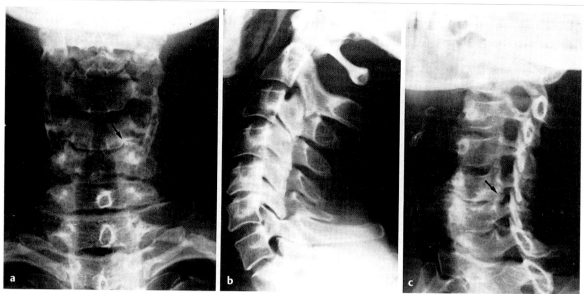

Fig. 9.14 a–c Anteroposterior (AP), lateral, and oblique radiographs of the cervical spine. The osteophytic reactions on the uncinate processes can be seen in the AP and oblique views (**a, c**); the lateral view (**b**) reveals narrowing of the C5/6 intervertebral space.

a kyphotic posture to open the intervertebral foramina in the affected motion segment as widely as possible. The associated dorsal widening of the disk space additionally counteracts discogenic nerve compression.

> ! In most cases, all motion segments above the site of the lesion are abnormally kyphotic (Güntz sign).

In acute cervical disk syndromes, generalized loss of lordosis and segmental kyphosis can also be seen on **functional (dynamic) lateral plain radiographs** obtained with maximal forward and backward bending of the neck. The abnormal findings on forward bending (inclination) include not only the dorsally convex arch of the cervical spine but also a mild ventral displacement of each cervical vertebra on the one below it, the so-called *staircase phenomenon*. This is seen mainly in younger individuals and may be more pronounced in a single segment where there is additional pathology of the intervertebral disk.

A further means of "objectifying" degenerative segmental slackening is provided by the radiological stretch test described by White and Panjabi (1978) and Panjabi (2004). Lateral plain radiographs and a neurological examination are carried out before and during Glisson traction of the cervical spine at one-third of body weight.

The evaluation of cervicobrachial and cervicocephalic syndromes should also include **oblique plain radiographs** of the cervical spine for visualization of the intervertebral foramina (**Fig. 9.14 c**). These may show osteophytes growing from the uncinate process and narrowing the foramen. The degenerative changes of the uncinate processes are seen on oblique radiographs as either sharp or blunt bony projections pointing laterally toward the foramen. The lower vertebral body end plate lying opposite often displays reactive sclerosis and osteophyte formation.

Our measurements in radiographic images and dissected specimens have revealed that the radiographs show only a part of the uncovertebral protrusion, i.e., its hard, bony, radiodense core (see **Fig. 9.12**). This core, however, is often covered by a tough connective tissue layer that is composed of remnants of the anulus fibrosus and the longitudinal ligaments and is therefore invisible on plain radiographs. Thus, the nerve root may be compressed within the foramen by encroachment of the uncinate process even in the absence of radiologically evident critical foraminal narrowing.

> ! Conversely, however, one often finds quite marked osteophyte formation from the uncinate processes, with marked radiologically evident narrowing of the intervertebral foramina, in the absence of any symptoms of nerve root compression. This is most often the case in older individuals.

Cervical intervertebral foraminal stenosis is of clinical significance mainly when it arises rapidly, so that the nerves and vessels have no time to adapt. Rapid decreases in foraminal size can be caused, for example,

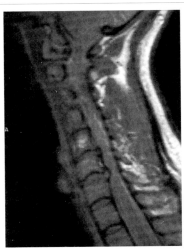

Fig. 9.15   Cervical spine MRI revealing C4/5 and C5/6 disk protrusions with well-hydrated (soft) sequestra. Conservative management.

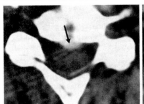 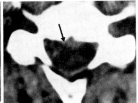

Fig. 9.16   Cervical spine CT revealing a broad-based median disk protrusion at C4/5, which lightly indents the dura mater in the midline (arrow). Conservative management.

by slackening of the motion segment, leading to a situation in which the relative position of the two adjacent vertebral bodies is constantly changing.

CT and MRI

These neuroimaging techniques enable the visualization of cervical disk prolapses. Myelography is only rarely needed for the exclusion of relevant types of neurological disease (**Figs. 9.15, 9.16**).

CT can be used to image the entire cervical spine or only the clinically relevant part of it, to limit radiation exposure. Cervical CT reveals the width of the vertebral canal and the extent of the osteophytic reaction at the uncinate processes. CT after the intrathecal injection of contrast medium enables visualization of the nerve root sleeves.

MRI enables visualization of the entire cervical spine and is particularly good for showing the intervertebral disks. Disk protrusions are best seen in the sagittal sections. Over-interpretation of MR images should be avoided (Siivola et al. 2002, Ullrich 2005).

> **!** MRI shows disk protrusions as being larger than they really are.

Neurophysiological Testing: EMG

Neurophysiological methods are useful for the differentiation of nerve root compression syndromes and cervical spondylogenic myelopathy from systemic diseases such as multiple sclerosis and amyotrophic lateral sclerosis, as well as from peripheral compression syndromes such as carpal tunnel syndrome. They also provide important information about the severity and extent of damage of the sensory and motor pathways. Preoperative neurophysiological assessment of the peripheral nerves (neurography, EMG), the pyramidal pathways (motor evoked potentials), and the afferent pathways of the posterior columns (somatosensory evoked potentials) is helpful not just to confirm the indication for a surgical procedure, but also as a baseline test that can be compared with postoperative follow-up studies (Dvořák 1996, 2002)

The more time-consuming motor and somatosensory evoked potentials play a less important role than conventional EMG in the diagnostic evaluation of cervical radiculopathy. Evoked potentials are very useful, however, in the evaluation of spinal stenosis with possible spinal cord compression.

EMG is a major aid to the objectification of cervical root dysfunction. The muscle action potentials, detected either at the skin or directly from muscle with needle electrodes, are amplified, displayed, and recorded to reveal the state of the muscle and of the nerves supplying it. EMG abnormalities can often be seen before any clinical signs such as paresthesia or muscle atrophy.

EMG technique. Muscle action potentials are recorded with a needle electrode at various positions and at various depths to ensure that a representative picture of muscle activity is obtained. The electrical activity of the skeletal muscle is recorded and analyzed. EMG requires the cooperation of the patient; it is time-consuming and, at times, painful. It should be done only in selected cases to answer specific questions (Dvořák and Haldeman 2004).

Indications. Nerve root compression not only causes segmental pain and paresthesia, but also impairs motor activity in the muscles that are mainly supplied by the root in question. EMG can thus be used to determine which nerve root is involved, with important therapeutic implications (e. g., for selective cervical root block procedures). The indications for EMG in cervical syndromes include the following:

- differentiation from carpal tunnel syndrome
- differentiation of isolated discogenic nerve root compression from a systemic neurological disease
- differentiation of radicular from peripheral nerve lesions
- determination of the severity of neural involvement
- assessment of the extent of re-innervation, if any.

Findings. Cervical nerve root compression usually causes no more than a mild slowing of motor and sensory nerve conduction. This is not surprising, as the speed of conduction is measured in the region of the forearm and hand, although the lesion is much more proximal. Only severe, chronic radicular compression syndromes are accompanied by muscle atrophy with reduced amplitude of muscle action potentials and by a low-amplitude or undetectable sensory nerve action potential. F-waves are often harder to generate, or their latency is prolonged (Dvořák 1996, Dvořák and Haldeman 2004). Comprehensive and detailed descriptions of EMG findings can be found in Conrad and Bischoff (1988), Hopf (1988), Dvořák (1998, 2002), Haig et al. (1998), Mumenthaler et al. (1998), Nargol (1998), Balague (1999), Hirayama (1999), Krämer and Nentwig (1999), Perlick et al. (1999), Colloca (2000), Greenough (2003), and Dvořák and Haldeman (2004).

General Differential Diagnosis

Cervical syndromes produce many different kinds of symptoms and signs and their differential diagnosis is correspondingly broad. Any type of cervical discogenic syndrome must be distinguished from similar clinical pictures due to other kinds of disease. A cervical syndrome can only be confidently diagnosed when all other possibilities have been ruled out.

! Cervical syndromes should be diagnosed by exclusion.

The high prevalence of disk disease must not tempt the clinician to diagnose a cervical syndrome, and then immediately begin treating it, after a cursory clinical examination of a patient complaining of pain in the shoulder and neck. Massage, traction, and manual therapy may have decidedly negative consequences in patients who are actually suffering from a vertebral metastasis or spondylitis. On the other hand, the primary battery of diagnostic tests should be chosen so as to avoid unnecessary expense. Thus, it generally suffices to carry out a thorough clinical examination, including a neurological examination, supplemented by a basic laboratory profile and a plain radiograph series of the cervical spine. The sudden onset and positional dependence of the symptoms are highly suggestive evidence of a discogenic syndrome. The age of the patient is a further diagnostic criterion (cf. age-related prevalence curves, **Fig. 9.1**). Unexpected features of the following types should prompt **further testing:**

- insidious onset
- persistent pain independent of position
- advanced age
- elevated erythrocyte sedimentation rate (ESR)
- bone destruction in plain radiographs
- fever
- abnormalities in the complete blood count, with differential.

Unclear neurological findings can be further investigated with MRI, CT, cervical myelography, EMG, and evoked potentials.

Classification of Cervical Syndromes

"Cervical syndrome, " as we have seen, is a general term covering all cervical spine problems due to the degenerative process rather than to a tumor, infection, or developmental anomaly. If the symptoms are limited to the cervical spine, the disorder is called a *local cervical syndrome,* and the patient is said to be suffering from *neck pain* (just as the patient with a local lumbar syndrome suffers from *low back pain*). Neck pain, in turn, is subdivided into two kinds, simple and complex. Simple neck pain regresses rapidly, whereas complex neck pain carries a risk of becoming chronic (for the danger signs, see **Table 9.2**).

Simple neck pain is usually mechanically induced, e. g., by an unthinking, sudden movement, but can also arise spontaneously, e. g., after a draft of cold air on the nape of the neck. The pain is typically motion-dependent, moderately severe, and short-lasting, with spontaneous remission in 3–6 days. A longer duration is likelier if there are complicating psychosocial factors (a danger sign!), if the pain is severe enough to disturb sleep, or if it has already lasted longer than a week. Par-

9

Table 9.2 Classification of degenerative diseases of the cervical spine (cervical spine syndrome) (from Krämer in Wirth and Zichner 2004)

Neck pain (local cervical syndrome)		Neck and arm pain (cervicobrachial syndrome)		Neck pain and headache (cervicocephalic syndrome)	Danger signs (red flags)
Simple	Complicated	Simple	Complicated		
		Proximal radiation	Distal radiation	Headache	Cervical myelopathy
Mechanically induced	Additional psychosocial factors	Mechanically induced	Additional psychosocial factors	Dizziness	Gait disturbance
Movement-induced		Movement-induced	Paresis	Auditory and visual disturbances, dysphagia	Paralysis
Moderate distress	Impaired sleep	Moderate distress	Impaired sleep		History of trauma, tumor, infection
Short-lasting (< 6 days)	> 1 week	Short-lasting (< 6 days)			Constitutional symptoms (feeling ill)
Age 20–60	Age < 20 or > 60	Age 20–60			Weight loss Laboratory abnormalities

Table 9.3 Major symptoms of local cervical syndrome

- Position-dependent shoulder and neck pain
- Restricted range of motion of cervical spine
- Tension of neck and shoulder girdle musculature

ticular attention should be paid to recurrent neck pain in adolescents or elderly people.

Similar considerations apply to the cervicobrachial syndrome, i.e., to pain in the neck radiating into the shoulder and arm, no matter whether it is of radicular or pseudoradicular type. Here, too, simple neck and arm pain, with proximal radiation, moderate severity, and brief duration, can be contrasted with complicated neck and arm pain, which is usually in a radicular distribution, radiating as far down as the hand, and sometimes accompanied by weakness.

The term "cervicocephalic syndrome" encompasses all pains in the head and neck with origin in the cervical spine, with or without associated dizziness, visual or auditory dysfunction, or dysphagia. Head and neck pain often arises after an acceleration–deceleration injury of the cervical spine (see Chapter 17).

Dangerous varieties of head and neck pain include the pain of cervical myelopathy (often accompanied by gait disturbance and weakness) and pain due to a tumor, infection, or malformation (see the section on differential diagnosis, p. 93).

Local Cervical Syndrome

Etiology and Symptoms

! Definition: the term "local cervical syndrome" refers to any combination of clinical manifestations that is confined to the neck and is the direct or indirect result of degenerative and functional disturbances of the cervical motion segments.

These conditions are characterized exclusively by position-dependent shoulder and neck pain, muscle tension, and restricted movement of the cervical spine (**Table 9.3**).

The symptoms are caused by degenerative and post-traumatic changes of the cervical motion segments, which produce **mechanical irritation** of the posterior longitudinal ligament, the intervertebral joint capsules, and the vertebral periosteum. The sensory fibers of the meningeal and dorsal branches are predominantly affected. Local cervical syndrome can be either acute or chronic. Any symptoms that can be shown to originate in the intervertebral joint capsules (e. g., by injection of local anesthetic) are designated as **cervical facet syndrome,** which is analogous to its lumbar counterpart. Clinical studies indicate that the facet joint is the origin of a good percentage of lumbar and cervical spinal pain. Studies using diagnostic blocks suggest that the incidence of cervical facet pain is higher than that of lumbar facet pain (Cavanaugh, 2006).

Local cervical syndromes are the most common disk-related clinical conditions of the cervical spine. Precise epidemiological data are impossible to obtain, because most individuals with local cervical syndromes probably have only mild symptoms and therefore do not seek medical attention. Furthermore, the condition is often self-limiting and responds well to traditional household remedies such as heating pads, hot-water bottles, etc.

Among the more prominent symptoms of local cervical syndromes is painful **muscle tension in the shoulder and neck.** The muscles in these areas are supplied by the dorsal branches of the spinal nerves. A precise segmental localization of the etiology of the pain is not possible, because each muscle is supplied by the dorsal branches of more than one nerve (the pattern of innervation of the ventral branches is more highly segregated). The onset of symptoms may be acute, e. g., after abrupt turning of the head, or gradual without any particular precipitating factor. Patients often mention a cool draft as a possible cause; another common precipitant is prolonged sitting in a hunched position with a kyphotic posture of the neck, e. g. while typing, reading, or working at a desk. Pain in such situations is not only discogenic but also partly due to muscular insufficiency.

On examination, the patient can localize the pain fairly precisely. Pain due to involvement of the upper cervical segments is localized to the territory of the dorsal branches of the spinal nerves *on the upper border of the trapezius muscle*, which stretches from the occiput to the acromioclavicular joint.

> **!** Irritation of the lower cervical motion segments causes pain between the shoulder blades.

In the latter situation, there is tenderness of the rhomboids and of the levator scapulae and subscapularis muscles.

In addition to the typical localization of the pain, examination also reveals a greater or lesser degree of spasm of the entire musculature of the shoulder and neck, with resulting restriction of neck movement. The pain may radiate into the shoulder and the dorsolateral portion of the arm; because it does not extend into the forearm and does not follow a radicular pattern, it is called "pseudoradicular brachialgia." Discography with a disk-distension test (see p. 121) can often provoke pain of this type.

Occipital neuralgia is a special type of local cervical syndrome. This is a local process in the nuchal–occipital region involving irritation of the greater occipital nerve, which lies just below the skin at the level of the external occipital protuberance (inion) and is tender to palpation at this point. The tender tendinous insertions of the upper portions of the trapezius muscles are immediately adjacent.

Local cervical disk syndromes have a chronic, recurrent course. Symptom-free intervals lasting months or even years alternate with bouts of very severe symptoms. Patients are often aware of their own individual precipitating factors (cooling, maintained unfavorable postures) and do their best to avoid them.

Differential Diagnosis

Tumors and infections can, depending on their precise location and extent, produce symptoms resembling those of a local cervical syndrome. Primary tumors of the cervical spinal cord, such as neurinomas of the spinal nerve roots and spinal meningioma, are rare compared to **metastases** into the cervical spine. The common sources of metastases include tumors of the bronchi, breast, thyroid gland, and kidney. The presence of a tumor may be suggested by the insidious onset of symptoms, abnormal laboratory findings, evidence of bone destruction on plain radiographs, or a deterioration of the patient's general condition (weight loss). These patients are also usually elderly. Their further diagnostic evaluation includes tomographic imaging of the cervical spine, bone scan, further laboratory tests, and, most importantly, a search for the primary tumor.

Infection (**spondylitis**) reveals itself in an elevated CRP and ESR, as well as fever. The loss of disk height that accompanies discitis can be mistaken, at first, for intervertebral chondrosis. Rheumatoid arthritis, too, commonly affects the cervical intervertebral joints.

The differential diagnosis of local cervical syndromes, like that of all other spinal diseases, must include **ankylosing spondylitis** (Bekhterev disease) (respiratory excursion, Schober distance). When this disease is suspected, plain radiographs of the sacroiliac joints should be obtained, even if there is no pain in these joints.

Sternal syndrome, as described by Brügger (1971), consists of pain arising in the sternum and sternoclavicular joints and leading to painful reflex contraction of the musculature of the shoulder girdle and neck. Pain due to excessive mechanical stress on the sternum usually comes about after prolonged sitting in a hunched position so that the weight of the head and shoulder girdle is transmitted through the clavicles and ribs to the sternum. Another set of conditions that must be distinguished from local cervical syndromes consists of **tendinopathies** affecting the spinous and transverse processes. Here, examination reveals radiating pain that can be reproduced by local pressure and intensified by muscle contraction. The diagnosis can be confirmed by infiltration with local anesthetic.

9

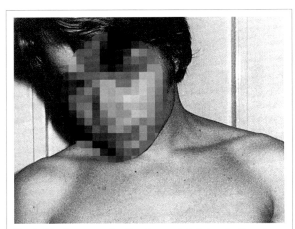

Fig. 9.17 Acute torticollis: the neck is laterally flexed, rotated, and markedly forward flexed.

Table 9.4 Typical clinical features of acute torticollis (wry neck)

- Sudden onset
- Fixed, abnormal posture
- Improvement with traction

Acute Torticollis (Wry Neck)

Etiology and Manifestations

 Acute torticollis is a variety of local cervical syndrome characterized by an abnormal posture and restricted mobility of the cervical spine.

It is most commonly seen in children and adolescents and is an *early variety of discogenic disease of the cervical spine.* Its causes are not completely understood.

This condition is evidently due to a specific biomechanical situation of the motion segment that mainly affects young people. At this age, anatomical studies reveal the presence of horizontal fissures and a very high mobility of the centrally located disk tissue, while the anulus fibrosus has already begun to lose some of its strength. Just as in acute lumbago, intradiscal tissue displacement causes irritation of the sensory fibers of the meningeal branch in the posterior longitudinal ligament. Myo- and arthrogenic symptoms arise secondarily. The skewed posture of the neck comes about as a

reflex; it places the intervertebral joint facets in an extreme position. The posture is maintained by lasting contraction of the muscles of the shoulder girdle and neck.

There seem to be no characteristic precipitating factors, though sometimes wry neck will arise in a child after rotatory movements of the cervical spine under stress, e. g., while playing (performing headstands, etc.). In other cases, acute torticollis is first noticed when the patient awakens in the morning, after sleeping with the head in an oblique position. Often, however, the history is noncontributory.

Inspection of the patient reveals a **grotesquely skewed posture of the head** (**Fig. 9.17**). Palpation reveals tension of the shoulder and neck musculature, more pronounced on one side. The abnormal posture of acute torticollis, like that of acute sciatica, is a protective reflex that prevents further intradiscal tissue displacement and reduces pressure on sensitive nerve fibers. Movements in any other direction, e. g., toward the neutral position or to the opposite side, are practically impossible. The cervical spine cannot be passively moved out of its abnormal posture except to a very limited extent and as a single, compact unit. There is hardly any pain, nor is there any neurologic deficit. Radiographs are often hard to interpret because of the abnormal posture, but in any case reveal no further abnormality.

The diagnosis is made in view of the sudden onset, fixed abnormal posture of the head, and improvement of symptoms on traction in the direction of the antalgic posture (see **Table 9.4**).

! Acute torticollis mainly affects children and adolescents and always takes a benign course.

The abnormal posture rapidly improves on treatment. In adults, the intradiscal tissue displacement may progress to a cervical disk protrusion, which is then associated with symptoms of radicular or spinal cord compression.

Differential Diagnosis

If there is any history of trauma, **bony injury** or **subluxation** of the cervical spine must be ruled out. This can be done with a series of plain radiographs of the cervical spine, including anteroposterior and lateral views and an open-mouth odontoid view. Tomographic views can be obtained in case of doubt.

Gradually developing, fixed, skewed postures of the head, as in wry neck of muscular, bony, or ocular origin, usually present no diagnostic difficulty. They are also associated with an asymmetry of the face. A suddenly arising skewed head posture may have a number of causes; the synonymous terms "wry neck" and "torticollis" merely refer to the chief manifestation, rather than to its etiology. **Spasmodic torticollis** is an extrapyramidal neurological disorder in which the abnormal posture is produced by tonic and clonic contractions of the sternocleidomastoid muscle and the deep muscles of the neck. So-called psychogenic torticollis often turns out, on detailed evaluation, to be discogenic. "Psychogenic" cases were diagnosed much more frequently in the past because their true cause was not recognized and objective findings were impossible to obtain.

Cervicobrachial Syndrome

> *!* The term "cervicobrachial syndrome" refers to a cervical syndrome with pain radiating into the upper limb.

Discogenic brachialgia is produced by lesions affecting the C5/6 and C6/7 motion segments. Cervicobrachial syndrome was, therefore, previously known as "lower cervical syndrome." It is characterized by pain and sensory disturbances that radiate from the cervical spine into the upper limb, in a more or less clear radicular pattern, i.e., in the distribution of the ventral branch of a spinal nerve. There may be both sensory disturbances in the cutaneous distribution of this branch (the dermatome) and motor disturbances in its muscular distribution (the myotome). Thus, one might alternatively designate cervicobrachial syndrome as "ventral branch syndrome." The patient simultaneously suffers from the symptoms of a local cervical syndrome.

The **topography** of the cervical dermatomes and myotomes is such that the myotome generally does not underlie the corresponding dermatome. Many of the muscles of the upper portion of the trunk are mainly supplied by the cervical nerve roots and are often affected in cervical syndromes. These muscles include the rhomboids, the supra- and infraspinatus muscles, and the deltoid, serratus anterior, and latissimus dorsi muscles. Patients often complain of pain between the scapulae; this is due to irritation of the dorsal branches of the lower cervical spinal nerves.

In our series of patients presenting with cervicobrachial syndromes for outpatient orthopedic treatment, 43% had objectifiable neurological abnormalities. Pain, sensory disturbances, or a motor deficit may be present, depending on which part of the ventral branch is most severely affected. In the initial phase, the main symptoms are usually neck pain and an abnormal posture of the neck.

> *!* The most common sensory abnormality is radiation of pain along a dermatome, sometimes accompanied by numbness or paresthesia within the dermatome.

Demonstrable hyperesthetic zones are found only in a minority of cases and only after persistent, massive nerve compression. It seems questionable whether discogenic nerve root irritation can really be the cause of dermatomal hypersensitivity to touch (hyperesthesia), but we have seen patients who complain of this.

> *!* Patients with cervicobrachial syndrome often also complain of a feeling of tension and swelling in the hand, without any corresponding objective findings.

Sometimes acrocyanosis and damp, cold hands indicate a concomitant disturbance of sympathetic function. A cervicobrachial syndrome can also limit the mobility of the shoulder; such cases should not be confused with subacromial syndrome.

Subacromial syndrome does appear to arise in many patients who also suffer from cervicobrachial syndrome, and the same is true of radial humeral epicondylitis. Yet there is no apparent causal connection between cervicobrachial syndrome and these two conditions, which are due to local degenerative changes in the rotator cuff and in the tendinous insertion of the extensor carpi radialis muscle.

The mechanism of cervicogenic shoulder stiffness is fundamentally different: the postural abnormality of cervical syndrome involves not only the neck, but also the shoulder girdle and shoulder joint. The shoulder is held somewhat higher on the affected side. The patient tries to move it as little as possible and holds the arm in an antalgic, adducted position. If a patient with chronic cervicobrachialgia does this for long enough, shoulder stiffness results (just as it does after prolonged wearing of a Desault bandage).

Muscle atrophy is rare in cervicobrachial syndrome, though it sometimes arises in the apparent absence of other symptoms. There is usually a history of pain radiating into the arm, at least at first.

> *!* Cervicobrachial syndrome can be caused either by a (soft) disk prolapse or by a (hard) bony constriction at the uncinate process.

These two different mechanisms produce distinct syndromes that differ in their manifestations and clinical course (**Table 9.5**). Their common feature is dermatomal cervicobrachialgia.

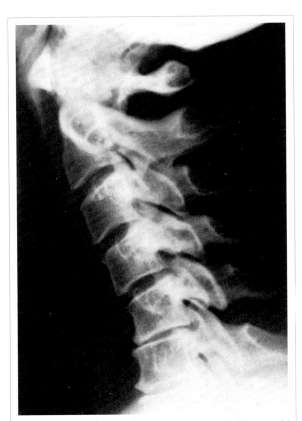

Fig. 9.18 Lateral cervical spine radiograph of a 34-year-old man 1 year after C5/6 disk prolapse. The disk space has collapsed to a narrow slit. The patient was treated conservatively and was free of symptoms thereafter, with a long follow-up. .

Brachialgia Due to Soft Disk Protrusion

Cervical disk protrusion or prolapse causing so-called "soft" nerve root compression is rare in comparison to lumbar disk protrusion or prolapse. Cervical disks protrude dorsolaterally and compress the nerve root, producing pain, postural abnormality, and neurological deficits. Protrusion represents displacement of disk tissue from the center of the disk toward the anulus fibrosus and then (under some circumstances) beyond it, perforating the boundary of the disk, resulting in *cervical disk prolapse.* Only in adolescents and young adults does the disk tissue possess the turgor pressure and the mobility (ability to be displaced) that are necessary for this to occur. Cervical disk protrusions and prolapses therefore occur most commonly between the ages of 30 and 45 and thus affect a much younger population of patients than compression syndromes due to uncovertebral osteophytes.

> **!** The symptoms begin acutely and consist of arm pain in a dermatome combined with a markedly abnormal posture of the head and a kyphotic posture of the cervical spine.

Motor disturbances and muscle atrophy arise only later. Coughing and sneezing worsen the pain. Plain radiographs reveal no abnormality beyond kyphosis of the cervical spine above the level of the abnormal disk (Güntz sign). Uncovertebral changes are usually absent, as the affected patients are mostly young. Follow-up radiographs obtained later may show collapse of the affected disk (**Fig. 9.18**).

Spondylosis and osteochondrosis at the affected level may not appear radiologically till years later, providing evidence of the end stage of the process that began with slackening of the intervertebral disk. Cervical disk prolapse can be seen directly by myelography, CT, and MRI. These studies should only be done, however, if a positive finding would be followed by surgical treatment.

Brachialgia Due to Uncinate Process Exostosis

Cervical nerve root symptoms due to osteophytic reactions on the uncinate processes are much more common than symptoms of disk protrusion or prolapse. These bony protuberances develop slowly and generally do not become large enough to impinge on nerve roots until the patient is at least 50 years old. As long as the nerves have enough room in the intervertebral foramina and the age-related fibrosis of the disks restricts excessive movement of the cervical spine, no symptoms will arise.

Table 9.5 Distinguishing clinical features of soft and hard cervical nerve root compression

	Cervicobrachialgia due to disk protrusion (soft compressive lesion)	Cervicobrachialgia due to uncovertebral osteophytes (hard compressive lesion)
Age	30–45	50–65
Onset	Sudden	Gradual
Leading symptom	Abnormal posture of neck	Brachialgia
Radiological findings	Loss of cervical lordosis due to muscle spasm	Uncovertebral osteophytes
Course	Acute	Chronic
Response to conservative treatment	Good	Poor

! Symptoms are usually produced by the combination of an uncovertebral osteophyte with local segmental slackening.

The treatment is designed accordingly. For symptomatic relief, it usually suffices to remove only one of these two factors.

The symptoms of cervicobrachial syndrome due to bony impingement on a nerve root arise gradually and generally consist of position-dependent arm pain in a dermatomal distribution. The abnormal neck posture and other signs of local cervical syndrome are not as marked as with "soft" protrusions. A typical complaint is pain at night combined with numbness and a pins-and-needles sensation (**brachialgia paresthetica nocturna**). Oblique plain radiographs demonstrate the bony spicules arising from the uncinate processes and projecting into the intervertebral foramina (**Fig. 9.14**). Though the clinical symptoms are related only to a single segment on one side, comparably severe uncovertebral changes are often found on both sides and at multiple levels. Thus, the presumption is that the symptoms have been precipitated by an additional factor of some kind, e. g., segmental slackening.

The direction of osteophyte growth is another determinant of the symptoms. *The nerve root can be compressed posterolaterally, but the vertebral artery can be compressed laterally* (cf. **Fig. 9.10**). In the former case, radicular symptoms (brachialgia) are produced; in the latter case, neurovascular symptoms (cervicocephalic syndrome, with circulatory insufficiency of the vertebral artery) (**Table 9.5**). Mixed syndromes with both types of symptoms are common.

Cervicobrachialgia due to uncovertebral osteophytes tends to recur chronically. Repeat attacks can be precipitated by external forces (acceleration–deceleration injury) or by prolonged maintenance of an unfavorable posture (working at a desk, watching television). Symptom-free intervals, often lasting months or years, alternate with periods of very intense pain.

! The symptoms only begin to diminish in intensity in old age, when the motion segments become increasingly immobile, despite the continued presence—or even the further enlargement—of the exostoses on the uncinate processes.

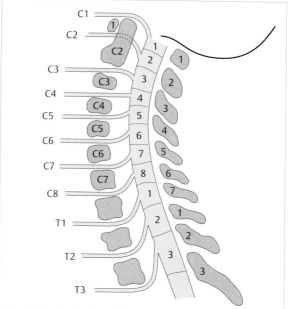

Fig. 9.19 Numbering of the cervical motion segments, spinal cord segments, and spinal nerve roots.

Segmental Syndromes

Anatomical Relationships and Determination of the Affected Segment

Anatomical relationships. The term "segment" can refer either to a motion segment (as we have been using it so far) or to the associated spinal nerve and its area of distribution. Each motion segment is named after the two vertebrae that encompass it, and each pair of spinal nerves is named after the spinal cord segment from which it is derived. There are seven cervical vertebrae and eight cervical spinal cord segments. Because of differential rates of growth during gestation and childhood, the motion segments and spinal cord segments are progressively more distant from each other as one proceeds down the spinal axis (**Fig. 9.19**). The difference is already evident at lower cervical levels: the lower cervical spinal cord segments lie one level higher than the correspondingly numbered spinous processes. The spinal nerve roots from the C4 level downward run caudolaterally to their site of exit from the spinal canal at the intervertebral foramen. Segmental syndromes are named after the affected nerve root; the number simultaneously designates the lower vertebral body of the affected motion segment. In C6 syndrome, for example, the C5/6 disk is involved; in C7 syndrome, the C6/7 disk. The C8 root passes through the C7/T1 intervertebral foramen.

9

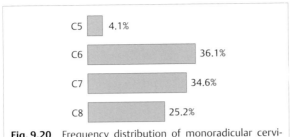

Fig. 9.20 Frequency distribution of monoradicular cervicobrachial syndrome.

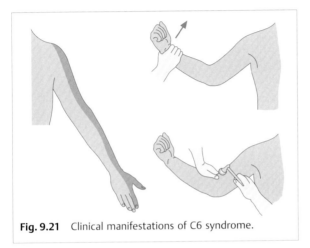

Fig. 9.21 Clinical manifestations of C6 syndrome.

! The syndromes of the lower cervical spinal nerve roots are the most clinically significant because of their high frequency.

Precise **localization of the affected segment** is important both for dorsal root blockade and for surgery. In recent years, discography, the distension test, and the many operative procedures that have been carried out for cervical syndrome have given us empirical knowledge of the area supplied by each of the spinal nerve roots. Cervical nerve root irritation syndromes are usually monoradicular. Overlapping or mixed symptoms may be due to anatomical variants, i.e., spinal nerve root anastomoses, which may be intradural (Marzo and Simmons 1987, Nobuhiro et al. 2002), or to the simultaneous irritation of multiple roots. In our series (Brux 1994, Knepel 1997), 28.4% of cases of cervicobrachial syndrome were multiradicular or difficult to classify by segment because of mixed symptoms.

The frequency distribution of monoradicular syndromes is shown in **Fig. 9.20**. C6, C7, and C8 are most commonly affected. In outpatients, the level of the lesion is usually inferred on clinical grounds. Only in ex-

ceptional cases, when surgery is considered, should supplementary tests such as electromyography, CT, or MRI be done.

In the cervical nerve root irritation syndromes, pain radiates down the upper limb into the hand in a dermatomal distribution. The distributions of pain due to irritation of adjacent nerve roots overlap to some extent in the arm and forearm. No matter which root is irritated, there is a dorsolateral band of pain and paresthesia in the shoulder and arm. In the forearm, the painful area in C6 syndrome is more on the radial side and that of C8 syndrome more on the ulnar side, with C7 syndrome in between. The distribution of pain in the hand is more reliable.

Nerve root irritation syndromes of C3 (C2/3 disk) and C4 (C3/4 disk) are very rare, making up only a small minority of cervical root irritation syndromes. Irritation of either of these roots produces pain and paresthesia in the neck and the proximal portion of the shoulder. Involvement of the diaphragm points reliably to these two roots. There are no other characteristic symptoms or reflex deficits.

C5 Syndrome

This is relatively rare (4.1% of all cervical nerve root irritation syndromes) and generally does not have any characteristic symptoms that point to the diagnosis. As in C6 syndrome, there is pain in the lateral portion of the shoulder and halfway down the arm, as well as biceps weakness and hyporeflexia (**Table 9.6**). There is no pain or sensory disturbance in the hand. Because the pain is largely limited to the shoulder region, C5 syndrome can easily be confused with humeroscapular periarthropathy (subacromial syndrome; see the section on differential diagnosis, pp. 93 and 103).

C6 Syndrome

The greatest percentage (36.1%) of monoradicular cervicobrachial syndromes is due to lesions of the C5/6 intervertebral disk. The C6 dermatome extends down the radial side of the arm and forearm to the tip of the thumb. Part of the index finger may be included as well. The boundary of the dermatome is not as sharp as that of the territory of a peripheral nerve. The pain sometimes radiates forward into the thorax. There is weakness of the biceps and brachioradialis muscles, and the biceps reflex is diminished or absent (**Fig. 9.21**).

The C5/6 motion segment is the most common site of origin of a cervical syndrome. If the segmental origin of a cervical syndrome cannot be definitively determined from the clinical examination alone and surgical treatment (anterior cervical discectomy and fusion) is under consideration, any discography or distension test should be done first at C5/6. The C5/6 disk is easy to puncture via an anterior approach.

Table 9.6 Cervical nerve root irritation syndromes

Nerve root	Disk	Peripheral dermatome	Indicator muscle	Reflex weakness
C5	C4/5		Deltoid	Biceps
C6	C5/6	Thumb, part of index finger	Biceps Brachioradialis	Biceps Radial periosteal reflex
C7	C6/7	Index and middle fingers, part of ring finger	Thenar muscles Triceps	Triceps
C8	C7/T1	Little finger, part of ring finger	Hypothenar muscles Finger flexors Interossei	(Triceps)

C7 Syndrome

This is the second most common type, accounting for 34.6 % of cervical syndromes. The C7 dermatome begins in the common dorsolateral pain field of the shoulder and forearm and proceeds down the midportion of the extensor surface of the forearm to the second, third, and (partially) fourth fingers. Pain and paresthesia are felt on the volar side of these fingers.

The C7 myotome includes the triceps brachii muscle, the pronator teres muscle, and the thenar muscles, i. e., the abductor pollicis brevis, opponens pollicis, and flexor pollicis brevis. Active extension of the elbow is weaker than normal, and the triceps reflex is weak or absent (**Fig. 9.22**). There may be marked atrophy of the thenar muscles, sometimes as the sole residual manifestation.

Mumenthaler et al. (1998) and Lang (1991) confirmed that the thenar muscles are innervated by the C7 root. C8 quadriplegics have intact thenar muscles while all of the remaining intrinsic muscles of the hand are atrophic; in C7 quadriplegics, the thenar muscles are atrophic as well.

Note that the region of the thumb is included in both the C6 *dermatome* and the C7 *myotome*.

C8 Syndrome

In C8 syndrome, which accounts for 25.2 % of cervical monoradicular syndrome, pain and paresthesia are felt in the fourth and fifth fingers. The painful and paresthetic areas of the arm and forearm overlap with those of the C7 syndrome.

There is weakness of the finger flexors, the interossei, and, above all, the hypothenar muscles (**Fig. 9.23**). In C8 syndrome, the affected dermatome and the motor weakness are located on the same side of the hand. The hypothenar atrophy is not as severe as the thenar atrophy of C7 syndrome. Diminution of the triceps reflex is not as common or as severe as in C7 syndrome.

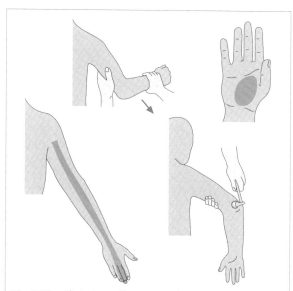

Fig. 9.22 Clinical manifestations of C7 syndrome.

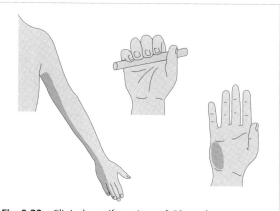

Fig. 9.23 Clinical manifestations of C8 syndrome.

Differential Diagnosis

Pain and neurologic deficits similar to those of cervicobrachial syndrome can also be caused by other diseases, such as the compression syndromes of the brachial plexus and the peripheral nerves of the upper limb. Disk-related nerve root irritation syndromes are usually very painful, but peripheral nerve lesions often cause slowly progressive neurologic deficits without much pain. **Sweating** is generally preserved in cervicobrachial syndrome but locally impaired in peripheral nerve lesions. In doubtful cases, special studies such as EMG and neurography can be helpful.

The brachial plexus and subclavian artery can be compressed in the scalene hiatus by an anomaly of the scalene muscles or by a cervical rib (**scalene syndrome**). The neurovascular bundle can also be compressed between the clavicle and the first rib (**costoclavicular syndrome**). In such cases, the patient suffers from pain on the ulnar side of the forearm and hand, and there is a position-dependent impairment of circulation to the arm. The longer the compression lasts, the more severe the neurologic deficit (lower brachial plexus palsy with weakness of the intrinsic hand muscles). Mumenthaler et al. (1998) state that this diagnosis is made much too often; it should not be made in the absence of objective findings. One such is a positive Adson test: the patient inspires deeply, leans the head back, and rotates it to the affected side. If the radial pulse disappears, this is evidence of a relatively narrow scalene hiatus. The examiner may also be able to hear a bruit by auscultation of the subclavian artery with the arm and head in various positions. The symptoms of costoclavicular syndrome worsen when the examiner presses down on the shoulders of a patient who is standing upright.

In **carpal tunnel syndrome,** the peripheral portion of the median nerve is compressed in the carpal tunnel under the flexor retinaculum (transverse carpal ligament). The causes include rheumatoid arthritis, other kinds of joint disease, or metabolic disorders causing narrowing of the carpal tunnel. The typical symptoms consist of pain, paresthesia, and swelling, which vary depending on the position of the wrist joint. The sensation on the first three digits and the radial half of the fourth digit is typically deficient. EMG reveals slowed conduction across the carpal tunnel. The pain often occupies a much wider area than the distribution of the median nerve itself and is felt not only at the site of compression, but also proximal to it. As carpal tunnel syndrome progresses, it leads to weakness of thumb abduction and atrophy of the lateral thenar musculature (abductor pollicis brevis). The symptoms can be temporarily relieved by injection of a mixture of cortisone and a local anesthetic into the carpal tunnel; relief simultaneously confirms the diagnosis, as cervicogenic pain in the hand cannot be alleviated in this way.

Other peripheral nerve lesions, e. g., *ulnar nerve compression* (cubital tunnel syndrome), can be differentiated from cervical radicular syndromes in analogous fashion.

Because cervical syndromes cause pain in the shoulder as well as in the neck, their differential diagnosis must also include **primary disorders of the shoulder,** above all the regressive changes in the subacromial juxta-articular region that produce the symptoms of subacromial syndrome. Complaints due to lesions of the supra- and infraspinatus tendons are called supra- or infraspinatus syndrome, or (more generally) subacromial syndrome. The major manifestations of cervical syndrome and humeroscapular periarthropathy are compared in **Table 9.7.** As already mentioned, humeroscapular periarthropathy can arise in a patient already suffering from a cervical syndrome and then develop independently to the point where it becomes the patient's major problem. In such cases, restricted mobility of the cervical spine, tension of the nuchal muscles, and stiffness of the shoulder are present simultaneously and must be treated in parallel.

Pancoast syndrome consists of a combination of pain and paresthesia in the upper limb with Horner syndrome and a deficiency of sweating on the upper quarter of the trunk on the same side. The cause is usually an apical lung tumor impinging on the medial cord of the brachial plexus, which passes closest to the apical pleura. The distribution of pain can easily cause confusion with a C7 or C8 syndrome.

Herpes zoster can, rarely, break out in a cervical segment, producing severe cervicobrachialgia. It often remains unrecognized and is treated as if it were a cervical disk syndrome until the typical cutaneous vesicles appear. Generally speaking, the history, physical examination, and laboratory findings ought to suffice for the diagnosis of herpes zoster radiculitis or *Borrelia* radiculitis (resulting from a tick bite).

Insertion tendopathies of the upper limb, such as radial or ulnar humeral epicondylitis, radial or ulnar styloiditis, etc., can be recognized by the characteristic local tenderness. Pain can also be induced by contraction of the muscles inserting onto the involved bone: for example, in lateral humeral epicondylitis, dorsiflexion of the wrist against resistance exacerbates the pain. The diagnosis can be confirmed by trial injection of local anesthetic.

Intractable segmental symptoms can also be produced by a **nerve root neurinoma.** This rare benign tumor widens the intervertebral foramen and has a typical hourglass or dumb-bell shape.

Cervicocephalic Syndrome

> **❗ Definition:** a cervicocephalic syndrome is a cervical syndrome associated with headache, dizziness, or (less commonly) visual or auditory disturbances or dysphagia.

Synonyms: Cervicogenic headache, head and neck pain.

History

Barré (1926) described a syndrome consisting of dizziness and auditory disturbances, which he attributed to irritation of the posterior cervical sympathetic chain by cervical spine pathology. He named it "le syndrome sympathique cervical postérieur." Bärtschi-Rochaix, in his monograph *Migraine cervicale* (1949), emphasized the importance of the uncinate processes in the pathogenesis of headache and dizziness. Kuhlendahl (1953) found the term "cervical migraine" potentially misleading and introduced the term "cervicocephalic syndrome" instead. He also pointed out the pathophysiologic significance of the vertebral artery.

More information on cervicogenic headache can be found in the articles by Clark et al. (2005), Hesselbarth (2005), Hülse (2005), and Hugger et al. (2006).

Etiology and Pathogenesis

Cervicocephalic syndrome is caused by impingement on the vertebral artery and the sympathetic chain in the region of the cervical spine. Contributory factors include abnormal positions of the joints at the craniocervical junction, deviations of the cervical spinal axis, apposition of neighboring vertebrae onto one another because of loss of disk height, and narrowing of the canal for the vertebral artery by lateral exostoses on the uncinate processes of C4–C7 (**Fig. 9.24**). Usually, more than one of these factors is at work.

The close topographic relationship of the vertebral artery, the cervical sympathetic chain, and the uncovertebral region has already been described.

> **❗** Structural and functional abnormalities in this critical area of the cervical motion segment produce not only local and segmental neurological deficits, but also cerebral dysfunction.

Thus, patients may suffer not just from the symptoms of a local cervical syndrome, but also from cerebrovascular and autonomic disturbances. Cervicocephalic syndromes can be further classified by their major manifestations—episodic headache (cervical migraine), dysphagia (pharyngoesophageal cervical syndrome), episodic dizziness, scintillating scotomata, or tinnitus, to name a few. The common feature of all cervicocephalic

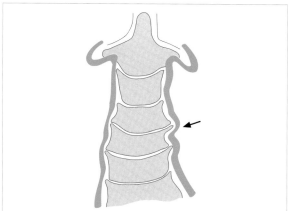

Fig. 9.24 Laterally projecting exostoses of the uncinate processes impinging on the vertebral artery.

Table 9.7 Differential diagnosis of cervical syndrome and subacromial syndrome

Cervical syndrome	Subacromial syndrome
1 Leading symptom: neurogenic pain. Pain along the dermatome in the neck, shoulder, and arm. Rest pain that barely increases with exertion. Reduced pain on cervical spine traction (Glisson test.)	1 Leading symptom: isolated shoulder pain. Only mild pain at rest. Free movements lead to severe pain limited to the shoulder joint and upper arm. Radiation into the hand is rare.
2 Leading symptom: attacks of pain at night, interfering with sleep.	2 Pain intensity independent of time of day. Pain at night only when the patient lies on the affected shoulder.
3 Leading symptom: peripheral segmental neurologic deficits (hypo- and paresthesia, diminished tendon reflexes).	3 No neurological deficit.
4 Possible severe limitation of passive and active mobility of the shoulder.	4 Leading symptom: abduction phenomenon. Most painful: abduction and internal rotation. Much less pain on abduction and external rotation. Passive mobility greater than active. Positive impingement signs.
5 Pressure tenderness of the corresponding spinous process and of the nuchal musculature on the involved side (myogelosis).	5 Pressure tenderness in the shoulder region (greater or lesser tubercle, intertubercular groove, middle of the deltoid muscle).
6 Not uncommonly, accompanying emotional and neurovegetative lability.	6 No emotional or neurovegetative abnormality.

9

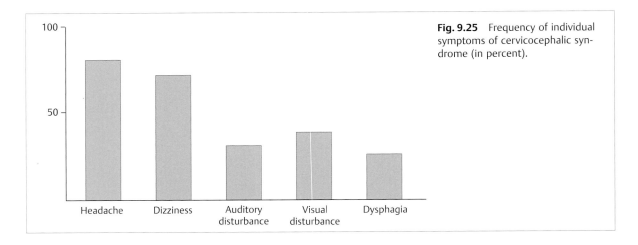

Fig. 9.25 Frequency of individual symptoms of cervicocephalic syndrome (in percent).

Table 9.8 Typical features of cervicogenic headache
■ Unilateral, or worse on one side
■ Positional dependence
■ Episodic, brief
■ Simultaneous symptoms of local cervical syndrome

syndromes is the positional dependence of the symptoms.

Blood flow in the vertebral artery varies depending on the position of the head even in the normal situation. For example, leaning back and turning the head to one side markedly reduces flow. When the bony canal for the vertebral artery is already narrowed by exostoses, such movements may cause temporary ischemia. Our own measurements of blood flow have revealed that perfusion in the vertebral artery is optimal when the cervical spine is mildly flexed (see p. 82).

Clinical Manifestations

The symptoms of cervicocephalic syndrome are listed by frequency in **Fig. 9.25**.

Some of the patients we have seen with cervicocephalic syndrome were referred to us after first presenting to other types of specialists (internists, ENT, ophthalmologists). All had more or less severe symptoms of a local cervical syndrome or cervicobrachialgia. Usually what pointed to the cervical origin of the cephalic manifestations was a restricted range of motion of the cervical spine, or a response of symptoms to orthopedic treatment (traction, cervical collar). The diagnosis of cervicocephalic syndrome was only assigned when all other causes had been excluded and after con-

firmation by sufficient follow-up. In accordance with the observations of Jung et al. (1974), Terrache (1984), and Evers and Schilgen (2006), our patients suffered mainly from headache and dizziness, but a few also complained of auditory and visual difficulties and dysphagia on close questioning.

The Cervicogenic Headache Study Group established the following criteria for the diagnosis of cervicogenic headache (Hesselbarth 2005):
- provocation of typical headaches by head movement
- maintenance of antalgic head posture
- marked partial relief, or total relief, of pain by diagnostic blockade.

Headache

In the International Headache Society classification, cervicogenic headache is category 11.2.1: "Headache associated with disorder of the cervical spine" (Greiner-Pert 1999). It occurs episodically and can be precipitated or worsened by certain positions of the head. It comes in a number of different clinical varieties (**Table 9.8**). It may be a migraine-like, hemicranial headache radiating into the forehead, for example, or a bilateral, neuralgiform nucho-occipital pain that is worse on one side. Some patients with cervicogenic headache also suffer from dizziness, subjective visual disturbances, and/or vestibular disturbances, which are sometimes objectifiable.

 Certain head movements can precipitate or worsen cervicogenic headaches; others can stop them.

For this reason, manual medicine often plays a prominent role in their treatment.

The diagnosis is confirmed, after other possible causes of headache have been ruled out, by improvement in response to treatment with a cervical collar and paravertebral blockades.

"School headache" (Gutmann and Biedermann 1984) is a special variety of cervicogenic headache that is induced by marked anteflexion of the head, due to fatigue, in the late hours of the school day. Its cause is thought to lie in an insufficiency of the transverse atlantal ligament.

Episodic Dizziness

Etiology. In cervicocephalic syndrome, dizziness and loss of balance can also be provoked by certain positions of the head: rotation of the head induces rotatory vertigo that usually lasts only a few seconds, or at most minutes. In some cases, dizziness is induced only by rotation to one side; frequently, it can be induced by hyperextension as well. Other patients report dizziness with any sudden movement of the head, particularly when rapidly looking upward. Fainting and prolonged loss of consciousness do not occur (**Table 9.9**). Cervicogenic dizziness may also arise from the proprioceptors of the joints of the craniocervical junction (Hülse 1983, 2005, Tilscher 1983, Terrache 1984).

The most important **diagnostic technique** for the evaluation of cervicogenic dysequilibrium is the investigation of cervical nystagmus (Boenninghaus 1984, Hülse 2005). This term refers to nystagmus that arises when the head is held in a fixed position, so that the labyrinths cannot be stimulated, while the body and neck are turned beneath it. The test is done in a dark room. The examiner holds the patient's head with both hands while an assistant rotates the patient's chair 60° in either direction, producing a pure rotation of the cervical spine without any movement of the head. The headache and dysequilibrium produced by this maneuver may either be mediated by the joint proprioceptors of the cervicocephalic junction, or they may be due to vertebral artery insufficiency. The *proprioceptive* cervical nystagmus seen in the former case arises immediately; the *vascular* cervical nystagmus seen in the latter case may arise after a delay of up to 50 s (Hülse 1983, 2005).

Auditory and Visual Disturbances and Dysphagia

Nearly one-third of all patients with cervicocephalic syndrome complain of **tinnitus**, which is episodic, low-pitched, and always unilateral. Most also suffer from hearing loss. There may also be **pain in the ear** (cervicogenic otalgia) due to neuralgia of the lesser occipital and great auricular nerves, which arise from the C2 and C3 roots and supply the skin and soft tissues around the ear. The characteristic feature of all of these symptoms is their positional dependence.

Table 9.9 Typical features of cervicogenic vertigo

- Induced by hyperextension and rotation of the cervical spine
- Brief duration
- Little or no objective correlate
- Simultaneous symptoms of local cervical syndrome

> **!** Cervicogenic tinnitus, hearing loss, and otalgia are precipitated or exacerbated by certain positions of the head. This is not true of auditory disturbances with other causes.

Cervicocephalic pain can also cause true **visual disturbances** in addition to the cervicogenic headaches that may radiate into the orbit. The most common types are short-lasting scintillating scotomata, blurred vision, and visual impairment during episodes of dizziness (seeing black). Cervicocephalic syndrome does not cause serious or lasting impairment of vision. The visual disturbances resolve once the cervicocephalic syndrome is successfully treated.

Degenerative changes of the cervical spine may cause **dysphagia** in various ways. Large spondylotic exostoses on the anterior surfaces of the cervical vertebrae may mechanically compress the esophagus (this can be demonstrated with a barium swallow, lateral view). Dysphagia after ventral fusion or cervical spine injury is also of mechanical origin. Traumatic dysphagia resolves spontaneously with resorption of the hematoma and regression of periesophageal edema.

Dysphagia can also be neurogenic. Patients complain of difficulty swallowing, a globus sensation, and abnormal sensations in the pharynx. This type of condition is due to mechanical impingement on the cervical sympathetic chain and the vertebral artery. The superior cervical sympathetic ganglion is connected, by way of the jugular nerve, to the inferior ganglion of the glossopharyngeal nerve, and by way of dorsal branches to the hypoglossal nerve.

Course. Cervicocephalic syndromes have the same course as local or brachial cervical syndromes: phases of very severe symptoms alternate with relatively or totally asymptomatic intervals. Progressive fibrosis and immobilization of the motion segments with advancing age limits the mobility of the cervical spine and renders impossible the movements of the head that induce the symptoms. The prognosis is, therefore, benign.

9

Table 9.10 Differential diagnosis of migraine vs. cervicocephalic syndrome

Migraine	Cervicocephalic syndrome ("cervical migraine")
Attacks begin spontaneously	Induced by specific positions of the head
Independent of position	Can be influenced by change of position
Each attack lasts for hours	Brief attacks (positionally dependent)
Nausea, vomiting	No vomiting
Full mobility of cervical spine	Restricted mobility of cervical spine, tension of nuchal musculature
Improvement with triptanes	Improvement with traction, soft collar

Table 9.11 Differential diagnosis of Ménière disease vs. Ménière-like symptoms of cervicocephalic syndrome

Ménière disease	Dizziness, auditory disturbances, and nystagmus in cervicocephalic syndrome
Attacks begin spontaneously	Induced by specific positions of the head
Independent of position	Can be influenced by change of position
Each attack lasts for hours	Brief attacks (positionally dependent)
Vomiting	No vomiting
Full mobility of cervical spine	Restricted mobility of cervical spine, tension of nuchal musculature
Improvement on infusion of 20% glucose solution and dehydration	Improvement with traction, soft collar

Differential Diagnosis of Cervicocephalic Syndrome

Differential diagnosis is important because headache, vertigo, auditory and visual impairment, and dysphagia are less commonly caused by cervical spine pathology than by other diseases. Most patients do not consult an orthopedist first, but rather the specialist responsible for the part of the body where the symptoms are felt.

Many diseases cause **headache**. The common causes of headache, such as *hypertension, metabolic disease,* and *visual disturbances,* should first be ruled out with simple diagnostic techniques.

! True migraine differs from cervicocephalic headache in the long duration of each attack (hours) as well as the typical accompanying symptoms—long-lasting scintillating scotoma, nausea, vomiting, and photophobia.

Cervicocephalic headaches, like migraine, are episodic and largely confined to one side of the head. The clinical features of each of these two types of headache are listed and compared in **Table 9.10**. A definitive diagnosis may be difficult when the symptoms and their course have been obscured by treatment. Patients with cervicocephalic headache, for example, can also suffer from nausea and vomiting with their headaches as a side effect of potent analgesics. Furthermore, disk-related symptoms are so common that a patient with true migraine may well have a cervical syndrome in addition. Observation over a longer period usually enables the correct diagnosis.

In general practice, **dizziness** is usually of circulatory origin. Patients complain of vertigo, light-headedness, seeing black, and spots before the eyes. They do not avoid certain positions of the head, as patients with cervicogenic dizziness typically do.

Any complaint of dizziness and dysequilibrium should prompt the suspicion of Ménière disease. In fact, orthopedists and ENT specialists often have the opportunity to collaborate in establishing this common diagnosis. The symptoms of Ménière disease include dizziness, vomiting, objectively demonstrable nystagmus, sensorineural hearing loss, and tinnitus. They appear episodically, suddenly and without any evident external precipitating factor. The proposed pathogenetic mechanisms include angioneurotic spasm of the labyrinthine arteries and elevated pressure in the inner ear.

Ménière-like symptoms are common in cervicocephalic syndrome, and indeed any symptom of Ménière disease may occur in a patient with cervicocephalic syndrome. The major distinguishing features of these two conditions concern the onset and course of the symptoms and their responsiveness to specific treatments (see **Table 9.11**). Axial traction or a Schanz bandage is effective in cervicocephalic syndrome, but not in Ménière disease, where an infusion of a hypertonic solution, or dehydration, can bring relief.

! Cervicogenic vestibular disturbances differ from those of other causes in that nystagmus can be provoked or worsened by movements of the cervical spine in certain directions (mainly reclination).

Deliberately provoked cervicogenic nystagmus often appears only after a delay of 10 s or more from the inducing movement. The major clinical distinguishing features of **cerebellopontine angle tumors** as a cause of dizziness include continuous dizziness of unvarying severity, continuous tinnitus, and cerebellar dysfunction of a type not seen in cervicocephalic syndrome.

In the differential diagnosis of **auditory and visual disturbances and dysphagia** it is particularly important to rule out organ-specific disease by consulting the appropriate medical specialists before initiating treatment for cervicocephalic syndrome.

Any hearing impairment produced by cervicocephalic syndrome is exclusively of the sensorineural type. Bilateral, symmetrical, high-tone hearing loss is probably not at all rare as a cervicogenic phenomenon, but a cervical cause can only be confidently diagnosed if the hearing loss is unilateral or markedly greater on one side. The sudden onset and fluctuating severity of hearing loss also suggest a cervicogenic process. In general, symptoms relating to the ears, nose, throat, and eyes are only rarely cervicogenic. Important differential diagnostic evidence for a cervical cause comes from the positional dependence of the symptoms and from their response to certain treatment measures, such as the application of a cervical collar or gentle connective tissue massage. These measures can be done diagnostically as well as therapeutically, as they are harmless if the symptoms are due to another cause.

Cervicomedullary Syndrome

! **Definition:** The term "cervicomedullary syndrome" refers to spinal cord manifestations caused by degenerative changes of the cervical spine.

Synonyms: Cervical myelopathy, cervical spondylotic (or spondylogenic) myelopathy.

Etiology and Pathogenesis

Spinal cord compression due to degenerative changes of the cervical spine usually occurs in the lower cervical motion segments. This is explained by two pathogenetic factors:
- Massive, space-occupying spondylotic exostoses and osteophytic reactions from the uncinate processes are more commonly found in the middle and lower regions of the cervical spine.
- The epidural space in the lower portion of the cervical spine is relatively narrow and contains little epidural fat.

Just as in the lumbar spine, stable, asymptomatic cervical spinal stenosis may decompensate and become symptomatic because of
- a new, additional disk protrusion
- activation of intervertebral joint arthrosis
- aseptic inflammatory changes of the soft tissues in the vicinity of the uncovertebral joints, or
- trauma.

Only a small number of systemic diseases are known to promote the development of cervical myelopathy: spondyloepiphyseal dysplasia, mucopolysaccharidosis, and ochronosis (Ohwada 1996).

Clinical Manifestations

Symptoms of spinal cord compression due to acute cervical disk prolapse tend to arise fairly suddenly. There is often a history of cervical spine trauma. In contrast, cervical spondylotic myelopathy generally has an insidious onset and course, dominated not by pain but by functional disturbances. Numbness and paresthesiae of the upper and lower limbs and gait disturbances are early signs of the disease. Physical examination may reveal pathological reflexes (involvement of the pyramidal pathway) or a dissociated sensory deficit (central cord involvement). Spastic hemi- or paraparesis may also occur. As the disorder becomes chronic, gait ataxia develops (Hohmann et al. 1985, Kretschmer 1989, Rubenthaler 2004, Houten and Errico 2005). Ohwada (1996) classified cervical myelopathy into the following clinical types:
- spastic quadriparesis with manifestations in upper and lower limbs
- spastic paraparesis due to compression above C6
- spastic quadriparesis with deltoid weakness
- atrophic form of myelopathic hand with long tract signs
- central cord syndrome in a patient with cervical spondylosis and history of trauma.

Any clinical suspicion of cervical myelopathy should prompt a comprehensive neurological examination, including neurophysiological testing, in order to determine the cause conclusively and enable a better assessment of the prognosis (Rubenthaler 2004).

Imaging studies. Plain radiographs of the cervical spine can rule out destructive masses impinging on the cervical spinal cord, but MRI is much more informative. Myelography used to be commonly done, but MRI has made it largely unnecessary (**Fig. 9.26**).

It is worth repeating the observation of multiple authors that local cervical syndromes, cervicobrachial syndromes, and cervicocephalic syndromes rarely progress to cervical myelopathy (Ohwada 1996, Matsumoto et al. 2001, Houten and Errico 2005, Zeidmann 2005).

Treatment

Simple cases of cervical myelopathy without progressive neurologic dysfunction can often be treated conservatively, particularly when the decompensation has been caused by a disk protrusion or by an inflammatory irritation and swelling of the soft tissue of the uncinate process or the intervertebral joint capsule. Local and

9

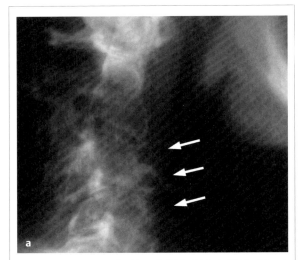

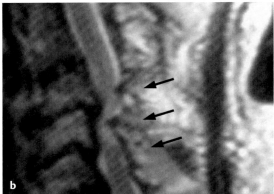

Fig. 9.26 a, b   The plain radiograph (**a**) shows marked degenerative changes of the entire cervical spine. The MRI (**b**) reveals mid-cervical spinal stenosis causing spinal cord compression (from Rubentaler et al. in Wirth and Zichner 2004).

systemic anti-inflammatory medication and resting of the affected motion segment with appropriate behavioral changes can stabilize the neurological findings or even enable them to regress. These treatment measures include neurophysiologically designed patient exercises, analgesics, physiotherapy, temporary wearing of a hard collar, and local infiltrations with local anesthetics and anti-inflammatories.

The patient should be closely monitored for progressive spinal cord damage due to persistent compression and should be referred promptly for surgical decompression if necessary (Dvořák et al. 1990). Decompressive surgery is the only way to prevent progressive spinal cord damage. The approach is either ventral (by discectomy, removal of spondylotic osteophytes, and fusion or disk replacement) or dorsal (extended laminectomy). The indications for operative

decompression of degenerative cervical spinal canal stenosis are solely clinical and should not be based on the radiological findings, even if these are very impressive.

Post-traumatic Cervical Syndrome

> **!** **Definition:** Post-traumatic cervical syndrome arises after injuries of the cervical spine.

"Injury," in this context, means damage restricted to soft tissue, due to a physically distorting traumatic event. The commonly used term in English-speaking countries is "soft-tissue neck injury." As has been pointed out (Moorahrend 1993), this term should be used only for noncontact injuries, i.e., those in which there has not been a blow to the head. Post-traumatic cervical syndrome differs from other degenerative disk-related conditions of the cervical spine only in its mode of onset and its course. The symptoms and treatment are the same.

Etiology and Pathogenesis

The position of the cervical spine between the head and the trunk exposes it to injury. If one of these two masses is accelerated or decelerated while the other remains stationary, the soft tissues of the cervical spine—including the disks—are exposed to strong forces of traction and compression (**Figs. 9.27, 9.28**). As long as the disks and ligaments that link the cervical vertebrae are still in their original, nondegenerated condition, their elasticity enables them to withstand even very large forces of these types. Common violent maneuvers, e.g., forceps delivery or a punch to the head in boxing, are well tolerated without injury. The most common type of post-traumatic cervical syndrome is acceleration–deceleration injury of the cervical spine, so-called "whiplash" (see Chapter 17).

The biomechanical situation of the cervical spine results in a particular pattern of distribution of cervical spine injuries. The C4/5, C5/6, and C6/7 segments are the most commonly injured. These are also the segments that exhibit the most marked degenerative changes. Thus, there appears to be a connection between pre-existing degenerative changes and the severity of traumatic injury. Head-turned rear impact causes significantly greater injury at C0–C1 and C5–C6, as compared to head-forward rear and frontal impacts, and results in multiplanar injuries at C5–C6 and C7–T1 (Panjabi 2006).

Where there is pre-existing monosegmental spondylosis and osteochondrosis, an applied traumatic force can cause tearing in that particular segment, with rupture of the spondylotic bridge. In our anatomical dissec-

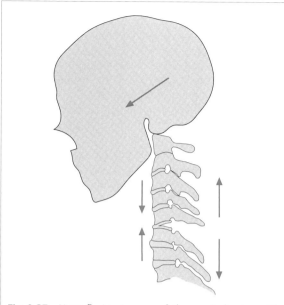

Fig. 9.27 Hyperflexion trauma of the cervical spine with ventral compression and dorsal distraction of the middle and lower cervical motion segments.

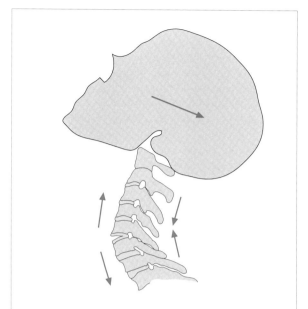

Fig. 9.28 Hyperextension trauma of the cervical spine with ventral distraction and dorsal compression of the middle and lower cervical motion segments.

tions of the cervical spine, we have repeatedly seen degenerated intervertebral disks that were still held together almost entirely by the outermost part of the anulus fibrosus and the longitudinal ligaments. The central portion of a degenerated disk is friable and, unlike that of a healthy young disk, can easily be grasped with forceps, displaced, and removed from its surroundings.

A cervical spine sprain or contusion, with ensuing cervical syndrome, can occur in many ways. Commonly, these problems arise during play or sporting activities, ejection of a pilot from an aircraft, diving head-first into a swimming pool, etc. Improper "therapeutic" manipulation of the cervical spine with hyperrotation is another cause of cervical spine sprain and can produce a post-traumatic cervical syndrome.

Clinical Features

Cervical syndrome due to cervical spine trauma takes a typical course. There is characteristically a symptom-free interval between the injury and the appearance of the first symptoms. In a simple sprain injury, these consist of nuchal and occipital pain and painful limitation of movement of the cervical spine—i.e., a **post-traumatic local cervical syndrome.** Unlike the usual types of cervical syndrome, post-traumatic cervical syndrome is associated with a worsening of symptoms in the first 2–3 days after their onset, similarly to other types of sprain injury, e.g., in the limbs. The intensity of the applied traumatic forces and the extent of the pre-existing degenerative changes will together determine whether

other components of the motion segment, or neighboring organs, will be affected as well. Depending on which structures are involved, the symptom complex that develops can be predominantly either cervicobrachial or cervicocephalic. Cervicomedullary syndromes with spinal cord compression can also occur.

Arm pain, i.e., a **post-traumatic cervicobrachial syndrome,** can be produced by nerve root irritation in the uncovertebral region due to a change in the relative positions of the spinal nerve and the degeneratively enlarged uncinate process. It can also be produced by direct pulling on the root, which is relatively immobile within the intervertebral foramen.

A **post-traumatic cervicocephalic syndrome** may present, for example, with intractable occipital pain of neuralgiform type. Unilateral or asymmetric nuchal and occipital pain may persist for several months (rarely more than 6 months). This type of traumatic syndrome is clinically no different from a purely degenerative cervicocephalic syndrome. The symptoms slowly resolve as the traumatically loosened motion segment gradually loses its mobility. Permanent damage is not expected unless the motion segment has been very severely injured.

Severe, traumatically induced kinking of the cervical spine can impinge on the spinal cord and cause a post-traumatic cervicomedullary syndrome. A central cord lesion is produced during retroflexion of the head by a pincer mechanism, in which the spinal cord is compressed between the lamina and ligamentum flavum dorsally and the vertebral body ventrally. The medullary injury is mainly ventral, i. e., it affects mainly the anterior horn cells and the more medial part of the corticospinal pathway. It follows that the clinical findings generally include flaccid paresis in the upper limbs with relative sparing of the lower limbs. Patients commonly complain of burning radicular pain in the C7 and C8 dermatomes. This is attributable to damage of the posterior horns and of the lateral portion of the posterior columns.

Differential diagnosis

Nuchal and occipital pain after an accident may also be due to a **brain concussion.** A concussion is not associated with any limitation of movement of the cervical spine or with tension of the shoulder and neck muscles, and the symptoms (pain) arise immediately, rather than after a delay. On the other hand, pure cervical spine injury does not cause loss of consciousness, vomiting, or retrograde amnesia. When the applied traumatic force is severe, the patient may suffer from a combination of brain concussion and cervical spine injury. The symptoms of the concussion are more prominent at first. Once these recede and the patient is mobilized, pain in the shoulder and neck develops, with limitation of movement of the cervical spine.

Post-traumatic brachialgia has the same differential diagnosis as cervicobrachial syndrome. Direct **injury to the shoulder and/or upper limb** should also be ruled out. If the localization of pain is not typically segmental, it may be due to muscular and ligamentous injuries that are not evident to superficial inspection.

Summary: Clinical Features of Cervical Syndromes

The collective term "cervical syndrome" denotes cervical spine symptoms of degenerative origin. Symptoms that are restricted to the cervical spine are called local cervical syndrome; neck pain in local cervical syndrome is analogous to low back pain in local lumbar syndrome. Neck pain can be either simple or complex. Simple neck pain resolves rapidly, but complex neck pain lasts longer and runs the risk of becoming chronic. The same is true of cervicobrachial syndrome, in which the pain radiates from the cervical spine into the shoulder and upper limb. Cervicocephalic syndrome comprises all pains in the neck and head that arise from the cervical spine, sometimes accompanied by dizziness, auditory or visual disturbances, or dysphagia. For all of these entities, the history is the key to clinical diagnosis: the most important feature is the positional dependence of the symptoms. A broad spectrum of other illnesses affecting the head and neck must be included in the differential diagnosis. It is therefore important to do a precise manual examination, with testing of the mobility of each segment (and of the potential generation of pain when it is moved).

Radiological findings in the cervical spine are important only when they have a clinical correlate. Far too much attention is paid to spondylotic and osteochondrotic changes of the cervical spine, such as disk protrusions with supposed narrowing of the spinal canal. Such findings may be visually impressive, but nevertheless asymptomatic. MRI exaggerates, particularly in the cervical spine.

Conclusion

The history and physical examination are more important than radiological studies in the differential diagnosis of cervical spine conditions.

■ Treatment of Cervical Syndromes

Overview of Treatment Methods

Despite their varying pathogenesis and manifestations, all cervical disk syndromes are treated with the same set of therapeutic techniques. The sequence in which these techniques are applied depends on whether the painful condition is acute or chronic. The spectrum of possible treatments for disk disease is broad, particularly in the cervical spine. It ranges from simple, conservative measures, such as heat application and analgesics, to complex operations.

_!_ In treating the multifarious manifestations of cervical syndrome, it is often useful to apply multiple treatment strategies simultaneously.

Treatment is aimed not just at the **primary** motor components of the condition but also at its **secondary** manifestations, such as muscle tension, abnormal posture, and emotional disturbances.

Etiological (cause-directed) and symptomatic treatments should be given in parallel. As described above, structural deformation, short-term postural changes,

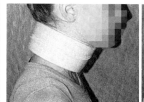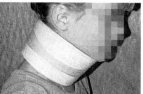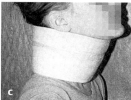

Fig. 9.29 a–c Cervical collars of even height all around, correctly and incorrectly fitted.
a Collar too narrow: the patient can still flex and extend the neck.
b Correct fit.
c Collar too wide: the collar extends the patient's neck, exacerbating symptoms.

and hypermobility produce clinical symptoms. The purpose of an etiological treatment is to eliminate one or more of these disease-producing mechanisms. Examples include isometric muscle-strengthening exercises, cervical support, and fusion operations.

Heat, electrotherapy, massage, and analgesics are intended to alleviate the secondary manifestations and break the vicious circle of pain, muscle tension, abnormal posture, and more pain. The relief of pain is of paramount importance, as pain is the reason why the patient is seeking medical help.

Conservative Treatment

Heat

Mechanism of action. The application of heat in its many forms is an important component of the treatment of cervical disk syndromes, particularly when the pain is acute. Heat exerts its beneficial effect through hyperemia and release of tension in the shoulder and neck muscles. This is followed by a comparable reflex effect in the corresponding motion segments. Deep heat alleviates local irritation of the ligaments and periosteum, such as commonly occurs during the process of disk degeneration. It also influences the speed of conduction of the motor nerves and the activity of the spinal α- and γ-motor neurons, so as to relax painfully tense muscle zones.

Application. Heat can be applied either directly, by the contact of a warm object with the patient, or indirectly, by radiant heat. Fango and mud packs are said to provide effective deep heat. Simple application of dry heat, e. g., with an infrared lamp or a hot air box, has also been found to be clinically useful. Immediately accessible home remedies include a heating pad, hot-water bottle, or hot bath. The patient can take advantage of endogenous body heat by wrapping a thick woolen scarf around the neck; this will also mechanically stabilize the cervical spine to some extent. Various types of radiation can also be used to induce heat, either directly or indirectly. References for the therapeutic effectiveness

of heat application are listed under "Conservative Treatment" in Chapter 11, p. 218. See also **Table 9.12**.

Soft Cervical Collar

The anatomy of the shoulder–neck region permits easy support and partial immobilization of the cervical spine with a soft cervical collar, a therapeutic device that is both simple and inexpensive. The collar should be of the same **height** all round, and the height must be right: a collar that is too large hyperextends the cervical spine, but one that is too small is ineffective (**Fig. 9.29**). Because the shoulder girdle is nearer to the mandible anteriorly than to the occiput posteriorly, a collar that is too large produces hyperlordosis of the cervical spine, perhaps exacerbating the symptoms. Most patients prefer a mildly kyphotic position of the cervical spine, as this opens the intervertebral foramina to the widest possible extent and releases pressure not only on the dorsal portion of the intervertebral disks, but also on the nerve roots. A properly fitted soft collar has three beneficial effects:

- immobilization
- warmth
- release of stress.

! A soft cervical collar eliminates all movements of the cervical spine that can lead to recurrent mechanical irritation of the nerve roots or of the sensory receptors in the posterior longitudinal ligament.

Pain can often be produced by movements of the head that the patient makes unthinkingly while awake or involuntarily when asleep; thus, it is particularly important for the patient to wear the soft collar even in bed. The collar can, however, be taken off for a short period (e. g., for showering), even in an acute cervical syndrome, as long as the patient concentrates on keeping the shoulder and neck muscles in the proper position during this interval. In post-traumatic cervical syndrome, the immobilization of the pulled and torn muscles and of the ligaments between the vertebrae is an important component of treatment. The soft collar should be worn for only a short time (1–3 days).

9

Table 9.12 Comparative studies on the conservative treatment of cervical syndrome (from Rubenthaler et al. in Wirth and Zichner 2004)

Author/Year	No. of patients (n)	Condition treated	Treatments compared	Study findings
Basmajian (1978)	83	Painful muscle tension	Cyclobenzaprine Diazepam Placebo	Better muscle relaxation with cyclobenzaprine
Barnsley (1994)	41	Cervical spine sprain	Facet injection with/without steroid	No difference
Brochgrevink (1998)	201	Acute cervical spine sprain	Post-trauma, 13 days of: No work + soft collar "Act as usual"	Better results in the "act as usual" group when followed up at 6 months
Castergnera (1994)	28	Cervico-brachialgia	Epidural steroid injection with/without morphine	No difference
Foley-Nolan (1990)	20	Acute cervical spine sprain	Soft collar for 12 weeks with one of the following: Pulsating magnetic field therapy NSAID Instructions for hourly exercises	No difference
Gennis(1996)	92	Acute cervical spine sprain	Strict soft-collar wearing for 2 weeks only relaxation and analgesia, without collar	No difference at 6–12 weeks
Goldie (1970)	73	Cervico-brachialgia	Isometric exercises Traction therapy	No difference at 24 weeks
Koes (1992)	256*	Nonspecific neck pain	Physiotherapy Manual therapy General care by family physician	Physiotherapy and manual therapy better than general care by family physician
Jordan (1998)	119	Nonspecific neck pain	Manual therapy Muscle training Physiotherapy	No difference
Lewith (1981)	26	Painful osteo-arthrosis of the cervical spine	red-light trigger point treatment placebo	No difference
Levoska (1993)	47	Cervico-brachialgia	Physiotherapy only Patient exercises	Patients who did exercises had better function and less pain at 1 year
Mealy (1986)	61	Acute cervical spine sprain	2 weeks of soft collar and rest Early mobilization	Early mobilization group better at 8 weeks
Nordemar (1981)	30	Acute neck pain	Soft collar TENS Manual therapy	Range of motion improved more rapidly with TENS; manual therapy no better than soft collar
Rubenthaler (2000)	57	Cervico-brachialgia	Spinal nerve analgesia with mepivacaine Placebo	Better than placebo after 14 days of treatment
Stav (1993)	42	Painful osteo-arthrosis and disk prolapse	Epidural steroids Paravertebral steroids	Epidural steroids better
Thomas (1991)	44	Painful osteo-arthrosis of the cervical spine	Acupuncture vs. placebo Diazepam vs. placebo	Acupuncture better than placebo medication
Trock (1994)	81	Nonspecific neck pain	Physiotherapy Manual therapy General care by family physician	Physiotherapy and manual therapy better than general care by family physician
Zylbergold (1985)	100	Cervico-brachialgia	Pulsating magnetic field therapy Placebo	Pulsating magnetic field therapy better after 1 month of follow-up

* Series includes lumbar spine.

! Furthermore, a soft cervical collar conserves the body heat of the shoulder and neck region, warming the muscles to reduce tension.

Release of tension on the affected motion segment is an important aim of treatment in discogenic syndromes. As discussed on page 84, the cervical disks are under considerable mechanical stress from the weight of the head (which is relatively large in humans). There are no other soft tissues or skeletal components to help bear this weight, unlike in the lumbar or thoracic regions; when an individual stands erect, the cervical spine alone must hold the head up, in an unstably balanced position. Any change of posture requires a re-equilibration of the head through a change in the tone of the shoulder and neck muscles.

Reduction of Mechanical Stress

A properly fitted soft cervical collar reduces the mechanical stress on the tense or overstretched neck muscles, and thus reduces pain. The collar takes part of the weight of the head off the cervical spine by transmitting it to the shoulder girdle. A further method of relaxing the cervical spine, if the pain is very severe, is horizontal positioning (bed rest).

A soft collar can also provide a mild degree of cervical **traction.** If the ventral neck muscles are symmetrically contracted, the cervical motion segments are lightly pulled apart, particularly dorsally (**Fig. 9.30**). This effect is reproduced each time the patient bends the neck forward.

Once the cervical spine has been immobilized and passively supported for a period of time, the partially inactivated muscles of the shoulder and neck must gradually resume their earlier functions. Patients can develop a feeling of insecurity or even painful muscular insufficiency if a soft collar that has been worn continuously for a long time is suddenly removed. The transition can be eased by removing the collar only intermittently at first, for a few hours at a time. Isometric muscle-strengthening exercises should be prescribed in parallel.

Patients in the **rehabilitation phase** should avoid all activities requiring a highly mobile cervical spine, e. g., driving in reverse or working above their head. They should preferentially adopt a "chin-down," partly flexed position of the neck. **Patient exercises** to strengthen the shoulder and neck muscles are not just part of the acute treatment of cervical syndrome, but also a major component of rehabilitation and prophylaxis.

Indications and Duration of Treatment

Many different kinds of cervical support used to be prescribed for prolonged periods of time to treat both degenerative and post-traumatic cervical syndromes.

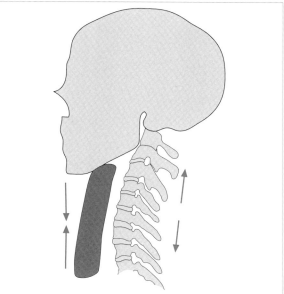

Fig. 9.30 Traction effect of a soft collar on the cervical spine.

Recently, however, a few comparative studies have shown that it makes no difference whether a patient with an acute cervical syndrome wears a soft cervical collar (Gennis 1996, Brochgevink 1998). Most authors nonetheless consider a soft collar to be advisable in the acute period, for the reasons explained above, and recommend that it be worn for a few days (Sandler et al. 1996, Hachemson and Johnsson 2000, Borenstein et al. 2004, Anderson et al. 2005, Clark 2005). The major factors for the success of treatment with a cervical support are (Bruns et al. 2004):

- an optimal fit
- wearing for a limited time only
- patient exercises to be performed in parallel.

It seems clear that cervical supports will continue to be used in the treatment of cervical syndromes, but not as the sole mode of therapy.

Medications (See Chapter 8)

The medical treatment of cervical syndrome is purely symptomatic and should be conducted in parallel with physiotherapy. There is no evidence that the drugs generally given influence the consistency or volume of disk tissue in any way. In view of the multiple pathogenetic mechanisms that are involved in cervical syndrome, it is not surprising that drugs with various mechanisms of action can be used to good effect. It should be remembered that the patient has come to see the doctor mainly for relief of the deep, severe pain in the shoulder and neck, or in the occiput.

9

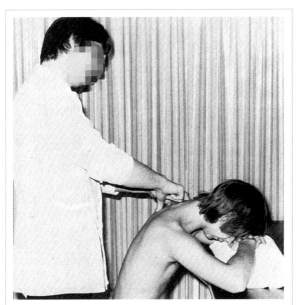

Fig. 9.31 Massage of the shoulder and neck muscles with the patient seated and the neck flexed (kyphosed).

9

! The treatment of severe pain should begin with the administration of a powerful analgesic.

Sedatives and tranquilizers can also be given, as combination or add-on therapy, for their indirect muscle-relaxing effect. Tranquilizers lessen the "nuisance effect" of mechanical irritation of the neural elements of the motion segment, thus breaking the vicious cycle of pain, muscle spasm, and more pain. Furthermore, in patients with chronic, recurrent cervical syndrome, the mainly nocturnal pain can produce such physical and emotional stress that psychoactive medication may be indicated for a brief period. Diazepam is valuable in this context as a barbiturate-free sedative, psychoactive drug and muscle relaxant that can be given as a supplement to other, parallel treatments.

Though the efficacy of these drugs has earned them a deserved popularity among physicians and patients alike, the beneficial therapeutic effect of a **thorough discussion with the patient** must not be forgotten. The physician should explain the condition concisely and intelligibly with the aid of an anatomical model, point out that it is benign and treatable, and, finally, **instruct the patient in the behavioral changes that need to be made, while emphasizing the importance of compliance with these instructions to bring about symptomatic relief.** Such a discussion goes a long way toward minimizing worry and setting the patient on the path to recovery.

Massage and Electrotherapy

These treatments are intended to reduce tension in the shoulder and neck muscles. **Massage** has wide application in the treatment of cervical disk syndromes. Reflexively increased muscle tension initially serves a useful protective function by immobilizing the abnormal motion segment, but it can then develop into a pathological state of spasm that itself causes further symptoms. Patients suffering from cervical syndrome often press and squeeze the tense muscles themselves in an attempt to gain relief. A properly performed massage is more likely to help, but should only be attempted after the acute pain has subsided.

! Massage may even worsen the pain of cervical syndrome in the acute stage, because any manipulation of the neck can irritate the nerve root in the loosened motion segment.

A gentle, rubbing massage can be used once the acute phase is over. The more severe the pain, the more cautiously massages should be introduced; the intensity of massage can be slowly increased as tolerated. If the muscles remain tensely contracted in chronic cervical syndrome, deep massage with kneading, shaking, and pressure on the muscles will be needed. The benefit of massage is derived both from its direct mechanical effect and from a reflex effect on the motion segment. Adhesions between muscles are separated, and the flow of blood and lymph is promoted. As muscle tension decreases, so, too, does the intradiscal pressure in the cervical disks. Any disk material that may have been displaced can return to its original position. The disturbed motion segment has the opportunity to heal.

Connective tissue massage is of value in the treatment of chronic, recurrent cervical syndrome. In this technique, strokes of a particular kind are carried out with the pad of one finger (usually the third or fourth digit) with the hand, arm, and shoulder in a gently springing posture. The strokes are made in a segmentally oriented direction.

! Segmental stroking of the shoulder and neck region can beneficially affect the reflex disturbance of the motion segment by way of the fibers of the dorsal branch of the spinal nerve.

The patient must be properly positioned for the massage. The simple prone position puts the cervical spine into excessive lordosis, placing excessive strain on the lower motion segments. The shoulder and neck muscles are best massaged with the patient sitting or lying and the neck in a mildly flexed position (**Fig. 9.31**). If the massage is to be done in the sitting position, the patient's head should be supported on a low table with the forehead resting on both hands, as shown in **Fig. 9.31**. This position relaxes the shoulder and neck muscles. If the patient is prone, the position of the hands and head is basically the same, with a cushion under the chest to raise it and ensure a properly flexed position of the neck.

The patient should feel better after the massage. If not, or if the pain is increased, then the position may have been wrong or the massage done too early. Patient exercises should only be initiated once the muscles have been properly conditioned with heat and massage.

Electrotherapy is another way of improving pain in the motion segment, particularly the muscles. It is described in further detail in Chapter 11. In patients with cervical syndrome, it may be difficult to apply the apparatus to the site to be treated, e. g., the occiput. The vacuum electrodes that form part of the equipment generally used today for interference-current therapy often leave cosmetically unappealing suction marks on the shoulder and neck, which can take weeks to resolve. This is why manual massage is generally preferred in the cervical region.

Traction

Changes in disk height are an important precipitant of disk-related symptoms. In particular, loss of disk height with narrowing of the intervertebral foramina can produce local and segmental cervical disk syndromes. The cervical disks normally shrink over the decades. Though this process is usually painless, pain may arise temporarily through fluctuations of cervical disk height and volume, e. g., in relation to the sleep–wake cycle. Traction brings relief.

> **!** Even minor changes of disk height can produce, or relieve, symptoms when a disk protrusion or uncovertebral osteophyte lies in the immediate vicinity of a nerve root

Effects of traction. The beneficial effects of traction on the motion segment are multiple. Traction
- widens the intervertebral foramen
- widens the intervertebral disk
- stretches the paravertebral muscles and ligaments
- re-positions abnormally situated intervertebral joints.
- Cervical spine traction with the neck in flexion *widens the intervertebral foramen* and reduces direct pressure on the nerve root. **Indirect reduction of pressure on the nerve root** is also promoted, because blood can flow out of the valveless paravertebral venous plexus, so that edema can recede.
- Cervical spine traction *stretches the inter- and paravertebral ligaments and the nuchal musculature,* thereby **reducing muscle spasm** and reducing pressure on the neural elements and blood vessels.
- Traction releases intervertebral joint facets that are tightly pressed into one another. *Joints that have been brought into an abnormal position by trauma* can **return to their normal, neutral position** by unloading of

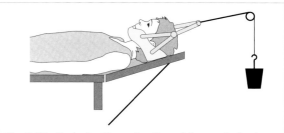

Fig. 9.32 Kyphotic Glisson traction of the cervical spine.

the cervical spine through traction. The applied traction must be strictly in the axial direction. Any additional rotatory or lateral component is harmful, particularly in patients whose motion segments have been loosened by a degenerative process.
- A reversal of fluid flow across the boundary of the disk, with *increase of disk volume,* can be achieved simply by positioning the patient horizontally. Traction lowers the intradiscal pressure still further; with strong traction, the intradiscal pressure actually becomes negative. The extra- to intradiscal pressure gradient promotes fluid movement into the disk. The **volume increase of the cervical disks** under traction is less than that of the lumbar disks, but only a fraction of a millimeter of increased height may be needed to relieve the pain arising from a nerve root compressed by a hard or soft disk protrusion.

Different types of equipment of varying degrees of complexity are available for cervical spine traction. The Glisson sling (**Fig. 9.32**) has long been used for both inpatient and outpatient treatment, and provides a gentle, easily adjustable pull. It must be well fitted to the head; it should not place any pressure on the chin or larynx, nor should it ever impede blood flow in the great vessels of the neck. For traction as for massage, proper positioning of the patient is very important. Glisson traction is generally carried out with the patient supine, rather than sitting, because less traction on the head is needed when the influence of gravity is eliminated. Lying also promotes muscle relaxation.

The spinal nerve roots are relaxed to the greatest extent when the arms are mildly abducted and elevated. Cervical spine traction in the sitting or standing position with the arms hanging down tends to exacerbate symptoms, because it stretches the roots instead of relaxing them. The direction of pull in Glisson traction should not be precisely along the body axis, but rather somewhat anterior, in order to produce mild flexion of the neck (the optimal position for the nerve roots).

> **!** Glisson traction should not be used for corrective realignment of the cervical vertebrae or to produce cervical lordosis.

9

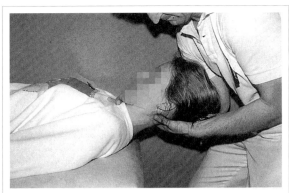

Fig. 9.33 Manual therapy of cervical syndrome with traction in the direction that relieves mechanical stress on the motion segments and brings them back to the neutral position.

Lordosis narrows the intervertebral foramina and also overstretches the anterior neck muscles. The principle of kyphotic traction likewise applies in step-positioning of the lumbar spine (see **Fig. 11.95**).

Cervical spine traction can be provided by a system of weights and pulleys, or intermittently with a motor. A cervical collar or other support must be applied immediately after each traction session so that the beneficial effect can be maintained. The traction should not be excessively prolonged, as a, extended reduction of intradiscal pressure may cause a rapid increase in disk volume, producing more pain.

The **indication** for cervical traction is a cervical syndrome that responds to a traction test (Glisson test, see p. 90).

Manual Therapy of the Cervical Spine

! Manual therapy is a technique in which the hands are used to diagnose and treat reversible functional disturbances of the musculoskeletal system.

Whereas in Glisson traction, for example, an external apparatus supplies the force used for treatment, by definition manual therapy uses the hands. As discussed in Chapter 4, pathoanatomical changes in the disk may lead to an abnormal position of the intervertebral joints beyond their normal range of motion. Changes in disk volume, consistency, and height alter the neutral position of the joints; certain movements, particularly reclination and rotation, can then lead to painful stretching of the joint capsules and compression of the joint surfaces. If simple heat application, relaxation, and repositioning do not result in a return to the functional neutral position, a brief dynamic impulse can be applied manually to the disturbed motion segment.

The goal of manual therapy of the spine is to return disturbed motion segments to their neutral position (**Fig. 9.33**). Generally, this involves pulling in the axial direction, as in the stretch test (see **Fig. 9.13**, p. 90).

Though manual therapy is primarily aimed at the joints, the disk is always involved too, as the intervertebral disk and joints form a functional unit. Brief, powerful pulling, the basic element of all chiropractic manipulations of the cervical spine, lowers the intradiscal pressure with a suction-like effect. Laterally or dorsally displaced portions of disk may return to their original position. The mechanism resembles that of traction with weights and pulleys. With a single pull, an experienced practitioner can achieve a therapeutic benefit that would otherwise require days of heat application, a cervical collar, and analgesics.

Indications and contraindications. Manual manipulation of the cervical spine, if it is to be done at all, must be strictly limited to *pure traction grips* (**Fig. 9.13**). Grips intended to produce marked rotation of the cervical spine seem dangerous, given the anatomical relationship of the vertebrae to the vertebral artery and the spinal cord. One must also bear in mind that the rotational stability of the disks may be impaired, even in younger patients, by horizontal fissures.

! Manual treatment of cervical syndromes is indicated for acute, painful (but not severely painful) restriction of movement of the cervical spine in an adolescent or young adult patient.

Under these circumstances, and in the absence of severe muscle spasm (which would contraindicate manual therapy), manual traction in the axial direction may be attempted. It can, at least, do no harm. The manipulations should not be too frequent, so as not to loosen the cervical motion segments.

In all other situations, manual therapy is contraindicated. In local cervical syndrome with spasm of the shoulder and neck muscles, the marked muscular resistance must first be overcome before the motion segment can be moved. The abnormal posture of torticollis is a typical example: here, muscle spasm is a reflexive mechanism serving to stabilize the abnormally loosened motion segment. Spinal manipulations aimed at reducing muscular tension would unnecessarily counteract this beneficial process. In addition, pulling on the patient's tense muscles will only increase the pain.

Likewise, segmental nerve root irritation in cervicobrachial syndrome can only be aggravated by manual manipulation, no matter whether the compressive lesion in the intervertebral foramen is hard or soft. The irritated nerve root needs rest.

All **symptoms due to disk prolapse,** whether cervicobrachial or cervicomedullary, are an absolute contraindication to manual therapy, because of the danger that the prolapse will be pushed further out of the disk, with resulting paralysis. In cervicocephalic syndrome, manual therapy is too dangerous because of the possible harmful effect on blood flow in the vertebral artery. Any relative narrowing of this artery by an exostosis from the uncinate process can be made worse by a shift or twist of the cervical spine. If the vertebral artery is atherosclerotic or has an aneurysm or other anomaly, grievous harm may result.

Age is the most important contraindication to manipulation of the cervical spine. The "benevolent" partial spinal immobilization of old age can be broken by chiropractic manipulation, leading to new hypermobility. So-called corrective manipulations will then be needed at ever-shorter intervals.

The same is true for patients who have suffered a traumatic neck sprain (post-traumatic cervical syndrome). The overstretched and partially ruptured soft tissues of the neck need rest in order to heal. Manual therapy of the cervical spine merely renews the trauma (**Table 9.13**).

There are many reports of the **results** of manual therapy for cervical syndromes, e.g., Goldy and Landquist (1970), Koes et al. (1992, 1993), Gross et al. (1996), Shekella and Coulter (1997). Often, different treatments are compared with one another. Only Koes et al. (1992, 1993) carried out a placebo-controlled study. Manual therapy was reportedly found to be more effective than placebo, but no more effective than physiotherapy.

Serious attention must be paid to reports of the adverse effects and complications of manual therapy, particularly when it is done in the face of the contraindications listed in **Table 9.13**. See Clark and Haldeman (1993), Dabbs and Lauretti (1995), Assendelft et al. (1996), Hurwitz et al. (1996, 2002, 2005), Senstadt et al. (1996), Haldeman et al. (1999, 2002), Barret and Breen (2000), Kraft et al. (2000), Rothwell et al. (2001), and Coulter et al. (2002), Haldeman et al. (2008).

Local Injections in the Cervical Spine

Indications and Anatomical Basis

If rest, heat, and analgesics fail to relieve the pain and muscle spasm of cervical syndrome, treatment with local injections may be considered. Such treatment is often provided initially, mainly in cases of acute cervicobrachialgia.

> **!** The local injection of analgesics and anti-inflammatories goes straight to the source of pain in cervical syndrome.

The principles of diagnostic and therapeutic local injection of local anesthetics and steroids in the lumbar spine, previously explained in Chapter 8, are also valid for the cervical spine.

Table 9.13 Contraindications for manual therapy of the cervical spine
▪ Segmental radicular symptoms or deficits
▪ Cervicocephalic syndromes
▪ Cervicomedullary syndromes
▪ Cervical spine sprain (status post acceleration–deceleration trauma)
▪ Age > 65

> **!** Therapeutic local anesthesia in the cervical spine is intended to break the vicious circle of pain, muscle tension, and more pain, at the precise site where it arises.

The trouble is usually located in the region of the intervertebral foramen, where the lateral portion of the uncinate process lies adjacent to the spinal nerve root and the vertebral artery (with its closely applied autonomic nervous plexus). This is the site of origin of local cervicobrachial and cervicocephalic syndromes. The intervertebral joints and the shoulder and neck muscles are secondarily affected.

Local Muscle Infiltration

The infiltration of painful muscle areas or the various types of *neural therapy* with *subcutaneous wheal injections* can be used routinely, in addition to heat application and massage, to interrupt the peripheral pain cascade. With the patient in the prone position, the joint area is infiltrated by introducing the needle two fingerbreadths from the midline, palpating along the transverse process medially and flooding the entire area with lidocaine. In occipital neuralgia, it has been found useful to infiltrate the upper border of the trapezius muscle with a mixture of lidocaine and cortisone crystalline suspension.

Painful spasms of the shoulder and neck muscles can be relieved by a stroking massage in combination with *muscle infiltration with lidocaine or other local anesthetics,* particularly at the upper border of the trapezius muscle and in the area of the rhomboid muscles. This treatment does not directly address the source of irritation in the motion segment. Muscle infiltration appears to be useless for the treatment of pain referred into the muscles from the irritated dorsal branch of a spinal nerve.

Cervical Sympathetic and Radicular Blockade

> **!** **Rationale:** Cervical spinal nerve analgesia (CSPA) is effectuated by the injection of a local anesthetic, sometimes mixed with steroids, through a posterior approach into the foraminoarticular region of the lower cervical motion segments.

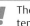
9

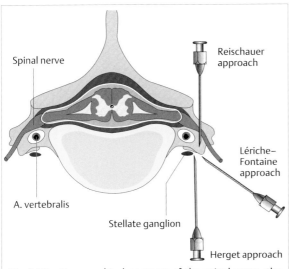

Fig. 9.34 Topographical anatomy of the spinal nerve, the vertebral artery, and the stellate ganglion, with three different approaches for percutaneous stellate ganglion block.

ments with the injecting needle; e. g., a ventral, lateral, or dorsal approach for a stellate ganglion block. The simplest and most reliable approaches are the direct ventral one of Herget (1943) and the ventrolateral one of Leriche and Fontaine (1934) and Mandl (1953). The main risk of either approach is an intradural injection if the needle is aimed incorrectly (obliquely). The dorsal approach for stellate ganglion blockade has been repeatedly described (Mandl 1925, 1953, Paraf et al. 1937, Reischauer 1956, 1961, Theodoridis and Krämer 2005); some authors recommend introducing the needle at C7, others at T1 (**Fig. 9.34**).

Indication for cervical nerve root blockade. Injections by the dorsal approach have been found useful in the treatment of cervical syndrome.

> *!* Cervicobrachial syndromes are the main indication, but local and cervicocephalic syndromes can also be treated in this way. The dorsal approach allows access to the cervical spinal nerves, part of the cervical sympathetic chain, and the area around the vertebral artery, without any risk of puncturing the dura mater or injuring the great vessels of the neck.

Targeted flooding of the cervical sympathetic chain with lidocaine, particularly the stellate ganglion and the associated nerve roots, has been found to be very effective in treating all forms of cervical syndrome. This technique strikes directly at the origin of nerve irritation in the motion segment.

> *!* The goals of this form of treatment are desensitization of the irritated spinal nerve root and temporary inactivation of parts of the cervical sympathetic chain, including its many interconnections in the vicinity of the vertebral artery.

Flooding with lidocaine lowers the irritability of the hypersensitive nerve structures.

It has been shown that the ability of cervical spinal nerve roots to generate neuropathic pain and other radicular symptoms can be greatly influenced by sympathetic blockade. The cervical spinal nerves play the role of an end organ of the sympathetic nervous system (Reischauer 1953, 1956, 1961, Schmitt 1955, Lang 1991, Bogduk 2000, Theodoridis and Krämer 2006). Thus, the success of treatment does not really depend on a full stellate blockade with Horner syndrome, despite frequent claims to the contrary. The important criterion is the infiltration of the irritated spinal nerve itself and of the sympathetic nerve fibers that join it at the same level. Infiltration of C7 and C8 simultaneously creates a stellate block; infiltration of C6 blocks fibers coming off the middle cervical ganglion. The sympathetic plexus around the vertebral artery is affected by infiltration of any of the lower cervical motion segments.

There are a number of ways of reaching the affected ventrolateral portions of the lower cervical motion seg-

Dorsal injection has the advantage that the patient is not frightened by the sight of the long needle and the related preparations. Furthermore, the neck flexion that this procedure requires is more comfortable for patients with cervical syndrome than the marked extension needed for an anterior or lateral approach. The same approach can also be used for the segments above the stellate ganglion. We refer to this injection method as "cervical nerve root blockade" because it is not intended to produce blockade of the stellate ganglion.

Technique for cervical nerve root blockade. The patient is seated, with neck maximally flexed, and arms hanging down by the sides. First, the puncture site is marked. The spinous processes of C6, C7, and T1 serve as landmarks for the definition of the midline. A detailed description of the technique is found in Theodoridis and Krämer (2006).*

Results of cervical nerve root blockade. Reports on cervical nerve root blockade for diagnostic and therapeutic purposes have been published by Bush and Hillier (1996), Grifka (1996), Rubenthaler (2004), Bogduk (2005), Eckardt (2005), Theodoridis and Krämer (2006), and Hanefeld et al. (2006). The Task Force on Neck Pain (Haldeman et al. 2008) summarized the literature with evidence for short-term improvement of radicular symptoms with selective nerve root injections.

Rubenthaler et al. (2004) conducted a prospective, randomized, double-blind study of cervical nerve root

---

* The English translation of this book is due to be published in 2009.

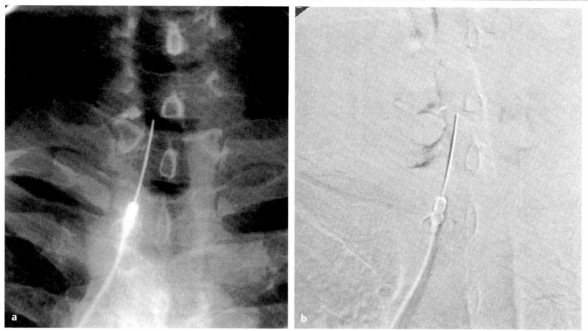

Fig. 9.35 a, b Cervical epidural injection. The solution of steroid in saline is injected between the laminae into the epidural space, in the vicinity of the spinal nerve roots.

blockade in a total of 57 patients with cervicobrachial-gia. They found that blockade with local anesthetic (mepivacaine, 28 patients) relieved pain significantly better than placebo (isotonic saline, 29 patients). The blinded patients and physicians judged the outcome of treatment after at least 3 days of injections. Ineffective initial treatment was followed by a single, combined injection of mepivacaine and triamcinolone acetate. After an average of 14 days of in-patient treatment, the patients were asked to rate their improvement on a scale of 1 (asymptomatic) to 4 (no improvement). The average value in the mepivacaine group was 2.15, and that in the placebo group was 2.54 (p = 0.038). Only two steroid injections were given after ineffective initial treatment in the mepivacaine group, as compared to 16 in the placebo group (p = 0.01).

Cervical Epidural Injection

! **Rationale:** Steroid medication in saline solution can be injected into the lower cervical epidural space through the interlaminar window.

The nerve root is bathed in the anti-inflammatory drug at the precise location where it can be compressed by osteophytes from the uncinate process, or by dislocated disk tissue, and consequently become edematous (**Fig. 9.35**). This local treatment of root edema decompresses the space around the nerve root enough to

enable outflow of static venous blood, which, in turn, permits the edema to subside still further.

These injection techniques must be accompanied by rehabilitation and physiotherapy, including Glisson traction, flexion positioning, and patient exercises.

Indications. Intractable cervicobrachial syndrome is the main indication for cervical epidural injection. Cervical nerve root blockade can be used in addition. Cervicocephalic and posttraumatic cervical syndromes also respond well to a combination of cervical epidural injections and cervical nerve root blocks.

Epidural injections carry an elevated risk because of the proximity of the CSF space and spinal cord and should therefore be used only when all other potential treatments have been ineffective. They can be carried out in the outpatient setting (Baric 1992).

Contraindications. Epidural injections should not be used in patients with underlying neurological illnesses, epilepsy, known reactions to contrast medium, skin infections at the intended puncture site, or other known contraindications to cortisone injection.

Technique of cervical epidural injection. The procedure is done under standby anesthesia, with an intravenous catheter in place, in a prone patient, with the neck mildly flexed to enable interlaminar access. The cervical epidural space is best reached through C6/7 or

9

9 Cervical Syndrome

C7/T1. For further details, see Theodoridis and Krämer (2006).*

The results of cervical epidural injection have been reported by Catchlove (1984), Warfield (1988), Wilson et al. (1988), Ferrante (1993), Nikkolai (1995), Bush and Hillier (1996), Grifka (1996), Willburger et al. (1998), Krämer and Nentwig (1999), Morcet et al. (1999), Klein and Vaccaro (2000), Lieberman et al (2003), Rubenthaler (2004), Klein and Vaccaro (2000), and Liebermann et al. (2003). All of these authors point out that this technique requires a great deal of care because the needle tip lies just posterior to the spinal cord. The correct position of the needle must be verified by epidural injection of radiological contrast medium under fluoroscopy (Renfrew et al. 1991). Stav et al. (1993) found epidural injection to be significantly more effective than intramuscular injection for the treatment of chronic pain syndromes. The addition of morphine to epidural cortisone made no difference.

The Task Force on Neck Pain (Haldeman et al. 2008) summarizes the literature that epidural corticoid injections in people with neck pain and radiculopathy can provide short-term relief, but that injections have unclear benefits in neck pain without radiculopathy.

Cervical Facet Infiltration

! **Rationale:** This technique uses local anesthetic for the temporary inactivation of sensory nerve fibers in the intervertebral joint capsules.

Indication. The indication for cervical facet infiltration is a cervical syndrome with pseudoradicular radiation of pain into the upper limb, i. e., pain radiation in a nondermatomal distribution. Pain arising from the dorsal branch of the spinal nerve and referred to the interscapular region responds particularly well to this form of treatment. Pain of this type is exacerbated by reclination of the head, which makes the intervertebral joints telescope into one another.

Technique. The injection can be done with the patient either seated or prone. The head should not be bent forward too far, so that the interlaminar window remains closed. More details can be found in Theodoridis and Krämer (2006)*.

There are very few published reports on the **results** of cervical facet infiltration. Rubenthaler (2004) states that there has bee only one randomized study in patients with chronic pain after cervical spine sprain (Barnsley et al. 1994). No difference was found between treatment with cortisone and treatment with local anesthetic.

* The English translation of this book is due to be published in 2009.

Operative Treatment

Indications and Preoperative Evaluation

Indications. Surgical treatment of a chronic, recurrent cervical syndrome with unbearable pain can be considered if all conservative methods, including nerve root blocks, have failed to bring relief. Though many patients with cervical disk syndromes are referred to us, we recommend surgery in relatively few cases.

Major neurologic deficits, such as are seen in cervicomedullary syndrome, require work-up with imaging studies such as myelography, CT, and/or MRI, followed by timely surgical treatment. In other types of cervical syndrome, an operation is indicated only late in the course of the disease. Transient successes with conservative treatment and the spontaneous remissions that occur in all disk-related conditions generally enable the patient and the treating physician to defer the decision to operate, particularly in view of the justifiable concern over possible surgical complications.

The physician who has been treating and observing the patient for years must also assess the patient's psychosocial situation before any operation is planned. There is no sense in operating on a patient who "needs" to suffer from shoulder–arm syndrome in order to alleviate unrelated occupational or familial difficulties. The best surgical candidates are patients with cervical disk prolapses, or chronic, recurrent cervicobrachialgia due to oncovertebral arthrosis, who no longer respond to conservative treatment. The deciding factor for surgery is a clear statement from the patient that they can no longer tolerate the symptoms and want an operation (**Table 9.14**).

Surgery may also be required when a motion segment that has been loosened by an acceleration–deceleration injury cannot be stabilized by conservative methods, as when a disk rupture fails to heal. Intractable symptoms, combined with clear radiological evidence of excessive opening of the segment on reclination, constitute the surgical indication. A disk-distension test is also done.

Table 9.14 Surgical indications and tests for confirmation of the diagnosis and determination of the affected segment in cervical syndrome

Indications	Tests to confirm the diagnosis or determine the affected segment
Cervical disk prolapse with myelopathy	MRI
Intractable cervicobrachial syndrome	Disk distension test, MRI
Unstable motion segment after cervical spine trauma	Functional images and disk distension test
Cervicocephalic syndrome	Digital subtraction angiography (DSA) of vertebral artery

Intractable headache and dizziness due to a cervicocephalic syndrome maintained by uncovertebral osteophytes may be an indication for uncoforaminectomy.

Cervical discography combined with a disk-distension test is the most important diagnostic method for determining whether the surgical treatment of a cervical syndrome is indicated (Caillet 1981, Grote 1986, Whitecloud and Scago 1987, Bhatia et al. 2004, Zeidman 2005).

The diagnostic information obtained from a contrast study of the cervical disks is not as useful as was once thought. The escape of contrast medium from the posterior border of a disk used to be taken as evidence that this particular disk was the site of the problem. Discography, however, merely provides a picture of the structural degenerative changes in the disks, without allowing any conclusion as to which disk is giving rise to the patient's symptoms. Many severely degenerated disks with a discontinuous anulus fibrosus cause no symptoms whatever. It has been found, however, that the injection of contrast medium under a moderate amount of pressure into the disk that is genuinely the origin of the patient's symptoms can reproduce the patient's typical pain syndrome. This phenomenon, called the disk-distension sign, is a more reliable indicator of the segment to be operated on than the mere image of the disk filled with contrast medium.

As discussed on page 87 above, the intervertebral foramen is narrowed not just by the bony projections that can be seen on a radiograph, but also by the overlying soft tissues, i.e., the dorsolateral portions of the anulus fibrosus and the posterior longitudinal ligament. In "soft" disk protrusions, it is these tissues alone that are responsible for nerve root compression.

! Temporary distension of the disk with fluid (contrast medium) intensifies the contact between the disk border and the nerve root.

The typical, segmentally radiating pain is produced or exacerbated by this maneuver (**Fig. 9.36**). It has the same effect when carried out on a degenerated lumbar disk that is causing lumbar disk syndrome.

! Diagnostic puncture of the lower cervical disks from an anterior approach can be a relatively simple and rapid procedure.

The patient lies supine with a cushion under the shoulders to enable maximum extension of the cervical spine. The head is turned slightly to the right. The patient should be asked to grip the sides of the table firmly and pull their shoulders downward, so that the lower cervical segments are well seen in the radiographic image. The skin is disinfected and infiltrated with local anesthetic, and then the left side of the neck is

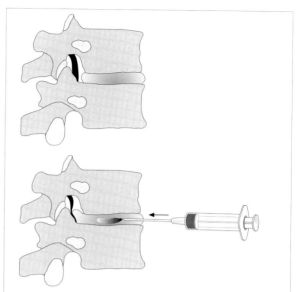

Fig. 9.36 Cervical disk distension test with provocation of typical symptoms (pain). The disk is distended with fluid so that the disk protrusion comes into greater contact with the nerve root.

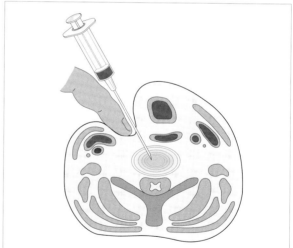

Fig. 9.37 Cervical disk puncture, ventral approach. The vessels and nerves are mobilized laterally under the examiner's finger; the trachea and esophagus are medial.

punctured with a needle (with stylet in place) at the medial edge of the sternocleidomastoid muscle at approximately the level of the cricoid cartilage. The index finger of the physician's free hand (**Fig. 9.37**) mobilizes the sternocleidomastoid muscle, the carotid artery, and the jugular vein laterally, while the trachea and esophagus lie medially. With this finger, the physician can palpate the spine. The needle is slowly introduced, under fluoroscopic guidance, through the anterior longitudinal liga-

9

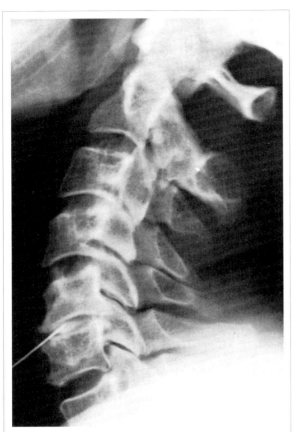

Fig. 9.38   Cervical discography and distension test at C5/6.

Asymptomatic disks should not be operated on even if they show very marked degenerative changes. The disk-distension test (**Fig. 9.38**) ought to provoke not only pain in the arm in the characteristic dermatomal distribution, but also pain in the scapula, mediated by the dorsal branch of the spinal nerve. If the intradiscal injection of fluid temporarily stretches the anulus fibrosus posteriorly in the midline, the patient may experience a transient sensation originating in the spinal cord, consisting of pain in both arms radiating down the back and into the lower limbs. All of these phenomena are reversible. No special positioning of the patient is required after the procedure.

Types of Operation and Their Objectives

The goal of surgery is to arrest or reverse the pathoanatomical and pathophysiological processes responsible for the degenerative changes in the cervical disks that lead to chronic, recurrent cervicobrachialgia. As discussed on page 87, instability and deformation of the motion segment are the major causes of cervical syndrome. Among the wide variety of possible surgical techniques, only a few meet both of the following basic conditions:

- the mechanically irritated neural element(s) should be freed from irritation
- the motion segment should be stabilized.

We will follow Weidner (2004) in classifying operations by approach, ventral or distal.

Ventral operative techniques involve ventral decompression and removal of the disk and the uncinate processes. The procedure is necessarily combined with a fusion operation or with the insertion of a disk prosthesis. Until a few years ago, the standard technique was to insert a plug of autologous iliac crest bone into the disk space. Attempts to obviate the need for bone harvesting and the attendant complications began with the use of bone cement as a placeholder (Grote et al. 1991). Later, metal (e. g., titanium) prostheses were developed for insertion into the disk space, and these are now generally accepted (Kaden et al. 1993, Kehr et al. 1993, Engelhardt et al. 2005). Empty metal placeholders, so-called "cages," can also be used. These need not be filled with autologous bone; unlike bone plugs, they are not designed to be incorporated into the bone structure, but to accommodate bone remodeling sufficient to provide stability (Payer et al. 2003, Weidner 2004). Many authors further recommend ventral osteosynthesis with metal plates and screws (**Figs. 9.39** and **9.40**).

The available reports of the **results of ventral fusion** must be interpreted with caution, because the methods of patient selection and outcome assessment are highly variable (Weidner 2004). Decompression followed by

ment in the midline and onward into the center of the disk.

The findings of the neurological examination determine which disk is to be punctured first. In case of uncertainty, C5/6 is punctured first and then C6/7, because these are the most commonly affected segments. Puncturing multiple disks in a single sitting presents no difficulty.

Once the fluoroscopic image indicates that the position of the needle is precisely correct, a small amount of normal saline is injected into the disk. As this sometimes requires a moderately high degree of pressure, we prefer to use Luer-lock syringes. In a normal cervical disk, 0.2–0.5 mL of fluid can be injected. If a greater volume is admitted, this is evidence for a degenerated disk, possibly with a dorsal anular tear. Contrast medium can also be injected, mainly for the purpose of documenting the level of puncture on a plain radiograph to be obtained immediately afterward. One can even inject methylene blue to facilitate exposure of the correct disk at surgery.

> **!** Provocation of the patient's typical pain by injection of fluid into the disk is of diagnostic significance.

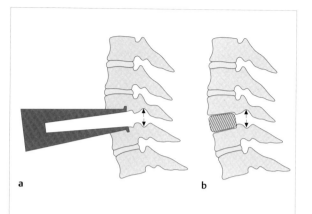

Fig. 9.39 a, b Ventral intercorporal fusion.
a The disk space is distracted.
b A bone plug of the corresponding size is inserted to maintain the distraction of the disk space and hold the cervical spine in this position. Ventral plating can be carried out after plug insertion.

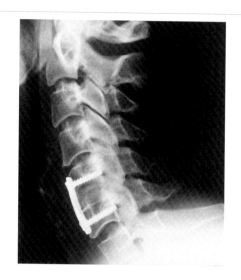

Fig. 9.40 Ventral spondylodesis with autologous bone plug and plating to secure it in place.

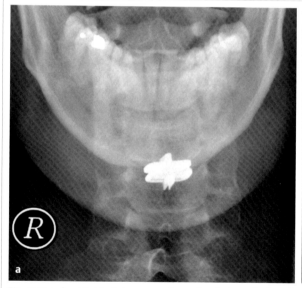

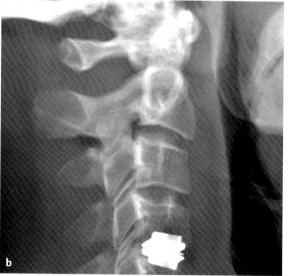

Fig. 9.41 a, b Mobile intercorporal prosthesis (so-called artificial disk) in the cervical spine.

spondylodesis with a bone plug is reported to improve symptoms in 81 % of cases. An additional osteosynthesis has little effect on the result (Zoega et al. 2000). The biomechanical studies of Wilke et al. (2000) showed that titanium cages may be a good alternative to bone plugs. These devices were studied with a special biomechanical method (Schmidt and Wilke 2005). The favorable findings have since been borne out by clinical experience.

More recent reports on the results of ventral operations on the cervical spine include those of Person et al.

(1997), Dunn et al. (1998), Grob (1998), Kadanka (2000), Kienapfel et al. (2004), Breidwell et al. (2005), Irwin et al. (2005), Schmidt et al. (2005), and Fischgrund (2005).

Artificial disks are inserted into the disk space in order to spare the neighboring motion segments the increased mechanical stress to which they would be exposed if a fusion were to be carried out. The various models developed to date generally consist of a titanium half-shell that is anchored in the vertebral body and glides over a synthetic surface. The titanium implant is well integrated into bone, as are titanium implants at other sites in the body, e.g., the hip. Disk prostheses have been in use for only a short time, and clinical follow-up studies are accordingly sparse (McAfee et al. 2003, 2004, Firsching et al. 2005, Phillips and Garfin 2005, Phillips and Garfin 2006). Comparative and long-term studies are lacking. It is not yet known how these mobile implants will behave when the patients age and their vertebral bodies soften from osteoporosis.

Dorsal operative techniques include foraminotomy, laminectomy, hemilaminectomy, and laminoplasty. Dorsal decompression is generally done without fusion. According to Weidner (2004), a medial disk prolapse should be operated on exclusively through a ventral approach, never dorsally, as any manipulation of the spinal cord will increase the risk of a postoperative neurological deficit. The main indications for the dorsal approach are lateral disk prolapses and compressive changes of the uncinate processes. In general, the dorsal approach is associated with fewer complications than the ventral approach. Loosening of any implanted plates and screws also has less severe consequences when it occurs dorsally, rather than ventrally. Whichever operative approach is used, however, the therapeutic success of the procedure and the absence of complications depend heavily on the experience of the surgeon (Weidner 2004). The available reports on the **results** of dorsal operations include those of Grumme and Kolodziejczyk (1994), Matsuyama et al. (1995), Aita et al. (1998), Borenstein et al. (2004), Klimo and Apfelbaum (2005), Lam et al. (2005), and Nagashima et al. (2005).

■ Special Patient Exercises, Rehabilitation, and Back School

Disk-related symptoms in the cervical spine take a fluctuating course, in which severe pain alternates with phases of little or no pain. The prevention of recurrences is of obvious importance.

Stabilisation. After successful initial treatment of a cervical syndrome, it is important for the good result to "hold."

! The repositioned motion segment must be kept in the neutral position as much as possible to prevent further intradiscal tissue shifting or abnormal positions of the intravertebral joints.

The irritated nerve roots must be allowed to recover while the nerve root edema subsides.

During the rehabilitation phase, **strengthening exercises for the shoulder and neck muscles** are also appropriate.

! Intradiscal tissue displacement and movements of the vertebral bodies and intervertebral joints against one another are less likely to occur if the motion segment is stably held from outside by powerful muscles than if the muscles and ligaments are slack.

The muscles can be strengthened, with long-lasting results, by the isometric muscle-tensing exercises done several times a day. These exercises involve no movement, i.e., the head and neck remain in the same position throughout (see **Fig. 9.42**). The cervical musculature can be conditioned in this way in a relatively short time. The efficacy of isometric muscle training has been demonstrated (Hettinger 1983). Doing the exercises shown in **Fig. 9.42** for 3 min twice a day is enough to strengthen the shoulder and neck muscles and keep them strong.

Isotonic muscle-contraction exercises, i.e., exercises associated with movement, are not appropriate for the rehabilitation of patients with cervical syndrome, because they often lead to irritation of the spinal nerves, particularly of the meningeal branch.

At first, isometric muscle-tensing exercises should be done with physiotherapeutic guidance and under a physician's orders. Massage and heat can be used immediately before the exercises to reduce any muscle tension that may be present. The exercises should be begun only after any excessive tension has been eliminated. Later, once patients are no longer under the care of the physiotherapist, they can perform these exercises independently and incorporate them into their daily routine.

Swimming is often recommended, but in fact only backstroke is appropriate for patients recovering from cervical syndrome. Breaststroke is associated with a lordotic posture of the cervical spine and tends to exacerbate symptoms rather than improving them.

The treating physician should give the departing patient at risk of recurrent cervical syndrome a set of **instructions for future behavior.** Marked rotation of the cervical spine (e.g., driving in reverse) should be avoided at first, and the patient should take care not to expose the neck to excessive cold. Patients who suffer from chronic, recurrent cervical syndrome should take a soft cervical collar along whenever they travel away from home, so that they can start wearing it immediately if symptoms should arise.

Prolonged maintenance of an unfavorable posture can also precipitate recurrent cervical syndrome and should be avoided. One example is keeping the head

Table 9.15 Behavioral guidelines (back school) for patients with recurrent cervical syndrome

- Take frequent breaks while reading, working with the hands, watching television, or driving.
- Avoid abruptly turning your head; turn your whole body instead.
- Avoid drafts. Wear a scarf or a soft cervical collar.
- Sleep with a small pillow and do not sleep lying on your stomach.
- When walking, keep your chin down. When bicycling, sit up straight.
- Do not work above your head. Use a ladder or a chair if necessary.
- In the theater or the cinema, sit toward the back rather than in the front rows.
- To drink from a can or bottle, use a straw.
- Wash your hair in the shower, rather than the sink.
- Do your neck exercises every day!

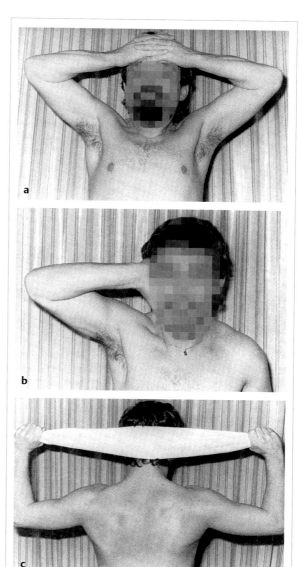

Fig. 9.42 a–c Isometric muscle-strengthening exercises for the shoulder and neck in the rehabilitation and prophylaxis of cervical syndrome.

bent forward while standing or sitting, e. g., while working at a desk. Patients should remember to reposition the cervical spine from time to time, and to support the head intermittently with the arms.

Unfavorable postures can also arise during sleep. A large pillow induces marked flexion in the cervical spine, which can, in turn, promote intradiscal tissue displacement. Sleeping prone causes lordosis and rotation of the cervical spine, which are also unfavorable. The best sleeping position is the supine or lateral decubitus position on a firm mattress, with support of the head and neck on a small pillow or neck roll.

Prophylaxis against acceleration–deceleration injuries in car accidents is provided by a neck rest that is firmly connected to the seat and is adjusted to sit immediately behind the passenger's occiput.

The important behavioral guidelines for patients at risk of cervical syndrome are listed in **Table 9.15** (back school, Krämer 2005).

■ Treatment Planning

Every physician who treats patients with disk problems should have a systematic concept of treatment to enable maximum efficiency while avoiding harm. The type and sequence of treatment measures to be applied depend, among other factors, on the severity of the symptoms and the age of the patient.

Table 9.16 outlines the treatment strategy that we have worked out in the last few years in our clinic, in cooperation with colleagues in private practice. Most patients with cervical syndrome are treated on an out-

patient basis with simple methods including heat, analgesics, anti-inflammatories, and a soft cervical collar. Local injections and physiotherapy are usually done only after referral to a specialist (if the treating physician is not a specialist). Outpatient treatment usually suffices for milder instances of chronic, recurrent cervicobrachialgia or cervicocephalic syndrome. If these methods fail to bring relief and the patient is repeatedly declared unfit for work despite the continuous use of analgesics, hospitalization may be necessary. The diag-

Table 9.16 Treatment scheme for cervical syndrome

- *Outpatient treatment* (for all types of cervical syndrome):

First-ever onset of symptoms: heat, analgesics
Chronically recurrent symptoms: massage, electrotherapy, local injections, traction
If severe symptoms persist despite treatment: CT, MRI, hospitalization for disk distension test

- *In-patient treatment:*

Cervicomedullary syndrome, intractable cervicobrachial syndrome, cervicocephalic syndrome
Conservative treatment: nerve root and stellate blocks, Glisson traction, sedatives
Operative treatment: ventral fusion, uncoforaminectomy, disk prolapse surgery, disk prosthesis
For rehabilitation: patient exercises, back school (see **Table 9.15**)

nostic tests listed in **Table 9.14** are used to establish the possible indication for surgery, but in-patient conservative therapy remains an option (Theodoridis and Krämer 2006)*. Daily stellate and nerve root blocks, followed each time by several hours of Glisson traction (see **Fig. 9.32**) under sedation, can often bring a surprising degree of relief, even to patients with apparently intractable cervicobrachial or cervicocephalic syndrome. One of the benefits of in-patient treatment is that the symptom-producing situations, such as desk work, television watching, and housework, are temporarily eliminated. For patients with any type of cervical syndrome, whatever measures have been found to bring relief in the in-patient setting should be continued over the longer term for rehabilitation and for prophylaxis against future attacks.

Treatment of Cervical Syndromes: Summary

The treatment of cervical syndromes, like that of lumbar syndromes, has changed in recent years. The passive treatments that were previously emphasized, such as massage, realignment, and cervical collars, have largely given way to active ones: gentle exercises and continued physical activity. Pain can be brought under control with properly chosen analgesics and local infiltrations at the site of origin of the pain. Cervical spinal nerve analgesia and epidural injections have also proved their worth in the treatment of cervicobrachial syndrome.

Surgery for degenerative disease should be used even more sparingly in the cervical spine than in the lumbar spine. Exaggerated importance should not be attached to the findings of imaging studies, especially MRI, in the absence of correspondingly severe clinical manifestations. In the cervical spine, any ventral decompressive procedure must be accompanied by a fusion of the intervertebral space, which is well known to have nega-

tive consequences for the neighboring motion segments. It remains to be seen whether mobility-preserving prostheses (so-called artificial disks) truly provide a long-term solution to this problem.

Before attempting an intervention of any kind on the cervical spine, the physician will do well to remember that this particular region of the skeleton naturally undergoes a beneficial partial immobilization in old age. Unnecessary manual manipulations and operations may get in the way of this process, and should be avoided.

Conclusion

The cervical spine is a complex structure. Disorders affecting it must be diagnosed and treated with the utmost care.

10 Thoracic Syndrome

■ Definition and Prevalence

! The term "thoracic syndrome" refers to all pathological clinical manifestations due to functional disturbances and degenerative changes of the thoracic motion segments.

Disk disease is far less common in the thoracic spine than in the cervical and lumbar regions. Thoracic disk disease accounts for only 2 % of all cases of disk disease and tends to be less serious than disk disease elsewhere in the spine. Thoracic nerve root irritation producing intractable intercostal neuralgia is a rare surgical indication. Massive disk prolapse resulting in spinal cord compression (occasionally even paraplegia) is also a rare event (Grote 1975, Awwad et al. 1991, Dietze 1993, Wilke et al. 2000, Borenstein et al. 2004, Endres 2005). Even though the degenerative process affects all disks in the spine, and the thoracic disks perhaps even more so than others, thoracic disk disease remains rare because of the special anatomical and biomechanical features of the thoracic motion segments.

■ Special Anatomy, Biomechanics, and Pathoanatomy of the Thoracic Motion Segments

Special anatomy. The thoracic disks become broader and higher toward the lower end of the thoracic spine. They are flatter than the cervical and lumbar disks in terms of the ratio of width to height. The thoracic spinal canal is relatively narrow, with only a thin epidural space between the spinal cord and the surrounding bone or disk. The canal is narrowest from T4 to T9.

The thoracic spine contains not only the intervertebral joints, but also the joints between the vertebral bodies and ribs, i. e., the costotransverse joints, which indent the lower portion of the intervertebral foramina; their upper portion is occupied by the exiting spinal nerve. Bony narrowing of the intervertebral foramina, such as is seen in the cervical spine, is hardly ever seen in the thoracic spine because the thoracic foramina are much wider.

In the thoracic spine, as in the cervical spine, the spinal cord segments become increasingly distant from the correspondingly numbered motion segments as one proceeds from cranial to caudal. This distance is the equivalent of two segments from T1 to T6, and of three segments from T7 to T10.

The ventral branches of the thoracic spinal nerves, i. e., the intercostal nerves, supply the wall of the rib cage: in particular, they supply the intercostal muscles, the costotransverse ligaments, the parietal pleura, and the skin. Irritation of a thoracic spinal nerve causes intercostal neuralgia.

Biomechanics and pathoanatomy. The dorsally convex curvature of the thoracic spine places the ventral portion of the thoracic motion segments under greater stress. The intradiscal pressure here is very high. In the lordotically curved cervical or lumbar spine an axial compressive force can be borne to a large extent by the intervertebral joints and interlaminar soft tissue, but in the thoracic spine the vertebral bodies and disks must

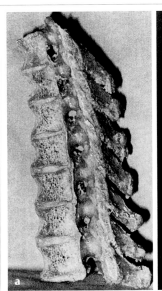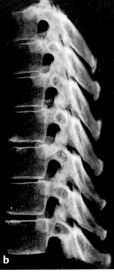

Fig. 10.1 a, b Parasagittal section of the mid-thoracic spine. The intervertebral foramina are not at the level of the disks, as in other regions of the spine (see **Figs. 9.12**, **11.3**), but rather at the level of the vertebral body.

- In the thoracic spine, as opposed to the cervical or lumbar spine, the intervertebral foramina are not located directly behind the disks, but rather at the level of the vertebral body (**Fig. 10.1**). Only a very large thoracic disk prolapse would be able to work its way upward or downward far enough to contact a spinal nerve root. In this rare event, the clinical manifestations of a thoracic disk syndrome may be produced, i.e., intercostal neuralgia.
- The thoracic motion segments move relatively little compared to the cervical and lumbar motion segments. Thus, the anatomical relationship of the sensitive neural structures to their surroundings, i.e., of the spinal nerves to the bone and connective tissue around them, remains relatively constant.

! Acquired deformities of the thoracic spine (scoliosis, Scheuermann disease) develop gradually, allowing the nerve roots enough time to adapt.

---

bear the entire burden. This explains the frequency of thoracic vertebral compression fractures and of protrusions of disk tissue through the vertebral body end plates into the spongiosa. The continuously high intradiscal pressure induces premature regressive changes, particularly in the middle and lower thoracic disks, often involving extensive spondylosis and osteochondrosis. These changes are usually noted incidentally on radiological studies and are all the more surprising because they are asymptomatic. In the thoracic spine even more than elsewhere, spondylosis and osteochondrosis can be quite advanced, radiologically speaking, but still clinically insignificant. Symptoms arise only when these processes take place in the immediate vicinity of a nerve root, and when the motion segment is unstable. These preconditions are not present in the thoracic spine.

There are essentially two reasons why clinically significant disk disease is less common in the thoracic spine than elsewhere:

A thoracic motion segment, even if it is slackened by intervertebral disk degeneration, remains splinted by the rib cage via the costotransverse joints, so that there can be no clinically significant displacement of the vertebral bodies.

Despite these favorable conditions, clinically significant disk disease of the thoracic spine does occasionally occur. The greater stress on the ventral portion of the intervertebral disk may cause central, mobile portions of the disk to become dorsally displaced, so that they cause the anulus fibrosus to bulge posteriorly, or even perforate it. A bulging or ruptured disk may compress the spinal cord and the intrathecal nerve roots. The compression can involve not only the neural elements themselves, but also the blood vessels that supply them. The most vulnerable vessel is the anterior spinal artery, which runs down the ventral surface of the spinal cord.

The sequestrated disk tissue often attains the size of a grape and, in the course of time, becomes adherent to the dura matter (Benson and Byrnes 1975). Central and ventrolateral disk displacements are about as common as lateral and posterior disk displacements. The T7–T12 segments are more commonly involved than the upper half of the thoracic spine (Kroll and Reiss 1951, Love and Schorn 1965, Benson and Byrnes 1975, Stillermann 1998, Endres 2005).

■ Classification

As in the other regions of the spine, degenerative thoracic syndromes can be classified as
- *local*
- *radicular,* or
- *pseudoradicular.*

Radicular thoracic syndrome is also known as intercostal neuralgia.

Degenerative thoracic syndromes can also be classified as simple or complicated, as in **Table 10.1**. One must also be aware of the danger signs indicating that a degenerative thoracic syndrome requires urgent treatment. Thoracic myelopathy, usually due to a disk prolapse, presents with gait impairment, weakness, and a sensory deficit.

Table 10.1 Classification of degenerative diseases of the thoracic spine (thoracic syndromes)

Simple thoracic spine pain (local thoracic syndrome)	Complicated thoracic spine pain	Danger signs (red flags)
Mechanically induced		
Movement dependent	Radiating anteriorly	Myelopathy
Moderate distress		Gait disturbance
Brief duration	Longer duration	Paralysis
Age 20–60	Age < 20 or > 60	Cardiovascular disturbances
		History of:
		– trauma
		– tumor
		– infection
		– constitutional symptoms (feeling ill)
		– weight loss
		– laboratory abnormalities

Clinical Features of Thoracic Disk Prolapse

Patients often give a history of axial compression of the trunk, e. g., a fall on to the buttocks or bending forward and lifting a heavy object. On presentation, almost all patients complain of pain localized to the motion segment involved, which worsens when they cough or increase the intra-abdominal pressure. Spinal cord and nerve root manifestations may or may not be present.

A medial thoracic disk prolapse produces spinal cord manifestations of varying types, reflecting more or less severe **partial functional transection of the spinal cord.** These manifestations can include sensory impairment below the level of the lesion, bladder and bowel dysfunction, hyperreflexia, and gait impairment. In most patients, the disease first manifests itself with weakness in the legs along with local tenderness to pressure, and pain on movement, in the affected thoracic motion segment.

Intercostal Neuralgia

Band-like pain in a thoracic dermatome is usually the sole symptom of intercostal neuralgia. There may be a mild accompanying abnormality of algesia. It should be noted that the dermatomal borders are not as well defined on the thorax as on the limbs.

Release of stress and extension of the spine improve the symptoms of intercostal neuralgia, but increased mechanical stress and certain rotatory movements worsen them. This has obvious implications for treatment.

> **!** An important diagnostic criterion for the causation of intercostal neuralgia by degenerative changes is its positional dependence, just as we have already seen in cervical syndromes.

Differential Diagnosis

Thoracic disk syndromes being relatively rare, symptoms in this area are more likely to arouse suspicion of a disease of the internal organs or (in the case of spinal cord dysfunction) of a primary disorder of the nervous system. A thoracic disk protrusion or prolapse is often found only after the other suspected causes have been ruled out. Patients with a partial spinal cord transection syndrome are often first thought to have multiple sclerosis or a spinal cord tumor until the correct diagnosis is revealed by a myelogram or MRI and then confirmed at surgery.

10

Intercostal neuralgia has a number of different causes. The most common causes of segmentally radiating pain are **herpes zoster** and the postherpetic neuralgia that can follow it. The typical cutaneous vesicles usually reveal the diagnosis, although, as Mumenthaler et al. (1999) point out, there may be very little or no skin eruption in some cases ("herpes zoster sine herpete"), or the eruption may be hidden under the breast or in the inguinal crease. Herpes zoster begins with general symptoms such as fatigue, headache, and pain in the limbs; the typical herpetiform rash appears only 3–5 days later.

Segmental pain can also be produced if a costotransverse joint compresses the nerve root in the intervertebral foramen. So-called costotransverse joint syndrome is due to inflammatory changes, arthrosis, or abnormal positions of the costotransverse joints. The symptoms may arise spontaneously but are often due to rib spreading for thoracic surgery, rib fractures, etc. Costotransverse joint symptoms can include the following (Hohmann 1968, 1985):

- diffuse pain along the course of a rib, worse on forced, deep breathing, sometimes with a feeling of constriction around the chest
- sudden, lightning-like, painful arrest of respiration, combined with a feeling of being unable to breathe.

Infections, tumors, and dilated arteries of the chest wall (collateral circulation) are further possible causes of intercostal neuralgia. In the differential diagnosis of pain on the trunk, the physician must bear in mind the possibility of **referred pain from the internal organs** (pain referred into the *zones of Head*) and rule out the diseases that might produce it.

In **Tietze syndrome,** the parasternal costal cartilage is painful and swollen. Spontaneous pain or tenderness between the scapulae is not due to pathology of the thoracic motion segments. As explained in Chapter 9, this pain arises in the rhomboid muscles and is due to a **cervical syndrome.**

■ Treatment

As long as none of the spinal cord danger signs listed in **Table 10.1** are present, thoracic disk syndrome should be treated conservatively. The mechanical strain on the disks can be reduced by horizontal positioning. Heat application, by any technique, brings welcome relief by relaxing the reflexive tension of the thoracic musculature, particularly the paravertebral extensors of the trunk, and by promoting circulation. Paravertebral infiltrations with local anesthetic are given concomitantly.

Intractable pain due to thoracic nerve root irritation (intercostal neuralgia) can be treated with thoracic spinal nerve analgesia (TSPA) (**Fig. 10.2**). If the patient's pain is rather of the local or pseudoradicular type, due to pathology of the thoracic intervertebral and costotransverse joints, thoracic facet infiltration or costotransverse block may bring relief. Details of these injection techniques can be found in Theodoridis and Krämer (2006).

Definite manifestations of spinal cord compression require **operative treatment.** The level of the lesion is determined by CT and/or MRI. Endres et al. (2005) recommend CT-guided marking of the segment to be operated upon if its intraoperative localization is expected to be difficult.

The disk prolapse can be reached by various approaches. The complication rate in thoracic disk surgery is relatively high because of the proximity of the spinal cord (Hulme 1960, Carson et al. 1971, Dreyfus et al. 1972, Benson and Byrnes 1975, Rothman and Simeone 1982, Kretschmer 1989, Todd and Haddad 1991, Fessler 1998, Wilke 2000). The approaches that have been favored in recent years are the dorsolateral approach via costotransversectomy and the ventrolateral approach via thoracotomy (Gilsbach 1975, Schirmer 1985a, 1985b, Simpson et al. 1993, Regan et al. 1995, Stillerman et al. 1998, Isaacs et al. 2005, Ohnishi et al. 2005).

Summary

Degenerative diseases of the thoracic spine are essentially of three kinds:
- benign spondylosis and osteochondrosis in the ventral portion of the thoracic motion segments
- disk prolapse into the epidural space with and without clinical signs of spinal cord compression

- structural and functional disturbances of the intervertebral and costovertebral joints.

Degenerative changes of the thoracic spine may be quite impressive in plain radiographs, CT, and/or MRI, but clinical manifestations requiring treatment are rare. Be-

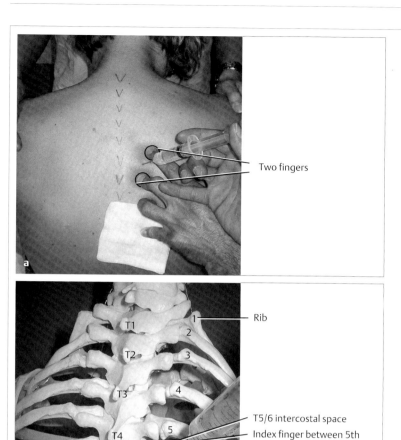

Fig. 10.2 a, b Injection therapy of the thoracic spine: thoracic spinal nerve analgesia.

Two fingers

Rib

T5/6 intercostal space
Index finger between 5th and 6th ribs
Right T6 transverse process
Middle finger between 6th and 7th ribs
T6/7 intercostal space
T7/8 intercostal space

10

cause of the favorable anatomical and biomechanical properties of the thoracic spine, even marked degenerative deformities are often asymptomatic. Yet, when a large thoracic disk prolapse compresses the spinal cord and causes weakness, surgical treatment is imperative. The transthoracic approach is currently preferred.

Most thoracic syndromes are due to degenerative changes of the form and function of the thoracic vertebrae and costovertebral joints, or to bony impingement on a thoracic spinal nerve in the intervertebral foramen. These syndromes can be treated conservatively, like the analogous syndromes in the lumbar spine. Manual diagnosis and therapy play the most important role. Local injections, including facet block, costotransverse block, and thoracic spinal nerve analgesia, have a high risk of

pneumothorax and should only be carried out by certified experts who specialize in these techniques and have a correspondingly large experience. Image guidance does not make these procedures any safer in inexperienced hands.

Nearly all thoracic syndromes, except disk prolapse with spinal cord compression, take a benign course and are self-limited.

Conclusion

Thoracic syndromes are rare, and they even more rarely require invasive treatment. Such treatments carry a high risk of complications.

11 Lumbar syndrome

■ Definition and Prevalence

> The term "lumbar syndrome" refers to disease manifestations caused by functional disturbances and degenerative changes of the lumbar motion segments.

These include local symptoms restricted to the lumbar spine (local lumbar syndrome) as well as pain radiating into the leg (lumbar root syndrome) and the symptoms and signs of deep, functionally transecting processes (cauda equina syndrome). The first two types of lumbar syndrome are very common.

> Nearly two-thirds of all cases of disk disease affect the lumbar spine.

One in 12 patients presenting to a general practitioner, and every third patient presenting to an orthopedic surgeon, seeks medical attention because of a lumbar syndrome. These figures include only the patients who need treatment. Not all patients with sciatica or exercise-related low back pain go to a physician. The overall prevalence of low back pain, and its relative prevalence as a fraction of all types of illness, are thus presumably much higher than these figures indicate.

Age and sex distribution. In general, lumbar spinal processes affect men somewhat more often than women. The predominance of the male sex is attributable not only to a greater degree of functional mechanical stress, but also to sex-specific factors that are not yet well understood.

Lumbar syndrome is not only an important medical entity but also has a considerable effect on society at large, both because of its high frequency and because it usually arises in middle age and thus strikes patients at the high point of their occupational productivity. The symptoms most often arise in the patient's late twenties and reach their highest age-related prevalence around age 40 (**Fig. 11.1**). This is also the age at which most operations for lumbar disk prolapses are required. As will be discussed in Chapter 12, the disks have a special biomechanical constellation at this age, in which the nucleus pulposus still has a high turgor pressure, but the mechanical resistance of the anulus fibrosus has already begun to decline. Because of these properties, centrally located disk tissue can become displaced outward. Further information on the point prevalence and the annual and lifetime prevalence of back pain (which can largely be equated with the epidemiology of lumbar syndromes) can be found in Chapter 3.

Etiology. The regularly observed statistical features of lumbar disk syndromes are few. Acute low back pain and sciatica often seems to develop spontaneously, without any recognizable external cause. The relationship between lumbar syndrome and heavy or light physical labor is discussed in Chapter 17. The incidence of certain other types of illness (e.g., ulcer disease) is known to vary seasonally; the incidence of lumbar syndrome is somewhat lower in the spring, but relatively constant at other times of the year.

> Symptoms arise largely because of the biochemical and biomechanical processes that occur autonomously within the disk tissue as part of the involutional process of normal aging.

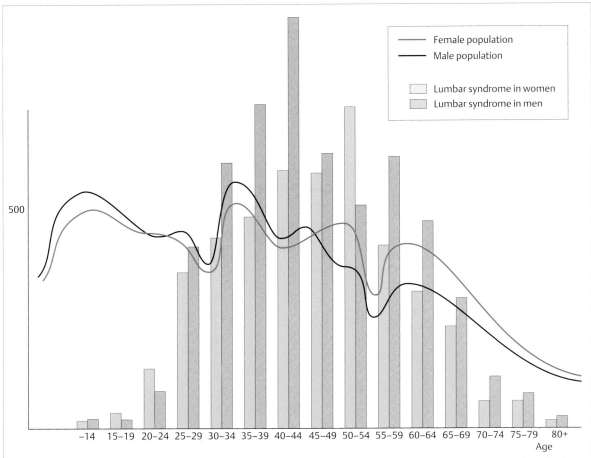

Fig. 11.1   The distribution by age and sex of outpatients treated for lumbar syndrome in Düsseldorf and Bochum (North Rhine-Westphalia, Germany) in comparison with the age distribution of the overall female and male population in the German state of North Rhine–Westphalia.

11

■ Special Anatomy of the Lumbar Motion Segments

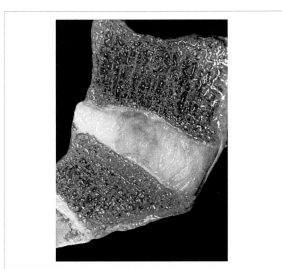

Fig. 11.2   Lumbosacral disk of an 18-year-old man.

Lumbar Disks

The lumbar spine generally has five freely mobile lumbar vertebral bodies, four lumbar intervertebral disks, and one disk each at the thoracolumbar and lumbosacral junctions. The lumbar disks increase in size from cranial to caudal, with the exception of the lowest (lumbosacral) intervertebral disk, which is about one-third thinner than the next disk above it. The biconvex shape of the disks is at its most pronounced in the lumbar region of the spine. The disks are higher ventrally than dorsally to an extent that depends on the degree of the lumbar lordosis. This ventral-to-dorsal difference is greatest in the lumbosacral (L5/S1) intervertebral disk, whose cross-section on a lateral image is trapezoidal in shape (**Fig. 11.2**).

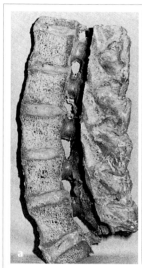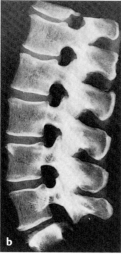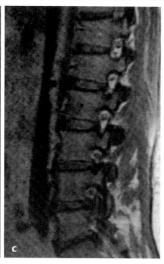

Fig. 11.3 a–c Lateral sagittal section through the lumbar spine.
a, b The intervertebral foramina are located at the level of the intervertebral disks.
c MRI: in the cranial portion of each intervertebral foramen, the exiting spinal nerve root can be seen in cross-section, appearing as a round dot.

Intervertebral Foramina

The **anatomical relationships** of the intervertebral disks and intervertebral foramina with the corresponding spinal nerve roots are of particular importance in the lumbar spine. As shown in **Fig. 11.3,** the intervertebral foramina are found at the level of the disk. The spinal ganglia and ventral roots lie more ventrally than in the thoracic region and are thus immediately adjacent to the disk. The bony border of the intervertebral foramen formed by the dorsolateral edge of the vertebra becomes more prominent superiorly, particularly in the upper portion of the intervertebral foramen, through which the nerve root travels. The caliber of the lumbar nerve roots increases as one moves caudally, with the L5 nerve roots being the thickest—approximately five times thicker than the L1 roots.

The intervertebral foramina of the lumbar spine are dorsally delimited by the facets of the intervertebral joints. The joint spaces of the L1–L4 joints are sagittally oriented, but the articular surfaces at the lumbosacral junction lie in the frontal plane, as in the thoracic spine. As a result, the lumbosacral intervertebral foramen is smaller than the rest. Variations and differences between the two sides are common. Changes at the joint facets and altered positions of the intervertebral joints can narrow the intervertebral foramen from its dorsal aspect.

! All of these anatomical properties create unfavorable initial conditions for the nerve roots of the lower lumbar motion segments. The roots are at risk of mechanical compression if the disk contour changes or if the vertebral bodies shift in position through slackening of the disks.

An increasing degree of importance is currently being ascribed to the **width of the lumbar spinal canal** in the frontal and sagittal planes as a contributing factor in the generation of low back pain and nerve root irritation. If the lumbar spinal canal is narrow, either congenitally or for an acquired cause, even a mild alteration of the contour of the intervertebral disks dorsally delimiting the canal can produce symptoms.

Ventral Epidural Space

The ventral epidural space is located between the posterior edge of the vertebral body and the dorsal border of the disk (forming the anterior border of the space) and the ventral dura mater (forming its posterior border). This space is divided into right and left compartments by connective tissue strands running between the dura mater and the vertebral body in the midline (Hofmann 1898). These midline connective tissue strands attached to the dural sac (also called the medial dural suspension) prevent the movement of large free disk fragments across the midline to the opposite side.

The ventral epidural space of the lumbar region, lying between the posterior edge of the vertebral body and the ventral dura mater, contains a thin peridural membrane that has veins running within it (Fick 1904, Dommisse 1974, Schellinger et al. 1990, Wiltse et al. 1993, Ludwig 2004). Extradiscal disk fragments (sequestra) can be displaced under this membrane; in such cases, discography reveals contrast medium occupying a round area in the epidural space, either cranial or caudal to the level of the disk, without any other epidural contrast medium. The MRI appearance is of a round shadow covered with a membrane. At operation, the surgeon

11

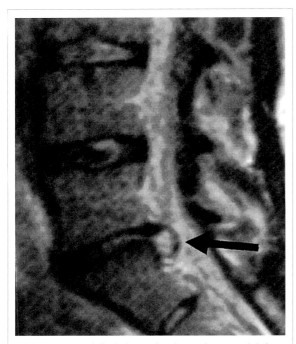

Fig. 11.4 A caudally dislocated, submembranous disk fragment (dislocation grade III) under the ventral epidural membrane (→).

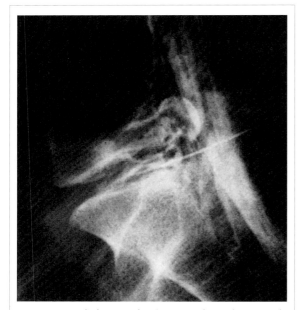

Fig. 11.5 Myelodiscography (i. e., myelography immediately followed by discography) at L5/S1. The discogram reveals a cranially displaced, submembranous fragment (dislocation grade III) that is still covered by a thin layer of tissue, the ventral epidural membrane. At surgery, a bean-sized fragment was found compressing the shoulder of the S1 root under the ventral epidural membrane. The membrane was easily perforated with a blunt dissector.

must open this membrane to gain access to the disk fragment (**Fig. 11.4**).

> **!** The medial dural suspension and the ventral epidural membrane determine the direction of displacement of lumbar disk prolapses as well as their clinical course and prognosis.

The space between the ventral epidural membrane and the posterior edge of the vertebral body is delimited medially by the relatively tightly adjacent posterior longitudinal ligament and laterally at infradiscal levels by the pedicle. At supradiscal levels its lateral boundary is formed by the adherence of the connective tissue layer to the vertebral body.

> **!** Submembranous disk fragments lie paramedially.

Hematomas can collect in the ventral epidural space and can be confused with submembranous disk fragments (Wiltse et al. 1993) (**Figs. 11.4, 11.5**).

Ligamentum Flavum

The *ligamentum flavum* (yellow ligament) is an important structure in disk surgery. It lines the posterior aspect of the spinal canal and runs from one vertebral arch to the next, spanning the intervertebral spaces. At surgery, it is easily separated from the vertebral arch and can then serve as an additional protective layer above the dura mater during a laminectomy or hemilaminectomy.

In the lumbar region, the ligamentum flavum has two layers (ventral and dorsal), which are separated by a cleft that can be demonstrated either during an anatomical dissection or at surgery. In a lateral (partial) flavectomy, the surgeon divides the dorsal layer of the ligamentum flavum sharply (i. e., with a scalpel) and the ventral layer bluntly (with a dissector) in order not to injure the dura mater, which lies beneath (Grifka et al. 1997, 1999).

The ligamentum flavum increases continually in thickness from the cervical spinal canal caudally. The ligamentum flavum and the interspinous ligaments help maintain the continuity of the posterior portions of the motion segment when the individual bends forward in maximum kyphosis or maintains an erect posture.

Venous System

The vessels of the vertebral **venous system** can also play a role in the generation or worsening of disk-related symptoms. The valveless veins of the spinal canal form an uninterrupted anastomotic chain running from the

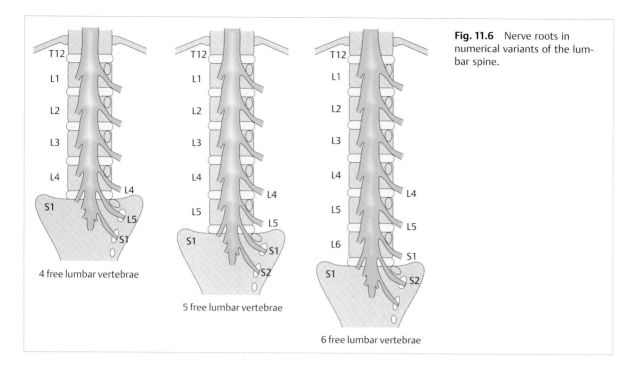

Fig. 11.6 Nerve roots in numerical variants of the lumbar spine.

4 free lumbar vertebrae

5 free lumbar vertebrae

6 free lumbar vertebrae

skull base to the sacrum. The degree of filling of the veins depends on the position of the body. The veins are tautly distended if the individual sits or lies prone. As our intraoperative measurements have shown, the degree of filling of the lumbar epidural veins depends on the central venous pressure (Ghazwinian and Krämer 1974). The degree of filling and the central venous pressure are lowest in the kneeling position. During lumbar disk surgery, the epidural venous plexus appears as a collection of flat strands containing only a small amount of blood; as a result, electrocoagulation is usually not necessary for hemostasis within the spinal canal. The studies of Clemens (1970) and Crock (1983, 1994, 2002) showed that the vertebral venous system not only plays a local role as the draining vasculature of the vertebral arches and the spinous and transverse processes, but also communicates with the interior of the skull by way of the emissary veins. The venous plexuses of the spine are also a venous pathway connecting the superior and inferior venae cavae. Together with the azygos system, they form a collateral venous circulation that operates beyond the local level, coming into play physiologically whenever the venous pressure is elevated in the thoracic, abdominal, or intracranial cavities—as when the individual coughs, sneezes, or presses. This partly explains why disk-related symptoms often worsen when these events occur.

! Elevations of pressure in the chest and abdomen worsen disk-related pain because they increase the degree of filling of the epidural veins.

Numerical Variations and Transitional Vertebrae

The clinical importance of malformations and developmental anomalies of the lumbar spine and their causative role in disk-related symptoms are generally overstated. Numerical variations are of practical clinical importance, e.g., in the designation and identification of segments. The number of ribless lumbar vertebrae above the sacrum should be counted. If there are only four, the term "sacralization" is often used; if there are six, "lumbarization." It is clear, however, that sacralization or lumbarization can only be determined from the enumeration of *all* vertebrae in a complete radiological image series. It is therefore preferable to avoid these terms and use only the designation "transitional vertebra." The numbering of the spinal nerve roots in numerical variations of the lumbar vertebrae is shown in **Fig. 11.6**. In such cases, one should count downward from L1—the first ribless vertebra—rather than upward from the sacrum. For example, if there are six free lumbar vertebral bodies, a disk prolapse between L5 and L6 produces an L1 syndrome. On the other hand, if there are only four free lumbar vertebrae, then a prolapse between the fourth vertebra and the sacrum usually produces an L5 syndrome.

11

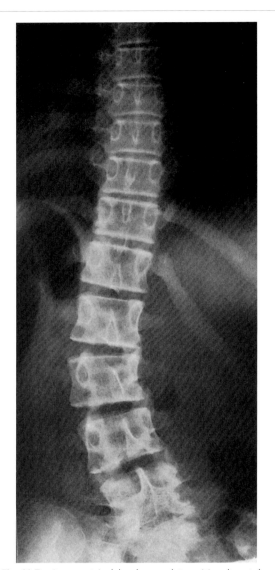

Fig. 11.7 Asymmetrical lumbosacral transitional vertebra in a 15-year-old girl with lumbar scoliosis.

! For the purposes of percutaneous intradiscal therapy or microsurgical discotomy, it is preferable to count the disks upward from the bottom, designating them (e. g.) as the last, second last, or third last vertebra (third vertebra from the bottom).
One should also be aware that rudimentary disks can appear differently in MRI and in plain radiographs.

Transitional vertebrae have characteristics of both of the neighboring regions. Lumbosacral transitional vertebrae may have free transverse processes, or they may be connected to the sacrum either rigidly or through joints. The intervertebral disk can take on many different transitional forms (**Fig. 11.7**).

As long as the transitional vertebra is symmetrical, having the same types of structures on both sides, no symptoms are to be expected. *Abnormal mechanical statics of the spine arise only when the transitional vertebra is asymmetrical,* e. g., when a free transverse process is present on one side and a rigid or articular connection to the sacrum is present on the other (**Fig. 11.7**). Asymmetrically shaped lateral masses of transitional vertebrae that have lumbosacral joints on both sides can also produce tilting of the transitional vertebra, resulting in a low-lying lumbar scoliosis. In such cases, the disks at higher levels are subject to an asymmetrical mechanical stress, by which they may become pathologically affected.

Topographical Relationships Between the Spinal Nerve Roots and Disks in the Lumbar Spinal Canal

The fact that most cases of lumbar root syndrome arise in the two lowest motion segments is due both to the high degree of mechanical stress affecting this region of the spine and to the close contact between the nerve roots and the disks at these levels. In the cervical spine, the clinically relevant degenerative processes take place mainly outside the spinal canal, but in the lumbar spine they much more frequently narrow the lumen of the spinal canal through dorsal disk protrusions and prolapses. The **lumbar spinal canal** is delimited ventrally by the vertebral bodies and disks and dorsally by the ligamentum flavum and vertebral arches (laminae). The lateral (articular) masses and intervertebral foramina are located laterally. The spinal canal is a cylinder whose shape and volume change with every movement of the trunk.

The contents of the lumbar spinal canal include the dural sac, the nerve roots, and the peridural tissues, which in turn consist of the veins and fat that surround the nerve roots. The nerve roots are thus protected from the bony borders of the spinal canal even in extreme movements of the lumbar spine.

The distance between spinal cord segments and their corresponding motion segments in the vertebral column is greatest in the lumbar spine. Because the spinal cord terminates at L1/L2, the spinal nerves, which exit the spinal canal at more caudal levels by way of their correspondingly numbered intervertebral foramina, must travel a considerable distance in the subarachnoid space. At levels below the conus medullaris, the nerve roots are mainly located laterally, so that they are generally not injured in the course of a medial lumbar puncture, myelography, or transdural disk puncture.

! Paramedian disk protrusions and prolapses can compress spinal nerves intrathecally and produce nerve root syndromes at lower levels than the level of the disk itself.

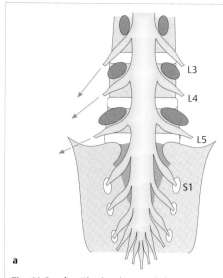

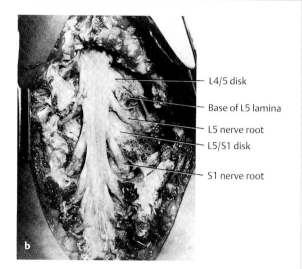

Fig. 11.8 a, b The lumbosacral dura mater and nerve roots and their topographical relationship to the disks.
a Schematic diagram.

b Dissection of the lumbosacral spine of a 32-year-old woman. The laminae have been removed as far laterally as possible (to the lateral masses).

The long caudal spinal nerves as they course through the lumbar spinal canal below L1/2, together with the filum terminale (the caudal continuation of the spinal cord, which extends to the second sacral vertebra), are known collectively as the cauda equina ("horse's tail").

The direction in which the **nerve roots** run after exiting the dural sac depends on the level of the segment. The further caudally the nerve root must travel to reach the corresponding intervertebral foramen, the more acute the angle it makes with the dural sac as it exits from it. It follows that the topographical relationship between the nerve root and the disk is different in each lumbar motion segment (**Fig. 11.8**). The origin of the L4 nerve root is found at the level of the L3 vertebral body. The L5 root, however, exits the dural sac at the level of the lower edge of the L4 vertebral body, and the S1 root at the lower edge of the L5 vertebral body. An L4/L5 disk prolapse generally impinges on the L5 nerve root. The L4 root is affected only if the prolapse is very large and laterally displaced, because the L4 root runs above the level of the intervertebral disk.

A lateral prolapse of the L5/S1 intervertebral disk can simultaneously impinge on the L5 and S1 nerve roots even if the prolapse is small. The L5 nerve root, as it passes through the upper portion of the L5/S1 intervertebral foramen, is immediately adjacent to the outer lamellae of the intervertebral disk. The root has very little freedom to move within the foramen. Only the lowest two lumbar nerve roots, which lie in the lowest two lumbar motion segments, are in direct contact with the corresponding intervertebral disks. It is here that the danger of compression by disk tissue is greatest.

Radiological/Surgical Subdivisions of the Lumbar Motion Segments

A topographical anatomical subdivision of the lumbar motion segments that takes the spatial relationships of the spinal nerves, disk, pedicles, and intervertebral foramina into account is a useful conceptual aid for the proper identification of anatomical structures and their pathological alterations in plain radiographs and CT and MR images, as well as for orientation in the operative field. The prognosis and clinical course of sciatica, too, depend not only on the size of a disk prolapse but also on its position in relation to its anatomical surroundings. Such spatial relationships are best assessed not just in the three conventional radiological anatomical planes—anteroposterior (frontal), lateral (sagittal), and transverse (horizontal, axial)—but also in a surgical anatomical perspective, with an oblique AP view of the spine. McCulloch (1989, 1998) analogized the motion segment to a three-storey house with the level of the disk constituting the first (lowest/most caudal), the infrapedicular level the second, and the level of the pedicles the third (highest/most cranial) storey. Wiltse et al. (1992) added a suprapedicular level to this subdivision. A subdivision with reference to the disk, rather than the pedicles, seems more practical, as the pedicles are not always precisely localizable in the operative field (Krämer 1995, Willburger et al. 2005).

11

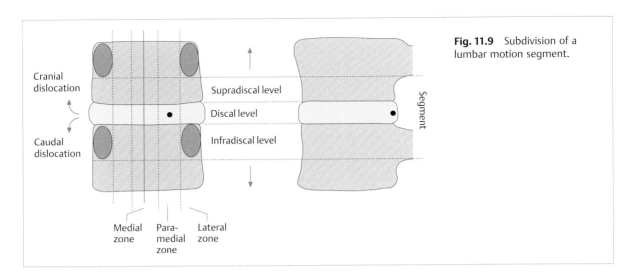

Fig. 11.9 Subdivision of a lumbar motion segment.

Frontal View (AP Projection)

The AP projection provides the best topographical overview of a lumbar motion segment. It also corresponds to the surgeon's view, albeit rotated by 90°. The successive transverse anatomical planes, from cranial to caudal, are called *levels*, and the successive sagittal planes, from medial to lateral, are called *zones* (**Fig. 11.9**).

Levels. The levels are defined from caudal to cranial in relation to the borders of the intervertebral space and the pedicles on the anterior wall of the spinal canal. Practically speaking, the intervertebral disk is the main orienting structure in radiology and disk surgery, because it is easy to identify both on radiological images and in the operative field.

- The **discal level** is delimited by the upper end plate of the vertebral body below the disk in question and by the lower end plate of the vertebral body above it.
- The **supradiscal level** is above the discal level and extends upward to the lower edge of the pedicles, i. e., to approximately the level of the middle of the upper vertebral body.
- The **infradiscal level** is below the discal level and extends downward to the lower edge of the pedicles of the lower vertebral body.

! A cranially dislocated fragment is supradiscal, and a caudally dislocated one is infradiscal.

Zones. The division of a lumbar segment as seen on a transverse radiological image (CT, MRI) into successive sagittal zones, from medial to lateral, differs depending on the craniocaudal level. At the **discal level,** the segment is divided into medial, paramedial, and lateral zones, without any further landmarks for orientation.

The medial zone has a right and a left half. The center of the paramedial zone corresponds to the central point of the interlaminar operative field after removal of the ligamentum flavum. All pathological findings in the immediate vicinity are described as paramedial, those nearer to the midline are medial and those further from the midline are lateral. The transition from the paramedial to the lateral zone is indicated by the medial border of the pedicles of the vertebral bodies above and below.

The same division is operative at **supra- and infradiscal levels.** The medial and paramedial parts of the vertebra lie between the pedicles, and the lateral part of the vertebra is the part lying lateral to the medial border of the pedicle. Thus, the pedicle itself and the infrapedicular zone corresponding to the upper portion of the intervertebral foramen lie in the lateral zone of the vertebra.

A disk herniation cannot lie in the lateral zone at the infradiscal level, because the lateral zone is occupied here by the pedicle. Lateral disk herniations at discal and supradiscal levels are located within the intervertebral foramen.

Frontal aspect, with roots. Myelography displays the dural sac and the roots exiting from it in a frontal view, projected over the vertebral bodies and disks. A similar view can be obtained by MRI. These views correspond to the view into the operative field at surgery.

In the lower lumbar motion segments, each root traverses an intervertebral disk before exiting the spinal canal through the intervertebral foramen under the pedicle of the segment below. Each lumbar interlaminar window contains two roots (**Fig. 11.10**):

- The **traversing** root lies in the paramedial zone at the discal level and is usually affected by paramedial disk prolapses and protrusions. The exiting root is found laterally, above (cranial to) the disk.
- The **exiting** nerve root is derived from the segment above and exits the spinal canal under the correspondingly numbered pedicle. Cranially dislocated

prolapses can compress the exiting root at the supradiscal (infrapedicular) level intraforaminally (i. e., in the lateral zone).

Extraforaminal prolapses are found further laterally at the discal and supradiscal levels.

Frontal view of the operative field. In a lumbar disk operation, the spine is seen lying transversely in front of the surgeon. After removing the ligamentum flavum laterally in the interlaminar window at either the L4/5 or the L5/S1 level, the surgeon encounters the **traversing** root and the paramedial zone of the intervertebral disk lying under it.

The **exiting** nerve root on either side lies craniolateral to the disk in the upper portion of the intervertebral foramen. This is where to look for cranially dislocated intraforaminal disk fragments; the intervertebral joint facets lying just above should be left undisturbed as much as possible. Disk fragments can migrate in practically any direction from the site where they perforate the anulus fibrosus in the paramedial zone of the disk.

! The exiting root always lies craniolateral to the disk.

For the purposes of description and documentation of radiological and intraoperative findings, not only the cardinal directions cranial, caudal, medial, and lateral but also the intermediate directions craniomedial, craniolateral, caudomedial, and caudolateral sheould be used. Directions can also be designated using clockface

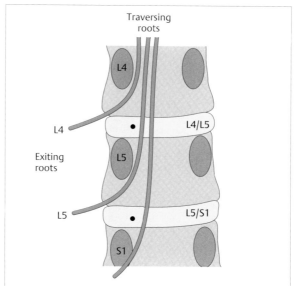

Fig. 11.10 Frontal view of lumbar motion segments, with roots.

notation (**Fig. 11.11**). In an operative report, not only the direction in which the disk fragment is located, but also its distance from the site of perforation should be mentioned.

! Most disk prolapses that require surgery migrate caudally (to the 9 o'clock position on the right side, or the 3 o'clock position on the left).

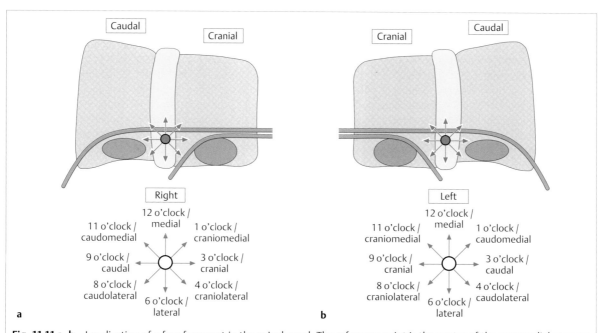

Fig. 11.11 a, b Localization of a free fragment in the spinal canal. The reference point is the center of the paramedial zone on the level of the disk.

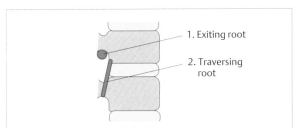

Fig. 11.12   Craniolateral displacement with compression of the exiting nerve root. Disk fragments lying at the level of the disk or displaced caudally to it impinge on the traversing nerve roots rather than the root that exits at that level.

The next most common direction of migration is cranial (to 3 or 9 o'clock). Craniolateral dislocation (to 4 or 8 o'clock), i. e., intraforaminal disk prolapse, is relatively rare, as is lateral prolapse (to 6 o'clock).

Even before surgery on a lumbar disk prolapse, the surgeon should know in which direction the spinal canal must be explored to find the fragment, to avoid opening the spinal canal any more widely than necessary. This important information is already visible on the CT or MRI scan.

Lateral View

Sagittal MRI sections give the best view of prolapsed disk tissue. The tissue may lie at the level of the disk, or else it may be cranially or caudally dislocated to a greater or lesser extent or lie behind the vertebral body. It is usually possible to tell from which disk the fragment originated (the "donor disk" or disk of origin). One can also determine the position of the disk fragment along the medial-to-lateral axis by viewing sagittal sections taken in different planes. Laterally and craniolaterally dislocated fragments lie within the foramen and compress the exiting root. Fragments that are dislocated in any other direction compress the traversing root (**Fig. 11.12**).

The lateral (sagittal) view is useful not only for prolapse localization, but also for **determination of the segment.** The radiographic image that is normally taken intraoperatively with a needle lying between two spinous processes must be correlated with the preoperatively obtained MR image showing the prolapse in order to

confirm that surgery is being carried out at the right level. Rudimentary and transitional disks look different in MRI than in a conventional lateral radiograph. Errors in counting can be avoided by using terms such as the "last" or "second last" disk, rather than "L5/S1," etc.

Overlapping laminae. The laminae cover the discal level to an extent that increases as one goes up the spine. This fact must be borne in mind when operating on the lumbar spine via an interlaminar approach, with a view of the spine from the side. Thus, while flavectomy at the L5/S1 level immediately exposes the level of the disk. Flavectomy exposes only the infradiscal level at L4/5 and even more so at L3/4, etc., so that that the discal level comes into view only after removal of the lower portion of the upper lamina (**Fig. 11.13**).

> **!** Cranially dislocated prolapses therefore often require removal of some of the lower portion of the upper lamina, or perhaps all of it (hemilaminectomy).

Transverse View

Transverse (axial, horizontal) sections of the lumbar motion segments are obtained by CT or MRI (**Fig. 11.14**). One can determine the level of any section from the sequential alternation of disks and vertebral bodies (or of pedicles and intervertebral foramina) across the series of transverse sections; reference to a lateral scout view ("topogram") is thus not necessary. The remaining posterior elements—joints, spinous processes, and transverse processes—have highly variable shapes and add nothing to segment localization except confusion. The two sides of a transverse section look different in the presence of scoliosis or if the section is improperly aligned (i. e., not really transverse).

A transverse section at the discal level displays the disk, possibly accompanied by partially sectioned portions of the upper and lower vertebral body end plates, as well as the intervertebral foramen. At the supradiscal level, the vertebral body and foramen are seen next to each other; an infradiscal section shows the vertebral body and the pedicle, but not the foramen.

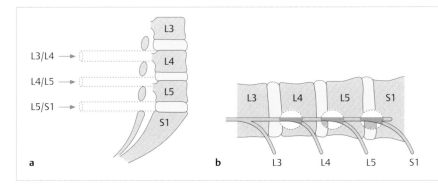

Fig. 11.13 a, b   A schematic view of the operative field in the interlaminar window at each of the lower lumbar motion segments. The level of the disk space is located between the laminae only in the L5/S1 segment. In successively higher segments, the lower edge of the upper lamina overlaps to an increasing extent with the level of the disk space.

At the supradiscal level, the exiting roots are seen laterally and the traversing roots are seen paramedially. The exiting roots are usually cut obliquely. Intraforaminal disk prolapses lie in the vicinity of the exiting roots and can be mistaken for them (the exiting roots, too, can be mistaken for disk prolapses).

At the infradiscal level, one sees the vertebral body and its continuous extension in the posterior arch (the pedicles and lamina). The lateral recess is found at the infradiscal level at the same position where one finds the intervertebral foramen at the discal and supradiscal levels. The lateral recess contains the traversing root next to the correspondingly numbered pedicle, e. g., the lateral recess of L5 contains the L5 root.

The division of the transverse sections at different levels into zones is the same as that described above for the frontal view (**Fig. 11.15**). The center of the paramedial zone is located between the midline and the lateral border of the disk and usually corresponds to the center of the operative field in the interlaminar approach. The medial edge of the pedicle, as seen in an infradiscal sec-

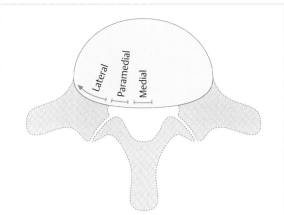

Fig. 11.14 Schematic view of a lumbar vertebral body and disk seen transversely, as in a CT or MRI scan.

tion (which contains the pedicle), defines the border of the lateral zone. Medial prolapses and protrusions can be more pronounced on either the right or the left side.

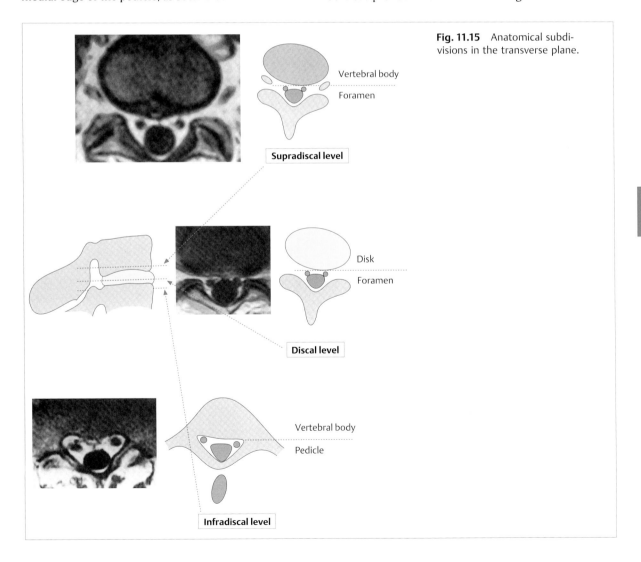

Fig. 11.15 Anatomical subdivisions in the transverse plane.

▮ Special Biomechanics of the Lumbar Spine

(H. J. Wilke)

Mechanical Stress on the Lumbar Disks

Beyond the general biomechanical properties of motion segments that were discussed earlier in Chapter 4, the lumbar spine has a number of special properties that are relevant to the causation of disk disease and to its prevention.

The human upright stance puts great stress on the lower spinal segments in particular. At these levels, the weight of the entire body above must be carried on a surface with an area of only a few square centimeters. Moreover, when the upper body deviates from the midline, the mechanical stress is multiplied many times over.

There are many ways of measuring the mechanical stress on the spine in different postures and when an individual lifts or carries heavy loads. Quantification is rendered difficult by the general impossibility of putting a measuring instrument directly into the spine in a living individual. Usually, therefore, we must resort to theoretical models or indirect measurements for most information of this type. Analytical models are used to determine the overall stress on the spine by calculating all of the individual forces that are placed upon it (**Fig. 11.16**). Stress on the spine is a complex matter, as the spine does diverse tasks and has a complicated mechanical structure. Muscles must exert force to counteract the forces acting upon the spine and keep the body mechanically stable.

These forces are the result of a complex interaction of many different muscle groups and individual muscle fibers acting in response to body position, movement, or the externally applied forces mentioned above. The degree of mechanical stress on the spine varies highly among individuals, depending on age, sex, stature, and physical condition. Further forces are said to be exerted on the spine by intra-abdominal pressure and muscle contraction (Grew 1980, Hemborg and Moritz 1980, Nachemson et al. 1986), yet the magnitude of such forces is unknown, nor is there even any consensus regarding their sign, i. e., whether they tend to compress or to distract the spine. It can be assumed that the complex structure of the normal spine is capable of providing adequate stability to the individual motion segments and to the spine as a functional unit, and thus of fulfilling its main tasks optimally, under physiological conditions. Injury, disease, or degeneration of part of the spine can, however, impair its stability.

The following sections outline the main methods of determining the stresses affecting the spine and present their advantages and disadvantages.

Methods of Measuring Stress on the Lumbar Motion Segments

Mathematical Models

Theoretical models provide a simple, analytic approach toward an initial rough estimation of the biomechanical condition of the spine under static or dynamic stress (Schultz and Anderson 1981, McGill 1992). Extensive calculations have been carried out using computer simulation models (Chaffin 1969, 1988; Nussbaum and Chaffin 1996, Parniapour et al. 1997). Finite element models can be used to obtain further information on specific parameters such as deformation, stretching or pressure in individual components of the motion segment (Shirazi 1991, Goel et al. 1993, Wang et al. 2000, Zander et al. 2001) (**Fig. 11.17**).

The complex overall system, with all of its individual components, can be modeled only in a simplified fashion because of the limitations of computing capacity. The input parameters of computational models must include anatomical, biomechanical, and biological data and materials constants; not all of these parameters can be adequately measured or estimated by other methods, and therefore not all of the inputs to computational

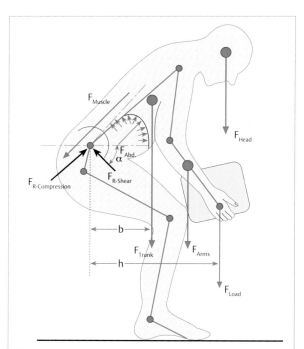

Fig. 11.16 Analytical models: forces determining the mechanical stress on the spine (including the force F resulting from the abdominal pressure P and the resulting reactive forces) (from Wilke 2004).

models can be considered reliable. The validity of such models, then, is limited by the simplifications and assumptions that they incorporate. The results of computation should always be checked against experimentally measured findings (**Fig. 11.18**).

In-Vitro Studies

In-vitro studies on anatomical specimens offer the opportunity to place measuring devices directly on to or into real structural components of the spine. Components such as the disk, the ligaments, or the vertebral body itself can be studied in isolation or as a functional unit. Thus, for example, the biophysical properties of a component of the spine can be tested in vitro to determine the maximum stress that it can tolerate. Moreover, special experimental apparatus can be used for the in-vitro study of the behavior of spinal component structures under well-defined conditions of stress. For example, the intradiscal pressure, stretching of ligaments, stress on an artificial implant, or movement of individual segments can be analyzed (Wilke et al. 1994, 1995, 1996).

In-Vivo Studies

In-vivo studies are done under much more realistic conditions, but they are feasible only to a limited extent, not just because of the greater technical difficulty of making measurements in the living organism, but above all for ethical reasons. In-vivo measurements in animals are of questionable applicability to humans, because the stresses on the spine in quadrupeds and bipeds are markedly different.

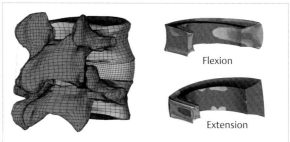

Fig. 11.17 An illustration of a finite-element calculation from our own research group. Left: complete model of an L4/L5 spinal segment, posterolateral view. Right: mid-sagittal section through the anulus. Comparison of the degrees of stretch in flexion and extension (from Wilke 2004).

Electromyography (EMG) provides information on individual muscle activity and also, if the experimental setup is held constant from muscle to muscle, a rough picture of the distribution of activity among different muscles. The surface electrodes that are usually used can yield no information about deeper muscles. Thin needle electrodes inserted deeply into the muscle yield direct information about the local situation at the site of the needle tip; thus, these electrodes, though much less commonly used in practice, are also much more informative. Andersson et al. (1974) reported the findings of intradiscal pressure measurements, some of which were made simultaneously with EMG. Unfortunately, it remains impossible to infer absolute muscle strength from the EMG data alone. This task requires more com-

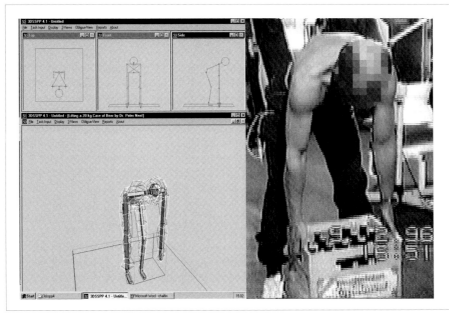

Fig. 11.18 Mathematical models such as the 3-D static model of Chaffin et al. at the University of Michigan (left) can be checked against disk pressure measurements obtained in vivo in certain body positions (right) (from Wilke 2004).

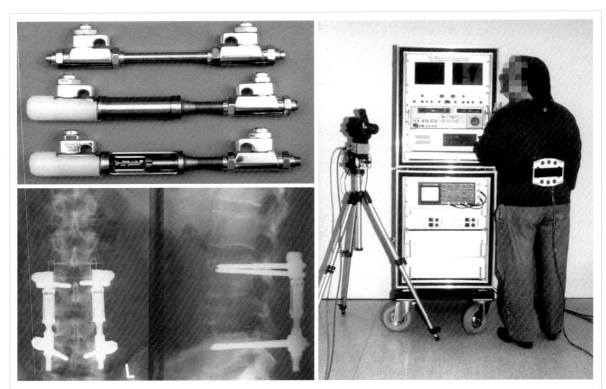

Fig. 11.19 Stress measurements with an internal fixator fitted with a measuring instrument. Within the measuring component, there are six load sensors consisting of semiconductor extension-measuring strips. A flat coil and a small receiver antenna were fastened to the patient's back for the measurement. When the fixator was removed as usual after solidification of the fusion, the measuring system was removed with it.

plex optimization algorithms, whose validity is still a matter of hypothesis (Parniapour et al. 1997). In any case, it has been conclusively shown with this method that a kyphotic sitting position requires less muscle activity then a consciously effected lordosis (Dolan et al. 1988, Betz et al. 2001).

Measurements with Instrumented Implants

Biomechanical measurements can be made indirectly in vivo with the aid of measuring devices located in implanted material, such as the implants used in fusion operations on the lower lumbar spine. These implants, when properly equipped, serve as measuring instruments in themselves. Such methods can be used only in a limited number of cases because of the enormous experimental effort required and the high demands that they place on the patient's readiness to cooperate. Measurements of this type on external fixators provided the first demonstration that these implants are not under any greater stress during sitting than during standing (Wilke et al. 1992). The experimental set-up was taken a step further with the fitting of measuring instruments on *internal* fixators (Rohlmann et al. 1999, 2000, 2001) (**Fig. 11.19**).

Rohlmann et al. (2004) report the measured stresses in the internal fixators of 10 patients in various bodily positions and during the performance of various activities. The stresses that were measured in the sitting position were approximately 10% lower than during standing and very much lower than during walking. The type of furniture that the patients sat on (stool, office chair, exercise ball, kneeling stool) made little difference with respect to stress. Office chairs with a backrest that could be inclined backward led to less stress on the implants than conventional office chairs. A comparison of the measured implant stresses with the intradiscal pressures measured in one of the experimental subjects revealed close agreement between these two variables for many activities, as long as the measured value of each variable in the standing position was used as a reference.

Intradiscal Pressure Measurements

The most reliable in-vivo data are derived from intradiscal pressure measurements of the type first reported by Nachemson and colleagues (Nachemson and Morris 1964, Nachemson 1966, Nachemson and Elfstrom 1970, Nachemson et al. 1986). These investigators inserted a needle with an integrated pressure-sensitive polyethylene membrane into the disk space and connected it to a measuring instrument employing the nanometer principle. The intradiscal pressure was usually measured in the L3/4 disk. The results were normalized to the intradiscal pressure in each subject while standing (which was assigned the value 100%). These measurements showed a marked increase of intradiscal pressure, by about 50%, when the subjects bent forward. If they additionally held weights in their hands, the pressure rose by a further 70–220% of the reference value.

These investigators obtained similar results with respect to the sitting position. Here, too, the intradiscal pressure was raised by forward bending, and even more so by holding additional weights in the hands. Pressure measurements in these positions were approximately 40% higher than during standing. Tensing the abdominal muscles (pressing) causes part of the weight of the upper body to be transferred from the chest cage to the pelvis by way of the abdominal air and fluid "balloon." The intra-abdominal pressure may rise as high as 140 mmHg (19 kPa) (Bartelink 1957, Eie 1962). Abdominal pressure maneuvers or an orthosis with abdominal support can reduce stress on the lumbar disks by about 30%.

More recent studies on disk stress in the lower lumbar motion segments have replicated Nachemson's measurements with updated measuring techniques and extended them to further positions and movements of the spine (Wilke et al. 1998, 1999, 2001, 2004). The intradiscal pressure was measured with a flexible pressure gauge with a constant diameter of 1.5 mm that was surgically inserted directly into the nucleus pulposus of the L4/5 disk under sterile conditions (**Figs. 11.20, 11.21**). Signals were transmitted through a wireless connection to a computer in order to allow the subjects full freedom of movement. Over a period of 24 h, pressures were measured during the following positions and movements, among others: various lying positions, sitting positions on a normal chair, in an armchair, and on an exercise ball (also called a gym ball, Swiss ball, or Pezzi ball), sneezing, laughing, walking, climbing stairs, lifting weights. The pressure changes taking place overnight because of hydration of the disks in the lying position was measured over a 7 h period.

The first measurements were made while the subjects were still on the operating table. When the subjects lay supine in a relaxed way with mildly flexed legs (ca. 20°), the lowest pressure values of all were measured, ca. 0.08 MPa (0.1 MPa = 1 bar). The pressure could not be reduced any further by using a knee roll or by having the patient lie in the step position. When the legs were extended, the pressure rose to 0.11 MPa; rotation into the lateral position raised the pressure only by a further 0.1 MPa, to 0.12 MPa. The intradiscal pressure in the prone position was intermediate between those measured in the supine and lateral positions, 0.11 MPa.

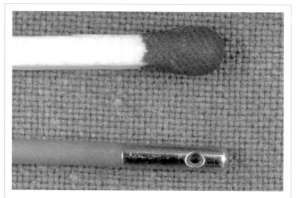

Fig. 11.20 Pressure sensor for intradiscal pressure measurements. The metal sheath, 7 mm long and 1.5 mm in diameter, was placed in the center of the nucleus pulposus of the L4/5 intervertebral disk.

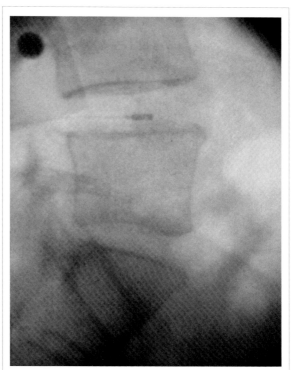

Fig. 11.21 Lateral plain radiograph of the pressure sensor after implantation at L4/5.

Sitting up from the prone position into the reading position by extending the back and propping the upper body up with the forearms doubled the pressure to 0.25 MPa. The turning maneuver itself (e. g., from supine to lateral) produced pressure spikes up to 0.8 MPa in magnitude. Coughing while supine produced pressures as high as 0.38 MPa, but hearty laughing raised the pressure only to 0.15 MPa.

11

11

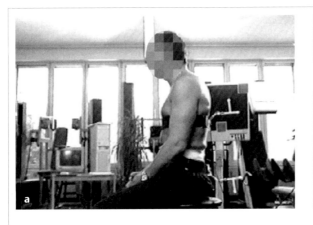
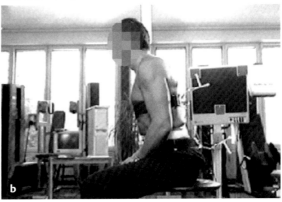
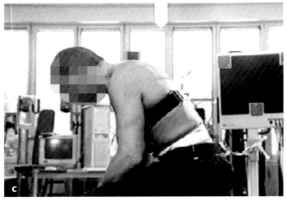
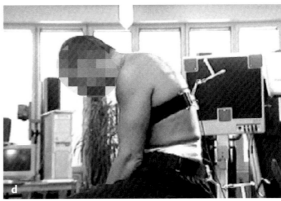
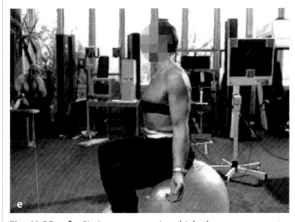
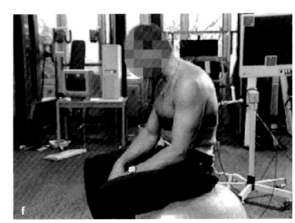

Fig. 11.22 a–f Sitting postures in which the arms are not supported on armrests (from Wilke 2004).
a Relaxed upright sitting: 0.45 MPa.
b Upright sitting, leaning forward: 0.63 MPa.
c Forward flexion with elbows on thighs: 0.43 MPa.
d Flexed, sitting upright: 0.90 MPa.
e Sitting on a Pezzi ball with straight back: 0.50 MPa.
f Sitting on a Pezzi ball with flexed back: 0.65 MPa.

Fig. 11.23 a–h Sitting postures in an armchair (from Wilke 2004).
a Relaxed upright sitting with supported back: 0.33 MPa.
b Stress-reducing sitting position (relaxed sitting): 0.27 MPa.
c Stress-reducing sitting position (relaxed sitting) with supported, extended legs: 0.38 MPa.
d Stress-reducing sitting position with arms folded across the chest: 0.36 MPa.
e Relaxed sitting without backrest (intermediate sitting position): 0.44 MPa. ▷
f Sitting in actively upright position (intermediate sitting position): 0.55 MPa.
g Relaxed standing: 0.48 MPa.
h Supporting the upper body, e. g., while standing up from a chair (bar supports): 0.10 MPa.

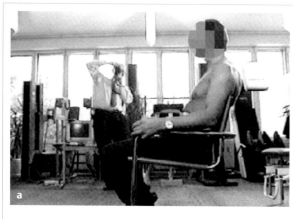
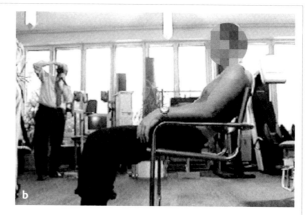
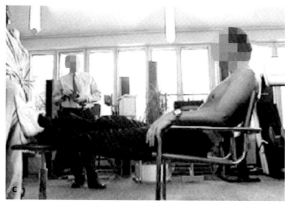
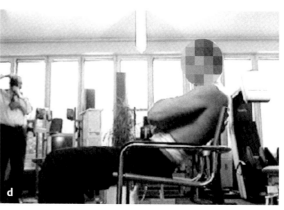
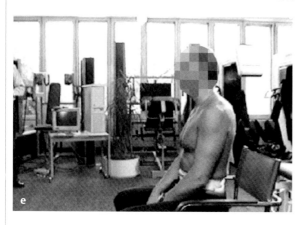
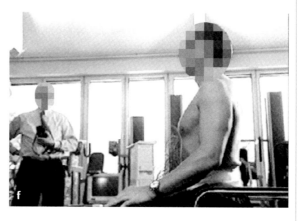
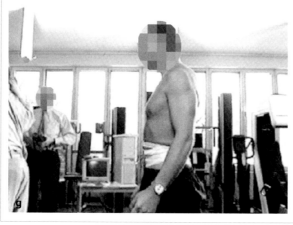
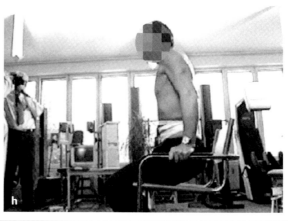

11

In relaxed standing, the pressure lay reproducibly between 0.48 and 0.5 MPa. Abdominal pressing raised it to 0.92 MPa and marked forward bending to 1.1 MPa.

In sitting, the pressure varied markedly depending on the degree of support from the back- or armrests (**Figs. 11.22, 11.23**). Sitting on a chair with a normal, straight back produced a pressure of 0.45–0.5 MPa. Active extension of the lumbar spine raised the pressure to 0.55 MPa. In the sitting position, too, forward bending produced a continual increase in pressure up to a maximum value of 0.83 MPa in maximal flexion, e. g., while tying shoelaces. Pressure in the sitting position could be markedly reduced by leaning back comfortably in an armchair. Relaxed reclining brought the pressure as low as 0.27 MPa.

In walking, the intradiscal pressure was measured at values between 0.53 and 0.65 MPa. The difference between slow and fast walking, or between walking in tennis shoes or barefoot, was small. In jogging, the pressure oscillated between 0.35 and 0.95 MPa. Jogging in tennis shoes lowered the pressure spikes by only a small amount, to 0.85 MPa.

The highest pressure values of all (2.3 MPa) were measured during biomechanically incorrect lifting of a full case of beer weighing 19.8 kg. Incorrect lifting in this case involved a rounded back and straight knees, rather than the correct method of keeping the back straight and bending at the hip and knee, as is taught in back school; correct lifting reduced the peak pressure during lifting to 1.7 MPa. When the case was held against the body at chest height, the pressure was 1.1 MPa; when it was held at the same height but at arm's length (ca. 60 cm) from the upper body, the pressure was 1.8 MPa (**Fig. 11.24**).

Conclusions. The findings of these more recent studies agreed with the results of Nachemson et al. (1964) with respect to the pressure values during standing, lying, lifting, and carrying. In particular, the pressure differences between lifting with a straight back and flexed knees vs. a rounded back and extended knees were reproduced with the newer methods. These important results of the older and newer studies measuring intradiscal pressure confirm rules 2 and 3 of back school (see **Table 14.1**): keep the back straight and kneel to lift. Incorrect lifting of a heavy weight, such as a 20 kg case of

beer, with rounded back and straight knees raised the intradiscal pressure to 450% of its initial value in the newer studies. This very high value was not matched even during trampolining. If the case was held correctly, however, with flexed knees and a straight back, as taught in back school, the intradiscal pressure rose only to 340% of its initial value. Finally, when the case, after being lifted, was held as close as possible to the body and the subject assumed a mildly lordotic posture, the pressure was only 200% of the value in normal standing.

On the other hand, the marked pressure differences that Nachemson et al. (1964) found in standing vs. sitting, or in lying in different positions, were not confirmed in the more recent studies. It could not be confirmed, for example, that comfortable (relaxed) sitting actually raises the intradiscal pressure by 40%. The current studies show rather that sitting in this position lowers the pressure by 10%; this could be demonstrated both with high-precision stadiometric measurements and with instrumented internal fixators (Rohlmann et al. 2000). The earlier finding that the intradiscal pressure was three times as high in the lateral decubitus position as in the supine position could not be replicated either; the current studies show only a small difference.

The new findings on the relaxed sitting position are of great importance. Relaxed sitting with diagonal positioning of the back and "deposition" of the upper body on the backrest lowers pressure markedly, and the subject also feels this reduction of pressure to be comfortable. As soon as the subject rose from the relaxed sitting position to the upright position, there was a marked increase of pressure in the lumbar disk (**Fig. 11.25**). Thus, even while seated, the individual can improve diffusion, and thus the nutritive process, within the intervertebral disks by regularly alternating between the upright and relaxed sitting positions (**Fig. 11.26**).

The differences between the newer measurements and those of Nachemson et al. (1964) are probably due to the different measuring techniques. Nachemson et al. (1964) integrated their measuring devices into a stiff cannula that could be bent, e. g., by muscle tension or displacement, which might have given rise to false signals and thus to incorrect measured values. The pressure gauges that are currently used cannot be bent out

---

Fig. 11.24 a–h Intradiscal pressure measurements during lifting and carrying (from Wilke 2004).

a Lifting a case of beer according to the rules of back training: straight back, bent hip and knee joints, case directly in front of body: 1.7 MPa.

b "Wrong" lifting of a case of beer: rounded back, extended knee joints, case far out in front of the truncal axis: 2.3 MPa.

c Gymnastic exercise with rounded back and extended knee: 1.6 MPa.

d Holding and carrying a case of beer next to the trunk with ▷ straight back: 1.0 MPa.

e Holding and carrying a case of beer about 60 cm in front of the trunk: 1.8 MPa.

f Carrying a case of beer with one arm: 1.0 MPa.

g Lifting two cases of beer, one with each arm: 2.1 MPa.

h Carrying two cases of beer: 0.9 MPa.

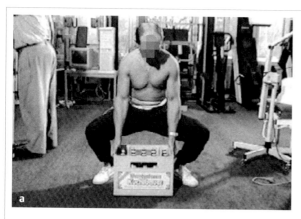

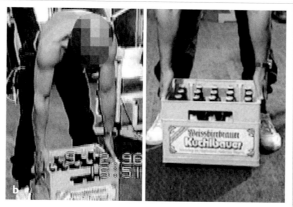

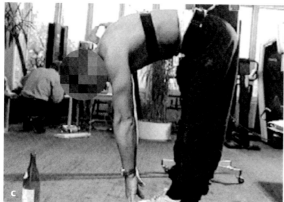

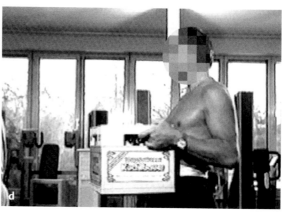

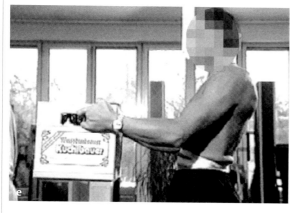

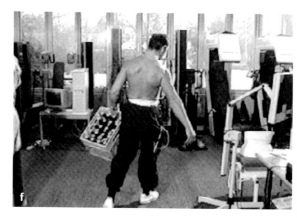

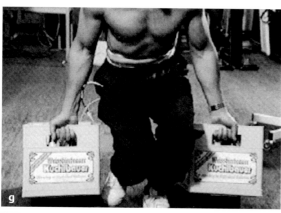

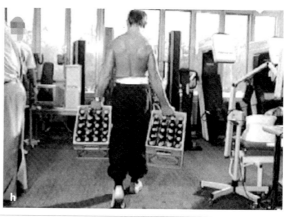

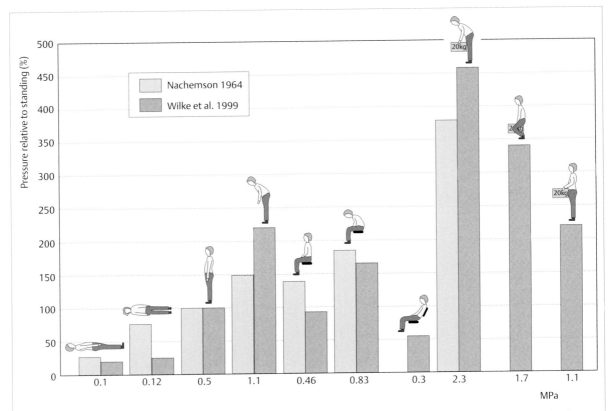

Fig. 11.25 Comparison of disk pressure measurements by Nachemson et al. (1964) with those of Wilke et al. (1992–2001). The absolute pressure values shown below the bars are from the newer measurements. The relaxed sitting position with reclined backrest, in which part of the weight of the upper body is supported by the backrest, yields a lumbar intradiscal pressure of 0.3 MPa and is thus associated with a significant reduction of stress on the lumbar disks. The low pressure allows fluid uptake into the disk even during sitting (see Chapter 4) (from Wilke 2004).

of shape, because they are flexible along their entire length. The only nonflexible element is the 7 mm metal tip, which, after implantation, is located completely within the nucleus pulposus, where it is exposed to hydrostatic and therefore equally distributed pressure. The new findings are confirmed by their excellent agreement with measurements made on external fixator implants (Wilke et al. 1992) and stadiometric measurements (van Deursen 2001).

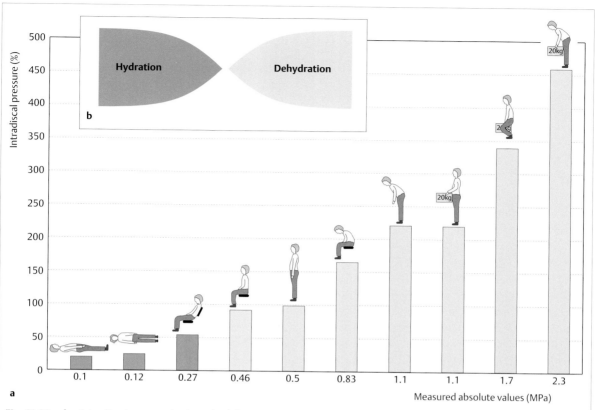

Fig. 11.26 a, b Intradiscal pressure in the L4/5 disk in various bodily positions (Wilke 20004) (**a**) and pressure-dependent fluid shifts at the edge of the disk (Krämer 1997) (**b**).

■ Special Pathological Anatomy and Pathophysiology

Protrusions and Prolapses

Terminology and Classification

The terms used in clinical practice should be well defined in order to convey precise information about the pathological anatomical changes that are present in so-called disk prolapse or disk herniation. Is the finding a bulging disk whose anulus fibrosus is still intact, or is it a prolapse with a free fragment of disk tissue lying outside the disk space? A wide variety of transitional states can occur, ranging from an intradiscal displacement of tissue to free sequestration of disk tissue in the spinal canal.

The current consensus in German-speaking countries is to use the terms *Protrusion* (protrusion) and *Prolaps* (prolapse), following the recommendation of the Working Group (now called the Section) on Degenerative Spinal Diseases of the German Society for Orthopedics and Orthopedic Surgery (Krämer 1983, Pharmaceuticals Commission of the German Medical Asso-

ciation 2006). These terms are used in the manner described in the relevant literature: DePalma and Rothman (1970), Rothman and Simeone (1982), Crock (1983), McCulloch (1989, 1998), Farfan (1996), Postacchini (1998), Nachemson and Jonsson (2000), Fardon (2001), Bendix (2004), Borenstein et al. (2004), Pearson et al. (2008).

Protrusion

A disk **protrusion** is a bulging of a disk whose anulus fibrosus is more or less well preserved. A disk **prolapse** is a disk herniation with perforation of the anulus fibrosus. Even in the case of a prolapse perforating the anulus fibrosus, the disk material outside the anulus may still be enclosed in a thin membrane. In the case of a disk protrusion, in which the disk tissue is displaced within the disk, the fibrous ring around it is largely intact (grade I or II dislocation) (see **Fig. 11.31**). Intradiscally injected contrast medium remains within the disk and

11

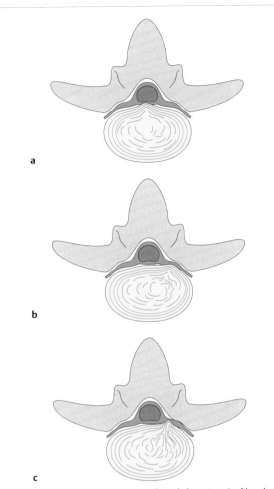

Fig. 11.27 a–c Protrusions (grade II dislocations) of lumbar disks. The anulus fibrosus is intact. There is a possibility for the displaced tissue to return to the center of the disk.
a Medial protrusion: lumbago.
b, c Paramedial protrusion: protrusion sciatica.

contrast medium is injected into the disk (discography), it fills the space occupied by the prolapsed tissue, which sometimes extends to supra- or infradiscal levels.

The disk tissue that lies outside the disk space, but remains covered, still remains in communication with the intervertebral space by way of its path of exit and is therefore in an exceptional situation from the biochemical point of view as well. The displaced disk tissue remains a part of the osmotic system of the intervertebral disk, i.e., it is still nourished by diffusion by way of the pressure-dependent fluid shifts within the disk. This tissue, therefore, does not shrink as rapidly as a fragment lying freely within the spinal canal, which is exposed to the enzymatic activity of the lymphatic fluid, among other influences. Furthermore, the still-covered disk tissue outside the intervertebral space continues to participate in the normal fluctuations of consistency and volume affecting the disk.

As long as there is still a strong layer of anulus fibrosus over the disk protrusion, the protruding tissue may still be able to find its way back into the center of the disk (unless it is a so-called incarcerated fragment). This possibility is exploited by a number of therapeutic techniques, e.g., traction, step positioning and movement therapy.

A distinction must be drawn between disk protrusion through outward displacement of the centrally located, mobile disk tissue and simple outward bulging of the anulus fibrosus in a totally degenerated disk (**Fig. 11.28**).

Anulus fibrosus bulges of this type are often found at multiple segmental levels simultaneously and become more pronounced with axial loading and backward bending. They play a role in the narrowing of the spinal canal in lumbar spinal stenosis, particularly when they are located at the level of the upper edge of the ascending facet.

does not flow into the epidural space. A protrusion (bulging) in this sense corresponds to the usual Anglo-American terms, "contained" or "bulging" disk (**Fig. 11.27**). Farfan (1996) calls it "intradiscal loose islands of disk material."

A *covered* prolapse (grade III dislocation, see **Fig. 11.31**) is one in which the displaced disk tissue has perforated the anulus fibrosus but is still covered by a thin membrane, the so-called ventral epidural membrane (Ludwig 2004). Fragments that find their way under this membrane or under part of the posterior longitudinal ligament, which becomes thinner laterally, are called submembranous or subligamentous sequestra (fragments) and correspond to the covered perforations found at surgery. The term "herniation" can also be used correctly in this situation, because the displaced tissue is still covered by a tissue layer. When

Prolapse

A disk prolapse involves complete perforation of the anulus fibrosus and the ventral epidural membrane. The dislocated disk tissue lies more or less free within the spinal epidural space; the perforation is no longer covered. Intradiscally injected contrast medium flows into the epidural space and distributes itself within it. The intraspinal fragment may still be contiguous with the disk (grade IV dislocation) and thus be located "half inside and half outside." A free fragment (grade V dislocation) lies free in the epidural space and has no connection to the disk.

Once it has perforated the posterior border of the disk, the dislocated disk tissue can travel in any direction. In general, the prolapsed material migrates laterally and caudally along the nerve root, compressing it from the ventral side. The root is thereby raised and pressed against the posterior wall of the spinal canal

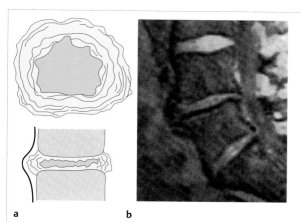

Fig. 11.28 a, b Rolling-out of the anulus fibrosus due to narrowing of the intervertebral space because of disk degeneration or surgical removal of the disk. The protruding tissue is the anulus fibrosus.

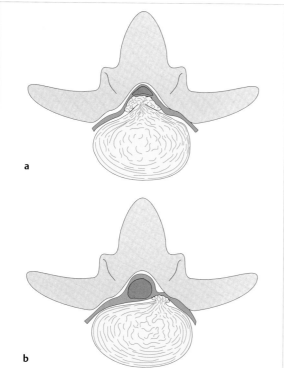

Fig. 11.29 a, b Medial and paramedial herniation (grade IV dislocation) of a lumbar disk. The anulus fibrosus is perforated. The displaced tissue cannot return to the center of the disk.
a Medial prolapse: cauda equina syndrome.
b Paramedial and lateral prolapse: prolapse sciatica.

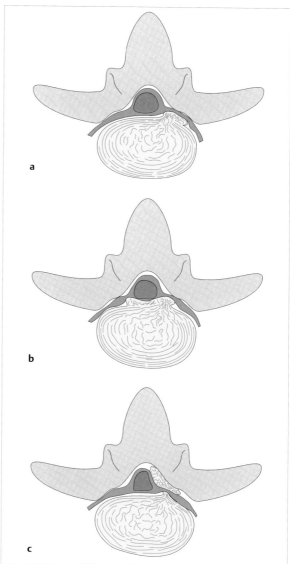

Fig. 11.30 a–c Different directions in which prolapsed disk tissue can migrate (grade V dislocation) at a single level.
a Laterally, with compression of the nerve root in the intervertebral foramen.
b Medially, with bilateral sciatica.
c Dorsally, with dorsolateral compression of the cauda equina.

(lamina, ligamentum flavum). The prolapsed tissue can also migrate cranially or further caudally to compress a nerve root at an adjacent level.

Every large operative series contains not just standard situations like these, but exceptional cases as well. If the prolapsed material migrates medially, the contralateral nerve root can be compressed: sciatica on alternating sides is the result (**Fig. 11.29**). The material can also migrate around the dura mater to compress the

11

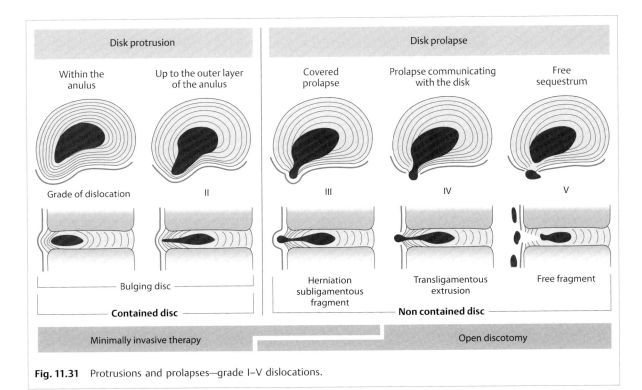

Fig. 11.31   Protrusions and prolapses—grade I–V dislocations.

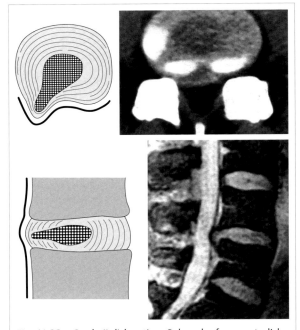

Fig. 11.32   Grade II dislocation. Subanular fragment; dislocated disk tissue has become displaced to the outermost layer of the anulus fibrosus and pushes this layer outward ("bulging disk," "contained disk"). The dislocated disk tissue can be reached at surgery only by incising the anulus fibrosus.

nerve root from the dorsal side (**Fig. 11.30**). Very rarely, hard sequestrated fragments can perforate the ventral dura mater of the lumbar sac and present as an intradural or intrathecal fragment. Such cases have been reported by Roda et al. (1982), Lee (1983), Griss (1984), Kasch (1986), Yildizhan and Okten (1991), McCulloch (1998), and Postacchini (1999).

Grades of Dislocation

The classification of disk protrusions and prolapses by grade of dislocation (I–V) is shown in **Fig. 11.31**. The grade of dislocation, together with the clinical findings, determines the most advisable form of treatment; intradiscal therapy may still be possible, or an open operation may be necessary (**Figs. 11.32–11.37**).

Spontaneous Changes of Disk Prolapse

Once the disk tissue has left its usual environment in the intervertebral space and entered the epidural space, it is subject to new metabolic conditions. It was originally nourished by diffusion through the normal, pressure-related fluid shifts within the disk, but it now lies more or less suddenly in a space surrounded by connective tissue where it is exposed to lymphatic fluid.

When the disk tissue is no longer subject to intradiscal pressure, it takes up fluid, according to the relation

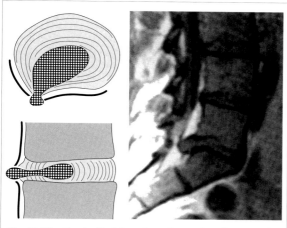

Fig. 11.33 Grade III dislocation. Covered prolapse at the discal level. The prolapsed tissue has completely perforated the anulus fibrosus and is only covered by a thin membrane (the ventral epidural membrane). This membrane can be bluntly perforated, e. g., with a 2 mm dissector. In general, the edge of the lamina will have to be resected for the prolapse to be reached.

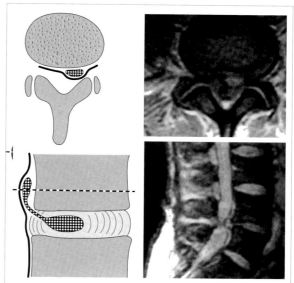

Fig. 11.34 Grade III dislocation. Covered prolapse at the supradiscal level. The dislocated disk tissue has emerged from the intervertebral space but is still covered by the ventral epidural membrane. The dislocated disk tissue can be reached only by opening the membrane with a blunt 2 mm dissector. In general, the lower edge of the lamina will have to be resected for the prolapse to be reached. A hemilaminectomy may be necessary.

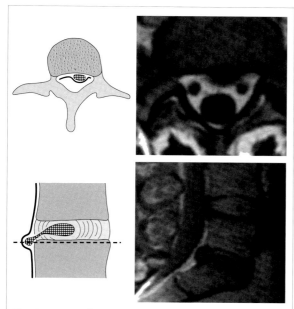

Fig. 11.35 Grade III dislocation. Covered prolapse at the infradiscal level. The prolapsed tissue is found under the ventral epidural membrane. After blunt opening of this membrane, e. g., with a dissector, the dislocated disk tissue is reached. The submembranous infradiscal prolapse can generally be reached by fenestration at L4/5 and L3/4. At the L5/S1 level, part of the sacral lamina may need to be resected.

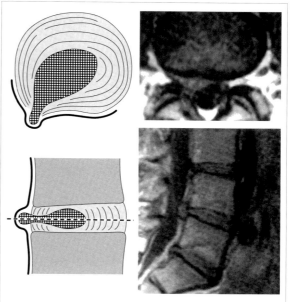

Fig. 11.36 Grade IV dislocation. The dislocated disk tissue is found partly inside and partly outside the disk. This situation generally obtains only at the discal level, when the ventral epidural membrane is also perforated at this level. Extensive removal of the dorsal portion of the disk is necessary to prevent recurrent disk herniation.

11

11

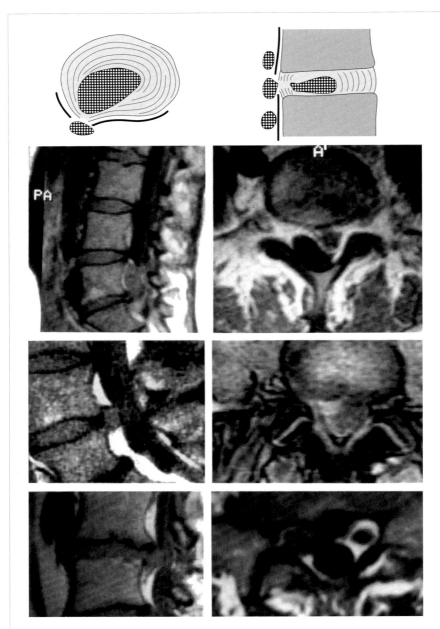

Fig. 11.37 Lumbar disk herniation, grade V dislocation. The prolapse is found as a free fragment in the spinal canal or the intervertebral foramen. When the prolapse is removed, the neighboring disk (donor disk) does not necessarily have to be emptied of disk tissue.

discussed in Chapter 4, thereby swelling up and increasing markedly in volume. This occurs because of the laws of osmosis and the intrinsic turgor of disk tissue. We have been able to show, in experiments on dissected specimens of disk tissue (Krämer 1973), that the volume of a disk prolapse induced by identical mechanical conditions is greater in hypo- or isotonic solution than in hypertonic solution. Nevertheless, neither this experiment nor others carried out on operatively removed disk tissue (Wittenberg et al. 1990) revealed any significant shrinkage of prolapsed tissue when exposed to hypertonic solution.

> **!** Increased pain and the progression of neurological deficits in the initial phase of discogenic sciatica are due, among other things, to spontaneous uptake of fluid by the prolapsed disk fragment (hydration), leading it to increase in volume.

Fluid uptake by prolapsed tissue can be demonstrated by MRI: on a T2-weighted image, the prolapsed tissue has higher signal intensity than the disk from which it emerged (**Fig. 11.38**).

Prolapsed disk tissue in the epidural space remains swollen for several weeks. As mentioned in the discus-

sion of the osmotic system in Chapter 4, the capacity for hydration and dehydration of disk tissue depends on its proteoglycan content. Nucleus pulposus tissue can take up more fluid than anulus fibrosus or cartilaginous end-plate tissue.

> ❗ After a period of hydration, the prolapsed disk tissue begins to become dehydrated and lose volume.

Its water content and volume decrease and the pressure on the nerves diminishes. Depolymerization and enzymatic degradation of the hydrophilic molecules in the disk fragment causes it to lose turgor. These processes can be verified at surgery: freshly prolapsed tissue (removed only a short time after the onset of symptoms) has more pronounced turgor than old extradiscal fragments, which are said in surgeons' jargon to be "pulpy."

Aside from osmotic swelling and shrinkage, extradiscal fragments are also enzymatically degraded.

> ❗ Disk tissue in the spinal canal induces a foreign-body reaction.

The disk and the nerve root are indeed part of the same motion segment, as far as their function is concerned, yet they are composed of very different types of tissue that arise from different primordial layers during embryonic development. The mechanical impingement and biochemical influence of disk tissue on epidural neural structures induce an inflammatory reaction that accelerates the degradation of the disk tissue. Small fragments are directly enzymatically resorbed by phagocytosis. It is therefore necessary, when a free fragment is to be surgically removed, to verify by a preoperative MRI scan that it is in fact still there. In some cases, persistent neurological deficits are not due to the persistence of compressive disk tissue but are rather the residua of past nerve compression.

Larger disk fragments are degraded by vascularization and connective-tissue organization from the surrounding epidural fat. Nucleus pulposus tissue is more easily degraded by macrophages and T cells than anulus fibrosus tissue. According to our own studies (Owczarek and Schmidt 1994) and others reported in the literature (McCulloch 1998, Postacchini 1999), once a disk prolapse has been spontaneously resorbed, follow-up CT and MRI scans reveal no significant degree of scarring or adhesion formation in the spinal canal.

> ❗ The time it takes for prolapsed disk tissue to be spontaneously resorbed depends on the mass and composition of the fragment as well as its position in the spinal canal.

Large fragments, i.e., those that occupy more than one-third of the cross-sectional area of the spinal canal, are less likely to be resorbed in an acceptably short period

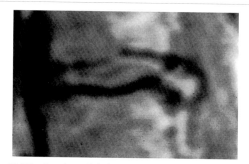

Fig. 11.38 Lumbar disk herniation, grade III dislocation. The extradiscally located tissue is brighter (contains more water) than the disk from which it was extruded.

of time than smaller fragments. Parts of the anulus fibrosus and the cartilaginous end plates are resorbed more slowly than parts of the nucleus pulposus. Hard disk fragments therefore more commonly require surgery and also cause more intense pain (Krämer, Herdmann, and Krämer 2005, Willburger 2005). Supra- and infradiscal fragments are resorbed more rapidly because they are surrounded by the well-vascularized ventral epidural membrane and the posterior wall of the vertebral body. The farther away the fragment is from the donor disk, the more likely it is to be spontaneously resorbed. If it is located in the concavity of the posterior surface of the vertebral body, the disk prolapse also exerts less pressure on the dura mater and nerve roots. The fragment has less of an opportunity to avoid impingement on these structures if the spinal canal is narrow and if the fragment is located within the foramen. Our group has published reports on the spontaneous course of lumbar disk prolapses that have been successfully managed conservatively, as observed in serial CT and MRI scans (Owczarek and Schmidt 1994, Krämer and Wilke 1988, Krämer, Hermann, and Krämer 2005), and so have many others (Koeller et al. 1984, Saal and Saal 1989, Hirabayashi et al. 1990, Saal and Herzog 1990, Yutaka et al. 1993, Donelson et al. 1997, Martikainen 1998, Trasimeni 1998, Fergusson 1999, Aelart 2004, Nakagawa 2004) (see also Chapter 12).

In some cases, total resorption of the prolapsed fragment is accompanied by complete remission of the clinical signs and symptoms; in other cases, the clinical findings regress partly or completely despite unchanged findings on CT or MRI. The prolapsed tissue usually becomes calcified. In such cases, the patient's condition tends to improve after a shorter or longer follow-up interval.

11

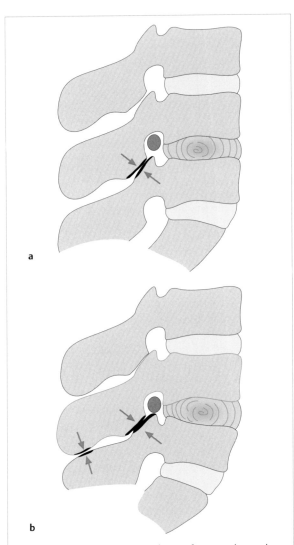

a

b

Fig. 11.39 a, b Symptom-producing factors when a lumbar disk is slack, and their accentuation by lordosis.

Disk slackening and instability do not necessarily imply the presence of clinical signs and symptoms. These conditions become clinically relevant only when pain and disability arise as a result of instability (see Chapter 6). If disk slackening and instability are present in combination with the associated clinical manifestations, the term "clinical instability" can be used (White and Panjabi 1978, Frymoyer et al. 1979, Kirkaldy-Willis 1984, Farfan 1996, Krismer et al. 1997). Instability leads to insufficiency of the lumbar erector spinae muscles, excess stress on the intervertebral joints, and sometimes manifestations of nerve root irritation. Disk slackening also plays a role in the pathogenesis of lumbar spinal stenosis.

In its initial stages, disk slackening can be compensated for by the abdominal and erector spinae muscles when the spine is under normal amounts of stress. If the functional reserve capacity of these muscles is exceeded, however, signs of insufficiency appear. The most commonly affected muscles are the deep and superficial erector spinae muscles of the lumbar motion segments, though the proximal muscles of the lower limbs can also be affected. Not just the muscles, but also the intervertebral joints are subjected to increased stress by disk slackening. The intervertebral joints of the lumbar spine already have a greater range of normal positions than those elsewhere in the spine because of the marked pressure and volume fluctuations of the lumbar disks (**Fig. 11.39**).

If the lumbar disks are also slack and subject to greater than normal fluctuations in volume, **abnormal and excessive stress on the lumbar intervertebral joints** can result, producing arthrogenic symptoms after long periods of mechanical loading followed by unloading. If the joints are subject to abnormal or excessive stress for a long time because of disk slackening, spondylarthrosis can develop (arthrosis deformans).

> Disturbances of the muscles, ligaments, and joints arising in the setting of lumbar disk slackening are the cause of arthroligamentous low back pain.

Displacement of the vertebral bodies with respect to one another can also come about because of disk slackening. Dorsoventral dislocation was called *pseudospondylolisthesis* in the nomenclature of Schmorl and Junghanns (1968)—"pseudo," because the articular facets are fully intact in this condition, as opposed to genuine isthmic spondylolisthesis. The most commonly used term in current clinical parlance is **degenerative spondylolisthesis.** Rotatory spondylolisthesis is usually due to disk slackening in combination with scoliosis, though it can also occur in the absence of scoliosis.

Sciatica can also be produced by slackening of intervertebral disks without any displacement of disk tissue (Benini 1976, Krämer, Herdmann, and Krämer 2005). In a slackened motion segment, the disk is of less than nor-

Disk Slackening and Instability

Not all symptoms arising from the lumbar motion segment are due to displacement of disk tissue. Apart from protrusions and prolapses, there are a number of other pathological structural changes that can be collectively designated by the term "disk slackening." Schmorl and Junghanns (1968) described a condition that they called "instabilitas intervertebralis."

> The term "disk slackening" refers to all phenomena that are due to progressive loss of water from the matrix of the disk and to the loss of fiber elasticity.

mal height and the lumbar vertebrae are displaced to some extent in relation to one another. The intervertebral foramina are narrowed, producing nerve root compression, mainly when the disk loses height dorsally and the vertebral body above is simultaneously posteriorly displaced with respect to the one below. The intervertebral foramen between them is then narrowed ventrally by the posterior border of the upper vertebra and by the upper portion of the articular facet of the lower vertebra. The lateral and oblique views of a myelogram or myelographic MRI scan will then reveal indentations in the column of contrast medium (spinal canal stenosis).

If a disk is slackened, low back pain and radicular symptoms tend to arise in particular positions and with particular movements, e. g., reclination of the trunk.

> **!** Hyperlordosis of the lumbar spine is an important symptom-provoking factor in slackening of the lumbar disks.

Returning the lumbar lordosis to its normal shape through relaxing positions and postures thus plays a major role in the treatment and prophylaxis of disk disease (**Fig. 11.40**).

Clinical course. Disk slackening and its clinical manifestations are present during a transient, though sometimes quite prolonged, phase in the course of disk degeneration. As the disks progressively dry out and become fibrotic with advancing age, the abnormal movements and displacements of the motion segment also diminish, so that the symptoms gradually disappear—unless the bony changes at the intervertebral joints have lead to narrowing of the spinal canal, i. e., **spinal canal stenosis.**

Bony Deformation

The types of bony deformation arising in spondylosis, osteochondrosis, and spondylarthrosis of the lumbar spine are not as clinically significant as those in the cervical spine, but they can nonetheless produce bony compression of nerve roots with symptomatic nerve root irritation. Ventral and lateral spondylotic osteophytes can often be very prominent in the lumbar spine yet are of no clinical relevance. They provide documentary evidence of disk slackening that has occurred in the past.

> **!** Of greater clinical significance are small osteophytes on the posterior border of the vertebral body, so-called retrospondylosis, particularly when they are dorsolaterally located and compress a nerve root.

Dorsal osteophytes can arise by appositional bone growth at the edge of the vertebral body. It is also

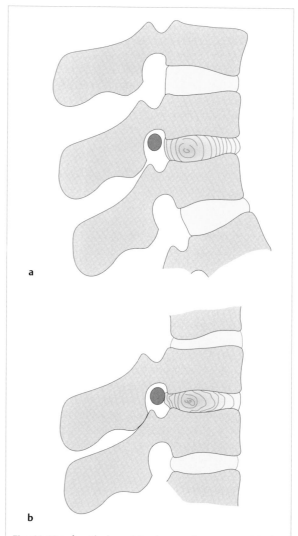

a

b

Fig. 11.40 a, b Slackened lumbar motion segment in kyphotic posture (**a**). When the patient rapidly leans back, the inelastic anulus fibrosus is rolled out posteriorly (**b**).

11

possible, however, for a small prolapse to harden by calcification and then become rigidly attached to the dorsal edge of the vertebral body.

In such cases, one speaks of a "hard prolapse." Though bony projections of this type develop slowly, giving the nerve root sufficient opportunity to adapt, they may be so sharply pointed that they repeatedly induce segmentally radiating pain. Inflammatory adhesions and bridging bands gradually form and finally encase the nerve root, maintaining it in a state of chronic irritation.

This situation is often not recognized because the objective clinical signs and changes on CT and MRI are not very pronounced. It can be remedied only by surgical removal of the osteophytes and freeing of the nerve roots from the surrounding tissue (rhizolysis). In **spondylarthrosis**, osteophytic reactions also arise at the edges of the intervertebral joints. If they jut into the spinal canal, they cause degenerative **spinal canal stenosis.** Because the lumbar intervertebral joints are part of the dorsal wall of the intervertebral foramina, spondylarthrosis can also cause foraminal stenosis. As mentioned above, bony deformation alone is not clinically relevant; symptoms are produced only when the segment is also slack.

In end-stage disk degeneration, fibrosis and osteophytes are still present, but there is no longer any segmental instability and the pain therefore improves. The lumbar spine has a markedly restricted range of motion in all directions. New protrusions and prolapses arise much less commonly in end-stage disk degeneration, but they sometimes occur even in individuals aged 70 or older.

Summary: Anatomy, Biomechanics, and Pathology of the Lumbar Motion Segments

In the lower lumbar spine, the intervertebral foramina and the spinal nerves traveling through them are situated at the level of the intervertebral disks, so that degenerative changes of the disks lie in the immediate vicinity of the spinal nerves. The traversing and exiting L5 and S1 nerve roots can be compressed by disk protrusions and prolapses in the anterolateral epidural space; from the dorsal side, they can be impinged upon by displacement or arthrotic enlargement of the L4/5 and L5/S1 articular facets. Local and radicular lumbar syndromes usually arise from these critical points in the lower two lumbar motion segments. Variations in the number of lumbar vertebrae and the possible presence of transitional vertebrae should be taken into account when planning treatments by local (epidural or foramino-articular) injection or open microsurgical procedures on the lumbar spine.

High intradiscal pressure in the lower lumbar intervertebral disks is the cause of intradiscal tissue displacement, leading to protrusions and prolapses. In children and adolescents, this produces extension stiffness of the hip and thigh; in adults, it produces lumbago. There is a continuous pathological spectrum ranging from disk protrusion to disk prolapse. Dorsal and dorsolateral displacements of disk tissue are clinically significant. These produce both low back pain and signs of nerve root irritation. The pattern of clinical symptoms is determined by the precise site of a lateral disk protrusion, i.e., whether it points more toward the midline, laterally, or fully outward (into the neural foramen). Protrusions and prolapses are classified according to the extent of the tissue dislocation and the amount of tissue that still separates the dislocated disk tissue from the neural structures in the epidural space. The therapeutic approach is determined by the major clinical manifestations rather than by the pathoanatomical finding alone.

Conclusion

The vast majority of cases of low back pain and sciatica arise from a circumscribed region of the lower lumbar spine characterized by a special combination of topographical, anatomical, and biomechanical properties.

■ Clinical Features of Lumbar Syndromes

Introduction

Just as in the cervical spine, the clinical symptoms and signs of damage to the lumbar disks are characterized by a wide variety of pathological manifestations. The range of symptomatic conditions ranges from mild low back pain to a deep spinal transection syndrome, with all possible transitional states in between. The spectrum of organs that can be directly or indirectly affected is not as wide as in cervical syndrome, but nevertheless the course, extent, and intensity of the symptoms in the back and the sciatic distribution are highly variable and their systematic classification is difficult. The same pathoanatomical substrate—e. g., a lateral disk protrusion—can produce symptoms that differ from patient to patient and that change over time in the individual patient as well. This variability is due to biochemical and biomechanical changes in the disk matrix and to individual differences in the responsiveness of the central and peripheral nervous systems to external stimuli.

At the onset of a lumbar syndrome, the symptoms produced by disk tissue displacement still correspond to well-defined clinical patterns (lumbago, sciatica). Later, as the secondary degenerative changes in the motion segment increase, it becomes increasingly difficult to ascribe the disease manifestations—e. g., chronic low back pain—to particular pathoanatomical states.

11

Diagnostic techniques that have been recently developed or improved (EMG, CT, and MRI) now permit better differentiation of the disease manifestations in lumbar syndrome. MRI images of the soft-tissue structures in the lumbar spinal canal are steadily improving in quality. Such images have already revealed that displacement of the dural sac and nerve roots by disk protrusions and deformation of the spinal canal play the most important role in the generation of low back pain and sciatica. The lower two lumbar motion segments are most commonly affected.

Lumbar syndromes are broadly **classified** according to the most prominent clinical manifestations of disease, with the use of generally recognized terms such as lumbago and sciatica. Some further specification is necessary, however, so that the clinician can draw the necessary therapeutic consequences; e.g, protrusion sciatica should be distinguished from prolapse sciatica. In the following sections, we present the general types of symptoms and signs that appear in all disk-related conditions of the lumbar spine. The specific findings of particular segmental syndromes will be discussed later on in the relevant sections.

Symptoms

Pain is the most important symptom of lumbar syndrome. What the patient says about the onset, development, and responsiveness of the pain provides important clues to the diagnosis. Objective signs are often mild or absent despite severe pain; thus, physicians often have difficulty assessing the situation correctly, especially (but not only) in the medicolegal setting. Moreover, the physician often sees the patient for the first time only after the pain has begun to diminish in intensity, or during an asymptomatic interval.

Table 11.1 Typical characteristics of the pain of discogenic lumbar syndrome

- Sudden onset
- Fluctuating course
- Positional dependence
- Intensification by coughing, sneezing, pressing

The patient can usually describe the localization and character of the pain so precisely that the diagnosis of "lumbar syndrome" can be given on the basis of the history alone. When objectifiable neurological deficits are lacking, the only evidence for lumbar root syndrome is the typical band of pain in the lower limb, whose precise location is also an important clue to the affected segment. The patient complains of numbness or *sensory irritative manifestations* such as a pins-and-needles sensation or the feeling that the limb has "gone to sleep." The severity of the pain is, in general, proportional to the pressure exerted on the nerve root, until the area supplied by the root becomes entirely anesthetic and analgetic when the nerve is maximally compressed.

Disk-related symptoms in the lumbar region generally develop over a short time; in most cases, their onset is sudden (**Table 11.1**). Many patients attribute the onset of the pain to a particular event, perhaps because of a natural desire for a plausible explanation. The events most commonly mentioned in medicolegal assessments are *faulty lifting* and *rotatory movements of the trunk*.

More than half of the patients who were interrogated by questionnaire in specialized practices and in our outpatient clinic (**Fig. 11.41**) reported **no particular event before the onset of the pain** to which the pain could be attributed. Their sciatica or lumbago appeared to strike

11

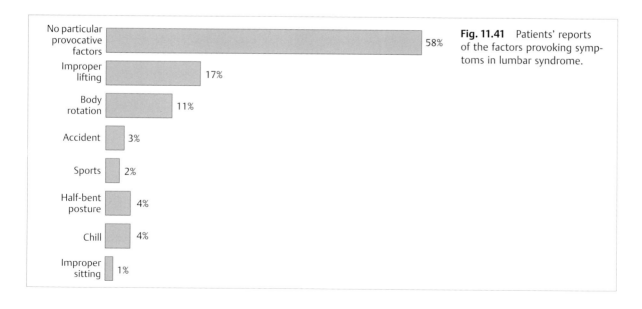

Fig. 11.41 Patients' reports of the factors provoking symptoms in lumbar syndrome.

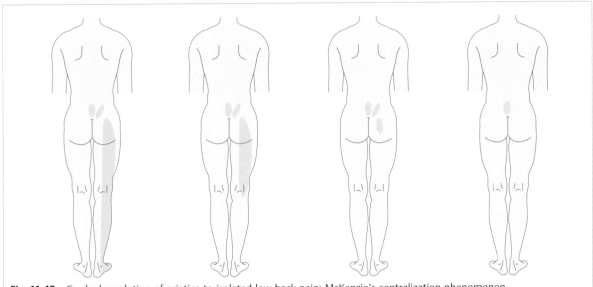

Fig. 11.42   Gradual resolution of sciatica to isolated low back pain: McKenzie's centralization phenomenon.

11

them out of a clear blue sky. Accidents and other mechanical forces of the types commonly discussed in medicolegal cases played a numerically insignificant role in this group of nonmedicolegal patients.

The character and radiation of the pain in lumbar syndromes are subject to continuous change: pain lying deep in the low back moves to one buttock or to the sacroiliac region on one side. Sciatica sometimes arises, too, initially only in the thigh, then later radiating all the way down to the foot. The low back pain may entirely disappear, leaving only sciatica in the lower limb (sciatica without low back pain). The reverse type of *varying course* is seen when the pain moves proximally, reflecting a centralization phenomenon (McKenzie 1987): sciatica changes to isolated low back pain (**Fig. 11.42**).

The **positional dependence** of disk-related symptoms is more pronounced in the lumbar region than anywhere else in the spine because of the marked fluctuations of intradiscal pressure and the changing relative positions of the neural structures and the posterior border of the disk that accompany postural shifts. Both low back pain and sciatica are functions of the position of the lumbar motion segments and the mechanical demands placed on them. This is also reflected in the circadian variation of symptoms. Aside from intradiscal pressure, another important question is whether the patient is able to assume a stress-reducing position. If this is not possible, the pain intensifies even when the patient lies down with a lordotic posture of the lumbar spine, e. g., in the prone or flat supine position. Forward bending or sitting in a chair raises the intradiscal pres-

sure considerably, though many patients are asymptomatic when they sit because this posture widens the intervertebral foramina. Only when the patient sits up, increasing the lumbar lordosis, does the slackened posterior portion of the disk get caught in the "nutcracker" of the posterior vertebral body edges and protrude toward the dura mater and nerve roots. This situation arises at night, too, when the patient shifts from the kyphotic lateral decubitus to the flat supine or prone position. Most patients are most comfortable when lying with flexed hip and knee joints, either on their back or on their side (the "fetal" position).

Other patients, however, say that they feel relief only when they are prone or bending backward. The asymptomatic, stress-reducing position thus differs from patient to patient depending on the site of the protrusion or prolapse.

The **exacerbation of pain** *by coughing, sneezing, or pressing* is a common feature of all disk-related symptoms in the lumbar region. The importance of the valveless epidural venous plexus in the spinal canal and its relation to intraabdominal and intrathoracic pressure has already been discussed in Chapter 4. Nachemson (1976), in his measurements of intradiscal pressure, found that abdominal pressing raises the pressure in the lumbar disks to a considerable extent. Patients are aware of, and fear, these elevations of pressure and assume all possible pressure-reducing positions when abdominal pressing is unavoidable. The dependence of the pain on position and on pressing is subject to change at different times of day and also over the course of the illness. Any reported bladder or bowel symptoms or sexual dysfunction can be an important clue to a possible partial cauda equine syndrome; any weakness of the dorsiflexors of the feet and toes, or of the gluteal and calf muscles, may indicate a motor disturbance of a type that often accompanies sciatica.

Some patients with S1 syndrome report **cramps in the calf muscles.** Motor dysfunction limited to the monosegmentally supplied muscles must be clinically distinguished from pain-related, reflexive "favoring" of an entire limb. Patients will often state that the limb seems to be "weak" or "paralyzed" even though the examination reveals no motor deficit; they are merely reflexively avoiding movement in order not to stir up additional pain.

At the initial examination, the physician must allow sufficient time to take a full history from the patient, because the symptoms that the patient relates often provide crucial clues to the diagnosis.

> **!** A physician who is a "history fanatic" has the best chance of diagnosing a disk syndrome correctly.

Findings of Clinical Examination

After taking the history, the physician should carry out a thorough physical examination, consisting of inspection, palpation, functional testing, and a directed neurological examination. Special tests for lumbar syndrome should be a routine part of the overall examination, to facilitate differential diagnosis. The examination should be structured in such a way that the patient needs to move as little as possible, because each change of position will be difficult and painful.

> **!** Thus, multiple tests (e. g., tests of range of movement and neurological function) should be carried out in each position of the body.

The first indication that a lumbar syndrome may be present is already evident on **inspection** of the patient when they enter the room. Their gait is inharmonious, cautious, and (if the patient suffers from sciatica) limping. The patient prefers to stand during clinical history-taking, or sits down hesitantly on the edge of a proffered chair. All movements, including sitting down, standing up, dressing, and undressing, are executed cautiously and appear stiff. The patient has great difficulty taking off shoes and socks, because this maneuver requires bending the trunk forward, which is painful. Postural abnormalities may already be noted while the patient is still dressed; they are most noticeable when the unclothed patient is viewed from behind.

Closer inspection reveals a marked bulging of the tense lumbar erector spinae muscles (lumbar spasm). Flexion of the lumbar spine to eliminate the lordosis makes this even more evident.

> **!** The presence of lumbar spasm and partial fixation of the lumbar spine are among the most important diagnostic criteria for lumbar syndrome.

The standing patient is first asked to bend forward and to the sides and to rotate the trunk actively, and then these same movements are tested passively. A *limited range of motion to one side* is found. Lateral bending is not as severely restricted as forward and backward bending. The abnormal posture and limited range of motion of the trunk may sometimes be only mild or even absent, e. g., in the asymptomatic interval of a lumbar syndrome or with a far lateral S1 disk protrusion. Painful limitation of motion of the lumbar spine is often not evident until the patient is asked to bend laterally while keeping the trunk bent slightly forward. If the physician suspects that a limited range of forward bending may have a nonorganic cause (e. g., in medicolegal situations or possible psychogenic overlay), a **kneeling test** can be done at this point (see Chapter 13): if the patient still cannot bend forward (at the hip joint) when kneeling on a chair, a position in which the sciatic nerves and ischiocrural muscles are relaxed rather than stretched, then the limited range of motion is probably of nonorganic origin.

Next, the patient is asked to stand, and to take several steps, when standing on tiptoe and then on the heels; this will reveal any possible weakness of the *foot dorsiflexors (L5)* or *calf muscles (S1).*

The remainder of the examination is carried out with patient lying down. Lumbar spasm often disappears when the patient is horizontal, because the trunk muscles no longer have a stabilizing, antigravity task to do. The supine position with mildly flexed hips and knees is usually the most comfortable position for the patient (the maximally stress-reducing position). Patients find it unpleasant to lie flat in the prone position.

With the patient **prone,** the physician should palpate the spinous processes and ascertain whether there is any tenderness of the affected motion segment to gentle shaking or percussion. Because the lumbar intervertebral joints are sagittally oriented, lateral shaking of the spinous process will always produce movement of the vertebral bodies above and below as well; thus, this part of the examination cannot be considered segmentally specific.

Paraspinous tenderness is more informative: in thin and not particularly well-muscled patients, one may be able to exert pressure on the ligamentum flavum and the nerve root lying directly under it by deep palpation with one finger. The soft tissues between the laminae may be depressed by this maneuver to such an extent that the nerve root is squeezed between them and a disk protrusion lying anterior to it in the spinal canal (**Fig. 11.43**), resulting in the provocation of the patient's

11

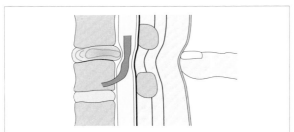

Fig. 11.43   Deep paravertebral palpation with pressure on the nerve root that is compressed by a disk herniation.

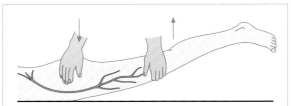

Fig. 11.44   Overextension of the hip causing femoral nerve stretch pain (the "reverse Lasègue sign") in a patient with an upper lumbar radicular syndrome.

typical local and sciatic pain. This pain on deep palpation is still more intense if it is evoked when the patient's back is in a lordotic posture, with flexed hip joints, in the kneeling, squatting, or lateral decubitus position, because these positions increase the height of the interlaminar window.

The result of this test is significant only when it is positive; it may be negative, for example, in the presence of a far lateral protrusion or of one located under a broad lamina, neither of which can be reached by deep interlaminar palpation.

The region of the sacroiliac joint on the affected side is also tender to palpation and percussion. This finding does not indicate an abnormal position or blockage of the sacroiliac joint but is rather a type of radiating pain corresponding to the dorsal branches of the affected spinal nerve. Intradiscal injections can provoke this type of pain in typical fashion.

Keeping the patient prone, the physician proceeds to test the ability of the hip joints to be hyperextended, checking for the provocation of pain on femoral nerve stretching, the so-called "reverse Lasègue sign" that indicates a disk protrusion at a higher level (**Fig. 11.44**).

> Just as the sciatic nerve is stretched when the patient lies supine and the lower limb is elevated, the femoral nerve is stretched when the patient lies prone and the hip joint is hyperextended.

Certain parts of the neurological examination can now be carried out while the patient remains prone, starting

with sensory testing in the dorsally located dermatomes. The physician asks the patient to tense the gluteal musculature and palpates for any difference in muscle tone that may indicate the presence of an S1 syndrome. The prone position is also suitable for testing of active knee flexion, which can be impaired in higher lumbar root syndromes.

The supine position.   After determining that the range of motion of all joints (including rotation at the hips) is free, the physician tests for the presence of the *Lasègue sign;* this can be done either by raising the straight lower limb or by extending the knee when the limb is already flexed at the hip.

No matter which of these two methods is used, Lasègue's test consists of hip flexion at a right angle combined with knee extension. If this provokes pain in the back radiating down into the sciatic distribution, the Lasègue sign is said to be positive; the clinician must differentiate among locally induced back pain, classic radicular pain, and the dull discomfort that accompanies stretching of the hamstrings. Lasègue (1864) was also the first to observe that patients with sciatica keep the foot in a plantar flexed position and complain of increased pain when it is dorsiflexed (**Fig. 11.45**). In common medical parlance, the term "positive Lasègue sign" can also refer to the provocation of pain by raising of the straight lower limb; this is the "straight-leg raising test" often mentioned in the Anglo-American literature. The provocation of pain by this maneuver was first described as a typical finding in sciatica by Forst, a pupil of Lasègue (cited in Finneson 1980).

Straight-leg raising displaces the L4, L5, and S1 spinal nerves by up to 5 mm and stretches them by 2–4% (Smith et al. 1993).

> Pain is induced by the same mechanism in the straight-leg raising test and in the test originally described by Lasègue (passive extension of the knee when the hip is in 90° of flexion): components of the sciatic nerve are stretched.

The straight lower limb can normally be raised to 70–90° by passive flexion at the hip, with some variability between individuals and depending on age. Limb raising is limited by a feeling of tension in the ischiocrural muscles, but no unusual feeling normally arises from the sciatic nerve during this maneuver. Sciatica is provoked only when the sciatic nerve is irritated or if it is less than normally mobile, or already under stretch, in the region of the nerve roots.

The sensitivity and specificity of the Lasègue sign have been investigated by Edgar (1995), Andersson and Deyo (1996), Hogen et al. (1996), Igarashi et al. (2004), and Summers et al. (2005). In their systematic review of the literature, Walter et al. (2000) concluded that the specificity of the Lasègue sign is low. Thus, pain on

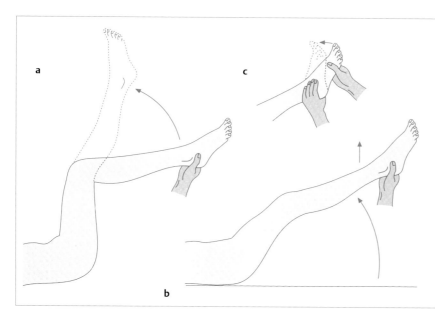

Fig. 11.45 a–c The Lasègue test.
a Pain on raising the flexed leg.
b Pain on raising the extended leg (straight-leg raising test).
c Additional dorsiflexion of the foot as a test of sciatica.

straight-leg raising should only be considered to be of diagnostic value in the context of other accompanying manifestations of lumbar syndrome.

Depending on the site of the displaced disk tissue, radicular pain may also be induced or intensified by raising of the contralateral lower limb, i.e., the one that is *not* painful (*contralateral Lasègue sign*). This is sometimes the case when the prolapse is medially situated and compresses the nerve from the caudal side (**Fig. 11.46**).

Straight-leg raising will also be painful in pathological conditions affecting the hip and sacroiliac joints. To rule out these potential sources of pain, one can do the *sciatic nerve test* (**Fig. 11.45c**): The straight lower limb is raised to the point at which pain begins to be felt and then lowered till the pain just disappears. If mild passive dorsiflexion of the foot at this point induces pain again, then it can be regarded as certain that a sciatic nerve syndrome is present. Dorsiflexion stretches the tibial nerve by about 1–2 cm. This maneuver does not induce pain originating in the hip or sacroiliac joints, because it causes no additional movement in these joints.

In the popliteal fossa pressure test, the straight leg is raised to the point at which pain begins to be felt, and then the knee is flexed and placed on the physician's shoulder. Pressure from the physician's thumb in the patient's popliteal fossa provokes sudden sciatic pain if the nerve is under tension (**Fig. 11.47**).

The pain-provoking effect of sciatic nerve stretch in patients with lumbar syndrome is also exploited in the straight-leg sitting test (see Chapter 13). The patient is unable to sit up on a flat surface, e. g., in bed or on an examining table, with the knees extended. This objective sign of the intensity of pain is of particular value in medicolegal assessment: because straight-leg raising is a

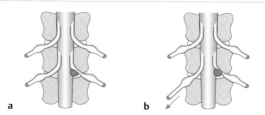

Fig. 11.46 a, b Paramedian disk prolapse in the axilla of the nerve root (**a**). Tension on the *opposite* root when the leg is raised increases the pressure exerted by the prolapse on the affected root (positive crossed Lasègue sign) (**b**).

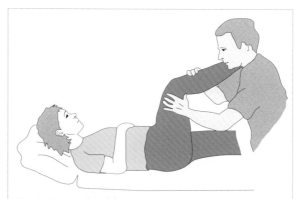

Fig. 11.47 Popliteal fossa pressure test in sciatica.

commonly known medical test, patients will often indicate the presence of severe pain when the leg is raised only to 20° or 30°, but will then be able to converse normally with the physician when sitting up in bed with

11

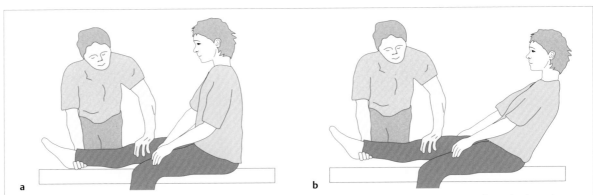

Fig. 11.48 a, b Positive reclination test: when the leg is extended at the knee and raised, the patient leans backward.

the knees extended. The same applies to the sciatic nerve stretching test in the sitting position, the so-called **"reclination test":** the patient sits up in a chair without leaning back and the examiner raises the patient's calf. If the patient then leans back because of pain, the test is positive (**Fig. 11.48**).

The remaining testing of sensorimotor and reflex function is carried out with the patient **supine**. The reflexes should be examined very carefully, with distracting maneuvers if necessary, because even slight *asymmetry of the reflexes* is of diagnostic value. The knee-jerk reflex is often influenced by antalgic tensing of the entire lower limb. The patient must first be brought into as pain-free a position as possible.

> **!** *Increased* reflexes are of no diagnostic value in lumbar syndromes.

The knee-jerk reflex is diminished in compression of the third or fourth lumbar nerve root.

If the Achilles reflex cannot be elicited with the patient supine, it should be tested with the patient in the kneeling position and performing a distracting maneuver, such as interlocking the hands and attempting to pull them apart (the Jendrassik hand grip).

> **!** Motor testing in lumbar syndromes focuses on the monosegmentally innervated muscles of the lower lumbar segments, because positive findings here are of the greatest diagnostic significance.

Some useful diagnostic evidence can already be obtained at the start of the examination when the examiner observes the patient during toe-standing, heel-standing, toe-walking, and heel-walking. The motor dysfunction may be so mild that the patient does not notice it. Fibrillation may be seen in affected muscle groups. The magnitude of the motor deficit is generally proportional to the pressure on the nerve root. Large muscles are only mildly weakened in monosegmental

lumbar irritative syndromes, even when a nerve root is massively compressed. The quadriceps, for example, is supplied by the L3, L4, and L5 nerve roots, but the extensor hallucis longus is supplied only by L5. An L3/4 disk prolapse compressing the L4 root produces quadriceps weakness that is evident only during active knee extension, but an L4/5 prolapse compressing the L5 root produces marked loss of strength of the foot dorsiflexors (i.e., a foot drop). Thus, the knee flexors and extensors should always be tested, but the most important tests are of the raw strength of the plantar flexors and dorsiflexors of the feet and, specifically, of the big toes (**Fig. 11.49**).

Although motor testing often yields unexpected findings for both the physician and the patient, the findings of sensory testing are often already partly implicit in the clinical history itself (complaints of numbness, etc.). Because disk-related nerve root syndromes generally impair sensation only superficially, sensory testing can be restricted to directed testing with a pinwheel, needle, cotton-wool pad, or similar object. Just as in motor testing, dermatomal overlap (particularly in the proximal portion of the lower limb) often precludes reliable assignment of a sensory deficit to a single segment.

Bradford and Spurling (1950) reported a surgical series of S1 rhizotomy (complete transection of the S1 root within its dural sleeve) on a number of patients. They found that this produced a different distribution of hypesthetic areas in the thigh and leg in each patient. The various dermatome charts that are available also differ from one another; the classic ones are those of Foerster (1933), Tilney and Riley (1938) and Keegan (1943).

> **!** The only reliable statement that can be made is that an area of the dorsum of the foot that includes the big toe belongs to the L5 dermatome, but the heel, the lateral edge of the foot, and the little toe belong to the S1 dermatome.

11

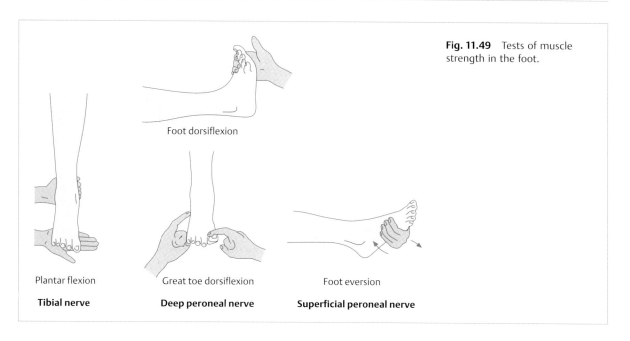

Fig. 11.49 Tests of muscle strength in the foot.

Foot dorsiflexion

Plantar flexion

Great toe dorsiflexion

Foot eversion

Tibial nerve   **Deep peroneal nerve**   **Superficial peroneal nerve**

Cutaneous sensation must also be tested in the perineal area in order not to miss the finding of *saddle anesthesia* in cauda equina syndrome.

Hyperesthesia is also a feature of lumbar nerve root irritation syndromes. It is due to an incomplete spinal nerve lesion, a common result of compression by a lumbar disk protrusion. If the examination reveals evidence of altered temperature sense or proprioception or other deficits that are not generally seen in lumbar syndrome, a neurologist should be consulted for a thorough neurological examination.

Precise history-taking and physical examination of a patient with lumbar syndromes usually reveals not only the diagnosis but also the specific level that is affected. Plain radiographs, blood and CSF analyses, myelography, EMG, CT, MRI, and other tests are used to confirm the diagnosis and exclude other diseases.

Neurophysiologic Testing—EMG

The general remarks on neurophysiologic testing on the cervical spine (Chapter 9) also apply to the lumbar spine. Because lumbar nerve root compression syndromes are common and often produce paresis of variable severity, neurophysiologic testing in the lumbar area can be very useful, particularly EMG. The physician and the patient want to know to what extent the nerve root is already damaged, how long this damage has been present, and whether it can be expected to improve. These questions arise particularly in the follow-up evaluation of patients with mild to moderately severe weakness, who now increasingly tend to be treated conservatively. In contrast to a routine primary diagnostic assessment

and clinical follow-up, EMG still involves a relatively invasive procedure with multiple needle-sticks. Muscle action potentials are recorded with two or more concentric needle electrodes inserted about 1 cm apart, in a transverse orientation with respect to the muscle fibers. Recordings must be made at various depths and at multiple insertion sites. EMG should therefore only be used in directed fashion and to answer specific questions (Dvořák and Haldeman 2004).

In the lumbar region EMG is most often used for the diagnostic assessment of dorsiflexor and quadriceps weakness, because the findings may imply the need for surgery. Patients suffering from nothing more than a pins-and-needles paresthesia and/or weakness of unimportant muscles, such as the extensor hallucis longus, should be spared the unpleasantness of an EMG and instead followed up clinically with serial assessment of muscle strength.

Plain Radiographs

Just as in the cervical spine, plain AP and lateral lumbar spine views mainly serve the purpose of **ruling out other diseases.** Disk protrusions, prolapses, and slackening all take place in the radiologically transparent intervertebral space and therefore can only be visualized with special techniques involving the injection of contrast medium.

Degenerative disk changes can be recognized by the narrowing of the intervertebral space and the bony reaction of the neighboring vertebral bodies. Plain radiographs of older patients reveal narrowing of the disk

11

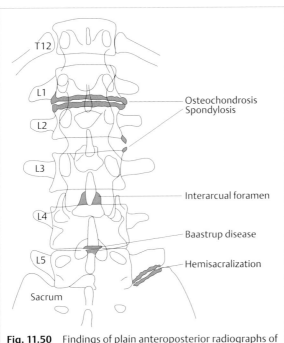

Fig. 11.50 Findings of plain anteroposterior radiographs of the lumbosacral spine.

Labels in figure: T12, L1, L2, L3, L4, L5, Sacrum; Osteochondrosis Spondylosis; Interarcual foramen; Baastrup disease; Hemisacralization

increased prevalence of degenerative changes in the upper lumbar segments in individuals over the age of 40 without any associated clinical manifestations.

Despite this, the interpretation of plain radiographs remains important, as it is necessary to recognize not just infection and tumors of the lumbar spine but also pre-discotic structural abnormalities such as axial deviation, asymmetrical transitional vertebrae, juvenile developmental anomalies, abnormalities of the laminae, and narrowing of the spinal canal, all of which predispose to the development of intervertebral disk disease.

In the **AP view,** one first counts the lumbar vertebrae and notes any transitional vertebrae, which are of clinical importance only in the case of an asymmetrically anchored lumbosacral vertebra causing asymmetrical stress on the disks lying above it (see p. 28). One should also note whether the upper and lower end plates are parallel, as they should be, and inspect the shape and location of the oval shadows representing the pedicles seen on end. In torsion scoliosis, for example, these are projected toward the concave side, and they may be blurry or absent if the pedicles are involved by a neoplastic or infectious process.

Disk collapse and lumbar hyperlordosis cause adjacent spinous processes of the middle and upper lumbar spine to touch one another, leading to reactive sclerosis and, sometimes, clinical symptoms (Baastrup disease) (**Fig. 11.50**).

The width and borders of the interlaminar windows are of importance for epidural and perineural injections and can be seen in their projections on an AP view, so that the physician can determine the optimal puncture site in advance. *Spina bifida occulta,* if present, should be mentioned in the radiography report for the sake of completeness but is of no biomechanical significance for the motion segment or for the generation of disk-related symptoms. The **lateral view** of the lumbar spine is more informative than the AP view (**Fig. 11.51**).

> **!** Loss of the normal lordosis (i. e. abnormal straightening) of the lumbar spine is called the Güntz phenomenon.

Just as in the cervical spine, straightening of the lumbar spine cannot always be interpreted as evidence of an acute disk syndrome, because the normal lordosis can also be abolished voluntarily. When radiographs are taken with the patient lying on one side and flexing the hip and knee joints, as is often done, the lumbar lordosis is often considerably reduced in any case. Findings of greater significance include marked *narrowing* of the intervertebral spaces in young adults; lateral, rotational, or dorsoventral displacement of the vertebral bodies with respect to one another without interruption of the articular processes (*pseudospondylolisthesis* in the terminology of Schmorl and Junghanns 1968); and exophytes on the posterior edge of the vertebral column.

spaces, which may be very marked, as well as osteosclerotic changes of the upper and lower end plates, with hook-like osteophytes at the vertebral body edges that fuse with one another to form bony bridges. These newly formed bony structures initially jut horizontally outward from the vertebral body margin for a greater or lesser distance and then take a vertical course; if a similar osteophyte grows from the vertebral body on the opposite side of the disk, the intervertebral space at this level can be bridged by bone. These bony struts are usually located ventrally and laterally. Only in exceptional cases does a dorsal osteophyte derived from an old disk prolapse protrude into the spinal canal or the intervertebral foramen.

> **!** Spondylotic and osteochondrotic changes are documentary evidence of earlier disk slackening rather than of a currently active disk syndrome.

Torgeson and Dotter (1976) obtained plain lumbar spine radiographs of more than 300 patients with lumbar syndrome and compared them with radiographs of a control group of asymptomatic individuals. The frequency of spondylosis was the same in the two groups. Wansor and Fleischhauer (1986), in our institution, came to the same conclusion. Other comparable findings in the literature include those of Bogduk (2000), Nachemson and Jonsson (2000), Jarvik and Deyo (2002), Borenstein et al. (2004), and Van et al. (2006). An evaluation of our patient population by Strickstrack (1983) revealed an

If such changes are found in the plain lateral radiographic view, one should proceed to obtain oblique, spot, and tomographic views. Particularly when there is a question of spondylolysis and spondylolisthesis, **oblique views** should not be omitted. These also show intervertebral joint arthrosis, with characteristic telescoping of the joints due to degenerative disk collapse (**Fig. 11.52**).

The notochordal remnants and juvenile developmental anomalies to which so much attention is often paid are actually clinically unimportant and imply nothing more than possible weakness of the structures bordering the intervertebral disks, which might create a predisposition to disk disease. Not every protrusion seen in the posterior silhouette of the vertebral column on a plain lateral radiograph is a dorsal osteophyte; a large lateral osteophyte may also be projected over the spinal canal (**Fig. 11.53**). This situation can only be clarified with a CT or MRI scan.

Lumbar Myelography

! Myelography is the visualization of the spinal subarachnoid space with contrast medium.

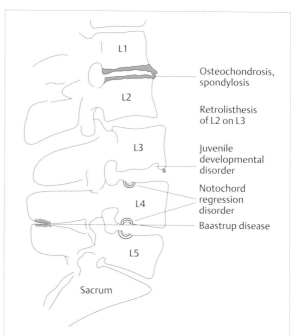

Fig. 11.51 Findings of plain lateral radiographs of the lumbosacral spine.

The lumbar subarachnoid space is a compartment filled with cerebrospinal fluid (CSF) that is contained between the arachnoid membrane lying just under the spinal dura mater and the pia mater surrounding the spinal cord and nerve roots. The space between the spinal dura mater and the arachnoid membrane is only virtual under normal circumstances. The dural sac containing the subarachnoid space extends caudally to the S2

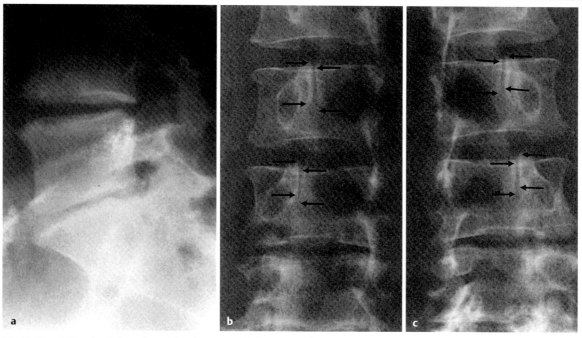

Fig. 11.52 Arthrosis of the spine with telescoping of the joint surfaces (arrows) due to disk degeneration.

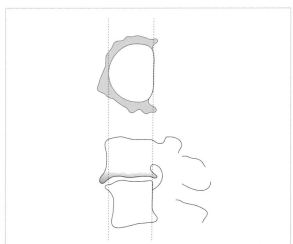

Fig. 11.53 Large lateral osteophytes mimicking a dorsal osteophyte in the lateral radiographic view.

Table 11.2 Indications for lumbar spine CT

- Trauma
- Spondylolisthesis
- Spinal canal stenosis
- Spondylitis
- Tumors
- Disk herniation
- Post-discographic CT

vertebral level. In the lumbar region, the *CSF of the subarachnoid space* surrounds the nerve rootlets of the cauda equina; CSF continues to surround the nerve roots in nerve root sleeves that extend into the intervertebral foramina.

Myelography has become a much less important diagnostic technique for the assessment of disk disease since the introduction of CT and MRI. It is now possible to display the CSF-containing spaces with MR myelography in much the same way that they were displayed with conventional myelography. Furthermore, MRI displays the soft tissues neighboring the CSF spaces, including disk protrusions and prolapses, which myelography does not. Thus, myelography is currently used only for a narrow range of indications, e. g., when a patient suffers from acute cauda equine syndrome and all lumbar segments must be examined radiographically but an MRI scanner is not available.

The combination of myelography with post-myelographic CT has also largely fallen out of use because of the improved display of intraspinal structures with MRI. Practically the only advantage that myelography has over other procedures is that CSF is always obtained as a part of the procedure and can be analyzed in the labora-

tory for the differential diagnosis of a variety of neurological diseases.

In conclusion, myelography has largely gone out of use, being supeseded by CT and MRI, in accordance with the MIRACLE principle stated in Chapter 1. In comparison with these newer techniques, it is more invasive, has a greater risk of complications, and generally provides less information, at least in the diagnostic evaluation of disk disease.

CT

! CT generates cross-sectional radiological images in the horizontal plane with the aid of computer technology. An roentgen ray tube rotates around the patient's body and obtains pictures from many different angles, which are then manipulated by computer to create a cross-sectional image.

Indications

Although CT is a noninvasive diagnostic technique it is quite expensive and exposes patients to ionizing radiation. A CT scan should therefore be obtained only when there is suspicion of a **space-occupying lesion** in the lumbar spinal canal and should be restricted to the region of suspicion, i. e., as few levels as possible. Thus, the radiologist should be informed at what level the pathological process is expected to be found. Patients with disk-related radicular sciatica usually have a lesion in the L4–S1 segments. Imaging of higher segments is indicated in patients with upper lumbar root syndromes, polyradicular manifestations, suspected tumor or spondylitis, or cauda equina syndrome. MRI displays lumbar disk prolapses and protrusions much better than CT; if MRI scanning is available, the remaining indications for CT include all bony changes of the lumbar spine, including fracture, infection (spondylitis), and bony tumors, which CT displays better than MRI.

In combination with discography ("disco-CT"), CT can still be used to advantage in the diagnostic evaluation of disk protrusions and subligamentous prolapses. A disco-CT can be helpful in differential diagnosis, particularly for the choice of the optimal intradiscal therapeutic technique (**Table 11.2**). Its main disadvantage is that the invasive procedure of disk puncture has to be carried out twice: once for diagnostic purposes and then later, after evaluation of the CT images, for therapeutic purposes in a second sitting. A CT scan of the lumbar spine can also be useful as part of a comprehensive assessment in medicolegal cases, if warranted by the clinical findings.

The findings of degenerative spinal change that are revealed by CT have the same significance as those revealed by plain radiographs and myelography: these radiological findings are of no pathological significance and do not imply a need for surgical intervention except when they are closely correlated with the patient's clinical manifestations.

> **!** Treatment of any kind, including surgical treatment, should never be based on radiological findings alone, and certainly not on the findings of myelography, CT, or MRI when these lack clinical correlation.

Technical Procedure

Positioning. A CT scan of the lumbar spine is obtained with the patient supine. Roentgen rays emitted by rotating tubes, oriented in all radial directions perpendicular to the long axis of the body, are sensed by detectors placed opposite the tubes. The resulting data are processed by computer to generate a cross-sectional image in the transverse (horizontal) plane. The lumbar spine should be as straight as possible, i. e., the lumbar lordosis should be reduced as much as possible, so that the planes of section will be parallel to the vertebral bodies and disks. This is achieved by positioning the patient with the knees flexed and the pelvis tilted backward (**Fig. 11.54**). This method of compensating for the lumbar lordosis is not adequate at the L5/S1 level, for which one can additionally tilt the imaging plane by 20° by tilting the gantry of the CT scanner.

Once the patient is properly positioned, the position must be maintained for the duration of scanning, which takes a few minutes, so that the individual cross-sectional images will correspond correctly to the planes of section indicated on the scout view or topogram of the lumbar spine that is obtained at the beginning. The planes indicated by lines in the scout view are numbered with the numbers of the corresponding transverse (horizontal) images in the study.

The sequence of cross-sectional images and their interpretation. The distance between cross-sectional images can be chosen at will; the images should be more closely spaced at levels near the intervertebral disks than elsewhere. The mid-level of the vertebral body at the height of the pedicles is generally not imaged, to reduce cost and radiation exposure, even though free fragments can be found at this level, just as at other levels.

The cross-sectional images generated by computer are always displayed in the same way (**Fig. 11.55**).

> **!** The CT images are always displayed as if one were looking at the patient from below, i. e., in the caudocranial direction.

Thus, the patient's right side is always seen on the left side of the image. Because the lumbosacral junction

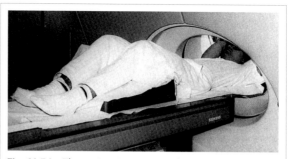

Fig. 11.54 The patient is supine with gently elevated legs to neutralize the lumbar lordosis for the lower lumbar CT scan.

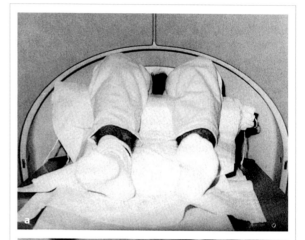

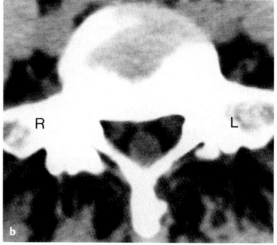

Fig. 11.55 a, b The lower lumbar CT scan is displayed as if one were looking at the patient from the feet upward, as seen in (**a**). Thus, the right side of the body appears on the left side of the radiological image (**b**).

contains structures that are visually distinct and easy to recognize (the sacrum and ilium), the sequence of images is generally best viewed from the bottom up, i. e., from caudal to cranial.

Further computer processing enables the reconstruction of a more familiar-appearing AP or lateral view of the spine from the horizontal CT sections. In principle, a reconstruction of the images in the sagittal or frontal planes can yield no further information than is already present in the horizontal images, from which the findings can be read directly. It therefore seems a better idea to get adequate practice in the interpretation of the cross-sectional horizontal images, rather than routinely obtain reconstructed views. The horizontal images are easy to interpret as long as they are displayed one after the other in sequence, from cranial to caudal or the other way round, and are adequately labeled. In any case, the pathological finding in question, generally a disk protrusion or prolapse, will only be clearly visible in two or three individual sections.

> ! It is advisable to refer to the L5/S1 disk seen in a CT scan as the "last" intervertebral disk and to the L4/5 disk as the "second-last" one to avoid any possible confusion, particularly when intradiscal therapy or disk surgery is to be performed.

Otherwise, the presence of transitional vertebrae may lead to inconsistent numbering. When the image intensifier is used in the operating room, it is safe and easy to image the sacrum first and then count the intervertebral spaces from the bottom up.

The Normal CT Scan

The interpretation of CT scans is similar to that of conventional **radiographs.** In a CT image, as on a plain radiograph, thick (cortical) bone appears white and fat or air appears dark. All shades of gray are possible in between. The vertebral body spongiosa has a salt-and-pepper appearance. Disk tissue, the dural sac, and the nerve roots usually all appear equally gray to the naked eye and can thus be told apart only by their configuration. They are separated from one another by the intervening epidural fat.

Before searching in detail for pathoanatomical findings in the spinal canal on a cross-sectional CT image, one must first ascertain the segment, and the **level** within the segment, that the image represents. The lateral scout view (topogram), on which the individual cross-sections are indicated and numbered, can be of assistance here, informing the examiner whether the plane of section passes through a vertebral body, a disk, or (in the case of L5/S1) both.

Even without looking at the scout view, however, the examiner should still be able to determine the level of a CT section of the lumbar spine within the particular segment at which it was obtained. Sections in which the intervertebral foramina are not seen can easily be distinguished from those in which they appear as lateral openings in the vertebral arch. The images displaying the intervertebral foramina are clinically important because they show the immediate vicinity of the intervertebral disk.

> ! On all sequences of CT images of the lumbar spine, it is important to follow the nerve root from its site of origin from the dural sac all the way to its exit from the spinal canal through the neural (intervertebral) foramen.

Displacement of the nerve root, or invisibility of the nerve root because of impingement from adjacent pathological structures, is of clinical significance. A disk protrusion that does not impinge on a nerve root cannot be the cause of sciatica.

The CT scan demonstrates the entire course of the nerve roots and clearly shows that protrusions and prolapses of the lower two lumbar disks can often impinge on the L5 and S1 nerve roots at the same time. Thus, for example, a large paramedian L4/5 disk prolapse can impinge on the L5 root from the medial side and simultaneously impinge on the S1 root from the lateral side just as it emerges from the dural sac, or while it still lies intrathecally. A similar situation arises with a lateral L5/S1 disk herniation, which can push the L5 root outward and the S1 root inward.

Anatomical variants, including conjoined roots and variable origin of the nerve roots from the dural sac, can produce unusual clinical and radiological situations. A preoperative imaging study—CT, myelogram, or MRI—is therefore essential in every case, even if the segmental symptoms and signs appear to be unequivocal.

Protrusions and prolapses of lumbar disks. Modern CT scanners have high enough resolution to enable displaced disk tissue in the spinal canal to be recognized and differentiated from the neighboring soft tissues. The contours of the disk are at their most pronounced where there is a large amount of epidural fat in the vicinity, e.g., behind the L5/S1 disk.

Disk protrusions and prolapses can be recognized in the lumen of the spinal canal either because of their typical localization and configuration or through the manner in which they impinge on and distort the neighboring dural sac, epidural fat, and nerve roots. Disk tissue is usually more radiodense than the lumbar CSF, though these two tissues sometimes appear isodense to the human eye. Isodense soft tissues in the spinal canal are more commonly seen in CT images produced by older scanners with poorer resolution, or else when the spinal canal is narrowed, so that the relatively radiodense rootlets of the cauda equina are not surrounded by much CSF, epidural fat is largely absent, and the dural sac is adjacent to the bony wall of the vertebral canal on all sides.

Signs of tissue displacement. Displaced disk tissue always pushes some of the ventral epidural fat aside, producing an asymmetrical configuration of the fat. It must be borne in mind, however, that epidural fat may be absent, e. g., because of spinal canal stenosis (see below), postoperative adhesions and scoliosis, or simply advanced age. The most important radiological finding is the displacement or loss of contour of a nerve root together with indentation of the dural sac. The differential diagnosis includes asymmetry of the nerve root origins from the dural sac and scoliosis causing the CT plane to be angulated rather than truly transverse in relation to the spine.

The site and extent of the dislocated disk tissue must be precisely specified with information in all three dimensions. Stating the level of the disk fragment specifies the horizontal plane in which it lies; its horizontal distance from the midline determines its location in the frontal plane; and the extent to which it protrudes into the spinal canal is its size in the sagittal plane. Inspection of the images at multiple levels reveals whether a prolapse is more displaced in the more cranial or more caudal direction. The precise depiction of the displaced disk tissue on the CT scan tells the surgeon how far to explore within the spinal canal to remove all of the expelled disk fragments.

An indirect sign of nerve root compression is thickening of the nerve root shadow at the affected level and at more caudal levels. Inspection of the course of the nerve roots in a series of transverse sections often reveals asymmetrical nerve root diameter over multiple levels.

When dislocated disk tissue protrudes into the spinal canal, the indication for surgery or intradiscal treatment depends to a large extent on whether the finding is a **protrusion** with a preserved anulus fibrosus or a prolapse perforating the outer layer of the fibrous border of the disk. Discography provides an unequivocal answer to this question, but CT can also be very helpful. Disk protrusions have a symmetrical base and a greater ratio of base width to height than prolapses; prolapses, on the other hand, jut further into the epidural space from

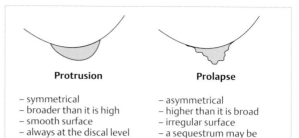

Protrusion	Prolapse
– symmetrical	– asymmetrical
– broader than it is high	– higher than it is broad
– smooth surface	– irregular surface
– always at the discal level	– a sequestrum may be
– moderate displacement	supra- or infradiscal
of dura mater and nerve	– marked displacement of
roots	dura mater and nerve roots

Fig. 11.56 CT criteria for distinguishing disk protrusions (with intact anulus fibrosus) from disk prolapses (with perforated anulus fibrosus).

a relatively narrow base and tend to have an irregular surface with a pointed tip, producing a triangular outline (**Fig. 11.56**).

The periphery of a protrusion may contain sickle-shaped areas of calcification representing the initial stage of ossification of the posterior longitudinal ligament. In a young patient, this finding represents the bony margin of the vertebral body, which has been undermined and lifted up by disk tissue.

A **prolapse** can be displaced cranially or caudally, either wholly or in part, and can be seen on transverse sections at vertebral body levels, but this is not the case for a simple disk protrusion.

The CT appearance of subligamentous fragments is intermediate between that of protrusions and prolapses. Subligamentous fragments can be treated by intradiscal methods.

Even very broad prolapses seen on CT do not necessarily require invasive treatment. Their management should always be based on the clinical findings (**Figs. 11.57–11.62**).

11

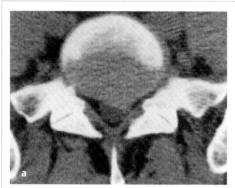
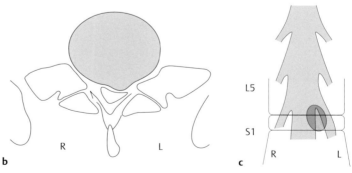

Fig. 11.57 a–c Clinical findings: 42-year-old man with S1 sciatica for the last 12 weeks, Lasègue sign positive on the left at 30°, crossed Lasègue sign positive on the right at 60°, pain and band-like hypesthesia in a left S1 distribution, diminished left Achilles reflex, no motor deficit. CT: broad-based protrusion of disk tissue (grade II dislocation) at the L5/S1 level, with left paramedial indentation of the dural sac. Treatment: conservative.

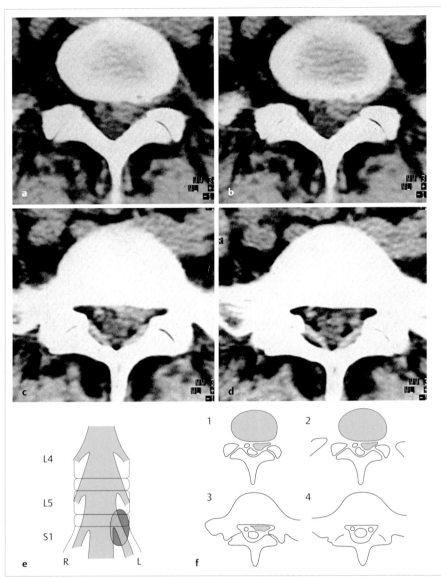

Fig. 11.58 a–f Clinical findings: 51-year-old woman with severe, persistent left-sided sciatica for the last 6 weeks, Lasègue sign positive at 40°, Achilles reflex absent on the left, pain and band-like hypesthesia in the left S1 distribution, grade 3 paresis of left plantar flexors. CT: a free fragment lying paramedially in the epidural space on the left side is seen at the L5/S1 level (dislocation grade V); it extends caudally to the upper edge of the S1 vertebral body. The two S1 roots can be seen again ventral to the dural sac only at the mid-S1 level; even here, the left S1 root is still somewhat dorsally displaced. Treatment: surgery. A caudally displaced free fragment, hard and bean-sized, was found in the axilla of the S1 nerve root (see **Fig. 11.58 e**).

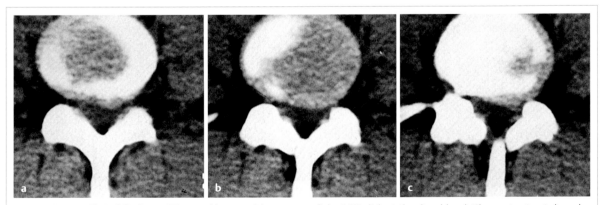

Fig. 11.59 a–c Clinical findings: 37-year-old man with massive contralateral sciatic postural abnormality for the last 5 weeks. Band-like pain in an L5 distribution, mild weakness of the left extensor hallucis longus. CT: broad-based protrusion of the L4/5 disk at the discal level. The protrusion is broader than it is deep and is mainly located paramedially on the left side. Disk protrusion, grade II dislocation. Treatment: conservative.

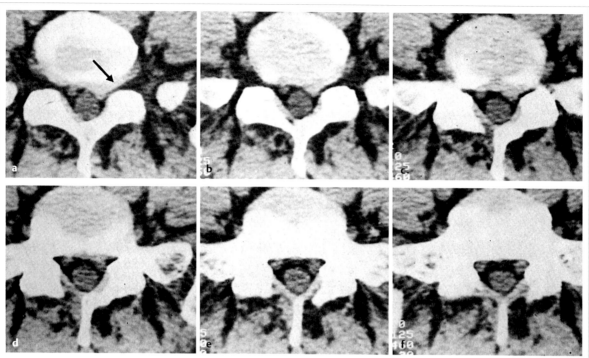

Fig. 11.60 a–f Clinical findings: 39-year-old woman with left S1 sciatica, diminished Achilles reflex on the left, positive Lasègue sign at 60°, band of pain and hypesthesia in a left S1 distribution, band-like pain partly in an L5 distribution as well. CT: broad-based L5/S1 disk protrusion extending into the intervertebral foramen (grade II dislocation), displacing the S1 root dorsally and also impinging on the exiting left L5 nerve root laterally in the foramen (→). In the more caudal images, the left S1 root is less severely displaced. This root is thickened in comparison to its counterpart on the right. Treatment: conservative.

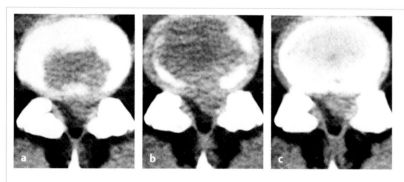

Fig. 11.61 a–c Clinical findings: 39-year-old man with L5 sciatica for the last 4 months and an acute exacerbation for the last 6 weeks. Grade III dorsiflexor paresis on the left, Lasègue sign positive at 20°, ipsilateral postural abnormality, absent left Achilles reflex, band of pain in an L5 and S1 distribution, hypesthesia of the entire dorsum of the foot, no cauda equina symptoms or signs. CT: large fragment at the L4/5 discal level obliterating the left L5 root and compressing the dural sac to half of its normal cross-sectional area. Treatment: immediate surgery. A prolapse the size of a fingertip, partly free and partly still under the posterior longitudinal ligament, was found deep in the axilla of the L5 root (grade IV dislocation).

Postoperative CT

Even though CT scanning technology is now quite advanced, **postoperative scans remain hard to interpret.** One reason is the limited experience that has been gathered in this area to date; another is the fact that a postoperative scan generally contains multiple isodense soft tissue shadows lying next to one another within the spinal canal that are poorly demarcated from each other. In the first few days after disk surgery, CT scanning may be necessary if the original symptoms persist or new ones have arisen. The cause may be a residual or newly expelled disk fragment, hematoma, abscess, or pseudomeningocele due to leakage of CSF from the dural sac.

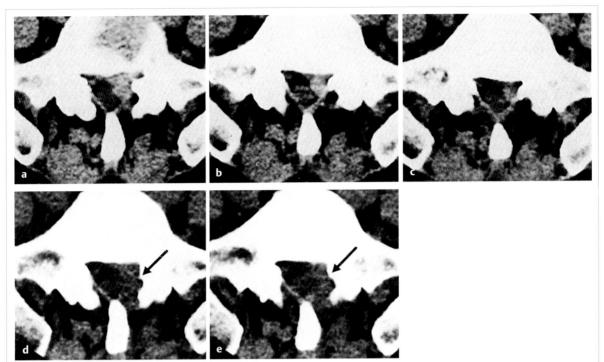

Fig. 11.62 a–e Clinical features: 46-year-old man with very severe left S1 sciatica for the past 5 weeks. Absent Achilles reflex, Lasègue sign positive at 30°, band of pain and hypesthesia in a left S1 distribution, ipsilateral postural abnormality. CT: extradiscal fragment (grade V dislocation) from the L5/S1 disk extending caudally, seen at its greatest extent in the section just below the L5/S1 disk. The left S1 nerve root is obliterated by the fragment. Additional finding: lateral spinal canal stenosis. Treatment: surgery. Immediately upon opening of the ligamentum flavum at the left L5/S1 level, sequestrated disk material came forward, having worked its way posteriorly past the dura mater and nerve root to just under the ligamentum flavum. Postoperative CT: status post prolapse removal and widening of the lateral recess (→). The patient has been asymptomatic ever since the operation. Collections of serous fluid in the wound, the dural sac, and the nerve root together create an isodense shadow on the left side of the spinal canal; this is a normal postoperative finding.

Collections of blood or CSF can usually be recognized by their rounded shape and distinguished from one another by density measurements in Hounsfield units: for example, the CSF-filled cavity of a pseudomeningocele has the same radiodensity as water.

Scar tissue in the epidural space is recognizable as a grayish mass with irregular borders adjacent to the disk, posterior edge or the vertebral body, and/or lamina. The configuration of the dura mater and nerve root is asymmetrical. Often, the nerve root can no longer be seen on the operated side, because it is enveloped in scar tissue. The most important sign of scar tissue is the absence of epidural fat.

After hemilaminectomy, the laminar contour is interrupted on one side. In this case, the scar tissue runs uninterruptedly from the dural sac to the muscles of the back.

When a fat pad has been placed in the wound before surgical closure, the postoperative scar tissue is interrupted by a more or less broad, rounded area that appears dark (i. e., with the density of fat). The CT findings after fat-pad insertion have been described by Schroeder (1982), Burton (1983), and Krämer and Köster (2001), among others.

The difficulty of interpreting postoperative CT scans lies in the fact that nerve roots, disks, and scar tissue all have similar radiodensity. Thus, a recurrent disk prolapse may hide within the apparently uniform gray shadow of extensive postoperative scarring. The extent of impingement can then only be recognized indirectly by the distortion of the dural sac.

A further means of distinguishing different types of soft tissue from one another in CT scans is the systemic (i. e., intravenous) administration of contrast medium. The theoretical basis for this is the fact that well-perfused tissue will take up contrast medium to a greater extent than tissue that is only poorly perfused or not at all, such as a **fresh disk prolapse.** Contrast-enhanced CT scans are mainly useful for the detection of recurrent disk prolapse within peridural scar tissue. Fresh, well-perfused scar tissue naturally takes up more contrast medium than old, fibrotic sheets of scar in which old disk-derived tissue has become incorporated.

In view of these difficulties, one should not be too quick to use postoperative CT to diagnose recurrent disk prolapses, in order not to cause further undue worry in patients who have just undergone disk surgery but still have symptoms. Most of these symptoms are due to scarring and adhesions rather than new prolapses. Every new operation only makes this situation worse.

Summary: CT

In CT scanning, roentgen rays are used to produce cross-sectional images in the transverse plane. A roentgen ray tube rotating around the patient obtains data in each plane of section that are then synthesized into images by computer. Even though CT does not distinguish different types of soft tissue as well as MRI, it is superior to MRI for the examination of bony structures. For example, it enables a clear differentiation of disk tissue from calcification or ossification (the latter may be the residua of old disk prolapses). In addition to its limited ability to tell different types of soft tissue apart, further drawbacks of CT include the imaging of only part of the lumbar spine and the associated radiation exposure, which is especially high in repeated so-called CT-guided injections of the lumbar spine.

Diagnostic Study of the CSF

Additional studies of other types are done mainly for differential diagnostic purposes. These include laboratory tests such as the complete blood count, CRP, and electrophoresis, which show no pathological changes in lumbar syndrome. Whenever myelography is carried out, CSF is obtained as a by-product and should always be sent to the laboratory for analysis.

! In patients with lumbar disk prolapse, the CSF is of normal appearance (clear) and flows rapidly through a thin spinal needle.

If blockage of CSF flow is suspected a Queckenstedt test can be done, but this is not part of the routine examination in lumbar syndrome. The CSF laboratory findings in lumbar syndrome are usually normal. When the lumbar nerve roots are subject to continuous, intense irritation from a large prolapse, or in post-discotomy syndrome, one may sometimes find a mildly *increased protein concentration,* though the cell count remains normal.

A markedly elevated protein concentration combined with a normal cell count and normal CSF opening pressure is called albuminocytologic dissociation. This is a classic finding in **Guillain–Barré syndrome** but can also be seen in spinal irritative conditions of many other types and is thus nonspecific. In such cases, both the total protein content and the colloid curves display high values.

The analysis of CSF contributes very little to the positive demonstration of a disk prolapse and is therefore used mainly for the exclusion of other potential causes of the clinical syndrome, e.g., infectious processes (herpes zoster, syphilis) or tumors.

Pathological elevation of the protein concentration and cell count, or obstructed flow as revealed by the Queckenstedt test, is an indication for further diagnostic testing.

Discography

After initial enthusiasm for this diagnostic technique (Erlacher 1949, Lindblom 1951, 1969, Witt 1951), lumbar discography fell into almost total disuse for a long period, because it was recognized that pathological configurations of contrast medium in the interior of the disk lacked clinical significance. Not every degenerated disk produces symptoms. Moreover, myelography with the newly developed contrast media proved to be much more informative. Only in the last few years have publications on lumbar discography begun to reappear, though each new publication seems to emphasize different aspects of the interpretation of the findings (Hugdins 1977, Crock 1983, Fraser et al. 1983, Park 1985, Sullivan 1985, Schleberger et al. 1986, Sachs et al. 1987, Mooney 1988, Weinstein et al. 1988, Braithwaite 1998, Ito 1998, McCulloch 1998, Carragee 1999, 2000, 2002, 2006, Lam 2000, Nachemson and Jonsson 2000, Herkowicz 2004, Böhm et al. 2005). A meta-analysis by Ahn (2006) shows that the role of discography remains controversial in the work-up of patients with low back pain and degenerative disk disease. A lumbar discogram is considered to be positive, with reference to the indication for surgery, only when the contrast medium that is injected into the interior of the disk flows out dorsally into the epidural space (reflux) or when a disk fragment is found in the dorsal portion of the anulus fibrosus, in some cases protruding out of it. All other discographic findings are designated as negative, even when severe degenerative changes are found.

! The interpretation of discograms focuses on the question whether a disk prolapse or protrusion is present.

The diagnostic accuracy of lumbar discography, when it is employed in this way, is 83% (Hudgins 1977) (**Fig. 11.63**). Discography is also a useful supplement to CT

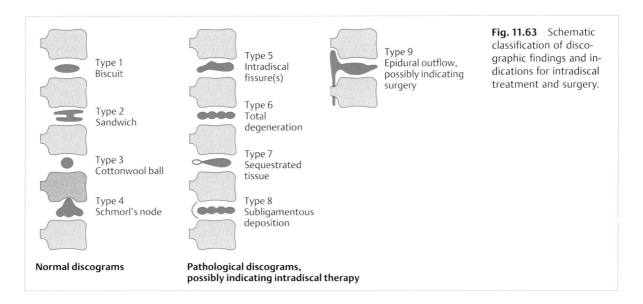

Type 1
Biscuit

Type 2
Sandwich

Type 3
Cottonwool ball

Type 4
Schmorl's node

Type 5
Intradiscal
fissure(s)

Type 6
Total
degeneration

Type 7
Sequestrated
tissue

Type 8
Subligamentous
deposition

Type 9
Epidural outflow,
possibly indicating
surgery

Fig. 11.63 Schematic
classification of disco-
graphic findings and in-
dications for intradiscal
treatment and surgery.

Normal discograms

**Pathological discograms,
possibly indicating intradiscal therapy**

11

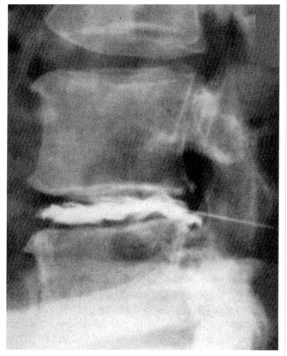

Fig. 11.64 Discography at L4/5 reveals a totally degenerated disk with a dorsally displaced fragment, type 7. No
epidural outflow of contrast medium. If this finding correlates with the clinical findings, intradiscal therapy is indicated.

closed (not perforated), the injection pressure and in-
jectable volume of fluid indicate the size of the intradiscal cavity system and the extent of disk degeneration
(**Fig. 11.64**). Injection of the affected disk generally re-
produces or intensifies the patient's typical radiating
pain, similarly to the cervical spine distension test
(**memory pain**).

The interpretation of contrast medium patterns. In
general, a lateral radiographic view suffices to show
whether the contrast medium injected into the disk remains in the center of the disk or flows out of it
through a narrow connecting pathway into the epidural space. To localize a fragment more precisely, additional oblique views are needed (**Fig. 11.65**). The contrast medium injected into the interior of the disk
spreads out in different patterns depending on the size
and type of the intradiscal cavity system. The contrast
medium depot may appear rounded or branch out ir-
regularly toward the periphery. These intradiscal contrast medium patterns are of little clinical importance,
however, because from a certain age onward nearly all
lumbar disks display degenerative tears and branching
of greater or lesser severity. The only findings that
should truly be considered pathological with reference
to a possible indication for surgery are contrast medium reflux into the epidural space and the presence of
a tissue fragment.

> A tissue fragment is defined as a piece of tissue around
> which contrast medium flows but which is not itself
> filled with contrast medium and lies at the dorsal edge
> of the anulus fibrosus, possibly protruding outward from
> it.

Such fragments are often covered by a thin layer composed of the outer lamellae of the anulus fibrosus, the

scanning in many cases, because it provides special information about the location and size of any dorsally
displaced disk fragments. Discography yields information about the disease process beyond the findings that
can be appreciated visually on radiographs: if the disk is

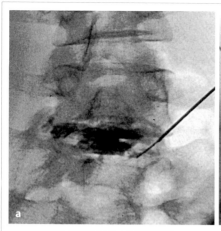
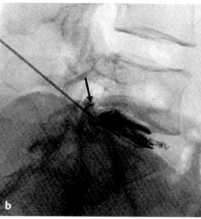

Fig. 11.65 a, b Discography at L5/S1 reveals a subligamentous (→) fragment, type 8. If this finding correlates with the clinical findings, intradiscal therapy is indicated. Even when the tip of the needle is placed at the edge of the disk, the intervertebral space can be filled with contrast medium, and thus also with the therapeutic agent.

posterior longitudinal ligament, and/or the ventral epidural membrane. The hernia-like sac around the fragment may take up so much contrast medium that the fragment itself can no longer be seen.

Corresponding to the diverse pathoanatomical operative findings in patients with lumbar disk prolapses, discography can reveal almost any conceivable pattern of contrast medium, a fact that makes interpretation rather difficult (**Fig. 11.66**). If the lateral and oblique radiographs after discography do not provide sufficient information about the site of a disk fragment, a CT scan of the affected segment can be obtained about 2 h later (so-called CT discography). This technique is especially suitable for the demonstration of intraforaminal protrusions (Jackson and Glah 1987, Kornberg 1987, Schultiz et al. 1988).

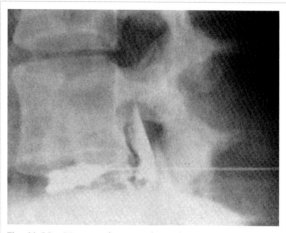

Fig. 11.66 Discography at L4/5 with type 9 findings. A large amount of contrast medium immediately flows into the epidural space.

MRI

Synonyms: MRT (magnetic resonance tomography), NMR (nuclear magnetic resonance).

> **!** **Physical principles underlying MRI.** When a strong external magnetic field is applied to the body, atoms within the body that have a magnetic moment orient themselves in the direction of the field. When the external field is then switched off, the "relaxation" of the atoms oriented along it is accompanied by the emission of electromagnetic radiation that can be detected and measured outside the body. The patient must lie still for a relatively long time inside a fairly narrow tube containing a strong magnetic field while the images are produced with the aid of computer technology. Images can be generated in any imaging plane. Unlike CT, MRI does not involve the use of ionizing radiation.

Technical procedure. Just as in CT, the patient lies supine with slightly flexed legs and must remain in the same position throughout the study. The scout scan and sectional images in the transverse plane are analogous to their CT counterparts. The patient's right side is always on the left side of the image (cf. **Fig. 11.54**, p. 173).

Advantages. MRI is the diagnostic imaging method of choice for lumbar disk disease because it enables imaging of the entire lumbar spine, in multiple planes of section, with better differentiation of various types of soft tissue from one another than CT. A particular advantage is the absolute harmlessness of the technique, which has now been fully documented.

> **!** MRI is the only technique used to diagnose lumbar disk prolapses that does not employ roentgen rays.

The advantage of MRI for disk surgery is that it can be used to generate images of all of the lumbar motion segments in a single study. It is thus much harder to over-

11

Table 11.3 Comparison of MRI and CT in disk herniation

MRI	CT
No ionizing radiation	Ionizing radiation
Time-consuming study	Quick study
All segments	Routinely only 2–3 segments
All planes	Only the axial plane
High contrast resolution for disk tissue	Low contrast resolution for disk tissue
Very expensive	Expensive

Table 11.4 Indications for lumbar spine MRI

- Disk herniation
- Post-discotic syndrome
- Differential diagnosis of other neurological diseases

Table 11.5 Comparison of imaging techniques in the lumbar spine

Question	MRI	CT	Myelography
Disk herniation	+++	++	(+)
Spinal canal stenosis	+++	+++	++
Post-discotic syndrome	+++	++	+
DD neurological diseases	+++	+	+++
Trauma	+	+++	+
Spondylolisthesis	+	+++	+
Spondylitis	+	+++	–
Tumors (metastases)	+	++	+

11

look dislocated disk fragments or simultaneous disk prolapses at other levels in an MRI scan as compared to CT, which is routinely used to image only two or three lumbar segments at a time.

The ability to show images in any plane of section at will (sagittal, coronal, horizontal, or selective demonstration of foraminal planes) permits the precise localization of dislocated fragments and osseous nerve root compression.

The resolution of the technique is such that prolapsed disk tissue and the dural sac are well demarcated from one another. The indentation of the dural sac by a disk prolapse resembles what is seen in a lateral myelographic image. Furthermore, the prolapsed tissue is seen in fine detail. Well-hydrated nucleus pulposus tissue has a high signal intensity, equivalent to that of CSF, in T2-weighted images. Portions of the anulus fibrosus, the cartilaginous end plates, and the posterior longitudinal ligament have a low signal intensity in all signal weightings because of their low water content (**Table 11.3**).

! The water content of the disk prolapse or protrusion is an important determinant of the optimal form of treatment, and of the prognosis.

A well-hydrated free fragment in the epidural space can be treated conservatively at first, as long as no major neurologic deficit is present, because it can be expected to shrink rapidly in volume now that the nucleus pulposus tissue within it is no longer in contact with the intradiscal osmotic system. On the other hand, hard, cartilaginous fragments, which usually produce severe pain, are unlikely to shrink over time and one should not wait too long before removing these surgically.

In addition, MRI enables quantitative assessment of degenerative changes of the disks, particularly their water content. We have found that the human intervertebral disk contains more water in the morning than in the evening. This finding reveals the operation of an osmotic system within the disks (see Chapter 4).

We know from pathoanatomical studies and clinical experience in discography that disk degeneration is not synonymous with disk-related symptoms. Findings on MRI within 12 weeks of the inception of serious low back pain are highly unlikely to represent any new structural change (Carragee 2006). Thus, it is wrong to attach too much importance to the radiological finding of degenerative dehydration of disk tissue with consequent bulging of the anulus fibrosus. On the contrary, the hypointense, poorly hydrated degenerated disks seen on an MRI scan ("**black disks**") bode fewer problems for the future than the bright, well-hydrated disks that still have a normal turgor pressure (see **Fig. 11.68**).

CT or MRI?

The indications for lumbar spine MRI in disk disease are determined mainly by considerations of availability and cost. The entire diagnostic spectrum can be covered by CT, occasionally supplemented with myelography (**Table 11.4**).

The special advantages of MRI have to do with the localization and differentiation of dislocated fragments in the epidural space. A surgeon should not operate on a disk without a preoperative MRI scan, particularly if microsurgery is to be done through a small incision. MRI is also much better than CT and myelography at distinguishing postoperative scar tissue from residual or recurrent prolapses. Likewise, it is better for the differential diagnosis of other neurological diseases in the lumbar region. All other questions, particularly those concerning bony structures, are better answered by CT (**Table 11.5**).

Findings in Disk Degeneration

The strengths of MRI are particularly easy to appreciate when MRI and CT scans of the same patient are compared. The surgeon obtains clear information about how

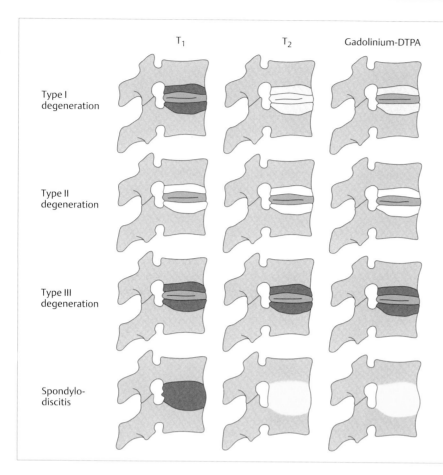

| | T₁ | T₂ | Gadolinium-DTPA |

Fig. 11.67 Modic classification, including differential diagnosis vs. spondylodiscitis (from Linhardt and Grifka in Wirth and Zichner 2004).

far and in what direction the spinal canal must be explored so that all sequestrated fragments can be removed. The designation of locations in the lumbar and epidural space with a conventional scheme of levels and zones enables radiologists and surgeons to communicate effectively and unambiguously about the MRI findings. In addition to precise localization, MRI also yields information about the consistency and water content of disk tissue. **When interpreting MRI scans, however, the clinician must be aware that the perifocal edema surrounding dislocated pieces of disk tissue makes the degree of impingement on neighboring structures appear more extensive, and more impressive, than it really is.** Medial protrusions and prolapses seen in sagittal MRI views often seem to occupy the entire spinal canal.

! MRI exaggerates the true findings in disk prolapse.

The clinical findings above all determine the choice of therapy, no matter how impressive the MRI findings may be.

The pathoanatomical changes in the intervertebral space are displayed better on MRI than on plain radiographs or CT scans. Loss of water within disk tissue,

leading to fibrosis and sclerosis, is revealed as loss of signal. Recent improvements in MRI technology make it possible to visualize individual structures within the intervertebral space, e. g., fragments that have lost their connection to the surrounding tissue, the outer lamellae of the anulus fibrosus, and ligamentous structures. Protrusions can be distinguished from prolapses. Discography is very rarely needed now to answer these questions.

The Modic Classification

Beyond the changes in the disk, there are also corresponding changes in the neighboring vertebral bodies, expressed not only as spondylosis and osteochondrosis, which can be seen even in plain radiographs or CT scans, but also as a variable appearance of the spongiosa. The MRI abnormalities of the bone marrow space of the neighboring vertebrae were classified by Modic (1985) into three types, representing stages that cannot always be sharply distinguished from one another (**Fig. 11.67**):

- Type I: ingrowth of vascularized, contrast-enhancing tissue into the neighboring bone marrow, with increased signal intensity on T2-weighted images and decreased signal intensity on T1-weighted images.

11

- Type II: fatty degeneration of the bone marrow with increased signal intensity on T1-weighted images and moderately increased signal intensity or isointense signal on T2-weighted images.
- Type III: increasing sclerosis and scarring of the bone marrow space with loss of signal in images of all signal weightings.

Type I degenerative changes of the vertebral bodies may resemble spondylodiscitis on MRI. Therefore, if the clinical manifestations and laboratory findings warrant it, conventional tomography, CT, and in some cases diagnostic tissue biopsy for infectious material should be carried out.

The clinical relevance of the degenerative changes classified by Modic is slight. Bone marrow changes are seen on MRI as a normal correlate of age-related, generalized intervertebral disk degeneration. A few publications have appeared in which the authors attempt to correlate the changes described by Modic with certain clinical symptoms (Pfirrmann et al. 2001, Kuisma et al. 2004, 2007, Albert and Manniche 2005, Jones et al. 2005, Kjaer et al. 2005, Modic et al. 2005, Linhardt et al. 2007, O'Connell et al. 2007).

Postoperative MRI

Relatively well-hydrated disk tissue can be more easily distinguished from postoperative scar tissue on a plain radiograph than on a CT scan. In T2-weighted MR images, disk tissue appears bright and thus different from hypointense, poorly vascularized scar tissue. As soon as some of the disk material is degenerated, however, it becomes isointense and is no longer so easy to distinguish from scar tissue. In such cases, intravenous contrast medium must be used, just as for a CT scan. Clinical experience has shown that diagnostic accuracy can be improved by comparing T1-weighted images obtained before and after the injection of contrast medium (Peters et al. 1990, Krämer and Köster 2001). Even this method, however, does not eliminate all differential diagnostic problems, because granulation tissue that is histologically identical to epidural granulation tissue may grow from the end plates into the disks as part of the degenerative process.

Further discussion of postoperative CT vs. MRI can be found on pages 286 ff. and 290 ff.

MRI Findings without Symptoms

Disk protrusions, signs of degeneration with black disks, signal changes in the vertebral bodies, and postoperative scarring on the MRI scan need not necessarily be accompanied by corresponding symptoms. Often, such MRI findings are found in segments neighboring a disk prolapse as radiologic correlates of asymptomatic disk degeneration, as the following ex-

amples will show. When a patient presents with a nerve root compression syndrome and the MRI scan shows abnormal findings in multiple segments, it is usually only one segment that is responsible for the clinical manifestations. Other diagnostic techniques in addition to MRI must be used to localize the origin of the pain, e. g., a discogram revealing "memory pain," a nerve root block, or an EMG.

Reports in the literature. There are many published reports of extensive degenerative changes seen on MRI in individuals who had no symptoms at all, or who at least had none at the time the MRI was obtained. Boden et al. (1990), for example, found a disk protrusion or prolapse in 20% of individuals under age 60 and 36% of those over age 60. In their longitudinal study of asymptomatic individuals, Borenstein et al. (1998) found that degenerative changes seen on MRI have no predictive value for future low back pain. Further studies documenting pathological radiological findings in asymptomatic individuals include those of Bozzao et al. (1992), Buirski and Silberstein (1993), Carragee et al. (2000), Krämer and Köster (2001), Krappel and Harland (2001), and Assheuer (2002).

Case Illustrations (from Krämer and Köster 2001)

1. L2/3 Protrusion and Prolapse, MRI and CT (**Fig. 11.68**)

Clinical presentation. This 44-year-old man reported feeling a sudden snap in his back while getting up from a low chair 4 weeks ago, and thereafter severe back pain radiating into the lateral aspect of both thighs. The pain persisted despite 3 weeks of conservative treatment, and he was admitted to hospital. Examination revealed a sciatic postural deformity with the torso inclined slightly to the right. There were no motor deficits, and the deep tendon reflexes were normal. The Lasègue sign was positive on the right at 30°.

MRI and CT. These study sequences are shown in **Fig. 11.68**.

Findings. The L3/4 and L5/S1 intervertebral discs are of markedly diminished signal intensity in the T2 image. There is a broad-based, asymmetrical posterior displacement of disk tissue of relatively high signal intensity at level L2/3 (**c,** →), which compresses on the dural sac (**a–c**). There is also a circumscribed posterior displacement of disk tissue in the median zone at the L5/S1 level (**a, b, d**), without compression the dural sac. The CT findings at L5/S1 are consistent with the MRI findings, but the CT additionally shows clear evidence of calcification or ossification (**e,** →).

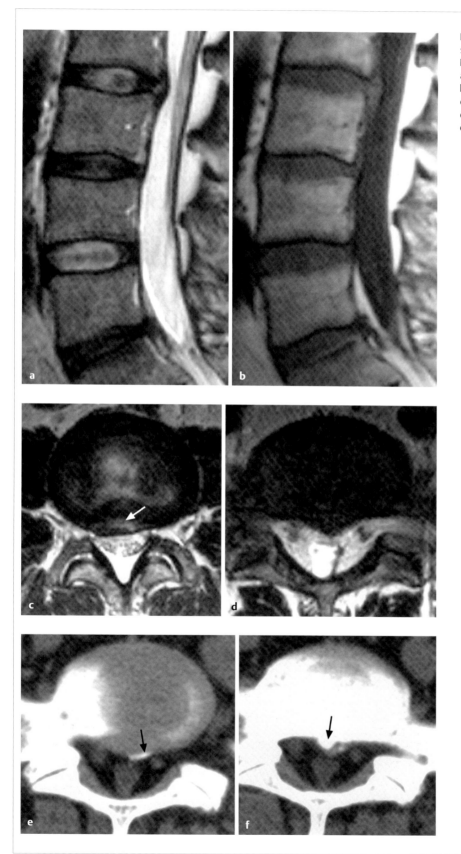

Fig. 11.68 a–f Study
sequences (from Krämer and
Köster 2001).
a T2 TSE, sagittal, median.
b T1 SE, sagittal, median.
c T2 TSE, axial, L2/L3.
d T2 TSE, axial, L5/S1.
e, f CT, axial, L5/S1 (**e**) and
superior end plate of S1
(**f**).

11

Diagnosis. Protrusion (grade II dislocation) of the L2/3 intervertebral disk and old medial prolapse of the L5/S1 intervertebral disk.

Note. Bony structures in the L5/S1 segment that are seen on the CT scan cannot be visualized by MRI with the sequences shown in this case.

Treatment. Hospitalization was recommended for conservative treatment consisting of relaxation supine with the hips and knees flexed, a flexion orthosis, and local injections.

Clinical course. The pain improved steadily under conservative treatment. After 3 months there was only mild residual sacral pain, without radiation into the legs.

Comments. The subligamentous paramedial protrusion in segment L2/3 produced the clinical symptoms in this case. Compression involved only the intrathecal portions of the spinal nerves, and for this reason the pain did not radiate further down the legs. The broad-based protrusion seen in the axial images is consistent with an intact anulus fibrosus. The protrusion at L5/S1 is not clinically significant: both CT and MRI show that it makes no contact with the neural elements.

2. L5/S1 Protrusion and Prolapse, Modic II Signs (**Fig. 11.69**)

Clinical presentation. This 40-year-old man complained of low back pain and left-sided sciatica of 3 months' duration. The band of pain corresponded to the left S1 segment. The pain was of moderate intensity; he was able to sleep at night, and he felt pain during the day only with certain movements. Examination revealed a diminished left Achilles tendon reflex and a positive Lasègue sign on the left at 60°.

MRI. The study sequences are shown in **Fig. 11.69**.

Findings. Disk degeneration is present in the last two segments, which are of diminished signal intensity and diminished height (**a, b**). Marked changes (Modic type II) are seen in the superior and inferior end plates at L4/5. The L4/5 disk and especially the L5/S1 disk (**a–c**) are posteriorly displaced, narrowing the left caudal intervertebral foramen (**e, →**). The subligamentous portions of the disk are of relatively high signal intensity in the T2 image (**e, →**). The left S1 nerve root is thickened (**a, b, f, →**).

Diagnosis. Broad-based disk protrusion at L4/5 (dislocation grade II) and prolapse at L5/S1 (dislocation grade V).

Treatment. Because the pain was relatively mild, conservative treatment was provided.

Clinical course. The treatment included epidural perineural injections on the left side in segment L5/S1, cube positioning (with hips and knees flexed), and physiotherapy. The symptoms improved, and the patient returned to his office job.

Comments. Neither the clinical findings nor the MRI findings are particularly severe. Some of the denser tissue in the left lateral recess of S1 corresponds to the left S1 nerve root, which is thickened because of edema. Modic type II changes of the upper and lower end plates of L4/5, of no clinical importance.

3. L4/5, Prolapse with Supradiscal Extension, Modic II Signs (**Fig. 11.70**)

Clinical presentation. This 61-year-old man had suffered from back pain, with occasional radiation into the legs, for several years. In the week leading up to presentation, the pain had become increasingly severe and radiated into the right leg in an L4 and L5 dermatomal pattern, with some radiation into the anterior aspect of the thigh as well. Physical examination revealed limping on the right side due to pain and a positive Lasègue sign on the right at 60°. The right Achilles tendon reflex and patellar reflex were slightly diminished.

MRI. The study sequences are shown in **Fig. 11.70**.

Findings. The last two intervertebral discs are of diminished height and signal intensity on the T1- and T2-weighted images, and there is a zone of increased signal intensity in the end plates (**a, b**). There is disk tissue lying posterior to the L4 vertebra (**a, b**, arrowhead) and retaining only tenuous contact with the intervertebral disk (**a, →**). This tissue fills the entire right L4 lateral recess (**c**) and masks the right L4 nerve root (**→** = left L4 nerve root). The MIP reconstruction (**d**) shows the topographic relationship of the prolapse (P), the L4 nerve root (**→**), and the L5 nerve root (**→**).

Diagnosis. Right paramedial L4/5 disk prolapse with supradiscal fragment (dislocation grade V). Osteochondrosis at L4/5 and L5/S1 with Modic type II bone marrow changes.

Treatment. Surgery was recommended because of the severe pain and the massive fragment, despite the absence of a motor deficit.

Operative findings. Half of the inferior margin of the L4 lamina was removed to reveal a massive free fragment compressing the intrathecal portion of the L5 nerve root medially and the exiting L4 nerve root laterally. The L4/5 intervertebral space was so narrow that it did not admit insertion of a disk rongeur.

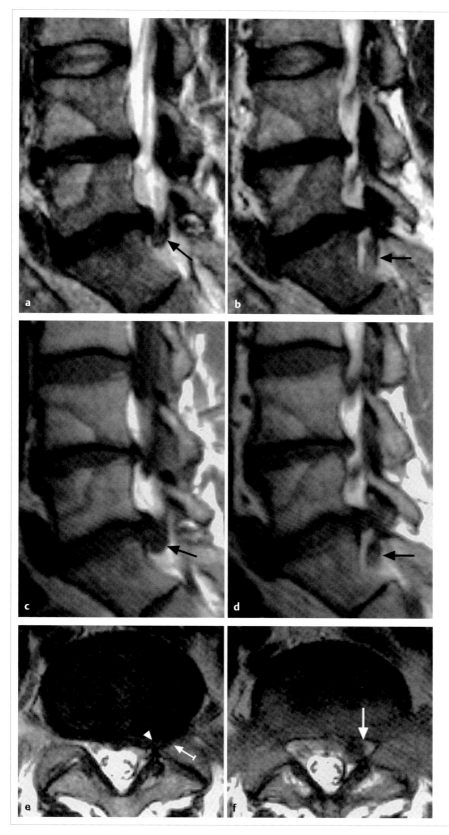

Fig. 11.69 a–f Study sequences (from Krämer and Köster 2001).
a, b T2 TSE, sagittal, left paramedian/paramedial (**a**) and left paramedial/lateral (**b**).
c, d T1 SE, sagittal, left paramedian/paramedial (**c**) and left paramedial/lateral (**d**).
e, f T2 TSE, axial, L5/S1 (**e**) and superior end plate (**f**).

11

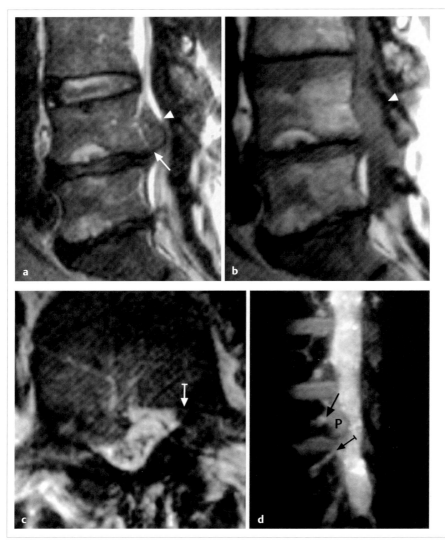

Fig. 11.70 a–d Study sequences (from Krämer and Köster 2001).
a T2 TSE, sagittal, right paramedial.
b T1 SE, sagittal, right paramedial.
c T2 TSE, axial, middle third of the L4 vertebral body.
d FISP 3D, oblique sagittal MIP reconstruction.

Clinical course. There was almost no leg pain after surgery. At the 3 month follow-up examination there was still no leg pain, but the back pain remained at its preoperative background level.

Comments. The massive fragment had separated from the parent disk at L4/5 and migrated craniolaterally, where it compressed both the intrathecal portion of the L5 nerve root and the exiting L4 nerve root. This produced a band of pain in the L4 and L5 dermatomes. Surgical intervention was deemed necessary because of the severe pain and the large size of the fragment.

4. L3/4, Prolapse with Supradiscal Extension and Modic I Signs (**Fig. 11.71**)

Clinical presentation. This 52-year-old man complained of severe back pain of 3 weeks' duration. The pain had initially radiated into the anterior aspect of his right thigh, but then radiated laterally in a band corresponding to the proximal portion of the right L5 derma-

tome. A marked ipsilateral sciatic postural deformity was present (i. e., the torso was inclined to the right). The Lasègue sign was positive at 30° on both sides.

EMG. There was evidence of nerve root irritation at the L3 and L4 levels, without any sign of florid denervation or a functionally relevant deficit.

MRI. The study sequences are shown in **Fig. 11.71**.

Findings. The lowest three intervertebral discs are of diminished signal intensity. A circumscribed subligamentous posterior displacement of disk tissue is seen at the L3/4 level, and the annuloligamentous complex (→) is well demarcated. The extruded disk tissue extends cranially as far as the middle of the posterior margin of the L3 vertebral body and is continuous with the parent disk (**a, b**). The dural sac is markedly compressed (**a–c**). A circumscribed edematous area in the posterobasal portion of the L3 vertebral body (**a, c,** →) is consistent with Modic type I bone marrow changes.

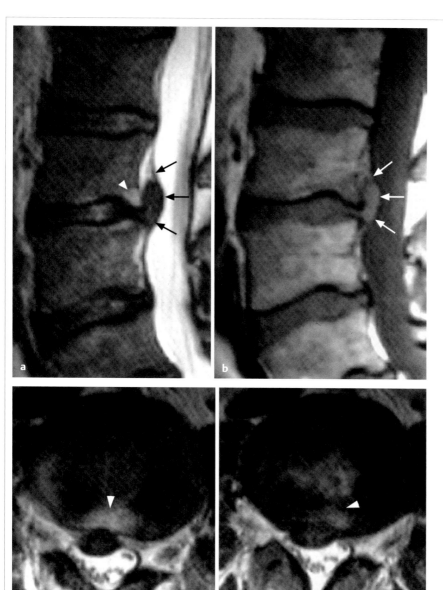

Fig. 11.71 a–d Study sequences (from Krämer and Köster 2001).
a T2 TSE, sagittal, median.
b T1 SE, sagittal, median.
c, d T2 TSE, axial, inferior end plate of vertebra L3 (**c**) and L3/L4 (**d**).

Diagnosis. Subligamentous medial and paramedial L3/4 intervertebral disk prolapse with supradiscal extension.

Treatment. Because there was no relevant functional impairment, conservative treatment was provided, consisting of relaxation supine with the hips and knees flexed, epidural perineural injections, physiotherapy, and back school.

Clinical course. Gradual resolution of symptoms with disappearance of leg pain, so that only sacral pain remained. The patient was discharged 2 weeks after surgery and fitted with a Discoflex torso orthosis. At follow-up examination 3 months later, the patient was nearly asymptomatic. Lumbar spine mobility was limited only at the end of the range of motion, and physiotherapy was not needed.

Comments. The L3/4 extrusion at disk level initially caused severe pain referable to the L3 and L4 nerve roots as it migrated into the concavity of the posterior wall of the vertebral body. The pain later became less severe. The extruded fragment was not sequestrated in the epidural space, but rather lay beneath the epidural membrane of the L3 vertebra, as can be seen from its relatively broad-based bulging into the epidural space, with a smooth margin (**Fig. 11.71c**). There are no nerve roots in the median and paramedian zones of the supradiscal level of the L3/4 segment; a disk prolapse at this level affects only the intrathecal nerve roots.

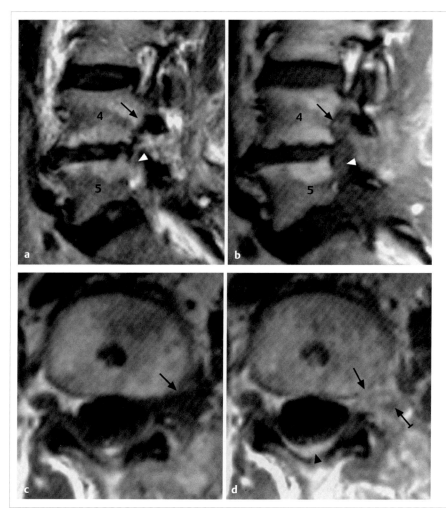

Fig. 11.72 a–d Study sequences (from Krämer and Köster 2001).
a T2 TSE, sagittal, left lateral.
b T1 SE, sagittal, left lateral.
c T1 SE, axial, inferior end plate of vertebra L4.
d T1 SE, axial, inferior end plate of vertebra L4, after IV injection of gadolinium.

5. L4/5, After Previous Surgery, Modic Type II Upper and Lower End-Plate Changes (**Fig. 11.72**)

Clinical presentation. This 58-year-old woman had undergone disk surgery 2 years previously. Pain in the left leg resolved after surgery, but returned 3 months later and persisted. The pain radiated into the L5 dermatome and occasionally also the S1 dermatome. The Lasègue sign was positive on the left at 30° and on the right at 60°. There was no neurologic deficit.

MRI. The study sequences are shown in **Fig. 11.72**.

Findings. There is soft tissue formation in the left L4/5 intervertebral foramen, with marked contrast enhancement (**c, d,** →). The spinal ganglion is only vaguely distinguishable in the contrast-enhanced images (**d,** →). There is marked dural enhancement, mainly posteriorly (**d,** →). The sagittal images show a lack of fat signal at the infrapedicular (**a, b,** →) and infradiscal levels (**a, b,** →). The L4/5 intervertebral disk is severely degenerated,

with accompanying Modic type II degenerative changes in the upper and lower end plates.

Diagnosis. Scarring and granulomatous changes due to previous surgery in the left L4/5 intervertebral foramen and on the posterior aspect of the dura mater. No evidence of recurrent disk prolapse.

Treatment. This patient suffered from postdiscectomy syndrome. Conservative treatment was initially provided, with epidural perineural injections, physiotherapy, and a flexion orthosis.

Clinical course. Conservative treatment yielded no significant improvement. As leg pain was the primary symptom, neurolysis was recommended.

Comments. This patient had a typical postdiscectomy syndrome. There was no evidence of recurrent disk prolapse. Extensive postoperative scarring was present, both in the spinal canal and in the paraspinous muscula-

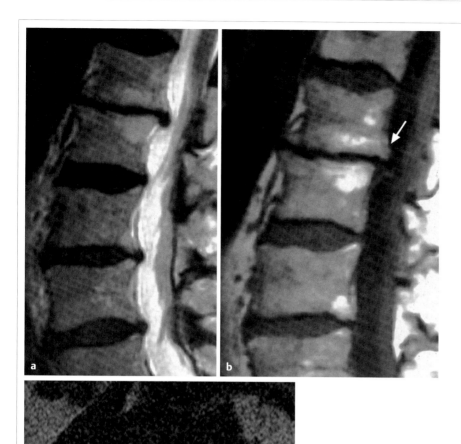

Fig. 11.73 a–c Study sequences (from Krämer and Köster 2001).
a T2 TSE, sagittal, median.
b T1 SE, sagittal, median.
c T2 TSE, axial, L1/L2.

11

ture. As the radicular symptoms were more prominent than the back pain, neurolysis and fat-pad insertion was preferred to spinal fusion as the surgical treatment.

6. L1/2, Protrusion, Multisegmental Degeneration with Modic Type II Changes (**Fig. 11.73**)

Clinical presentation. This 60-year-old man had suffered from back pain for 20 years. There had been recurrent episodes of severe low back pain, occasionally radiating along either the anterior or the posterior aspect of the thighs.

MRI. The study sequences are shown in **Fig. 11.73**.

Findings. All of the lumbar intervertebral discs are of markedly diminished signal intensity, with varying reductions in height and disk protrusions of varying severity. There is a marked reduction of disk height at L1/2, where mild retrolisthesis and posterior osteophytes (**b**, →) are also seen. There are circumscribed areas of Modic type II degeneration in the upper and lower end plates. There is a broad-based posterior displacement of the disk, most severe in the lateral zones, causing marked bilateral stenosis of the intervertebral foramina, while the posterior surface of the disk remains concave (**c,** →) and the dural sac and the conus medullaris within it are, therefore, not compressed.

Diagnosis. Chronic, broad-based, bilateral disk protrusion at L1/2 with accompanying multisegmental degenerative disk disease.

Treatment. Conservative treatment was recommended, consisting of flattening of the lumbar lordosis (relaxation supine with the hips and knees flexed and a flexion orthosis), epidural injections, and facet infiltrations.

Clinical course. Only moderate improvement under conservative treatment.

Comments. There is disk degeneration in almost all of the lumbar segments; L1/2 is the most severely affected, with protrusion of the anulus fibrosus, but without disk prolapse. Surgical decompression is not advisable, because the symptoms are not localizable to any particular level. Further conservative therapy is recommended. Gradual spontaneous improvement can be expected over the next few years.

Summary: MRI

MRI is a noninvasive imaging technique, not employing roentgen rays, that can be used in the diagnostic assessment of degenerative changes in the spine. Multiplanar visualization and differentiation of different types of soft tissue are the major advantages that have led MRI to be widely adopted in place of certain types of invasive imaging study that were previously used, i. e., discography and myelography. MRI truly provides "all-in-one imaging."

The precise localization of the pathoanatomical changes causing pain makes precisely directed treatment possible, including directed injection techniques (the province of the pain specialist) and microsurgical removal of the responsible lesion through a small incision. The MRI findings are of clinical importance only when correlated with the patient's symptoms and signs.

Conclusion

Assessed in terms of the MIRACLE principle (see Chapter 1), MRI is a noninvasive and risk-free but costly diagnostic study that provides much important information.

■ Clinical Syndromes

Classification of Lumbar Syndromes

Lumbar syndromes can be classified into three categories (**Table 11.6**): simple low back pain, back and leg pain, and alarming spinal syndromes (Nachemson and Jonsson 2000, Waddell 2004, German Back Pain Guidelines 2006). This threefold classification corresponds to the scheme of the Spine Working Group (now called the Spine Section) of the German Society of Orthopedics and Orthopedic Surgery, which divides lumbar syndromes into local lumbar syndrome, lumbar root syndrome, and differential diagnoses with alarming manifestations (Krämer 2004).

In accordance with this threefold classification, the following sections will deal with
■ local lumbar syndrome
■ lumbar root syndrome
■ the differential diagnosis of low back pain, with discussion of the serious conditions, both intrinsic and extrinsic to the spine, that can cause it.

No precise epidemiologic data are available on the relative frequency of simple and complicated low back pain, back and leg pain, and alarming spinal symptoms. Waddell (1993) estimated that 93 % of patients suffer from low back pain alone, 5 % from back and leg pain, and 2 % from alarming symptoms; similar estimates were given by Bogduk (2000), Casser (2001), and Nachemson (2004). Nonspecific low back pain should not be viewed as a homogenous condition. Outcomes can be improved when subgrouping is used to guide treatment decision-making (Brennan 2006)

Local Lumbar Syndrome, Low Back Pain

! **Definition:** Local lumbar syndrome consists of all clinical manifestations that are directly or indirectly caused by degenerative and functional disturbances of the lumbar motion segments and that are restricted to the lumbar region.

Table 11.6 Classification of lumbar syndromes

Low back pain (local lumbar syndrome)		Low back and leg pain (lumbar root syndrome)		Alarming spinal symptoms (red flags)	
Simple	*Complicated*	*Simple*	*Complicated*		
Mechanically induced	Yellow flag	Mechanically induced	Yellow flag	Neurological	Cauda equina syndrome Severe weakness Further neuro-logical symptoms
Movement-dependent	Persistent inability to flex the spine	Movement-dependent	Paresthesiae and mild weakness	History	Tumor Trauma Steroids and other medications Malaise Loss of weight Positionally dependent, continuous pain
Short-lasting	Longer-lasting	Radiating into the buttock and thigh, short-lasting	Reflex asymmetry	Clinical findings	Bony destruction on imaging studies Abnormal laboratory tests Fever
20–60 years	Deformities		Radiating into the calf and foot, longer-lasting		
	< 20 years old > 60 years old				

Local lumbar syndrome is largely analogous to local cervical syndrome in terms of its etiology, pathogenesis, and clinical features. All transitional states are possible in local lumbar syndrome, ranging from acute lumbago that suddenly arises and then rapidly abates to chronic, recurrent low back pain. It would be terminologically imprecise to refer to all of these conditions as "lumbago," as lumbago is only one of the possible manifestations of local lumbar syndrome.

Local lumbar syndrome is characterized by positionally dependent low back pain, spasm of the lumbar erector spinae muscles, and restricted range of motion of the lumbar spine. There is no segmental radiation of pain into the lower limbs (**Table 11.7**). The symptoms arise from degenerative changes of the lower lumbar motion segments leading to mechanical irritation of the posterior longitudinal ligament, the intervertebral joint capsules, and the spinal periosteum. The sensory fibers of the meningeal and dorsal branches of the spinal nerve are mainly affected. Reflex spasm of the erector spinae muscles of the back is unpleasant and painful. These muscles are innervated by the dorsal branches of the lumbosacral spinal nerves. It is not possible to identify the particular segment that is involved when pain arises through irritation of a dorsal branch, unlike when it arises through irritation of a ventral branch (sciatica).

Table 11.7 Major manifestations of local lumbar syndrome

- Positionally dependent low back pain
- Spasm of the lumbar erector spinae muscles
- Painful limitation of motion of the lumbar spine
- Pain on percussion and shaking of the lumbar spinous processes

Local lumbar syndromes are by far the commonest type of disk-related symptom in the entire spine. They are even more frequent than local cervical syndromes. Patients with only mild local lumbar syndrome (so-called simple low back pain) rarely consult a physician because their symptoms resolve spontaneously in a short time and respond well to treatments that are commonly known to the general public, such as the application of heat of any type and suitable positioning. Only when the pain is very severe, lasts longer than usual, or recurs frequently and at ever shorter intervals does the patient start to worry and seek medical help.

Classification. Local lumbar syndromes are subdivided into acute and chronic types based on the pattern of major symptoms. It is of therapeutic importance

11

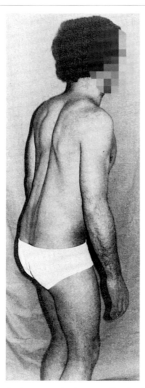

Fig. 11.74 Typical postural abnormality in lumbago. Mild inclination of the trunk (antalgic kyphosis). Marked spasm of the paravertebral muscles limiting movement of the lumbar spine.

whether the patient is suffering from discogenic lumbago or from chronic low back pain of arthroligamentous origin. The most important clues to the diagnosis are to be found in the clinical history, as in all disk-related conditions.

Lumbago, Discogenic Back Pain

! Lumbago is an acute type of local lumbar syndrome. All of the major symptoms of local lumbar syndrome are accentuated and appear suddenly.

The history often includes an unexpected mechanical stress on the spine, such as **bending** and lifting; heat and dampness are often also mentioned. Immediate-onset low back pain usually leads to instant immobility of the low back, which freezes in a characteristic abnormal posture. In order to maintain this locked position, which is the only position in which the pain is reduced, there is reflexive, strong contraction of the lumbar erector spinae muscles. Any attempt to move actively or pas-

sively out of the locked abnormal position causes severe pain. The patient fears and avoids any movement and also reports that coughing, sneezing, or pressing worsens the pain.

The main cause of lumbago is **intradiscal tissue displacement** with irritation of the posterior longitudinal ligament (cf. **Fig. 11.27 a**). The **main zone of pain** is located in the lower lumbar region and over the sacrum, either in the midline or somewhat lateral to it. The pain may also spread diffusely, on an autonomic basis, in the ventral or cranial direction. There may be *pseudoradicular radiation* of pain to the thigh muscles (cf. **Fig. 8.5**). In addition to lumbago of sudden onset associated with a particular movement, there is also a rarer form that gradually increases in severity and that takes a few hours to reach its peak.

The major finding on clinical examination is the abnormal, rigidly held posture of the lumbar spine (**Fig. 11.74**). Flexion of the trunk is impossible; any flexion that the patient may be able to carry out occurs only at the hip joints, while the lumbar spine remains completely rigid. The patient can rise from the examining table only with a characteristic lateral rolling movement, using the buttocks as a fulcrum.

The lower lumbar spinal processes are tender to deep pressure and percussion. Straight-leg raising in the supine position worsens low back pain. There are no positive neurological findings.

The *abnormal posture* depends on the site of the lesion; it may consist of a rigid extension (kyphosis) of the lumbar spine combined with inclination to the right or left side. This abnormal posture is also the only positive radiological finding. When stress is taken off the low back, i. e., when the patient lies with the hips and knees lightly flexed, the pain is usually absent and the abnormal posture disappears.

It is mainly **younger patients** who suffer from lumbago, because their intervertebral disks are more likely to undergo intradiscal tissue displacement.

The attacks of pain are usually of brief duration at first and *tend to resolve spontaneously*. Their **further course** is unpredictable. Attacks of lumbago in youth and middle age may remain the only manifestation of disk degeneration. Often, however, they represent the beginning of a chronic, recurrent lumbar disk syndrome that expresses itself in its further course with frequent attacks of low back pain and sciatica.

Low Back Pain of Arthroligamentous Origin

Characteristics and etiology. Long-lasting and recurrent low back pain constitutes the chronic form of local lumbar syndrome. The major symptoms of local lumbar syndrome are often of only mild intensity, arise gradually, and subside slowly. Low back pain of arthroligamentous origin can be regularly provoked by certain positions, e.g., prolonged sitting, standing, or sometimes even lying, and ameliorated by changes of position. Lumbago, in contrast, is of sudden onset and is not induced or ameliorated by positional changes. Chronic, recurrent low back pain is usually thought to be due to changes of the elasticity and volume of the lumbar disks with secondary effects on the joints, ligaments and muscles. Because these manifestations arise only when disk degeneration has reached an advanced stage, chronic low back pain generally arises only after age 35–40. Depending on the position that induces it, the pain can be designated as low back pain in flexion or in extension, or else as lumbar kyphosis pain or low back pain in hyperextension (facet syndrome).

Facet Syndrome

! Facet syndrome is low back pain arising mainly from the lumbar intervertebral joint facets. It may radiate into the lower limbs, but not in a radicular pattern.

Symptoms arising from the intervertebral joints were comprehensively described as early as 1936 by Lange in his monograph entitled *Die Wirbelgelenke* ("the intervertebral joints") (Lange 1936). The condition was usually referred to as "spondylarthrosis" in the German-speaking countries till the adoption of the term "facet syndrome," which was coined by Mooney and Robertson (1976) and then entered into international use (Schwarzer et al. 1994, 1995, Bogduk 2000, Herkowicz 2004, Jerosch and Steinleitner 2005). Neuroanatomical studies on the subject were carried out by Kiessling (1993) and by Murata et al. (2000).

Most facet syndromes are stress-related, with symptoms worsening over the course of the day. The pain disappears when the patient lies flat with mildly flexed hips and knees (Helbig and Lee 1988). In many individuals, postural weakness while standing leads to hyperlordosis of the spine that becomes painful in a very short time. In this position, the facet joints are subject to excessive stress, and the spinal canal and the intervertebral foramina are relatively narrow. The low back pain may even be associated with radicular symptoms (see **Fig. 11.39**). Low back pain in hyperlordosis arises after prolonged walking and standing, particularly when the individual wears *high-heeled shoes,* indirectly producing *forward tilting of the pelvis* and hyperlordosis of the spine. The pain of hyperlordosis can also be induced or exacerbated when the lumbar lordosis is increased by *downhill walking* or by activities requiring the individual to *lean backward,* e.g., hanging up laundry, looking at pictures, or any type of work above the head.

Other types of stress-related pain are due to gradual loss of height of the intervertebral disks and fatigue of the truncal musculature over the course of the day. The disks become less elastic as they shrink. The remaining components of the lumbar motion segments, mainly the intervertebral joints and ligaments, are subject to excessive or inappropriate stress and give rise to pain mediated by the meningeal branch of the spinal nerve.

The pain of facet syndrome originates in the lumbar intervertebral joints and is felt in the low back with radiation into the buttocks, groin, lower abdomen, thighs, and occasionally the scrotum. Patients describe it as diffuse and widespread and demonstrate its localization by laying the hand flat over the affected area, unlike patients with radicular syndromes, who can draw the borders of the affected dermatome with one finger. Examination reveals tenderness to shaking and percussion over the affected segments. Not all of the intervertebral joints are affected to the same extent, and the diagnostic assessment must therefore include segmental examination, with testing for pain on rotation, flexion, and extension of the lumbar spine (**Fig. 11.75**).

The Sacroiliac Joint and Sacroiliac Joint Syndrome

The sacroiliac joint can be considered functionally and neuroanatomically as the lowest pair of facets. Kiessling (1993) studied the neuroanatomy of the sacroiliac joint and found a pattern of innervation resembling that of the lumbar intervertebral joints. Spontaneous pain and tenderness to pressure can be found on the iliac crest, at the greater trochanter, and in the groin over the origin of the iliopsoas muscle.

A special test of the sacroiliac joint consists of palpation of the posterior iliac spine during movement to check for the so-called **forward bending phenomenon.** Normally, the two posterior iliac spines are at the same height both before the patient bends forward and afterward. A difference in height at the end of forward flexion is considered pathological (**Fig. 11.76**).

The diagnosis of facet pain or sacroiliac joint pain is strongly suggested by the generation of pain in the low back and leg with the so-called "figure 4" maneuver, in which the lumbar spine is passively brought into lordosis when the examiner maximally abducts and externally rotates the patient's hip (**Fig. 11.77**). The diagnosis is further confirmed by the reduction or elimination of the pain upon injection of local anesthetic into the capsule of the affected joint (facet infiltration, see p. 243).

Facet syndrome and sacroiliac joint syndrome with stress-related low back pain have a fluctuating course. The frequency and intensity of the pain depend on bodily activity and posture: patients can largely pre-

11

11

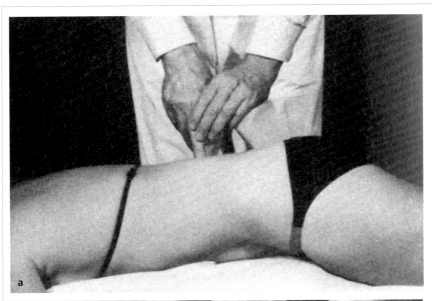

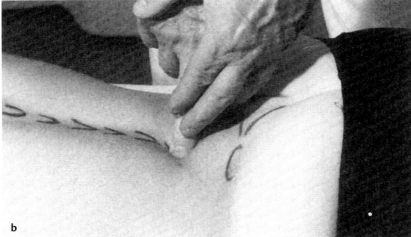

Fig. 11.75 a, b The search for a segmental irritation point in the lumbar spine (kyphosis sensitivity) (**a**). Testing for functional segmental irritation in the lumbar spine with testing of lordosis sensitivity (**b**) (Bischoff 1994, from Rubenthaler et al. 2005).

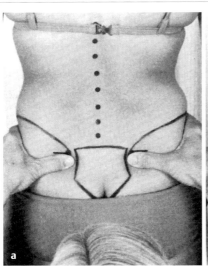
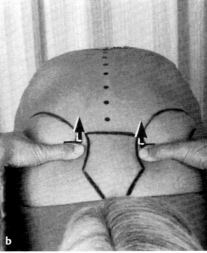

Fig. 11.76 a, b Palpation of the sacroiliac joints in motion, with forward bending phenomenon (Frisch 1998) (from Rubenthaler et al. 2005).

vent the emergence of symptoms by regularly alternating between sitting, standing, and lying positions and avoiding abrupt movements. On the other hand, biochemical and biomechanical involutional processes in disk tissue that are still poorly understood can cause the symptoms to arise and subside suddenly and unpredictably, because any change in the disk necessarily brings about an altered position of the intervertebral joints.

Back Pain in the Lying Position

Stress-related pain arises when the patient stands erect and disappears when the patient lies down, but the reverse is true for some patients, who have pain only in the lying position. Many disk patients have low back pain after prolonged lying, thus mainly in the **early morning hours.** As soon as they stand up (which they find very difficult), the pain reaches its maximal intensity. The clinical picture resembles lumbago, with an abnormal posture, considerable limitation of movement of the lumbar spine in all directions, and lumbar muscle spasm. Patients have to assume grotesquely distorted postures to put on their shoes and socks. This type of pain becomes markedly worse on coughing, sneezing, or pressing.

Unlike lumbago, this type of pain disappears within half an hour of the patient's standing up, as does the limitation of movement, so that the patient *can move fully normally during the day.* For this reason, this condition is not evident when the patient is in the doctor's office; the clinical history, rather than the physical examination, contains all of the relevant information.

The cause of low back pain in the lying position is **slackening of the intervertebral disks,** leading to loss of elasticity of the intervertebral ligaments and to abnormal fluctuations of the volume of disk tissue.

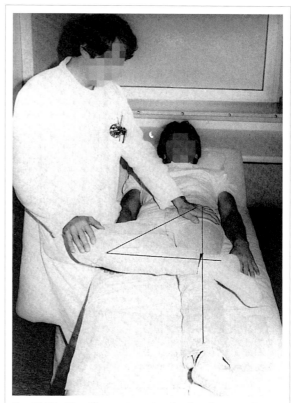

Fig. 11.77 The "figure 4 sign" in lumbar facet syndrome: the legs form the Arabic numeral 4. Pressing downward on the bent knee causes lordosis and torsion of the lumbar spine. Intervertebral joint pain is intensified or provoked by irritation of the joint capsule.

11

! The reduction of postural muscle tone in the lying position, particularly during sleep, enables the components of the motion segment to assume a nonphysiological position in relation to one another.

! After prolonged lying, the disks are tensely filled with fluid and press up against the pain-sensitive posterior longitudinal ligament, placing it under tension.

This produces neural irritation, particularly of the fibers of the meningeal branch.

A further mechanism by which pain can arise in the horizontal position is the involuntary change, during sleep, from the fetal position (lying on the side with rounded back) to the flat supine or prone position, with **hyperlordosis** of the spine, which often produces symptoms. If the intradiscal oncotic pressure is increased (i. e., if the disk tissue can take up more fluid), as is often the case in middle-aged individuals, then the reduction of mechanical stress on the spine in the horizontal position leads to **increased fluid uptake** into the disks.

Once the hydrostatic pressure is raised by an axial stress on the spine (i. e., when the patient stands up), a new equilibrium is rapidly established, and the symptoms disappear.

The optimal therapeutic and prophylactic measures, particularly with regard to proper positioning, have to be determined in each patient depending on the origin of low back pain upon lying in the individual case, i. e., whether it arises from increases or decreases of mechanical stress on the spine, from lumbar kyphosis, or from hyperlordosis.

Table 11.8 Risk factors for low back pain becoming chronic (yellow flags) (German Back Pain Guidelines 2006)

- Dissatisfaction with one's occupation
- Low work qualifications
- Inability to cope with psychosocial demands
- Emotional problems (depression, anxiety)
- Passive attitude
- Inappropriate illness model
- Operant factors (gain from illness), smoking
- Poor physical condition
- Current back pain for > 8 days
- Other types of pain of uncertain origin aside from back pain

Imaging Studies in Patients with Low Back Pain

A plain radiograph of the lumbar spine need not be obtained for every patient with simple low back pain (Nachemson and Jonsson 2000, Waddell 2004, German Back Pain Guidelines 2006). Waddell (2004) found that only 1 % of plain radiographs obtained in such cases reveal a finding that explains the patient's symptoms. Before a diagnosis of simple low back pain can be made, a careful history must be taken and the patient must be thoroughly examined. If the symptoms have persisted for a long time, if the patient remains unable to bend forward, if the clinical examination reveals structural abnormalities, and especially if alarming symptoms (**red flags**) are present, an imaging study (at least a plain radiograph) must be done for further diagnostic evaluation. According to Waddell (2004), the diagnostic usefulness of plain radiographs rises to 34 % if the patient complains of pain that has persisted for a long time and the ESR is greater than 25 mm/h. A plain radiograph is also recommended if one or more of the factors predisposing pain to become chronic (**yellow flags**; **Table 11.8**) are positive, if only to make it clear to the patient and the health insurance provider that no serious medical problem is present. Further imaging studies, such as MRI, CT, discography, and bone scanning, are required only if there are special questions that need to be answered or if low back pain remains intractable. The main reason for ordering such tests is to exclude other possible diagnoses.

Persistent discogenic pain can be diagnosed and distinguished from pain arising from other sources with two types of diagnostic test:
- discography
- MRI.

In discography, the physician doing the test tries to reproduce the patient's typical pain. A positive finding is 73 % sensitive and 89 % specific for discogenic pain (Guyere and Ohnmeiss 1995).

An MRI scan, evaluated according to the Modic criteria (see above, p. 183), is less invasive and considerably more informative, particularly with regard to the detection of spondylodiscitis.

Transition from simple to chronic low back pain (see also Chapter 8). Basic molecular research has not yet yielded any evidence suggesting that the transition from simple to chronic low back pain occurs at a clearly definable moment. Prospective studies have extensively documented the fact that psychosocial mechanisms predict the transition much more accurately than biological or somatic factors (Pfingsten and Schöps 2004; Hildebrand, Müller, and Pfingsten 2005). The risk factors for low back pain becoming chronic lie mainly in the domain of the psyche. If one or more such factors (yellow flags) are present, the physician should be alert to the fact.

The most important factors are included in a short questionnaire used to assess the risk of back pain becoming chronic (Neubauer and Schiltenwolf 2002), which can be given to the patient in the waiting room before the examination. The total score indicates the magnitude of the risk. If the risk appears to be high, then the psychosocial factors predisposing to pain should be treated along with the purely medical condition right from the beginning. When these yellow flag risk factors are present, interdisciplinary treatment of the patient should be initiated early with the consultation of, for example, a psychologist and a specialist in occupational medicine.

Differential Diagnosis of Low Back Pain

The "low back," or sacral region, is the part of the back that lies at the level of the sacral bone. In humans, this area has a cross-shaped depression in its center. Local pain arising in the lumbar motion segments attains maximum intensity here.

> **!** Lumbar disk disease is by far the most common cause of low back pain.

Aside from the major symptoms of lumbar syndrome, a positive extension test (cf. **Fig. 11.93**) points to the intervertebral disk as the source of the pain.

The term "low back pain" is also often used to designate pain in higher or lateral areas of the back. This entity therefore has a wide differential diagnosis.

Low Back Pain of Extraspinal Origin

There are many pathological conditions located *outside* the spine that are commonly thought to cause "low back pain." These conditions must be included in the differential diagnosis of low back pain, even though the pain that they produce is mainly not located in the sacral region itself, but rather in its vicinity or at more distant sites. Gynecological, urological, and a small number of internal medical conditions are included in this category. They are usually associated with types of pain radiation and other clinical phenomena that are not compatible with the diagnosis of lumbar syndrome.

Low back pain in women was, in past decades, often thought to be of gynecological origin; this was assumed, for example, by Martius (1944) in his extensive monograph on the subject. It is now known that most cases are actually due to problems in the lumbar motion segments, just as in men, so "gynecological low back pain" is rarely spoken of now.

 46 % of pregnant women have low back pain.

Low back pain in pregnancy originates, not in the pelvic viscera, but in the slackened ligaments of the lumbosacral region. Use of oral contraceptives leads to hormonal changes resembling those of pregnancy, which can also cause slackening of the pelvic ring and the intervertebral disks, giving rise to low back pain. In the second half of pregnancy, anterior loading of the trunk leads to static changes including hyperlordosis of the lumbar spine and tilting of the pelvis. Only 1 % of pregnant women suffer from sciatica (Ostgaard and Andersson 1991).

 The genuine gynecological causes of low back pain include space-occupying lesions of the female reproductive organs in the pelvis, such as ovarian cysts, uterine fibroids, and malignant tumors.

The resulting pains in the back, including the lower back, are diffuse; when asked to point to the site of the pain, the patient indicates a broad area with her entire hand (Martius 1944), whereas local, disk-related pain is usually indicated precisely, with one finger, at the site of the affected segment.

Today, the routine use of directed screening tests often leads to the early detection of diseases of these kinds before they reach the stage where they can cause back pain.

Endometriosis and altered positions of the uterus are less frequent causes of low back pain than is commonly thought.

These entities must, however, be considered in the differential diagnosis when the pain is dependent on the menstrual cycle. Pfau (1968) pointed out that descent and prolapse of the vaginal walls and the uterus can be associated with low back pain. It is typical for this type of pain to worsen over the course of the day and to disappear at rest, or when a pessary is applied. In general, the frequency of gynecological low back pain is very low among the vast number of women with low back pain. Gynecological evaluation in these patients mainly serves the purpose of ruling out a gynecological origin for the pain.

Pain due to **urological conditions** is seldom restricted to the sacral region. *Ureteric and urethral conditions* (stone, tumor, infection) are usually associated with spontaneous tenderness to percussion of the lateral lumbar region. The pain in these conditions is also usually of the colicky type, which discogenic pain never is. Diseases of the bladder (tumors with unilateral or bilateral obstruction of the urinary pathways, infiltrative tumor growth) or the male reproductive organs can also cause low back pain. If urinary obstruction is suspected as the cause of low back pain of unclear origin, further diagnostic testing is required (urography, ultrasonography). Retroperitoneal and pelvic *tumors* can cause either lumbago or sciatica, but of a persistent character, not responsive to changes of position.

A few **internal medical diseases,** too, can cause pain in the region of the spine; these include diseases of the *stomach, gallbladder, and pancreas,* among others. The pain is usually not in the low back, but rather in the mid-back, in the visceral pain projection fields (zones of Head) located mainly around the level of the thoracolumbar junction (**Table 11.9**).

Low Back Pain Arising from the Vertebrae

Degenerative disease of the lumbar motion segments is by far the most common cause of low back pain arising from the vertebrae. This category includes secondary phenomena such as the rubbing together of adjacent spinous processes **(Baastrup disease)** and signs of muscle insufficiency causing pain in the lower back. Painful manifestations of **muscle insufficiency in the back** accompany all static axial deviations of the spine in the frontal and sagittal planes but also arise as the result of poor posture or malpositioning of the pelvis. There are many processes in the lumbosacral spine other than lumbar syndrome that can give rise to low back pain. Some of them can cause sciatica as well.

Spondylolysis and **spondylolisthesis** may be entirely asymptomatic, but may also cause refractory low back pain and sciatica. Pain arising from these entities generally cannot be distinguished from discogenic pain on clinical grounds alone. Spondylolysis and spondylolisthesis are often accompanied by slackening or prolapse of a lumbar disk. Physical examination some-

11

Table 11.9 Differential diagnosis of low back pain

	Cause	Pain limited to the low back	May be associated with sciatica	Position-ally dependent	Restriction of move-ment of the lumbar spine	Muscle spasm	Traction test	Confirmation of the diagnosis (initial measures)
Vertebral	Disk degenera-tion	++	+++	+++	+++	+++	+++	Plain radiographs, CT, MRI
	Spondylolisthe-sis	++	+++	+++	+++	+++	+	Plain radiographs
	Spondylitis	+++	+	–	+++	+++	+	CT, MRI, lab tests
	Tumor (metastasis)	+++	+	–	+++	+++	+	CT, MRI, lab tests, scintigraphy
	Ankylosing spondylitis	+	–	+	+++	++	–	Plain radiographs, lab tests
	Baastrup dis-ease	+++	–	+++	+	+	+++	Local anesthesia, plain radiographs
	Muscle insuffi-ciency	+	–	+++	–	++	–	Local injection
	Osteoporosis	–	–	–	+++	+++	–	Plain radiographs
	Fracture		+	+	+++	+++	+	Plain radiographs
	Coccygodynia	+++	–	+++	–	–	–	Local anesthesia
Extra-vertebral	Gynecological causes	–	+	+	–	–	–	Lab tests, gyne-cological exami-nation, ultrasono-graphy
	Urological causes	+	+	–	–	–	–	Lab tests, ultra-sonography
	Bowel, stomach, pancreas, gall-bladder	+	–	–	–	–	–	Lab tests, ultra-sonography, en-doscopy

times yields a clue to the diagnosis in the form of a sliding vertebra, which can be recognized by forward slippage of its spinous process when the patient flexes the trunk; the spinous process is sometimes relatively loose and tender to deep palpation. The diagnosis is es-tablished by plain radiograph. In doubtful cases, ob-lique radiographs or tomographic views should be ob-tained, to display the pars interarticularis better. Among other types of deformities and developmental anomalies, spinal canal stenosis and asymmetrically anchored transitional vertebrae can also cause low back pain at rest.

In this context, too, it is important to point out that imaging of the lumbosacral region may yield visually striking findings that are not the cause of the pain, or indeed of any symptoms whatever. These in-clude, for example, symmetrical transitional verte-brae, incomplete closure of the laminae (spina bifida occulta), block vertebrae, and Schmorl's nodes. If the symptoms persist, other causes of pain should be sought.

Specific or nonspecific lumbosacral **spondylitis** causes severe low back pain, sometimes combined with symptoms of radicular irritation. The ESR and a plain radiograph are the most informative tests for this con-dition. The diagnosis, once suspected, is confirmed with tomography, further laboratory testing, and possibly tissue biopsy. The AP plain radiograph of the lumbar spine may reveal *widening of the psoas shadow,* an im-portant sign of a psoas abscess, which will also be vis-ible by CT or MRI. Spinal tumors can arise from the spine itself or, less commonly, from structures within the spinal canal. Tumors of the spinal cord and meninges are very rarely the cause of isolated low back pain, because they usually produce neurologic deficits as well. Localized low back pain has rarely been re-ported as an isolated finding due to an *ependymoma or spongioblastoma* of the cauda equina, or a neurinoma. Such tumors can sometimes be suspected from the plain radiograph if the interpedicular distance is widened, indicating a space-occupying lesion lying within the spinal canal, or if *the intervertebral foramen* *is widened*, indicating an intraforaminal tumor (neurinoma).

Plasmacytoma is an important type of tumor arising from the vertebral bodies themselves. It can be solitary, affecting only a single vertebral body. Typical signs of the disease include marked elevation of the ESR and the presence of paraglobulins that can be detected by electrophoresis and in the urine. When an elderly patient presents with low back pain, *metastases* should always be ruled out. The pain is persistent rather than episodic. The metastatic tumors that most commonly cause low back pain include carcinomas of the prostate gland, breast, kidneys, thyroid gland, or lung. A bone scan aids in the diagnosis.

If a tumor has been conclusively ruled out as the cause of severe back pain in an elderly patient, **osteoporosis** is the next most probable cause (more likely than disk disease). Osteoporosis causes diffuse pain and restriction of motion not just in the low back, but in other parts of the spine as well. There is no specific diagnostic criterion for osteoporosis; it is radiologically characterized by increased radiolucency and rarefaction of the bones, but these findings are evident only in advanced stages of the disease. Acute low back pain in osteoporosis is often caused by the collapse of a lumbar vertebra. Osteoporosis with low back pain can also arise in younger patients. Its causes include

- idiopathic juvenile osteoporosis
- hyperthyroidism
- Cushing disease
- Cushing syndrome after prolonged treatment with cortisone
- renal and intestinal osteoporosis.

A less common cause of low back pain is **Paget disease,** which is characterized by accelerated bone remodeling (both generation and resorption). The thoracic and lumbar regions of the spine are preferentially affected. The disease is diagnosed by the elevated alkaline phosphatase concentration and by the involvement of other parts of the skeleton, particularly the pelvis and femur.

Among the noninfectious inflammatory conditions that can affect the spine, the one that most commonly causes low back pain is **ankylosing spondylitis** (Bekhterev disease). This condition should always be thought of when the pain arises at night. The low-lying pain in the back arises from the sacroiliac joints, which are usually the first part of the skeleton to be affected. The pain is less positionally dependent than discogenic pain, nor does it worsen on coughing, sneezing, or pressing. An elevated ESR, increased respiratory excursion, and abnormal-appearing sacroiliac joints in the AP plain radiograph of the lumbosacral spine should prompt further diagnostic testing for this condition.

The defining manifestation of **coccygodynia** is pain that is situated very low in the back, radiating from the coccyx to the sacrum. Pressure on the coccyx is painful, e. g., when the patient leans slightly backward while sitting. This condition is diagnosed by palpation and by temporary elimination of the typical pain by the injection of a local anesthetic.

Most of the important causes of low back pain that need to be considered will become evident through comprehensive history-taking and physical examination. The laboratory tests and radiological studies that can be used to confirm the diagnosis of these conditions are listed in **Table 11.9**. If these tests and studies are normal, as is true in the overwhelming majority of cases in routine clinical practice, the only remaining etiologies of low back pain that must be considered are disk disease and muscle insufficiency. These two entities are more or less equally common; they can be differentiated from one another (if this is required) only by subtle questioning and examination, and above all by the extension test. The treatment and prophylaxis of both is essentially the same. In such cases, the correct diagnosis can be made by observing the further course of the symptoms and their responsiveness to treatment. Discogenic low back pain of acute onset usually subsides spontaneously in a few days and can be mitigated by measures that reduce the mechanical stress on the spine.

Red Flags in Low Back Pain

> **Definition:** "Red flags" are alarming disease manifestations in patients with low back pain that call for immediate referral to a specialist, and usually for hospital admission. There is a wide range of conditions originating in the spine and outside it that must be included in the differential diagnosis of low back pain and that announce their presence with "red flag" symptoms and signs.

The following disease manifestations are alarming in patients with low back pain:

- **Abnormal laboratory values,** e. g., in spondylitis, neoplasia, and metabolic disease.
- **Weight loss,** e. g., in tuberculosis, neoplasia, and metabolic disease.
- Other **neurological manifestations** (many neurological diseases, including Parkinson disease and multiple sclerosis, can cause low back pain).
- **Bone destruction** revealed by radiological studies can be a sign of neoplasia, osteoporosis, or infection.
- A positive history for conditions such as cancer, use of steroid medication, HIV infection, etc.

11

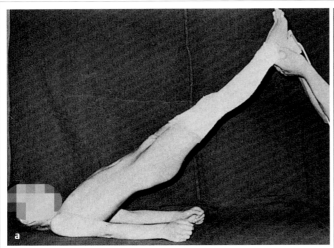
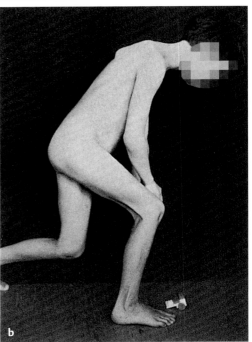

Fig. 11.78 a, b.
a The "board sign" in extension stiffness of the hip and thigh.
b A fixed lumbar spine.

Table 11.10 Major symptoms of discogenic hip and thigh extension stiffness
▪ Board sign
▪ Fixed lumbar spine
▪ Shuffling gait

Discogenic Hip and Thigh Extension Stiffness

> ! Discogenic hip and thigh extension stiffness is a constellation of clinical findings, the most prominent of which is the so-called "board sign": when the examiner lifts up the extended legs of the supine patient by the heels, the entire body, including the trunk, is lifted up in board-like fashion.

The hip joints cannot be passively flexed because of reflex contraction of the ischiocrural and erector spinae muscles. The legs and trunk form a board-like unit (**Fig. 11.78**). This sign is usually present on both sides and even persists under general anesthesia. When only unilaterally present, or more prominent on one side than the other, it is often associated with sciatica.

Spasm of the lumbar erector spinae muscles produces fixation of the lumbar spine that cannot be over-

come even with forward flexion of the trunk. A characteristic finding is a "shoving" gait, with slightly flexed hip and knee joints, resembling the type of gait seen after fusion of the hip joint (**Table 11.10**).

This condition mainly affects *younger patients* during the pubertal growth spurt. They often complain of only mild pain despite the impressive physical findings; the pain is usually limited to the low back, though some patients have sciatica as well. There are generally no positive neurological findings. Occasionally, there may be reflex asymmetry, muscle weakness, or a sensory deficit reflecting a nerve root syndrome.

The *cause* of this condition has been the subject of many different hypotheses. Schramm (1941) described it as "inflammatory lumbar lordosis." Fürmaier (1951) considered it the result of pachymeningitis of the spinal nerve roots. Other authors attributed it to specific (Hipp 1967) or nonspecific (Idelberger 1964) inflammation of the lumbosacral spine, or to tumors affecting the cauda equina (Hauberg 1957). The case series of Bösch (1977) included patients with disk calcification, discitis (metastatic), tumors, Calvé disease, juvenile ankylosing spondylitis, and spondylolisthesis, among other diagnoses, but these diseases are unlikely to be the cause of hip–loin extension stiffness, except in rare cases.

Our own observations and those of other authors lead us to conclude that hip–loin extension stiffness is usually due to **protrusions** of lumbar disks, which are by no means a rare occurrence in children and adolescents

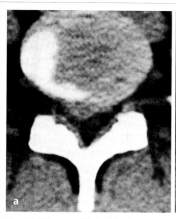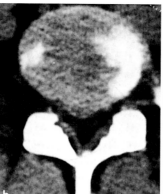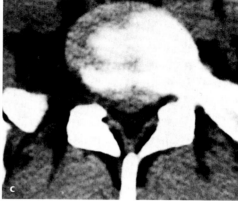

Fig. 11.79 a–c Clinical findings: 18-year-old man with extension stiffness of the hip and thigh for the past 5 months. Positive right Lasègue sign at 30°, positive left Lasègue sign at 50°. Band of pain in a right S1 distribution down to the calf and in a left S1 distribution to the thigh. Diminished right Achilles reflex. No sensorimotor deficit. CT: broad-based central protrusion at L5/S1, more prominent on the right. The protrusion is broader than it is deep (grade III dislocation). Treatment: intradiscal chymopapain injection. The patient is free of pain immediately after the injection and remains so. The Lasègue signs and the extension stiffness of the hip and thigh gradually resolve thereafter.

(Matzen and Polster 1959, Hipp 1967, Polster and Buesenez 1972, Bernbeck and Dahmen 1976, Stolke and Seifert 1984, Hähnel and Pfeiffer 1989, Mellerowicz et al. 1995, Salminen et al. 1995, Kayser et al. 1999, 2005, Balague 2001, Schlenzka 2001). Hip–loin extension stiffness can be considered a variant of lumbar syndrome that affects younger patients (**Fig. 11.79**).

> ! The special topographical size relationships of the lumbar spine during the growing period are the reason why lumbar syndrome expresses itself in the special form of hip–loin extension stiffness in children and adolescents.

The clinical picture of hip–loin extension stiffness arises when the normal mobility of the spinal nerve roots in the lumbosacral region is impeded for whatever reason. Flexion of the hip with an extended knee causes the S1 nerve root to slide more than 5 mm caudally out of the intervertebral foramen. During the growth period, the spinal canal is displaced gradually closer to the bony wall of the spinal canal. In neonates, the conus medullaris terminates at L3; in adults, at L1. Every growth spurt shortens the spinal cord, dura mater, and nerve roots in relation to the bony spinal canal.

The increasing use of CT and MRI in recent years has led to the recognition that disk protrusions cause many cases of hip–loin extension stiffness. In younger patients, the nerve roots are so short (in relation to the spinal canal) that they are placed under tension even by the mildest impingement from the side. When the nerve roots are stretched, the motor fibers for the ischiocrural and erector spinae muscles react the most sensitively.

The clinical examiner's main task is to exclude tumor and inflammation/infection, which are the most important dangerous conditions in the differential diagnosis of hip–loin extension syndrome. Oblique plain radiographs of the lumbar spine should always be obtained so that pathological changes of the posterior arches (laminae) can be recognized. As soon as the diagnosis of "discogenic hip–loin extension syndrome" has been made (by exclusion, as it were), **conservative treatment** should be initiated, just as for any other discogenic condition in the lumbar region.

As long as no neurologic deficit arises, conservative treatment can be continued for long periods of time. Time works in the patient's favor by normalizing the relative sizes of the neural elements and the bony spinal canal as the growth phase comes to an end.

Lumbar Root Syndromes

Etiology and Overview of Syndromes

The clinical manifestations of local lumbar syndrome are mediated mainly by the meningeal and dorsal branches of the spinal nerves, but those of lumbar root syndrome mainly arise in the area innervated by the ventral branches.

> ! Mechanical irritation of the L5 and S1 nerve roots, and sometimes of the L4 or S2 nerve roots, produces pain radiating into the leg, which, in combination with other neurological disturbances, is termed "sciatica."

11

Table 11.11 Major manifestations of sciatica
▪ Segmentally radiating pain
▪ Local lumbar syndrome
▪ Positive Lasègue sign
▪ Sciatic postural abnormality
▪ Segmental sensory deficit
▪ Reflex asymmetry
▪ Motor deficit

Sciatica is pain in the distribution of the sciatic nerve. Its most common **cause** is degenerative change of the lower two lumbar disks. Lumbar root syndromes arising at higher levels because of pathological changes of the L1/2 through L3/4 disks do not involve the sciatic nerve, but rather mostly the fibers of the femoral nerve; *femoral neuralgia* (a rarely used term) is thus the upper lumbar equivalent of sciatica.

It is remarkable that such a clearly defined pathological–anatomical entity as lumbar disk prolapse went long unrecognized as the most common cause of sciatica. As recently as 40 years ago, inflammations of various kinds were postulated as the cause of "sciatic neuritis." A clear demonstration of the relation between dorsal displacement of disk tissue with clinical low back pain and sciatica was provided by Mixter and Barr (1934), Dandy (1943), Bradford and Spurling (1950), Lindblom (1969), and others.

Not only protrusions and prolapses, but also deformations of other kinds produced directly or indirectly by disk degeneration, can cause a lumbar root syndrome. These include slackening and volume changes of the disks, osteophytes on the posterior margins of the vertebral bodies, and sliding of the vertebral bodies with respect to one another, as well as other changes within the lumbar spinal canal that can produce sciatica in the absence of a disk prolapse.

Lumbar root syndrome presents with the typical clinical manifestations of local lumbar syndrome and, in addition, the typical signs and symptoms of sciatica, including a positive Lasègue sign, segmentally radiating pain, dermatomal sensory disturbances, reflex asymmetry, and motor dysfunction. Among the **main clinical manifestations of sciatica** (**Table 11.11**), some are more common, others less so.

! The most important symptom of sciatica, which gives this constellation of signs and symptoms its name, is pain radiating into the area supplied by the affected spinal nerve root.

The intensity and extent of this pain varies from patient to patient, as well as over time for each patient. Its quality ranges from sharp and pulling to dull and aching, but the patient nearly always describes it as unbearably intense. The band of pain begins in the proximal part of the dermatome and may spread distally over the further course of the condition. Sometimes, however, the pain remains proximal and only radiates into the peripheral part of the dermatome when certain movements are carried out, or when the patient coughs, sneezes, or presses. In addition to the typical pattern of spread within a dermatome, there are also cases in which the pain is concentrated on a single point. Such points are usually located on the anterolateral shin (when the L5 root is affected) or on the heel and lateral edge of the foot (when the S1 root is affected) (**Table 11.1**). The manifestations of local lumbar syndrome are present in the great majority of patients with sciatica, but there are occasional exceptions, i. e., cases of sciatica without low back pain, which can pose a difficult problem in differential diagnosis. This type of pain is often restricted to the area over the sacroiliac joint or to part of the foot along the course of a dermatome. It does not change much in response to changes of position; often, it is only revealed to be discogenic as a result of a traction test (p. 213) or a CT or MRI scan. Residual sciatica with circumscribed areas of pain and hypesthesia or low back pain is also a feature of the postoperative state after lumbar disk surgery.

Whether or not the other clinical manifestations of sciatica will arise depends on the location and extent of the mechanical impingement on the nerve root. Individual signs and symptoms may fluctuate in prominence as components of the overall clinical picture. If pain and abnormal posture are the most pronounced manifestations at first, they will give way, in the further course of the illness, to paresthesiae and motor dysfunction. If the root is totally compressed, the pain disappears entirely, the affected dermatome becomes anesthetic, and a segmental motor deficit arises, e. g., a foot and big toe drop with compression of the L5 root. In such cases, immediate surgery is indicated.

The severity of the **postural abnormality of sciatica** depends on the patient's age. It tends to be most marked in younger patients, who also tend to have an early Lasègue sign (i. e., positive with only a few degrees of straight-leg raising) and a proximal band of pain. In older patients, the peripheral pain predominates, the postural abnormality is only moderately severe, and the Lasègue sign appears only as the leg is raised toward 90°. We infer from this age-related pattern of disease manifestations that younger patients suffer more commonly from protrusion-related sciatica, older ones from prolapse-related sciatica. Older patients also more commonly have intraforaminal fragments, which tend to produce peripheral rather than proximal symptoms.

Protrusion Sciatica or Prolapse Sciatica?

For treatment and prognosis, it is important to determine whether the patient's lumbar root syndrome is due to a disk protrusion or a disk prolapse.

! Sudden impingement on the nerve root by the protrud-
• ing posterior portion of the intervertebral disk—a structure that normally lies next to it—exposes the root to
different mechanical and biochemical effects than contact with disk prolapse material, which is a type of tissue
with very different properties.

It is likely that most cases of sciatica are induced by disk
protrusions. The usual finding is a taut, elastic out-
pouching of the posterior border of the disk, covered by
a membrane of variable thickness consisting of the
outer lamellae of the anulus fibrosus and the posterior
longitudinal ligament.

It can be disconcerting for the surgeon, particularly
when operating on a younger patient, to find that the
anulus fibrosus remains intact over a broad-based disk
protrusion, and that it must therefore be incised to gain
access to the "fragment." After the anulus has been
opened and the disk space has been subtotally emptied,
a new situation emerges in which further problems may
arise.

On the other hand, continuing to treat a complete or
incarcerated disk prolapse conservatively can be a fruit-
less and time-wasting exercise. Disk tissue lying free in
the epidural space will continue to cause symptoms
until it is surgically removed.

! The chance of a spontaneous cure is much better with a
• disk protrusion than with a disk prolapse.

The dislocated disk tissue in a protrusion may return to
its original position inside the disk, restoring the initial
anatomical situation. This cannot occur with a disk prolapse.

The history and the patient's current signs and symptoms provide a number of clues as to whether a prolapse
or a protrusion is responsible (**Table 11.12**). Prolapse sciatica is the more severe of the two clinical syndromes.
The pain and postural abnormality are of sudden onset
and worsen within a few hours as the disk tissue swells
within the spinal canal. Prolapses usually compress the
nerve root more severely than protrusions; the root is
tightly squeezed between the prolapse and the lamina
or ligamentum flavum. Thus, prolapses are more likely
to cause a motor deficit, dermatomal anesthesia, and a
reflex abnormality. Protrusions, on the other hand, often
produce no more than a proximal band of pain.

The **course of illness** also differs depending on
whether a protrusion or prolapse is responsible.

! The displaced disk tissue in a protrusion remains in con-
• tact with the intradiscal osmotic system and continues to
undergo physiological changes of volume and consistency.

The results are stress-dependent changes in the
patient's pain, paresthesiae, and abnormal posture.

Table 11.12 Differences between protrusion sciatica and prolapse sciatica

Protrusion sciatica	*Prolapse sciatica*
Gradually increasing pain	Lightning-like onset
Fluctuating postural abnormality	Constant postural abnormality
Mainly proximal band of pain	Distal pain and paresthesiae, motor deficit
Easily controlled with medication	Difficult to control with medication
High counterpressure felt during discography	Low counterpressure felt during discography
Discographic contrast medium remains in intervertebral space	Discographic contrast medium flows out into the epidural space

For differences visible in CT and MRI scans, see **Fig. 11.56**, p. 175.

General measures and medications that tend to reduce
disk swelling are also effective. A prolapse, on the other
hand, produces symptoms that are relatively unchanging and difficult to influence. The patient cannot find relief in any position.

As in all discogenic diseases, it is difficult to generalize
about the course and prognosis of sciatica due to disk
protrusions and prolapses. The differentiating features
listed in **Table 11.12** serve merely as rules of thumb.

Myelography generally cannot be used to distinguish
prolapses from protrusions. Only when the column of
contrast medium is massively indented can one state
with a fair degree of certainty that a prolapse is present.
The distinction is more likely to be made by CT or MRI:
prolapses jut further into the epidural space than protrusions and have a narrower base. Fragments can also
be seen above or below the disk space if the extruded
disk tissue has migrated. In the last analysis, the physician needs clinical skill and experience with disk syndromes to diagnose and treat disk protrusions and prolapses appropriately.

There are some disk protrusions and prolapses that
take a completely different course than the typical course
described in **Table 11.12**. A large protrusion with a thin
membrane and an incarcerated fragment can produce a
clinical picture closely resembling that of a prolapse.

! A small prolapse can migrate into a corner of the spinal
• canal where it no longer compresses any of the neural elements, so that all symptoms suddenly disappear.

The only means of distinguishing fairly reliably between
prolapses and protrusions before surgery is by discography or intradiscal injection. A protrusion has a markedly
higher resistance against injection than a prolapse.
When a prolapse is present, an arbitrary amount of fluid
can be injected into the disk, because it all flows out

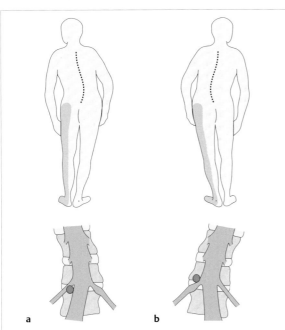

Fig. 11.80 a, b
a Ipsilateral sciatic postural abnormality due to a paramedian disk prolapse: the patient bends toward the side of
the sciatica.
b Contralateral sciatic postural abnormality due to a lateral
disk prolapse. The patient bends away from the side of
the sciatica.

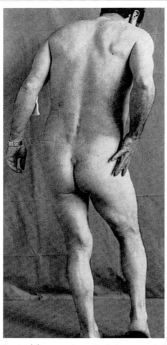

Fig. 11.81   Typical leg posture in intense sciatica: the hip
and knee joints are mildly flexed, and the patient stands on
his toes on one side. Right sciatica with rightward bending
of the trunk: ipsilateral sciatic postural abnormality.

again into the epidural space. In discography, the contrast medium flows out of the disk into the epidural
space (**Table 11.12**).

Sciatic Postural Abnormality

A positive Lasègue sign, pain on stretching of the
femoral nerve, and a sciatic postural abnormality are all
segmentally nonspecific signs of lumbar root syndrome,
each of which is more or less pronounced depending on
the site and extent of the disk protrusion or prolapse.
The positive Lasègue sign and postural abnormality are,
generally speaking, more severe in L4 or L5 syndrome
than in S1 syndrome, because of the immediate proximity of the L4/5 disk to the dura mater and nerve
roots.

Extension (hyperlordosis) of the lumbar spine and
mild forward bending of the trunk are characteristic
signs of lumbago that are also a part of lumbar root syndrome, in which the trunk is usually inclined to one side
as well. The precise type of sciatic postural abnormality
that arises depends on whether the nerve root is compressed from the cranial, caudal, or ventral side. The postural abnormality can be understood as a reflexive deviation that takes the stress off the nerve root (**Fig. 11.80**).

> **!** The trunk of a standing patient involuntarily assumes the
> posture in which nerve root compression by the displaced
> disk tissue is least (or even absent).

For this reason, many patients with postural abnormalities, even extreme ones, have very little pain. Pain arises
only when active or passive movements are made to
bring the trunk back to the neutral position. When there
is a large medial prolapse, inclination to one side is usually not seen, because it does not reduce the mechanical
stress on the affected nerve roots at all.

Types of abnormal posture. Abnormal postures are
designated by the direction in which the lumbar spine is
scoliotic (convex) and by the position of the trunk. Lumbar scoliosis may be convex on the normal or the diseased side. The lateral inclination of the upper body is
easier to recognize.

> **!** If the patient bends toward the side of the leg affected
> with sciatica, this is said to be an *ipsilateral* sciatic pos-
> tural abnormality; bending to the other side is a *con-
> tralateral* sciatic postural abnormality.

In severe sciatica, the patient puts less weight on the affected lower limb and keeps the hip and knee joints on
that side somewhat flexed. Plantar flexion of the foot
also releases tension on the sciatic nerve. Weight can be
put on the affected lower limb only for a short time, if at
all, with the patient standing on the ball of the foot
(**Fig. 11.81**).

The sciatic postural abnormality becomes more severe when the patient bends forward, because this position increases the contact of the nerve root with the disk prolapse or protrusion. In mild cases, the sciatic postural abnormality is only evident when the patient bends forward (**Fig. 11.82**) and almost disappears on lying or standing. Certain **regularly occurring configurations** can be recognized when one correlates the types of postural abnormality that are encountered with the site of the disk protrusion and prolapse as revealed by CT, MRI, or open surgery.

In the lumbar motion segments, the dorsal edge of the disk has a special topographical relationship to the nerve roots. Because the nerve roots take an oblique course from medial to lateral as they travel downward, circumscribed protrusions of the posterior disk contour come into contact with different nerve roots at different points. The site at which the nerve root traverses the disk space is different in each motion segment.

For the purpose of communication between physicians, it is useful in everyday clinical parlance to consider the dural sac as a trunk and the two nerve roots of a segment as arms exiting from it. This terminology enables easy visualization of the special anatomical relationships of these structures. The site where a nerve root exits the dural sac is its "shoulder," and the inferior surface of the root as it exits the dural sac is its "axilla." Disk prolapses may found behind or over the shoulder of the nerve root, or in the axilla (**Fig. 11.83**). Lateral bending of the lumbar spine moves the part of the disk on the convex side cranially in relation to the nerve root. If there is a protrusion impinging on the shoulder of the root, this movement moves it away from the root; on the other hand a protrusion impinging on the axilla of the root will press harder against it when this movement is performed.

When there is a lateral disk protrusion, the patient inclines to the normal side (contralateral sciatic postural abnormality); when there is a medial protrusion, the patient inclines to the side of the protrusion (ipsilateral sciatic postural abnormality) (**Fig. 11.84**). If the protrusion lies behind the shoulder of the root, no more than mild sciatic scoliosis is seen when the patient stands erect. Only when the patient bends forward does the root slide medially or laterally over the protrusion.

Aside from these standard situations, there are also **combined and transitional forms**. For example, a large prolapse can impinge on the roots from two adjacent levels—one cranially, one caudally—producing a combined type of postural abnormality. A broad-based medial protrusion can put the nerve root of the other side under tension. The mild forward flexion of the trunk seen in sciatic scoliosis is not a universal finding, either. There are patients who feel a certain degree of relief only when they bend backward (hyperlordosis), most commonly when the problem is a protrusion or prolapse of an upper lumbar disk.

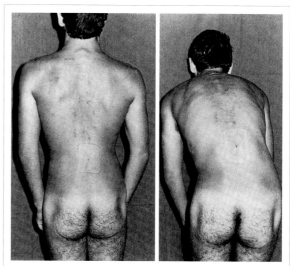

Fig. 11.82 a, b   A 19-year-old man with a right L4/5 lateral disk herniation. The contralateral sciatic postural abnormality is seen only when the patient bends forward.

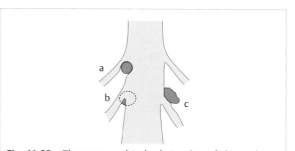

Fig. 11.83   The topographical relationship of the prolapse and the nerve root: (**a**) in the axilla, (**b**) behind the shoulder, (**c**) on the shoulder.

Sciatic postural abnormality is an important diagnostic criterion for lumbar root syndromes, both in clinical practice and in **medicolegal assessment.** The characteristic twisting of the trunk, with increasing asymmetry when the patient bends forward, is difficult to imitate voluntarily; nor can it be voluntarily suppressed if present.

Even after the causative lesion has been surgically removed, the typical postural abnormality of sciatica often persists for a long time, perhaps even months. Intensive **patient exercises** are then required.

Monoradicular Lumbar Syndromes

Frequency

Only about one-half of all cases of lumbar root syndrome are clearly monosegmental. In the remaining cases, the clinical manifestations either cannot be unequivocally attributed to a particular root or else reflect

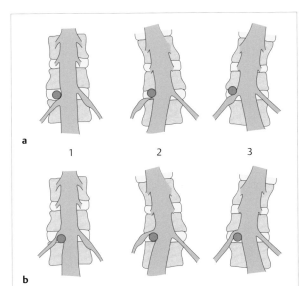

Fig. 11.84 a, b　Intensification and relief of pain by rightward and leftward bending, depending on the site of the prolapse.
a Lateral prolapse:
　1 Midposition.
　2 Bending toward the side of sciatica: pain worsened.
　3 Bending away from the side of sciatica: pain relieved (contralateral sciatic postural abnormality).
b Paramedian prolapse (in the axilla):
　1 Midposition.
　2 Bending toward the side of sciatica: pain relieved (ipsilateral sciatic postural abnormality).
　3 Bending away from the side of sciatica: pain worsened.

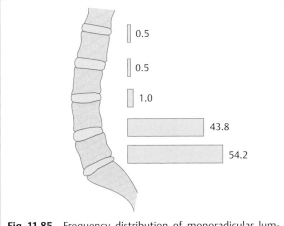

0.5	
0.5	
1.0	
	43.8
	54.2

Fig. 11.85　Frequency distribution of monoradicular lumbar syndromes.

the simultaneous involvement of more than one root (cf. **Table 11.13**). The vast majority of cases of monoradicular lumbar root syndrome (98 % in our series) affect the L5 or S1 root (43.8 % and 54.2 %, respectively). Clear-cut, monoradicular involvement of the L4 root is

seen in only 1 % of cases, and the remaining 1 % affect the L1, L2, and L3 roots (**Fig. 11.85**). This distribution accords with published data from the series of Bradford and Spurling (1950), Lindemann and Kuhlendahl (1953), Armstrong (1965), Rothman and Simeone (1982), McCulloch (1998), Borenstein et al. (2004), and Herkowitz et al. (2004). Although upper lumbar root syndromes are much rarer than L5 and S1 sciatica, they are very important clinical entities because of the difficulty they present in differential diagnosis. They are also quite common in absolute terms, because they represent a small percentage of cases of a very common disorder.

L1 and L2 Syndromes

The L1 and L2 nerve root syndromes are difficult to assign to the correct segment on the basis of the clinical neurological examination alone. The sole clinical manifestation pointing to a syndrome of either of these roots is a band of pain and hypesthesia from the upper lumbar spine to the groin. There are no motor or reflex deficits. The Lasègue sign is always negative, but there may be pain on stretching of the femoral nerve (a "positive reverse Lasègue sign") (**Fig. 11.86**).

Pain in the groin might be due to any of a large number of conditions, so the correct diagnosis of L1 and L2 nerve root syndromes requires special attention to their segmentally nonspecific symptoms. These include the usual manifestations of local lumbar syndrome, positional dependence of groin pain, and changing symptoms on a traction test.

L3 Syndrome

Evident manifestations of femoral nerve involvement are typical of the L3 nerve root syndrome. The zone of pain and hypesthesia occupies the anterolateral surface of the thigh, never reaching the knee or shin (**Fig. 11.87**).

The raw strength of the quadriceps is markedly reduced, and the knee-jerk reflex is diminished or absent. An L3 syndrome that has been present for a long time produces quadriceps atrophy. Total paralysis of the quadriceps, as seen after a femoral nerve injury, does not occur in L3 syndrome. The Lasègue sign is negative, but the femoral nerve stretch test, with the patient prone, is positive in many cases. Patients are often most comfortable with the lumbar spine in hyperlordosis.

L4 Syndrome

The band of pain and hypesthesia in L4 syndrome is lateral to that of L3 syndrome and, in distinction to it, also includes the knee, the anteromedial shin, and the medial edge of the foot. The knee-jerk reflex is diminished (**Fig. 11.88**).

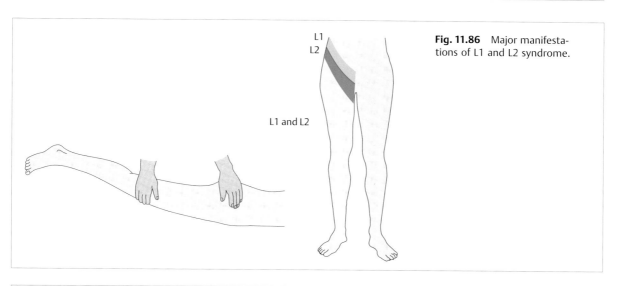

Fig. 11.86 Major manifestations of L1 and L2 syndrome.

L1
L2

L1 and L2

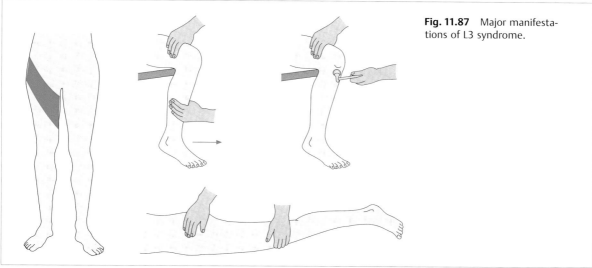

Fig. 11.87 Major manifestations of L3 syndrome.

11

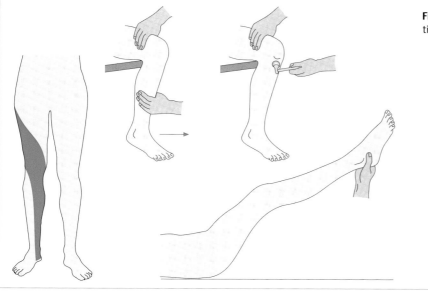

Fig. 11.88 Major manifestations of L4 syndrome.

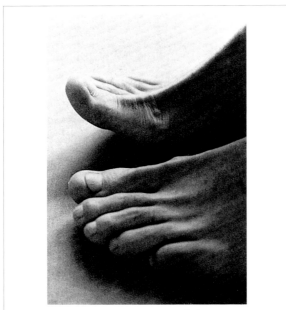

Fig. 11.89 Weakness of extension of the great toe in L5 syndrome.

ways associated with forward bending of the trunk. The pain radiates from the lumbosacral region across the posterolateral portion of the thigh and the anterolateral portion of the leg toward the lateral malleolus, where it is usually most severely felt. L5 syndrome is easiest to differentiate from the S1 syndrome by the area of pain and hypesthesia on the foot, which is on the dorsum of the foot on side of the big toe in L5 syndrome.

The most common and most important motor deficit in any type of disk disease is a **foot and toe drop** (**Fig. 11.89**). Because a persistent deficit can lead to a permanent abnormality of gait, motor function must be carefully tested in each patient. The extensor hallucis longus muscle is always monosegmentally innervated by the L5 nerve root (Schliack 1973), and weakness of this muscle is already easy to note on inspection of the foot (**Fig. 11.90**). Its chronaxie time is relatively easy to measure.

If the L5 root has been compressed for a long time, the tibialis anterior is also weak, resulting in weakness of dorsiflexion. The shin muscles may be mildly atrophic. There is no reflex abnormality in L5 syndrome.

Quadriceps weakness and atrophy, if present, are not as pronounced as in L3 syndrome. The tibialis anterior is also weak. About one-half of all patients with L4 root syndrome have a positive Lasègue sign; this indicates that the L4 nerve root already contains some fibers of the sciatic nerve.

L5 Syndrome

L5 syndrome makes itself obvious on initial inspection in the form of a markedly abnormal posture, almost al-

S1 Syndrome

S1 syndrome accounts for most cases of sciatica. Its segmentally nonspecific manifestations, including the Lasègue sign and the sciatic postural abnormality, are not as marked as in L5 syndrome because of the relatively wide space between the dural sac and nerve roots and the dorsal edge of the disk at the L5/S1 level. Most cases of sciatica without low back pain are also due to S1 nerve root syndrome.

The band of pain and hypesthesia lies dorsal to that of L5 syndrome, on the posterior surface of the thigh and

11

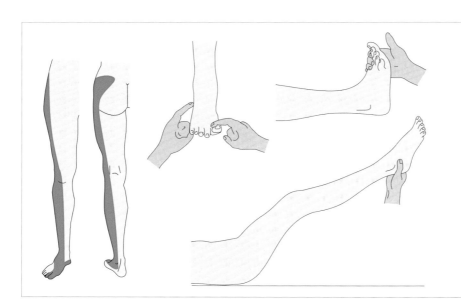

Fig. 11.90 Major manifestations of L5 syndrome.

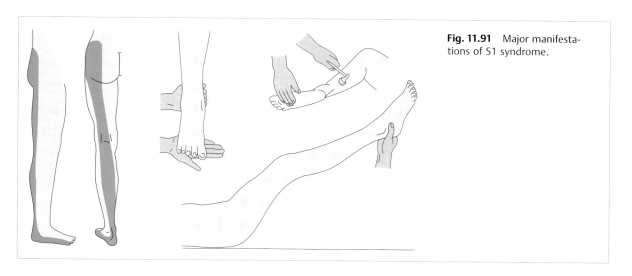

Fig. 11.91 Major manifestations of S1 syndrome.

leg (**Fig. 11.91**). Involvement of the S1 nerve root is indicated by pain radiation into the heel and lateral edge of the foot, including the third, fourth, and fifth toes. Weakness of the triceps surae muscle is evident as reduced raw strength of plantar flexion. The gluteal muscles, too, may be paretic. A characteristic finding is diminution of the Achilles reflex, which is seen even when the S1 nerve root is only mildly compressed. Stronger compression abolishes the reflex entirely; in such cases, the reflex usually does not return after surgical decompression of the root.

Severe S1 nerve root compression produces a characteristic gait abnormality because the patient cannot lift the heel on the affected side. Gluteal muscle weakness leads to the typical Trendelenburg limp. Because the triceps surae muscle is innervated by multiple nerve roots, the motor deficit of S1 syndrome is less severe over the long term than, for example, the foot drop of L5 syndrome. The patient can plantar flex the foot again after a period of adjustment and training. Atrophy of the calf muscles, however, is permanent.

S2–S5 Syndrome

The function of the S2 roots is, broadly speaking, auxiliary to that of the S1 roots. The S3–S5 roots provide sensory innervation to the perineal region (thus, a lesion produces saddle anesthesia) and motor innervation to the urinary and anal sphincters. These roots are affected in cauda equina syndrome.

Segmental Syndromes

Pathoanatomical changes in a lumbar motion segment, such as a disk prolapse or bony narrowing, only rarely produce isolated, monoradicular manifestations. Usually, the manifestations arising from the particular segment affected are combined with others relating to the nerve roots of neighboring segments. Manifestations of the latter type sometimes dominate the clinical picture. One reason for this is that space-occupying lesions in the lumbar spinal canal do not always impinge only on the exiting nerve roots that lie laterally at a given level, but can also affect the traversing nerve roots that are still intrathecal at this level and that run downward to supply lower segments. Meanwhile, pathological processes that lie laterally at disk level irritate not just the traversing root of the same segment, but also the exiting root of the next one above. The following segment-specific clinical constellations may be found:

L1–L3

Disk tissue displacement or spinal canal stenosis in the upper portion of the lumbar spine causes impingement on the dural sac, which, at this level, contains all of the spinal nerve roots of the segments below. Depending on the severity of the impingement, nerve root syndromes of the lower-lying segments may arise, ranging all the way to complete cauda equina syndrome. Paramedial disk herniations produce unilateral manifestations. Intraforaminal disk herniations of the upper lumbar segments produce symptoms referable to the roots of the next segment above.

Segment L3/4

Disk herniations at the discal level compress the still intrathecal, descending roots of the lower-lying segments, either medially (producing bilateral manifestations) or further laterally (producing unilateral manifestations). For example, a paramedial right L3/4 disk prolapse can produce right L5 or S1 sciatica, possibly accompanied by

11

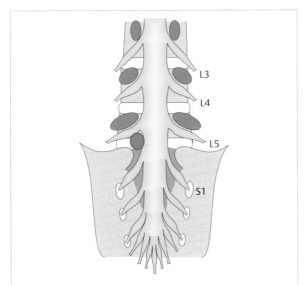

Fig. 11.92 Lateral L5/S1 disk herniation with lateral compression of the S1 nerve root and intraforaminal compression of the L5 nerve root. Clinical manifestations of L5 and S1 root compression.

pain in the groin or upper thigh because of additional involvement of the L4 root. A lateral, i. e., intraforaminal L3/4 prolapse causes isolated compression of the exiting L3 nerve root in the intervertebral foramen, with purely monoradicular manifestations.

Segment L4/5

Medial and paramedial prolapses and protrusions in the L4/5 segment impinge on the L5 nerve root, which still lies within the dural sac in this segment, at discal and supradiscal levels and produce the corresponding manifestations of L5 syndrome. A paramedial lesion can also impinge on the exiting L4 nerve root at the supradiscal level. At the discal and infradiscal levels, either a medial or a paramedial sequestrum can compress the S1 nerve root intrathecally. Thus, for example, a prolapse located in the axilla of the L5 root at an infradiscal level can produce an L5 root compression syndrome, with a foot drop, combined with mild S1 manifestations, e. g., diminution of the Achilles reflex and pain on the lateral edge of the foot. A lateral, intraforaminal prolapse of the L4/5 disk produces an L4 root compression syndrome at discal and supradiscal levels. If the prolapse is large, it can also compress the L5 nerve root intrathecally. The low back pain is relatively mild in comparison to the severe leg pain when there is a fragment at this location in the L4/5 segment. Far lateral, extraforaminal L4/5 disk herniations produce a pure L4 syndrome.

Segment L5/S1

Medial and paramedial protrusions and prolapses of the L5/S1 disk produce uni- or bilateral S1 nerve root syndrome, depending on their size. Peridural fibrosis (postdiscotomy syndrome) at this level can displace the scarred dural sac, exerting a pull on the higher-lying nerve roots. A massive medial disk herniation can cause cauda equina syndrome. The involvement of the S1–S5 roots can also be only partial. The chief symptom is pain radiating into the genital and sacral region.

Lateral L5/S1 disk protrusions and prolapses can produce additional manifestations relating to the L5 root, depending on the extent of their contact with this root at discal and supradiscal levels. If the lesion is more lateral, a pure L5 root syndrome can result (**Fig. 11.92**).

Bi- and multisegmental syndromes

The classification of a clinical syndrome by segment is more important than its classification by nerve root, particularly with regard to the indications for surgery and the question of the proper level for decompression. If pathological changes in a single segment, such as a lateral disk herniation, affect two or more nerve roots symptomatically at the same time, a mixed clinical picture can result. A typical clinical example would be an L3/4 prolapse causing both L4 and L5 root manifestations, whereas, in the same patient, an L5/S1 protrusion causes S1 manifestations of greater or lesser severity. A hitherto asymptomatic L5/S1 protrusion can become symptomatic when additional tension is placed on the entire dural sac by an L3/4 prolapse; intrathecal compression of the S1 nerve root at the level of the L3/4 prolapse is also conceivable. In either case, the S1 symptoms would improve after surgery on the L3/4 prolapse. In such situations, the surgeon should definitely refrain from carrying out additional surgery on the second affected disk.

! Some rules of thumb for the clinical assessment of multiradicular manifestations:
- Multisegmental surgery elevates the risk of post-discotomy syndrome.
- If there are pathological changes in multiple segments, the proper segment to operate on should be determined by interdisciplinary cooperation between the neurologist, radiologist, and surgeon.
- When decompressive surgery is indicated because of acute nerve root symptoms with severe neurological deficits and pain, the pathology responsible is usually to be found on a single level.

Table 11.13 Major manifestations of lumbar root syndromes

Segment	Peripheral area of pain and hypesthesia	Motor deficit (index muscle)	Reflex deficit	Nerve stretch sign
L1/L2	Groin	–	–	(Femoral stretch pain)
L3	Upper outer thigh	Quadriceps	Knee-jerk reflex	Femoral stretch pain
L4	Upper outer thigh, inner calf, foot	Quadriceps	Knee-jerk reflex	(Positive Lasègue sign)
L5	Outer calf, medial dorsum of foot, great toe	Extensor hallucis longus	–	Positive Lasègue sign
S1	Back of calf, heel, lateral edge of foot, third through fifth toes	Triceps surae, glutei	Achilles reflex	Positive Lasègue sign

Differential Diagnosis of Sciatica and Sciatica-Like Symptoms

Diagnostic Techniques

In the differential diagnosis of pain in the lower limbs, the clinician must first determine whether sciatica-like pain or true sciatica is present, and, if the latter, whether it should be classified as radicular pain or as neuralgia of a peripheral nerve.

! Most cases of true sciatica are discogenic and are caused by degenerative changes of the two lowest lumbar motion segments.

The same is true of the femoral nerve pain arising from pathology in the upper lumbar motion segments. Among the major symptoms of sciatica, the positional dependence of the pain is a clue to a discogenic nerve root syndrome. Sciatica and femoral nerve pain of other causes are generally not positionally dependent. The positional dependence of the pain can be demonstrated clearly by the **lumbar spine traction test,** which corresponds to the Glisson test in the cervical spine. Brief extension of the lumbar spine reduces the contact between a disk protrusion and the adjacent nerve root in such a way that the intensity and extent of radiation of sciatica or femoral nerve pain can change.

The traction test for the differential diagnosis of a lumbar root syndrome employs a traction bandage. The patient pushes against his or her own pelvis using handgrips attached to a belt, producing traction on the lower lumbar segments (**Fig. 11.93**).

! Brief, intense traction on the lumbar spine changes the quality and quantity of pain in a discogenic nerve root syndrome: the patient can also bend further forward.

If the underlying problem is a mild disk protrusion, sciatica and the sciatic postural abnormality disappear entirely under traction. Usually, though, the pain is only partially relieved and moves to another location: lateral pain becomes more medial. Sharp nerve root pain gives way to aching back pain. Sciatica is no longer felt in the distal portion of the dermatome, but in its proximal portion: the pain is centralized, as can also be observed later after successful treatment. Sometimes the pain becomes more severe under traction and radiates further down the limb. This can happen, for example, when traction creates a shearing movement of the root across part of the prolapsed disk, or when it causes a prolapse to bulge further outward.

The traction test can also be used to determine whether traction might be an appropriate treatment for the patient. In rare cases, the traction test can be positive in nerve root syndromes of nondiscogenic origin. Lower limb pain of extravertebral origin, e. g., due to diseases of the hip joint or the circulatory system, is important for differential diagnosis and is not influenced by the traction test.

11

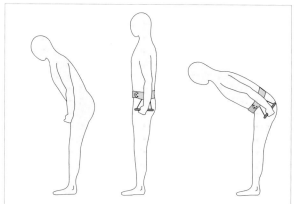

Fig. 11.93 Traction test with traction bandage for the differential diagnosis of leg pain: traction relieves disk-related pain and enables the patient to bend farther forward.

Table 11.14 Differential diagnosis of hip pain from lumbar root syndrome

	Hip pain	Lumbar root syndrome
History	Insidious onset, pain on standing and walking, improvement on sitting	Sudden onset, pain while sitting, improvement with standing and walking
Clinical findings	Limited range of motion of the hip (particularly internal rotation)	Full range of motion of the hip
	Sciatica test negative, lumbar spine traction test negative	Sciatica test positive, lumbar spine traction test positive
Confirmation of the diagnosis	Plain radiographs, intra-articular injection of local anesthetic	CT, MRI

Extravertebral Causes

Pain originating in the hip joint is often mistaken for the pain of a lumbar root syndrome, mainly because both conditions are very common and produce pain radiating into very similar regions in the hip and thigh region. The main distinguishing factor is hip pain in incipient arthrosis and necrosis of the femoral head. Massive coxarthrosis and coxitis are unlikely to be misdiagnosed. A lumbar root syndrome may be difficult to diagnose if some of the typical manifestations are lacking (**Table 11.14**). As mentioned above, sciatica may be unaccompanied by back pain, i.e., the main symptom of local lumbar syndrome. The neurologic deficit, too, may be very mild or absent. The Lasègue sign and the reverse Lasègue sign are of limited usefulness in differential diagnosis, because the elicitation of either involves passive movement of the hip. Only the sciatic nerve test is of differential diagnostic value for true sciatica (see **Fig. 11.45**). Conversely, testing the range of motion of the hip always produces some degree of movement of the lumbar spine, which may irritate a nerve root. The most reliable evidence of hip disease is an asymmetrical range of internal rotation.

Close attention should also be paid to the patient's complaints. If the patient relates that the pain is positionally dependent, and particularly that it changes during the traction test, then a nerve root syndrome is probably present.

A presumptive diagnosis of early coxarthrosis can be confirmed with a trial intra-articular injection of local anesthetic and with plain radiographs in multiple planes, possibly including tomographic views. Helpful tests to confirm a presumptive diagnosis of nerve root syndrome include CT, MRI, and sometimes myelography. Inflammatory or degenerative diseases of the **sacroiliac joint** can produce symptoms in the same area as the proximal projection field of sciatica; clues to the correct diagnosis include a Mennell sign on physical examination and positive findings on plain radiographs, tomography, and scintigraphy of the sacroiliac joint.

Pain in the hip region in the absence of pathological findings in the hip joint or the lumbar spine should raise suspicion of **trochanteric bursitis.** This diagnosis, too, is confirmed with test infiltration of the trochanteric area with a local anesthetic.

Extraspinal tumors arising in the rectum, uterus, or prostate gland must reach an advanced stage before they can impinge on the nerves of the lumbosacral plexus.

An **aneurysm of the common iliac artery** occasionally causes sciatica; the diagnosis is made by duplex ultrasonography and MRI. In our outpatient clinic, we have seen many patients referred to us by the vascular clinic who complained of leg pain of unclear origin and in whom the differential diagnostic question concerned discogenic root syndrome vs. **peripheral ischemia.** The latter generally presents with pain that worsens on walking, which is not the case for sciatica. A negative traction test and the positional independence of the pain serve to rule out lumbar root syndrome. Finally, **diseases of the sciatic nerve itself** must be included in the differential diagnosis. At one time these were wrongly held to be the most common cause of sciatica, but we now know that intrinsic sciatic nerve lesions are quite rare. Types include herpes zoster infection, alcoholic neuritis, leprous neuritis, tick-borne radiculitis, and polyneuropathy manifesting itself most severely in the sciatic nerve due to diabetes mellitus or periarteritis nodosa. Diabetic neuropathy should always be considered in an older patient complaining of neuralgia-like pain in the lower limbs.

Medicolegal consultants are often asked to make the differential diagnosis between **injection injury of the sciatic nerve** and discogenic sciatica, which was often the reason why the intramuscular injection was given. In injection palsy, there is circumscribed tenderness at the injection site; pressure here also induces the typical projecting pain. As described in Chapter 8, nerve root injuries in the lumbar spine, unlike plexus and peripheral nerve injuries, are not accompanied by any abnormal autonomic manifestations.

Direct injury to the sciatic nerve distal to the nerve roots causes a disturbance of sweating in exactly the same area as the sensory deficit. Nerve root lesions never cause loss of sweating, even when a total sensory deficit of a hand or foot occurs as the result of a multiradicular syndrome (Mumenthaler et al. 1998).

Table 11.15 Differential diagnosis of sciatica and symptoms resembling sciatica

	Cause	Segmental band of pain	Neurological deficits	Lumbar spine symptoms	Lasègue sign	Traction test	Confirmation of the diagnosis (initial steps)
Vertebral	Discogenic sciatica	++	++	++	+++	+++	CT, MRI
	Spondylolisthesis	++	++	+++	+++	(+)	Plain radiographs
	Spondylitis	++	++	+++	+++	(+)	CT, MRI, lab tests
	Tumor	++	++	+++	+++	(+)	CT, MRI, lab tests, scintigraphy
	Spinal canal stenosis	++	(+)	(+)	–	+	CT, MRI
Extra-vertebral	Coxalgia	–	–	–	(+)	–	Plain radiographs, local anesthesia
	Sacroiliac joint pain	(+)	–	–	+	(+)	Local anesthesia
	Trochanteric bursitis	(+)	–	–	–	–	Local anesthesia
	Retroperitoneal tumors	++	++	++	++	–	Lab tests, CT, MRI
	Peripheral vascular disease	–	–	–	–	–	Duplex ultrasonography, measurement of pedal pulses
	Diabetic neuropathy	++	++	–	++	–	Lab tests
	Injection injury to sciatic nerve	+++	+++	–	+++	–	Sweating test, neurophysiological testing
	Aneurysm	–	–	(+)	–	–	Duplex ultrasonography, MRI

When the pain and sensory disturbance are located in the groin and the anterior surface of the thigh, the cause may be **meralgia paresthetica** rather than an L3 nerve root syndrome. This disorder is caused by injury to the lateral femoral cutaneous nerve. Unlike L3 syndrome, meralgia paresthetica is not associated with a diminished knee-jerk reflex. For this condition, too, local infiltration and a traction test are helpful in differential diagnosis.

Vertebral Causes

Though discogenic nerve root syndromes are by far the most common cause, many other diseases affecting the lumbar motion segments can produce neuralgia of the femoral or sciatic nerve. These are essentially the same vertebral causes that must be considered in the differential diagnosis of low back pain (**Table 11.15**).

Sciatica in **spondylolisthesis** is usually bilateral and difficult to influence with changes of posture or a traction test. In this condition, nerve root irritation is due to fibrous overgrowth in the interlaminar window and to stretching of the roots over the posterosuperior edge of the vertebra below the sliding vertebra.

If **spondylitis** extends posteriorly, nerve root manifestations appear that are unchanged by a traction test or by changes of position. Pain at night is characteristic. Because spondylitis begins ventrally, sciatica is a late manifestation. The same is true of **tumors affecting the vertebral bodies,** which are usually metastases (**Fig. 11.94**). Here, too, nerve root manifestations arise only when the tumor mass extends into the spinal canal or when pathological fractures occur. In such cases sciatica is very severe and consists of persistent, positionally independent pain with dermatomal radiation, together with bilaterally positive Lasègue signs.

Vertebral body metastases are relatively common; *primary neoplasia in the motion segment* is rarer but can also occur, most commonly in the nerves. Primary tumors, too, cause constant, positionally independent neurological manifestations as well as CSF changes.

Paget disease and **fluorosis** are rare causes of sciatica. Appositional bone growth in these conditions can narrow the spinal canal and the intervertebral foramina.

The sciatica associated with **spinal canal stenosis** is usually indirectly discogenic as well. Patients with spinal canal stenosis, unlike those with purely discogenic sciatica, have less pain when sitting and more when

11

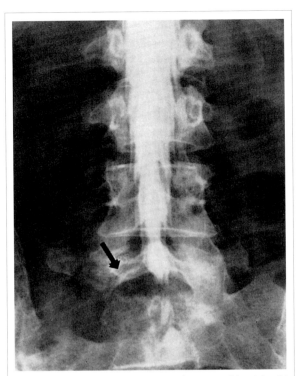

Fig. 11.94 64-year-old woman with intractable right S1 sciatica. The anteroposterior plain radiograph shows an indentation of the column of contrast medium on the right with nerve root cutoff, as well as partial destruction of the right sacrum by a tumor (breast cancer metastasis).

Table 11.16 Major manifestations of cauda equina syndrome

- Saddle anesthesia
- Bilaterally absent Achilles reflexes
- Bladder and bowel dysfunction

standing or walking. Neurologic deficits are rare. The diagnosis is made by CT or, better, MRI.

Cauda Equina Syndrome

Cauda equina syndrome is a special type of multiradicular lumbar nerve root syndrome. The nerve roots of the cauda equina in the lumbar spinal canal are compressed by a large, medial disk herniation, with resulting neurologic deficits of the lower lumbar roots and, later, all of the sacral roots as well. Pain, in the form of bilateral sciatica, is more or less severe depending on the extent and level of compression. The **typical manifestations** include *saddle anesthesia*, bilaterally absent Achilles reflexes, *weakness of the calf muscles*, and *diminished urinary and*

anal sphincter tone (**Table 11.16**). Sexual potency is also often affected. Involvement of the S4 and S5 roots produces a characteristic, narrowly circumscribed sensory deficit centered on the tip of the coccyx, which can be palpated externally. Sphincter function is affected by bilateral involvement of the S3 roots.

Higher lesions can additionally produce foot and toe drop, loss of the knee-jerk reflexes, and quadriceps weakness. Mumenthaler et al. (1998) point out that in cauda equina syndrome sweating remains intact on the soles of the feet even if they are totally anesthetic, because the autonomic fibers are not involved. Acute cauda equina syndrome is usually caused by **massive L3/4 or L4/5 disk prolapses in the midline.** Intense local and radicular pain precedes the complete neurologic deficit. As soon as the stage of paralysis is reached, the local lumbar symptoms disappear (which hardly ever happens in lumbar disk herniation without cauda equina compression). The *initial sciatica*, which provides an important clue to the diagnosis, resolves when the disk prolapse is surgically treated.

> ❗ Discogenic cauda equina compression is usually an acute event that demands immediate surgical treatment.

The prognosis of cauda equina syndrome depends on the time of intervention: 25% of patients operated on within 48 h will have a complete recovery of cauda equina function (McCulloch 1998). Patients operated on later than that will have an improvement of sphincter function and partial improvement of their motor deficits. The degree of recovery also depends on the extent of the initial deficit. According to the meta-analysis of Ahn (2000), the results are no different if surgery is carried out in the first 24 h or the second 24 h after the onset of symptoms. Nonetheless, as soon as the diagnosis is made, the patient should be operated on without delay.

In distinction to cauda equina syndrome caused by a massive disk prolapse, **cauda equina compression by a tumor** is an insidiously progressive process. Bladder and bowel dysfunction may continue to be normal for a long time. Patients initially suffer from intractable sciatica and gradually lose the knee-jerk and ankle-jerk reflexes. It is thus possible to intervene surgically before the full-blown clinical syndrome develops. The tumors that can compress the cauda equina include *neurinoma, epidermoid tumor, menigioma, ependymoma of the cauda equina,* and *glioma,* as well as *metastases* of various kinds of primary tumor that seed the vertebrae and extend into the lumbar spinal canal (Jochheim et al. 1961, Pia 1977, Herkowicz 1994).

As the clinical manifestations of cauda equina syndrome are pathognomonic, the only question in **differential diagnosis** is the nature of the causative lesion. Discogenic origin is suggested, as usual, by the sudden onset and positional dependence of the symptoms, together with normal laboratory values and plain radiographs. When the cause is a tumor affecting the cauda equina, the symptoms do not change with mechanical loading and unloading of the spine. Laboratory values, CSF findings, CT, MRI, and myelography aid further in the diagnosis.

Examination of the CSF is usually not necessary; the finding of *blocked CSF flow* indicates mechanical compression but is of no help in differential diagnosis. Even normal CSF findings and free flow of CSF in the Queckenstedt test do not exclude cauda equina compression at a level below the lumbar puncture. The most important diagnostic studies are CT, MRI, and myelography. Even these techniques do not provide a histological diagnosis, but this is not a problem, because surgery must follow immediately in any case.

Red Flags in Lumbar Root Syndromes

Alarming manifestations in true lumbar root syndrome or other conditions resembling it are known as "red flags" (see **Table 11.6**, p. 193). They include the alarming manifestations of nerve root compression itself, e. g., urinary and fecal incontinence and saddle anesthesia in cauda equina syndrome or severe weakness, as in an acute foot drop. Other conditions that may enter into the differential diagnosis of a lumbar root syndrome, including an extraspinal tumor, an aneurysm of the common iliac artery, peripheral ischemia, and tumor-associated pain, call for immediate further diagnostic or therapeutic measures.

Summary: Clinical Features of Lumbar Syndromes

The clinical manifestations of degenerative conditions of the lumbar spine are classified according to their localization and radiation as either local lumbar syndrome or lumbar root syndrome. Most cases of local lumbar syndrome are accounted for by so-called simple low back pain, whose cause can only be elucidated by thorough history-taking and physical examination with the aid of manual examining techniques. Its pathogenesis involves irritation of nociceptors in the disk itself (discogenic low back pain) and in the posterior portion of the motion segment (arthroligamentous low back pain). Imaging studies have little or no role in the diagnostic assessment of local lumbar syndromes, particularly simple low back pain: the history and physical findings already provide all the information needed for diagnosis and treatment.

Pain radiating into the leg can usually be attributed to a particular segment. Psychosocial factors (yellow flags) should be considered in the diagnostic assessment. Alarming spinal symptoms and signs (red flags), caused by discogenic disease or other conditions that may mimic it, should always be sought and ruled out.

MRI is rapidly becoming the imaging method of choice to display degenerative changes in the lumbar spine. Plain radiographs provide little information about changes in the intervertebral space. Spondylosis and osteochondrosis are of little clinical significance. Therefore, when assessing a patient with simple back pain, the physician should at first refrain from ordering plain radiographs of the lumbar spine in two planes, although this used to be the standard practice.

Discography and myelography have also largely given way to MRI. CT is cheaper than MRI, but considerably less informative in the diagnostic assessment of discogenic conditions. A further disadvantage of CT is radiation exposure.

Electrodiagnostic studies, however, have become increasingly important in recent years because of the trend toward conservative treatment of nerve root compression and the resulting need of the physician and the patient alike for a reliable means of monitoring the extent and course of neural damage over time.

11

Conclusion

Every pain in the low back or lower limb has a diagnosis.

■ Treatment of Lumbar Syndromes

Classification of Treatment Methods

The international literature has traditionally classified the methods of treating lumbar syndromes as conservative vs. operative, or as operative vs. nonoperative. This distinction is clearly useful as a demarcation between widely differing techniques, such as heat application and positioning, on the one hand, and open disk surgery on the other. In recent decades, however, new methods of treatment have arisen that occupy a place on the spectrum between conservative management and open surgery and that are designated as "minimally invasive." Because the origin of the pain in lumbar syndromes lies well beneath the surface, e. g., in lumbar root compression syndrome, and because open surgery is therefore impossible except by a relatively difficult surgical approach, many new methods have been developed by which the anterolateral epidural space and the foramino-articular region can be reached with the aid of special needle techniques and endoscopic instruments. The common feature of all minimally invasive measures is a percutaneous approach in which the instruments are introduced without a skin incision (except for a minimal stab wound).

A classification of the various methods of treating degenerative diseases of the lumbar spine is given in **Table 11.17**. Minimally invasive procedures are listed between conservative and operative methods and are themselves subdivided into paravertebral injections, intradiscal therapy, and endoscopic techniques.

All of the conservative methods of treating disk disease, and some of the minimally invasive ones, leave the osmotic system of the intervertebral disk undisturbed.

! Patients with disk protrusions should be treated with all possible methods that preserve the integrity of the disk.

The classic **conservative** measures include physiotherapy, heat application, positioning, and analgesia. Additional ones are local injections such as trigger point infiltration, intracutaneous injections, and muscle infiltration **(superficial needling techniques).**

Paravertebral injections are deep needling techniques involving infiltration of the epidural space or the foramino-articular region and are included among minimally invasive methods. These injections require directed needle introduction, often under imaging guidance. Because the target sites for injection are immediately adjacent to the nerve root sleeves and the dural sac, with the possibility of subarachnoid injection, paravertebral injections require circulatory monitoring during the procedure and post-procedural monitoring afterward. The application of medications in the epidural space is done either as a single shot or as a longer-lasting infiltration through a temporarily implanted percutaneous catheter.

Intradiscal techniques use either special needles (e. g., chemonucleolysis) or percutaneously introducible instruments, some of which are inserted under endoscopic guidance.

Purely endoscopic operations for the removal of lumbar disk herniations are done either transforaminally, i. e., through the intervertebral foramen, or by the interlaminar route, i. e., through the ligamentum flavum.

Open operations are defined as those requiring a skin incision of 3 cm or longer and are subdivided into microscopic decompressive methods with use of an operating microscope and more extensive approaches, with or without use of a microscope. Microsurgery enables precision to within a millimeter in a narrow operative field. Special instruments are needed. The conventional, more extensive approach generally involves a partial or total removal of the lamina (hemilaminectomy or laminectomy). When decompression is extensive and includes a partial or total resection of the intervertebral joint (facetectomy), a fusion operation is usually carried out in the same sitting. Fusion operations are classified as dorsal, ventral, or combined (dorsoventral).

Replacement of the entire disk by a moveable artificial disk is called disk prosthesis surgery.

Conservative Treatment

! **Definition:** The term "conservative" comes from the Latin "conservare," meaning to keep or preserve. Unlike surgical treatment and to some percutaneous minimally invasive procedures, the aim of conservative therapy is to improve the patient's symptoms while preserving the integrity of the disk.

Stress-reducing Positioning, no Bed Rest

There are no universally valid guidelines for the optimal bodily position for disk-related symptoms in the lumbar region. For every anatomical or functional disturbance in the motion segment, there is an optimal position of the spine in which the pain is less intense than in other positions. This optimal position may be the upright position or the horizontal position, in bed, in practically any conceivable posture, depending on the exact cause of the pain. In general, patients feel best in the supine or lateral decubitus position with the hip and knee joints flexed. For other patients, however, the optimal position

Table 11.17 The treatment of lumbar syndromes

Conservative		Paravertebral injections, PRT	Minimally invasive Intradiscal	Endoscopic	Surgical Decompression	Fusion
Heat Positioning Physiotherapy Analgesics Injections (superficial) Orthoses	Manual therapy Special patient exercises Back training	Epidural LSPA Facet infiltration Catheters	Chemo-nucleolysis Percutaneous nucleotomy Percutaneous laser Percutaneous thermotherapy	Transforaminal Interlaminar Intradiscal	Microdiscotomy Conventional Laminectomy	Dorsal Ventral Dorsoventral fusion Disk prosthesis

is standing bent forward, supporting the upper body with the arms.

> ! Mechanical stress on the lumbar disks is at a minimum in the so-called step position, i. e., horizontal with flexed hip and knee joints (**Fig. 11.95**).

All biomechanical factors of the step position lead to a minimization of contact between the disk protrusion and the spinal nerve. When disk tissue is displaced within the disk, but the anulus fibrosus is intact, there is a good chance that conservative management in the step position will result in a return of the displaced tissue to the center of the disk.

A stress-reducing position should only be assumed temporarily, e. g., during or after other therapeutic measures such as heat application, electrotherapy, progressive muscle relaxation, etc.

Prolonged bed rest is counterproductive in lumbar disk disease, even when the patient assumes a stress-re-

ducing position. Many controlled studies (**Table 11.18**) have shown that patients with lumbago and sciatica have more symptoms after prolonged bed rest than patients in a control group who are allowed to be mobile and continue to go to work (Hagen et al. 2004, Becker et al. 2006).

> ! Return to work is therapeutic (Nordin 2004).

The probability of returning to work decreases very rapidly with increasing duration of sick leave.

Heat Therapy

Patients with lumbar disk disease experience relief with heat in all its forms, whether through local heat application or simply through a **warm climate.** Cold, on the other hand, provokes symptoms even in the absence of other mechanical influences. The causal mechanism for this has not yet been fully explained. Patients with

11

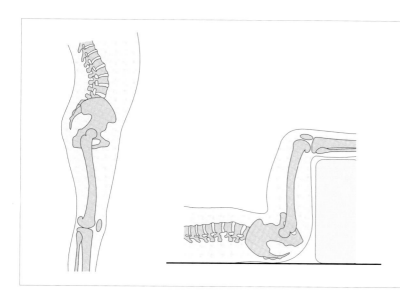

Fig. 11.95 Step positioning: a stress-reducing position with the patient lying on their back and the hip and knee joints in flexion. This results in low intradiscal pressure, widening of the intervertebral foramina, relaxation of the intervertebral joint capsules, flattening of dorsal disk protrusions, widening of the spinal canal, relaxation of the sciatic nerve, and reduction of stress on the sacroiliac joints.

Table 11.18	Randomized controlled studies on the effectiveness of bed rest for lumbar disk disease		
Author	*Year*	*Study*	*Result*
Postacchini et al.	1986	2–6 days of bed rest vs. remaining mobile	Bed rest worse
Spalski and Hayez	1992	7 days of bed rest vs. 3 days of bed rest	No difference
Malmivaara et al.	1995	2 days of bed rest vs. remaining mobile with physiotherapy	Bed rest worse
Wilkinson	1995	2 days of bed rest vs. remaining mobile	Bed rest worse

chronic, recurrent low back pain and sciatica avoid situations that may lead to cooling; they tend to wear warm underwear or corsets.

Warmth and pain relief can also be obtained through the use of **external agents** such as capsaicin plasters or ointments containing salicylic acid derivatives, vasodilator substances, or essential oils. These agents cannot be expected to exert a deep effect that alters the biochemical processes in the lumbar motion segment. The local anesthetic effect of deep heat is attributable to blood volume shift in the deep musculature, reduction of muscle tone, and the transport of inflammatory mediators away from the local area by the circulation. The therapeutic effect is increased by hyperemia, the improved elasticity of collagen fibers, and the resulting relaxation of the tense musculature and activation of inhibitory fields. When heat is applied, care should be taken that the patient is in the appropriate position. The prone position is inadvisable, as it is associated with lumbar hyperlordosis. **Heat application is contraindicated** in patients with thromboses and florid infectious or inflammatory processes. The patient's response to heat is thus a differential diagnostic criterion as well: patients with tumors or infectious/inflammatory processes have worse pain, due to hyperemia, when heat is applied.

Results. Aside from textbook data, the efficacy of heat in the treatment of low back pain is discussed in the treatment recommendation of the European Guidelines (2006) and the German Pharmaceuticals Committee (2007) as well as by Borenstein et al. (2004) and by Nachemson and Jonsson (2006), but only in general terms. The only controlled studies ore those of French et al. (2006) and Hochschuler (2006). In all the RCTs examined in the Cochrane Review, heat therapy had a modest advantage over comparison interventions (French 2006). Not enough attention has been paid to the different results of heat vs. cold application.

Electrotherapy

 Definition: The term "electrotherapy" covers all techniques in which electrical energy is used for healing purposes.

Principle. The pain-relieving and muscle-relaxing effect of heat can also be obtained with electrical apparatus. Constantly flowing **galvanic** (direct) current, e. g., in a galvanic bath, is said to relieve pain, among other effects. **Diadynamic** current, which is low-frequency alternating current of changing frequency and intensity, is also said to relieve pain.

In **interference current therapy,** two biological, non-irritating currents of intermediate frequency are applied to the body, each of them through two electrodes. The frequencies of the two currents differ by up to 100 Hz. The superposition of these two currents creates an amplitude- and frequency-modulated current within the body at a low, and therefore biologically active, frequency. In degenerative diseases of the spine, interference currents can be used to reach the deeper truncal musculature and the affected motion segment itself.

Pulsating signal therapy (PST) uses pulses of direct current administered through a specially adapted coil system. The diseased tissue is treated with currents of 1–30 Hz and a field strength of 12.5 G.

Results. The positive results reported in **retrospective case series** (Pärtan 1953, Wolf 1956, Hansjürgens 1974, Böhlau 1975, Milanowska 1983, Waddell 1998, Nachemson and Jonsson 2000, Moffett 2005) have not yet been validated by any well-designed randomized studies. For this reason, electrotherapy with various types of current and at various frequencies is principally used as a supplement to other treatments for lumbar syndrome whose effectiveness has been proven.

Transcutaneous Electrical Nerve Stimulation

Transcutaneous Electrical Nerve Stimulation (TENS) is a special form of electrotherapy designed specifically for the treatment of pain, using battery-powered stimulators and electrodes that are are taped or glued to the skin. It involves electrical stimulation of the A fibers of peripheral nerves through the skin, inhibiting the posterior horn of the spinal cord and thereby lessening the activity of the C fibers at the same segmental level. Stimulation may be either continuous or discontinuous; its goal is to influence nerve fibers electrically without inducing muscle contractions or pain. The effect of TENS varies considerably from one patient to another and must be adapted to suit each individual.

Results. Most studies have shown that the results tend to be markedly better in the first few weeks than in the ensuing months or years. A number of placebo-controlled studies of TENS for chronic lumbar syndrome can be found in the literature (Alcoff et al. 1982, Lehmann et al. 1983, Deyo et al. 1990, Marchand et al. 1993, Moore and Shurman 1997, Khadilkar et al. 2005).

Massage

> **Definition:** Massage is a special type of manual physiotherapy that aims to stimulate the skin, subcutaneous tissue, and deeper tissues in a nonspecific way through pressure, pulling, repositioning, and vibration.

Aside from such classic massage techniques as stroking, gentle kneading, and wringing, there are further measures that may be of use in the treatment of lumbar syndromes, e.g., underwater pressure massage with streams of warm water. A tangentially applied stream at a pressure of 100–200 kPa (1–2 atm) can be applied to treat spasm of the entire paravertebral erector spinae musculature without pressing the lumbar spine into lordosis, as can occur with forceful manual massage. Attention should be paid to proper positioning of the patient both for cervical spinal massage and for lumbar spinal massage. Massage in the prone position is contraindicated because the associated lumbar hyperlordosis is harmful and the pressure of massage only worsens the problem. The best position is the "upside-down step position," with the hips and knees flexed over large foam-rubber cubes of the type used for the normal step positioning with the patient lying on their back.

Results. Massage is recommended in various textbooks (Nachemson and Jonsson 2000, Heysel 2004, Borenstein, Wisely, and Borden 2004), but its efficacy in lumbar disk disease has yet to be demonstrated in any randomized controlled studies.

> The pleasing hand contact is certainly a factor in the popularity of any manual treatment of low back pain (Farfan 1996).

Manual Therapy

Synonyms: Chirotherapy.

> **Definition:** Manual medicine, or chirotherapy, is a method of diagnosing and treating functional disturbances of the organs of posture and movement with special hand grips (**Fig. 11.96**).

Manipulation is locating the lesioned segment and restoring axial alignement (Farfan 1996).

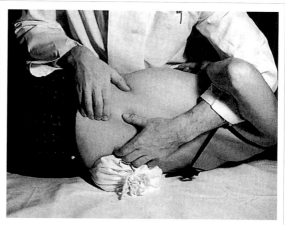

Fig. 11.96 Manual diagnosis and treatment of a segmental functional disturbance in the lumbar spine.

The **indications** for manual therapy in degenerative diseases of the lumbar spine, particularly disk protrusions and prolapses, are limited. One **contraindication**, for example, arises from the fact that the lumbar motion segments, which are already slackened by the degenerative process, can be further slackened by this form of treatment. There is also a risk that the symptoms of a protrusion may worsen because of further displacement of disk tissue. Physiotherapy for lumbar syndromes is, therefore, based on the principle of stabilization rather than mobilization. Manual therapy primarily involves manipulation with traction handgrips in an axial direction of pull. Spinal manipulations should be carried out only by experienced manual therapists, once tumors and inflammatory processes have been excluded.

Results. In a number of systematic reviews and meta-analyses of the putative efficacy of manual therapy, it has been pointed out that only a few of the clinical studies of this topic to date have been of adequate methodological quality (Shelkelle 1994, Assendelft et al. 1996, Koes et al. 1996, van Tulder 1997, Nachemson and Jonsson 2000). Although only limited conclusions can be drawn from the available data, it seems that patients with acute back pain but no radicular symptoms (within the first 4–6 weeks of onset) probably stand to benefit the most from manual therapy (Shekelle 1994, 1998, Kendall et al. 1997, Hildebrandt and Pfingsten 1998, Hurwitz et al. 2006, European Guidelines 2006).

11

Table 11.19	The goals of physiotherapy in the rehabilitation and prophylaxis of lumbar syndrome

- Muscle strengthening
- Transition from partial to full weight-bearing
- Training of disk-friendly movements
- Restoration of the original mobility of the affected spinal segments

Physiotherapy

Synonyms: Physical therapy, patient exercises.

> **Definition:** Physiotherapy consists of exercises ordered by a physician for the treatment of a number of conditions including musculoskeletal deformities, injuries and their consequences, or abnormal organic and/or mental function. In general, physiotherapy is a method of "healing by movement" (**Table 11.19**).

Physiotherapeutic exercises in lumbar syndrome serve the purposes of treatment, rehabilitation, and prophylaxis against recurrences. Rehabilitative physiotherapy can be begun only after the pain has largely subsided.

The most important aspect of rehabilitation and recurrence prevention is strengthening of the musculature. The truncal and proximal appendicular muscles are among the functional components of the motion segments in that they guide and stabilize the spine. When a motion segment is firmly stabilized by the surrounding muscle, disk tissue displacement and sliding of the vertebrae with respect to each other are far less likely to occur than when the segment is slack. **A sturdy "internal corset" composed of strong muscles can turn the trunk into a solid cylinder when the patient lifts and carries.** Activation of the abdominal muscles can lower lumbar intradiscal pressure by roughly 30%.

After prolonged immobilization, e. g., after sciatica with or without surgery, the phylogenetically older postural muscles—including the erector spinae muscles—tend to contract and become shorter, and the phasic muscles—such as the abdominal muscles—become atrophic, overstretched, and hypotonic. With step-positioning of the patient, the origin and insertion of each muscle can be brought closer together, and the tone can be increased by exercising. Thus, in physiotherapy, just as much attention should be paid to the abdominal and proximal appendicular muscles as to the erector spinae muscles.

Like massage, muscle-strengthening exercises should be conducted while the patient is in the stress-minimizing position and should be done as isometrically as possible, in order not to cause any additional irritation of the nerve root (**Figs. 11.97–11.98**).

Physiotherapy for degenerative diseases of the lumbar spine is carried out at varying intensities over the course of treatment. Once the pain has subsided, the goal of physiotherapy is no longer to reduce pain, but to prevent recurrences through a medically designed muscle-training program. The antalgic posture, with mild lumbar kyphosis to take stress off the posterior elements of the motion segment, must be reconverted to a normal posture and cannot be allowed to become permanent. The stress-minimizing kyphosis that has enabled the displaced disk tissue to return to its original position must gradually be brought back to a physiological lordosis ("eulordosis"). In an evenly distributed lordosis, the lower spinal segments have an optimal ability to bear axial loads.

Once the asymptomatic state has been achieved, exercises can be done cautiously in various positions, with gradually increasing lordosis. Extreme excursions under stress should be avoided, even later in the course of the training program (**Fig. 11.99**).

Results. Many randomized and controlled studies have documented the **efficacy of physiotherapy** in disk disease. The control groups in these studies usually underwent passive treatments such as massage, electrotherapy, or therapy with apparatus of various kinds. Treatment measures directly involving another person as therapist have been found, in general, to be superior to those involving apparatus (Lindstroem and Zachrisson 1970, Martin et al. 1980, Deyo et al. 1990, Turner et al. 1990, Lindstroem et al. 1992, Hansen et al. 1993, Risch et al. 1993, Sachs et al. 1994, Frost et al. 1995, Nachemson and Jonsson 2000, Borenstein et al. 2004, Herkowitz et al. 2004, Hildebrandt et al. 2004, Staal et al. 2005, European Guidelines 2006, Goldby 2006, Critchley et al. 2007).

There are special types of physiotherapy that have their own names and adhere to a specific concept; one of these is medical training therapy.

Medical Training Therapy

> **Definition:** Medical training therapy is a dynamic form of strength training that is considered to be an objectively based treatment method within the framework of manual therapy.

The basis of medical training therapy (MTT) is a body of scientific knowledge gained from the experience of trainers of active, healthy athletes. The repetition method of training is used; the number of sets and repetitions are set according to the deficits that are present. Before training starts, a functional admission interview is carried out so that any functional disturbances, such as muscular imbalances, can be detected. The content and goals of MTT include joint training, muscle training, and coordination training, just as in sports.

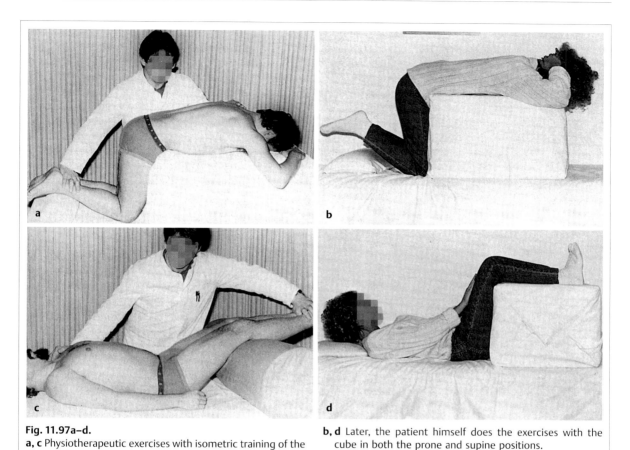

Fig. 11.97a–d.

a, c Physiotherapeutic exercises with isometric training of the truncal and proximal appendicular musculature from stress-reducing positions, both prone and supine.

b, d Later, the patient himself does the exercises with the cube in both the prone and supine positions.

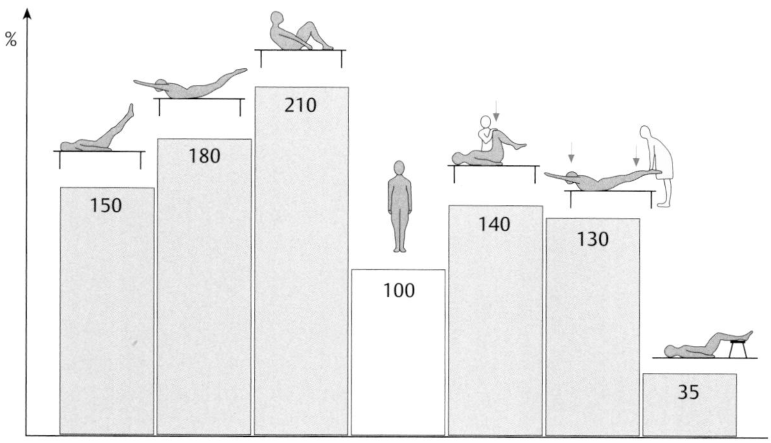

Fig. 11.98 Relative changes of stress (pressure) in the L3/4 disk when various physiotherapeutic exercises are performed (from Nachemson, 1966).

11

Kieser Training

! **Definition:** Kieser training is a dynamic form of strength training by the repetition method, done almost exclusively using apparatus.

The special features of Kieser training are its strict methodology and training by the clock. It is defined as a kind of MTT, so it is also used by healthy individuals who want to do something positive for their health in the form of preventive medicine.

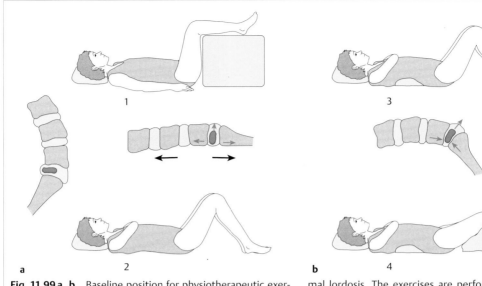

Fig. 11.99 a, b Baseline position for physiotherapeutic exercises, starting with reduction of the lumbar lordosis in the step position and then proceeding to restoration of the nor-

mal lordosis. The exercises are performed from these positions.

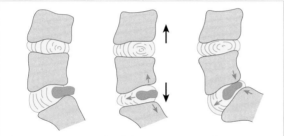

Fig. 11.100 Return of a disk protrusion into the intervertebral space on traction of the spine. Repositioning of the disk protrusion requires not just traction, but also kyphosis of the lumbar spine (step positioning).

Results. The efficacy of MTT and Kieser therapy, like that of other mainly apparatus-oriented methods, e. g., MedX therapy (Miltner 2001) or the FPZ concept (Denner 1998, Morgenstern et al. 2005), has not yet been scientifically evaluated. The common feature of all of these methods is the principle of movement and muscle strengthening. As this principle is well founded in biomechanics and easily accepted by patients and therapists alike, these methods seem to play a positive role in the treatment and prevention of disk-related symptoms in the lumbar region.

Traction

Traction exerts its therapeutic effect at multiple sites in the motion segment. Extension of the spinal column widens the intervertebral spaces and thereby stretches,

and removes mechanical stress from, all of the motion segment's functional elements. It also increases the volume of the intervertebral disks (Krämer 1973, Farfan 1996).

> ! The main effect of traction on the lumbar motion segment, however, is to reduce the intradiscal pressure. This allows disk tissue that has become displaced, either in an intradiscal displacement or as a disk protrusion, to return to its original position at the center of the disk.

De Sèze and Levernieux (1952) showed that a pulling action on the intervertebral disk during traction causes discographic contrast medium to be aspirated centrally into the nucleus pulposus. Mathews (1968) studied the contours of the posterior surfaces of the vertebral bodies and intervertebral disks during traction with epidural injections of contrast medium. The disk protrusions that were seen became much smaller during traction (**Fig. 11.100**).

A traction effect on the lumbar spine can be achieved with a wide variety of **exercises** and **apparatus**. Reischauer (1949) recommended treating acute lumbago and disk-related sciatica by shaking the trunk with the patient suspended from a set of gymnastic wall-bars or from the horizontal bar of a carpet-beating frame. A stable *doorframe* is a suitable alterantive. The same effect can be achieved by suspending the patient head downwards in special apparatus of a type that is now widely available. In mild cases, it also helps to have the patient lifted up by another individual. These methods can scarcely do any harm, except for possibly reinforcing any coexisting emotional disturbance.

Traction can be delivered continuously with small weights, for brief periods with a strong tractile force, or intermittently with a force that rhythmically increases and decreases. A large number of devices that were once primarily used to treat abnormal curvature of the spine, of varied etiology, have since been used to provide spinal traction. Now that the pathoanatomical basis of back pain and sciatica has been worked out over the last few decades, there has been no lack of attempts to treat the abnormal intervertebral disk with complicated traction devices of newer types.

We use a **traction bandage** to exert traction on the lumbar spine. The development of this apparatus was motivated by the observation that disk patients whose back has been under stress for any length of time tend to place their hands on their iliac crests and push downward. The traction bandage (**Fig. 11.101**) consists of a band modeled around the iliac crests with adjustable handgrips on either side. The patient pushes downward on the handgrips and thereby exerts an axial pulling force on the lumbar and lower thoracic spine.

The tractile force can be measured with a tension gauge placed between the handgrip and the band of the traction bandage (Krämer 1970). In this way, we were able to observe how the tractile force increases and decreases as the individual pushes down on the handgrips. The forces measured in the standing position in the test subjects (mostly lumbago patients) were unexpectedly high: a mean of 65 kg for women and 112 kg for men. Even patients whose muscular strength was no more than moderate could keep up a maximal tractile force for 10 s without difficulty.

Plain radiographs obtained before and during this type of traction revealed a measurable widening of the intervertebral spaces. Rhythmically pushing downward on the pelvis through the handgrips of a traction bandage, while the patient assumes a stress-reducing position, meets all criteria for effective traction for the treatment of lumbar disk-related symptoms. It is the task of the orthopedic technician to fit the polypropylene band perfectly to the patient's iliac crests and to position the handgrips at the proper height to assure an optimal transfer of force.

Before a traction bandage or any other form of treatment is ordered, a **traction test** should be carried out (see **Fig. 11.93** and the discussion on p. 213). If the test transiently relieves pain, then traction is indicated. The pain usually changes only qualitatively. Laterally situated pain moves toward the midline, sharp radicular pain turns into dull back pain, or sciatica is no longer felt in the foot and calf, but only in the buttock (centralization) (after McKenzie 1987).

Treatment with a traction bandage seems to be particularly effective for younger patients with intradiscal tissue displacement. If the patient's attacks of lumbago are not very severe, a preliminary warming treatment can be administered (e. g., fango packs or a hot bath),

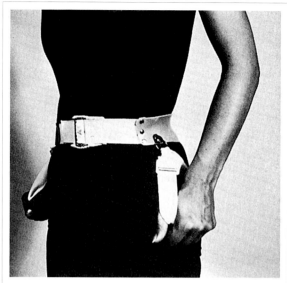

Fig. 11.101 Traction of the lumbar spine with a traction bandage (Teufel, Stuttgart).

while the patient assumes a stress-reducing position (usually the step position). Traction can then be applied rhythmically for 10 min. The maximal tractile force should be maintained for 10 s each time.

Results. Many authors have reported good results from the use of traction as the sole method of treating lumbar disk-related symptoms (Erlacher 1949, Papernitzki 1953, Wyss and Ulrich 1953, Judovich 1954, Neuwirth 1954, Amman 1955, Crisp 1955, Miehlke 1955/1956, Scott 1955, Endler 1956, Hoening 1957, Kohlrausch 1957, Parson and Cumming 1957, Lawson and Godfrey 1958, Cyriax 1959, Stoddard 1961, Harff 1963, Chrisman et al. 1964, Worden and Humphrey 1964, Hood 1968, Kendall and Jenkins 1968, Mathews 1968, Neugebauer 1969, Dethloff 1970, Ulrich 1974, Küsswetter and Bade 1983, Burton 1984). In more recent literature, however, the effectiveness of traction for the symptoms of lumbar disk disease has judged less enthusiatically (Nachemson and Jonsson 2000, Herkowitz 2004, Waddell 2004, European Guidelines 2006). In their review of the literature, Nachemson and Jonsson (2000) arrived at the same conclusion that we have, namely that **traction is an effective treatment for the acute symptoms of lumbar disk disease,** but not for chronic lumbar syndrome.

11

Table 11.20 The goals of truncal orthoses in the treatment of degenerative diseases of the lumbar spine

- Removing pressure from the intervertebral disks
- Flattening the lumbar lordosis
- Preventing movements that induce pain
- Supporting the truncal musculature

Orthoses

Synonyms: Corsets, braces.

> Orthoses are orthopedic aids that support and correct the curvature of the spinal column.

Orthoses come in two varieties. On the one hand, *rigid* orthoses, i. e., apparatus and corsets, assume the mechanical supportive functions normally carried out by the musculoskeletal system, sparing these bodily structures the mechanical stress that is usually placed on them. Stress-reducing apparatus and spondylitis corsets are orthoses of this type. *Dynamic* orthoses, on the other hand, exert a corrective, healing function. In the treatment of degenerative spinal diseases, the supporting and corrective functions of truncal orthoses are exploited equally. If the patient's muscles are out of condition and there is a high risk of recurrent disk disease, the unaided musculoskeletal system will be inadequate to promote healing. A temporary truncal orthosis will be needed until the body's own organs of mechanical support and movement can reassume their normal functions.

The aim of treatment with supports and braces is restoration of function and activity with regained movement and freedom from pain (Kirkaldy-Willis 1988). The orthosis should take mechanical stress off the affected disks, flatten the lumbar lordosis, limit movements that induce pain, and support the postural function of the truncal and proximal appendicular muscles (**Table 11.20**).

> The relief of pain, which patients often report from the use of a corset, is secondary to the increased intra-abdominal pressure and the resultant decreased load on the disk (Wiltse 1977).

Truncal orthoses based on the flexion principle. The orthosis may be chosen to have a mainly dynamic and corrective, or else a mainly static and supportive function, depending on the severity of the preceding illness and on the currently manifest functional disturbance of the motion segment. Orthoses of the latter type include the enveloping, firm synthetic corset of Hauser's flexion jacket (1945), which was further developed by Morris, Lucas, and Raney (1961). The concept of a synthetic shell was taken further in the flexion corset described by Torklus (1982).

> The position of the lumbar spine that works best is the flexed position (Farfan 1996).

Because many patients do not tolerate firm, closely fitted shells of synthetic material, we have applied the flexion principle to the Hohmann bridging corset (Krämer 1981), fitting it with an abdominal cushion and a kyphosing back element. This semirigid type of construction underlies the Lumboflex and Discoflex dynamic flexion orthoses. The flexion principle should be applied for only a limited period of time in patients with lumbar disk disease; thus, as the transition to the normal state with physiological lumbar lordosis proceeds, flexion orthoses of these types need to be replaced. The need to change the orthosis can be avoided with the use of a newly developed modular system (T-Flex) whose components can be added or removed to adapt it optimally to the patient's current condition.

Mechanism of action of flexion orthoses. To consistently lessen the lumbar lordosis and take stress off the lumbar spine, the cushion should not be placed on the patient's back, as in the common types of low back support systems, but rather on the abdomen. An elastic, suprapubic abdominal cushion presses the abdomen toward the lumbar spine. Counter-pressure is exerted by a straight back element that makes contact with the upper and lower ends of the lumbar spine, as in the Hohmann bridging corset. The back element, which can be perfectly straight or even somewhat kyphotically curved, must provide adequate space for dorsal excursion of the lumbar spine and must not be too close to the skin. When the patient is standing, the examiner should be able to insert a hand comfortably between the midportion of the back element and the patient's back. The abdominal cushion should be situated just above the pubic bone and exert an evenly distributed pressure on the lower portion of the abdomen. The dynamic flexion orthosis makes use of the three-point principle to flatten the lumbar lordosis (**Figs. 11.102, 11.103**). Unlike a rigid orthosis, a dynamic orthosis allows the patient some freedom of movement while exerting a corrective influence. Only backward bending of the trunk, which would induce pain, is prevented.

Under the constraint of the dynamic three-point system, any posture assumed or movement undertaken by the patient follows the path of least resistance and brings the patient into the lumbar stress-reducing position, with mild forward flexion of the trunk, backward pelvic tilt, and flattening of the lumbar lordosis. Reduction of the lumbar lordosis and minimization of pressure have the same effect as step positioning: the intervertebral foramina are markedly widened, and the dorsal protrusions of the anulus fibrosus are flattened. The washboard pattern of dorsal disk protrusions is no longer seen in the myelogram or myelographic MRI (**Fig. 11.104**).

11

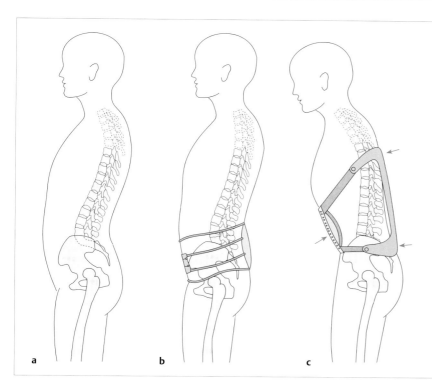

Fig. 11.102 a–c
a Without corset.
b Mild flattening of the lumbar lordosis and abdominal compression with a sacral support corset.
c Accentuated flattening of the lumbar lordosis in the three-point system of a flexion orthosis.

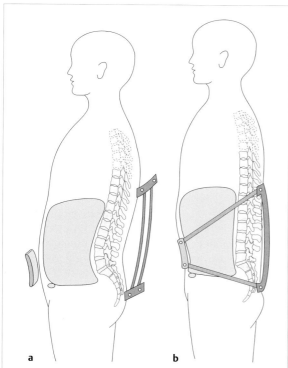

Fig. 11.103 a, b Mechanism of action of abdominal compression by flexion orthoses with an abdominal cushion. The lumbar lordosis is flattened and the lumbar spine can move posteriorly.

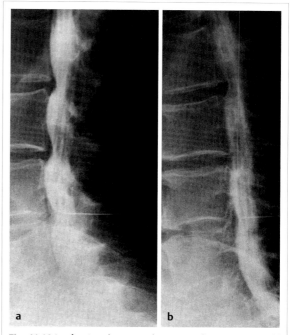

Fig. 11.104 a, b Lumbar myelogram of a 66-year-old woman with clinical evidence of spinal canal stenosis (low back pain in hyperlordosis, spinal claudication). The lateral myelographic image (**a**) shows indentations of the column of contrast medium at the level of the disks; these disappear when the patient assumes the kyphotic position (**b**). The sagittal diameter of the dural sac at the discal level increases in kyphosis. These findings are an indication for flexion therapy with an antilordotic orthosis, in addition to physiotherapy exercises in the step position.

11

Table 11.21 The effect of dynamic flexion orthoses

- Dynamic reduction of the lumbar lordosis:
  - enlargement of the intervertebral foramina
  - flattening of dorsal disk protrusions
  - repositioning of telescoped facet joints
  - widening of the spinal canal
- Reduction of intradiscal pressure
- Increasing the effectiveness of the truncal musculature

Table 11.22 Indications for flexion orthoses

- Lumbar disk disease:
  - nerve root compression syndrome
  - facet syndrome
  - discogenic low back
  - pseudoradicular syndrome
- Postoperative:
  - after lumbar disk surgery
  - after decompressive surgery for spinal canal stenosis

The intervertebral joints, previously telescoped into one another because of degenerative or postoperative disk collapse, are brought back into their functional, neutral position, and their overstretched capsules are relieved of tension. Our experimental studies have shown that reduction of lumbar lordosis, or lumbar kyphosis, also results in marked widening of the spinal canal (Däne 1976).

Elastic traction belting of the suprapubic abdominal cushion markedly reduces lumbar intradiscal pressure, by ca. 30% according to Nachemson and Morris (1964). Abdominal compression converts the abdominal cylinder into a taut, elastic bubble that assumes some of the weight-bearing function of the trunk. The analogous effect exerted by well-conditioned abdominal muscles can be enhanced by the wearing of a snugly fitting abdominal binder.

Indications and contraindications. The indications for orthoses are implicit in their mechanism of action. In principle, any painful lumbar syndrome can be supportively treated with an appropriately fitted dynamic flexion orthosis, if the body's own mechanical supports (muscles and ligaments) are inadequate for the task. This is the case above all for **pseudoradicular syndromes with hyperlordosis** and for **spinal canal stenosis,** but flexion therapy should always be tried in protrusion-related sciatica as well (**Table 11.21**).

An important indication for treatment with a dynamic flexion orthosis is the **postoperative state** after discectomy either by open surgery or by percutaneous intradiscal methods. Continuously elevated intra-abdominal pressure serves to take some of the mechanical load off the affected disk until it is replaced by scar tissue that is capable of bearing weight. In this intermediate phase, the lumbar intervertebral joints must also be protected from excessive strain by a reduction of the lumbar lordosis. The same holds for the postoperative state after decompressive surgery for spinal canal stenosis (**Table 11.22**).

Regaining of physiological lordosis (eulordosis) through the reduction of lumbar lordosis. A reduction of lumbar lordosis is recommended in the acute phase of disk disease and of spinal canal stenosis, spondylolysis, spondylolisthesis, and osteoporosis. The *goals of treatment* are widening of the intervertebral foramina, reduction of mechanical stress on the lumbar motion segments, flattening of disk protrusions, widening of the spinal canal.

The main goal of flattening the lumbar lordosis to achieve the desired biomechanical effects should not be pursued permanently, because physiological lordosis is part of the normal static state of the vertebral column. Once the patient's symptoms remit, the normal state should be restored. The transition from reduced lordosis to eulordosis should not be undertaken abruptly, with removal of the flexion orthosis in an "all-or-nothing" manner, but rather in small steps, with the appropriate accompanying physiotherapy. On the other hand, the reduction of pressure in the motion segments with an abdominal binder that raises the intra-abdominal pressure can be maintained for a longer time, till the patient's reconditioned muscles are able to assume their normal task once again. **An incremental transition from reduced lordosis to eulordosis can be effected with the application either of a graded series of orthoses or of a single, modularly constructed orthosis, which can be made progressively more lordotic by the removal of successive components.** Conversely, in case of a recurrence with reappearance of acute symptoms, the modular orthosis can be reconfigured to lessen the lordosis once again.

Results. Many studies of the biomechanical effects of truncal orthoses on the lumbar spine have documented their clinical benefits, particularly with respect to raising the intra-abdominal pressure and the more or less intentional restriction of the range of motion, with a supportive effect on the lower lumbar motion segments (Chang and Pope 1998, Cholewicki and Panjabi 1998, Havey et al. 2000, Hodges 2000, Giorcelli 2001, Shirado et al. 2004).

Poppel and Koes (2000), in a systematic review, found that most types of truncal orthosis are biomechanically effective. Nonetheless, there has not yet been adequate proof, through clinical studies, of the effectiveness of orthoses in achieving a lasting remission of symptoms (Ludwig et al. 2004). According to Nachemson and Jonsson (2000), the evidence for a clinical benefit of orthoses in the treatment of chronic, recurrent back pain is limited. Recent studies from Martimo et al. (2007) and Pepijn et al. (2007) conclude that lumbar

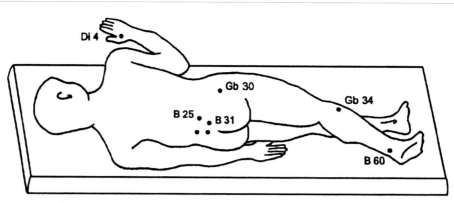

Fig. 11.105 An acupuncture program that can be used to treat sciatica. The patient lies in a relaxed lateral decubitus position with the hip and knee joints mildly flexed and the painful side uppermost. Needles are inserted, beginning at the feet, one after another at depths ranging from 2 to 15 mm and are removed 15 min later. The acupuncture points mainly lie in the area of the pain and the sites to which it radiates (acupuncture points after Stux 1993) (from Krämer and Nentwig 1999).

supports (back belts) may offer a benefit to workers with a history of low back pain, so Schoene and Nelson (2007) propose taking a second look at back belts.

Acupuncture

> **!** **Definition:** Acupuncture is the insertion of needles in certain areas of the skin with the intention of activating the body's own pain-inhibiting mechanisms.

The analgesic effect of acupuncture is probably due to endorphin release. As theorized by Pomeranz (1981), a painful stimulus in the periphery can exert an analgesic effect through a mechanism that operates on three levels. In accordance with the model proposed in Chapter 8 (**Fig. 8.7**), the noxious stimulus of needle insertion (1) stimulates the nociceptors (2), and the resulting nociceptive impulses are conducted over afferent fibers (3) to the posterior horns of the spinal cord (4). Here, the impulses are conveyed through a synapse to a second neuron, which sends them onward to the thalamus and, finally, to the cerebral cortex (5), where nociceptive impulses must arrive if they are to be consciously felt and localized. Endogenous opioid peptides (endorphins) inhibit nociceptive transmission at the synapses of the nociceptive system at both spinal (4) and cerebral (5) levels. The neurons that secrete endogenous opioids as inhibitory neuromodulating substances can be viewed as part of an antinociceptive system that might be activated by acupuncture (Stux 1993). Acupuncture is derived from **traditional Chinese medicine,** where it is performed by the insertion and warming of needles. The acupuncture points that are defined on the body surface are also sometimes called "acupuncture holes," because they are said to lie in the vicinity of an aperture in the deep fascia that is traversed by a nerve, a vein, and an artery (**Fig. 11.105**).

Indication. Classic acupuncture can form an adjuvant treatment as part of the overall therapy of pain due to disk disease. It should be carried out with the patient in the most relaxed position possible, i. e., in a position that minimizes stress on the lumbar spine and puts the intervertebral joint capsules under a minimum of tension.

Results. We carried out a comparative study on the usefulness of acupuncture in the treatment of pain, in which the acupuncture points were not chosen individually for each pain patient, but rather standardized across all patients (Grifka and Schleuss 1995). In this study, we were able to show that acupuncture at the classic acupuncture points is superior to placebo acupuncture at randomly chosen points. After 14 treatments, patients who had undergone classic acupuncture had markedly lower maximum and overall pain scores that those who had undergone placebo acupuncture. Nonetheless, the patient's individual responsiveness to acupuncture makes a major difference to its effectiveness (Grabow 1992). A meta-analysis of 75 studies revealed a positive effect of acupuncture as a component of pain therapy, particularly in lumbar syndromes (Molsberger 1997).

Despite the large number of randomized controlled studies that have been published, in a review of the literature Nachemson and Jonsson (2000) found no compelling evidence for the effectiveness of acupuncture as a treatment of back pain. Because of the uncertain state of the data, a controlled study on the safety and effectiveness of acupuncture for the treatment of various conditions, including back pain, has been carried out in Germany (German Acupuncture Study [GERAC]; Haake et al. 2003, 2007). This was a three-armed prospective multicenter study that was double-blinded for

11

acupuncture. "Verum" acupuncture, according to the concepts of traditional Chinese medicine, was compared to a type of "sham" acupuncture that was invented for the study, as well as to standard therapy without acupuncture. In sham acupuncture, needles were inserted at points other than the traditional Chinese acupuncture points. The study arrived at the following conclusions for acupuncture in the treatment of back pain:

- Verum acupuncture is more effective than standard therapy without acupuncture.
- Sham acupuncture is also more effective than standard therapy without acupuncture.
- There is no significant difference between verum and sham acupuncture.

In conclusion:

> **!** Acupuncture is useful in controlling pain, but science does not understand how or why it works (Farfan 1996).

Local Injections

> **!** **Principle:** The injection of analgesic, anti-inflammatory, and antiedematous medications at the site within the motion segment where nociception arises is a means of exerting a direct effect on the primary disturbance, without taxing the rest of the body with medications any more than necessary.

The treating clinician decides where to inject on the basis of the patient's history and the findings of a specialized manual-medical examination. Local injections can also be used for directed, diagnostic local anesthesia or for diagnostic pain provocation, either with saline solution or with radiological contrast medium, with the intention of reproducing pain in the patient's typical radiating pattern (memory pain). Local anesthetics, steroids, or both can be given as a therapeutic local injection, depending on the purpose of the intervention.

Therapeutic local anesthesia (TLA) is an important type of therapeutic local injection. A few milliliters of a dilute solution of local anesthetic (0.5–1.5%) suffice to switch off sensitized nociceptors and nerve fibers that have been transformed into nociceptors (see Chapter 8). This results in

- reduction of pain
- reduction of nerve excitability
- an increase of local perfusion.

Local anesthetics infiltrated into tissues reversibly inactivate both nociceptors and afferent fibers, i. e., they locally and reversibly reduce the excitability of the nociceptive sensory end organs as well as the conducting ability of the sensory nerve fibers. Because the effectiveness of local anesthetics is inversely related to the diameter of nerve fibers, they block sensory nerve fibers first, and motor fibers only at higher concentrations.

Therapeutic local anesthesia is directed at the sensory nerve fibers. Local anesthetics lower the membrane permeability to cations, particularly sodium ions, which, in turn, reduces nerve excitability.

The use of higher concentrations of local anesthetic causes total anesthesia and paralysis and is not necessary in local infiltrative treatment. The goal is reduced excitability and elevation of the stimulus threshold.

The neurophysiological basis of therapeutic local anesthesia lies in the lack of a close correlation between muscle tension and nociceptor activation (Zimmermann 1993). Nociceptor or nerve block reduces pain and nerve excitability and raises local perfusion for the duration of the local anesthesia that it produces, i. e., 3–8 h. In our experience, the pain-relieving effect actually tends to last longer than might be expected from the typical duration of effectiveness of the local anesthetic used, particularly if it is given repeatedly. A state of low excitability persists; thus, a series of 8–12 infiltrations on consecutive days can have a lasting effect.

Repeated infiltration of local anesthetic into the nociceptor field with the afferent fibers that proceed from it leads to desensitization of the hyperactive neural elements. The frequency and intensity of the nerve impulses that lead to pain and to motor and autonomic reactions are reduced.

Repeated therapeutic local anesthesia helps to prevent the development of chronic pain in the musculoskeletal system. If the pain has already become chronic, therapeutic local anesthesia helps break the vicious circle of abnormal posture—nerve irritation—muscle tension—pain—abnormal posture by diminishing nerve irritation (**Fig. 11.106**).

The desensitization of nociceptors and afferent fibers and the raising of their thresholds make the same mechanical stimulus produce less pain. This is the phase in which causal treatment should be provided, with stress-reducing positioning, physiotherapeutic exercises, etc.

In chronic pain syndromes of the musculoskeletal system, repeated application of therapeutic local anesthesia at the site of the nociceptors and afferent fibers lessens pain perception and pain processing (Zieglgänsberger 1986) (**Fig. 11.107**). The reactive inflammatory changes of the nerves and nerve roots, e. g., those due to disk prolapses, were studied by Rydevik (1990), Olmarker (1993), Hunt et al. (2000), Onda et al. (2000), and Kobayashi et al. (2005). These authors showed that chronic compression causes inflammation and edema that can be largely counteracted by lidocaine injection (Yabuki 1996).

Most local anesthetics also have a vasodilating effect and thereby markedly enhance perfusion in the infiltrated area. This also has the consequence that the local anesthetic itself is removed more quickly from the local area by the circulation. The additional injection of a vasoconstrictor is usually not indicated in local anesthetic treatments of pain in the musculoskeletal system.

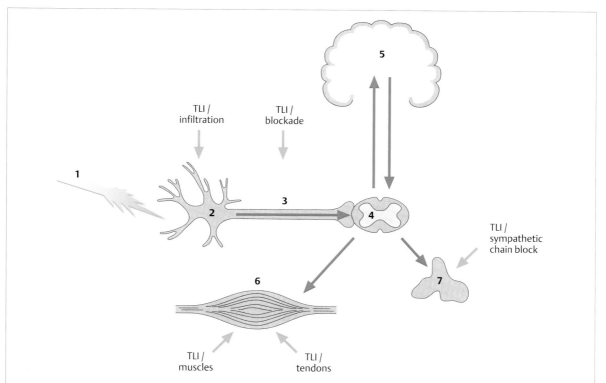

Fig. 11.106 Therapeutic local infiltration (TLI): the effect of TLI on nociception in the musculoskeletal system. Switching off of nociceptors and afferent fibers by local infiltration and nerve block (**2, 3**). Interruption of the vicious circle of nociception, muscle spasm, and abnormal posture (**2, 3, 4, 5, 6, 1**) by therapeutic local infiltration of the muscles and tendinous insertions. Switching off of the autonomic response (**7**) by sympathetic chain block (see **Fig. 8.8**, p. 74).

The specific **side effects** of local anesthetics include allergic reactions and cardiovascular complications due to overdoses. Both of these problems are very rare.

In order to avoid excessively high blood levels, no more than 10 mL of a 0.5–1 % solution of local anesthetic is injected during each treatment session. Intravascular injection is avoided by aspirating continuously while inserting the needle. The following substances have proved useful for local injection therapy:

Local anesthetics

- **Lidocaine** is a local anesthetic with rapid onset and long-lasting effect.
- **Bupivacaine** is preferred for very long-lasting local anesthesia. It is a lipophilic local anesthetic that can produce lasting analgesia in concentrations up to 0.25 % without substantially affecting motor transmission.
- **Ropivacaine** has a particularly favorable profile of sensory vs. motor effect.

Steroids. In pain therapy with local injections, steroids are repeatedly injected along with local anesthetics, both initially and in the further course of treatment. The target of steroid treatment is the inflammatory reaction

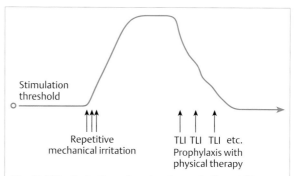

Fig. 11.107 Reduction of nociceptor and afferent fiber excitability by repetitive therapeutic local anesthesia (up to 12 sessions). The irritative threshold of the nociceptors and afferent fibers has been elevated by repetitive harmful stimulation and can be lowered again by repetitive local anesthetic infiltration. The effect is intensified by concomitant physiotherapy, with proper positioning, patient exercises, and heat application.

that accompanies nociception and that is found in the vicinity of the afferent fibers. Steroids neutralize pain-producing prostaglandins and leukotrienes (Wehling 1993).

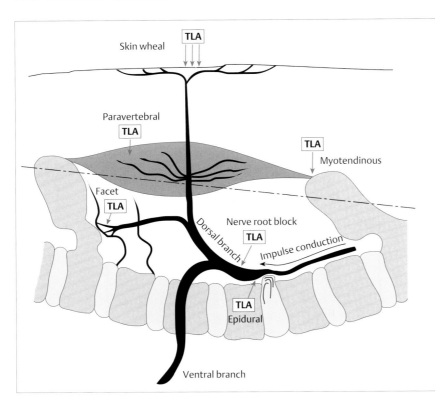

Fig. 11.108 Local anesthetic injections in the lumbar spine are classified as nonsegmental (i. e., superficial) or segmental (i. e., deep) infiltrations. Infiltration of the skin, paravertebral muscles, or tendinous insertions is considered nonsegmental (above the hatched line), whereas epidural injections, nerve root blocks (spinal nerve analgesia), and facet infiltrations are considered segmental (below the hatched line).

Steroids thus not only reduce inflammation but also relieve pain. Types of steroid with a high receptor affinity, e. g., triamcinolone, are preferred. An effective pharmacodynamic effect of steroids on local inflammatory processes is possible only if the steroid concentration is high enough in the immediate vicinity of the irritated structures.

Systemic medication, e. g., with orally administered steroids, is thus not indicated in pain therapy, except in unusual cases. The steroid concentration at the site of origin of the pain should be maintained for a long time, and the systemic steroid concentration should simultaneously be held to a minimum to avoid additional pharmacodynamic stress to the overall organism. These requirements are best met by the use of glucocorticoid depot preparations in the form of crystalline suspensions. We thus prefer to treat acute and chronic radiculopathy mainly with triamcinolone diacetate and triamcinolone acetonide. Our studies (Barth 1990) have shown that the local application of 5–10 mg of these steroid preparations saturates all steroid receptors in the surrounding tissue. If this is done 1–3 times as a treatment cycle for a pain syndrome, major side effects such as lasting suppression of endogenous cortisol production are not expected to arise. Allergic reactions to the carrier substances of steroids and local anesthetics can occur, as they can with any medication.

Classification of Local Injections in the Lumbar Spine (Fig. 11.108)

Intrasegmental–Extrasegmental

Injections in the lumbar spine are either **intra-** or **extrasegmental**. The latter type includes trigger point infiltrations, intracutaneous injections, paravertebral muscle infiltrations, and infiltrations of the muscular and ligamentous attachments to the spinous processes.

Extrasegmental superficial infiltration usually requires a needle that is no longer than 6 cm. Because superficial infiltrations do not go near important neural elements such as the dura mater and nerve roots, they are considered to have a relatively low risk and thus no special cardiovascular monitoring is required.

Intrasegmental local injections in the lumbar spine (**Fig. 11.109**) target an area immediately adjacent to the spinal canal, or within it, and are considered a type of minimally invasive treatment. A needle that is at least 12 cm long is needed to reach the spinal canal, or its vicinity, through a dorsal approach. In the course of this type of injection the dura mater or the nerve root sleeves may be punctured, and the risk of complications is accordingly higher than with extrasegmental injections. For example, there may be an internal CSF leak, causing an intracranial hypotension syndrome. Periinjectional circulatory monitoring, at least with a pulse oximeter, is mandatory.

Diagnostic–Therapeutic

Another way to classify lumbar spinal injections is by their purpose (**Fig. 11.110**). A **diagnostic** local injection is done as a test. Normal saline is injected first to provoke the patient's typical pain, and then, in some cases, contrast medium is injected under radiological guidance to localize the site of injection. One can then proceed to relieve the pain with the injection of a local anesthetic: this diagnostic local anesthesia can then be converted to **therapeutic** local anesthesia. When local anesthetic is injected to localize the origin of pain, no more than 1–2 mL should be injected at a time, because greater amounts can easily spread to, and anesthetize, the neighboring segments. In therapeutic local injections, a local anesthetic is used either alone or combined with a steroid. Another possible combination is normal saline with steroid but without local anesthetic, e. g., for cervical epidural injections; we consider it too dangerous to inject local anesthetics epidurally so close to the cranial cavity.

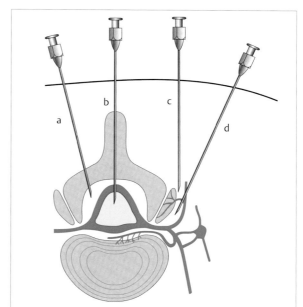

Fig. 11.109 Types of segmental local injection for the treatment of lumbar syndrome.
a Epidural.
b Intrathecal.
c Facet infiltration.
d LSPA.

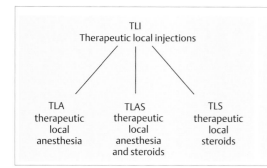

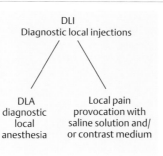

Fig. 11.110 Local injections in the spine.

11

Case Illustrations (from Krämer and Köster 2001)

1. Monosegmental Disk Disease (**Fig. 11.111**)

Clinical presentation. This 22-year-old woman complained of deep sacral pain of 3 days' duration, without radiation into the legs. Movement of the lumbar spine was painful at the end of the range of motion in every direction, and backward bending was markedly limited. Patrick's four-part sign was positive, there were no significant neurologic findings, and the Lasègue sign was negative on both sides. The clinical diagnosis was lumbar facet syndrome.

MRI. The study sequences are shown in **Fig. 11.111**.

Findings. The nucleus pulposus and anulus fibrosus are of normal signal intensity in the T2 image, with a slight posterior height reduction and minimal posterior bulging in the L3/L4 disk (**a, b**, →). The concavity of the posterior surface of the disk is preserved (**c**). The dural sac is of normal width.

Diagnosis. Mild degenerative disk disease at L3/L4, with a disk protrusion of grade I dislocation and otherwise normal findings.

Clinical course. The patient's condition improved markedly over the next few days after treatment with heat and analgesics (aspirin).

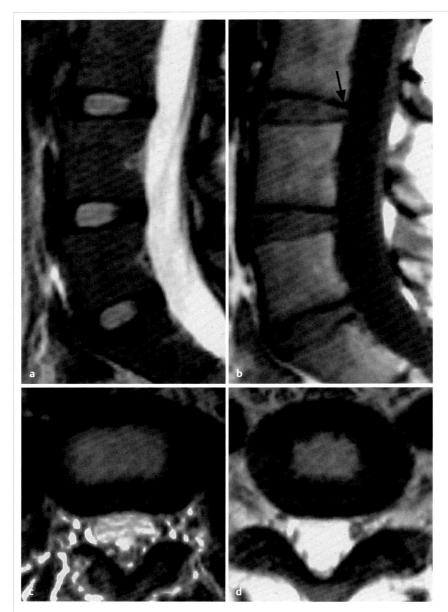

Fig. 11.111 a–d Study sequences (from Krämer and Köster 2001).
a T2 TSE, sagittal, median.
b T1 SE, sagittal, median.
c, d T2 TSE, axial, L3–L4 (**c**) and L5–S1 (**d**).

Comments. The clinical findings suggest that this patient's back pain is arising from the facet joints of the lower lumbar segments. This is a facet syndrome. MRI is useful for differential diagnosis, but provides no positive findings contributing to the diagnosis, although it rules out inflammatory and neoplastic processes in this area of the spine. For young patients in whom such processes need to be excluded, MRI should, in future, be considered the imaging study of choice.

2. Protrusions in Segmental Degenerative Disk Disease (Fig. 11.112)

Clinical presentation. This 58-year-old man complained of low back pain of 3–4 years' duration and the recent onset of pseudoradicular pain radiating into the posterolateral aspect of both legs. Shortly before the images were obtained, the pain had increased, with paresthesiae in both legs and feet when walking, and pain on bending backward, primarily on the left side.

MRI. The study sequences are shown in **Fig. 11.112.**

Findings. The signal intensity is markedly diminished in the two lower disks, with only a slight reduction in height (**a, b**). There is mild posterior displacement of disk tissue at L4/L5 and L5/S1, with only mild impression of the dural sac at L5/S1 (**d**) but with a relatively intense signal in the posterior periphery of the disk (**a**, →). The bone marrow is of normal signal intensity.

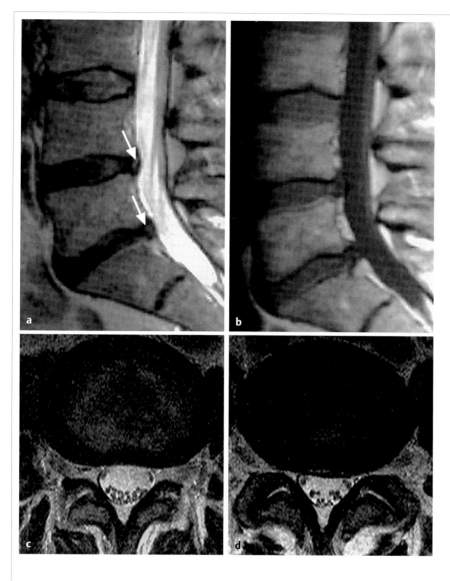

Fig. 11.112 a–d Study sequences (from Krämer and Köster 2001).
a T2 TSE, sagittal, paramedian.
b T1 SE, sagittal, paramedian.
c, d T2 TSE, axial, L4–L5 (**c**) and L5–S1 (**d**).

Diagnosis. Disk degeneration with mild protrusions (grade II dislocation) in the two lower motion segments.

Treatment. Conservative outpatient treatment to flatten the lordosis, facet joint infiltration, abdominal muscle training, step positioning, and Discoflex bandage.

Clinical course. The symptoms improved slightly under conservative therapy.

Comments. The protrusions extend only to the outer layer of the anulus fibrosus and do not constitute an indication for invasive treatment, especially in light of the mild symptoms. Therapeutic measures to flatten the lumbar lordosis are indicated.

3. Erosive Osteochondrosis at L4/L5 (**Fig. 11.113**)

Clinical presentation. This 47-year-old man complained of low back pain of 2 years' duration, which did not respond satisfactorily to conservative treatment. The patient was afebrile, and the laboratory findings were normal.

MRI. The study sequences are shown in **Fig. 11.113.**

Findings. The noncontrast T1 and T2 images reveal markedly increased signal intensity in the L4 and L5 vertebrae, but the fat-saturated T1 images after gadolinium injection reveal markedly decreased signal intensity in portions of these vertebrae (**a–c**). The L4/L5

11

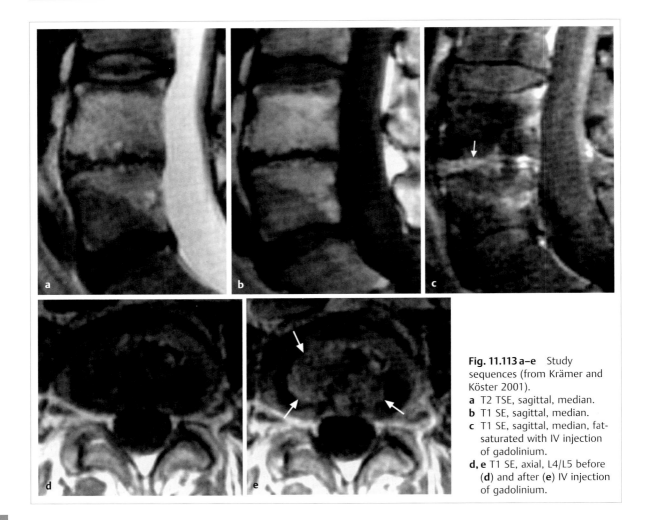

Fig. 11.113 a–e Study sequences (from Krämer and Köster 2001).
a T2 TSE, sagittal, median.
b T1 SE, sagittal, median.
c T1 SE, sagittal, median, fat-saturated with IV injection of gadolinium.
d, e T1 SE, axial, L4/L5 before (**d**) and after (**e**) IV injection of gadolinium.

11

intervertebral disk is markedly narrowed, and there are contour irregularities of its delimiting end plates (**a, b**). Marked, inhomogeneous contrast enhancement is seen in the L4/L5 intervertebral disk (**c, e,** →) and, to a lesser extent, in the upper half of the L5 vertebral body.

Diagnosis. Active, erosive osteochondrosis in segment L4/L5, with Modic type II bone marrow changes. There is no evidence of disk prolapse or protrusion.

Note. The findings of this study are unchanged in comparison with a study carried out 1.5 years earlier. Laboratory parameters of inflammation are negative. Spondylodiscitis is ruled out on MRI by the absence of bone marrow edema, the intact marginal ridges of the upper and lower end plates, and the minimal or absent contrast enhancement in the vertebral bodies. Enhancement of the L4/L5 intervertebral disk is consistent with erosive osteochondrosis.

Treatment. Conservative therapy was provided, rather than disk aspiration for putative spondylodiscitis, be-

cause of the negative laboratory findings and the unequivocal exclusion of spondylodiscitis by the plain radiographs and MRI. The patient declined to undergo a fusion procedure or the implantation of a disk prosthesis.

Clinical course. Conservative treatment, with physiotherapy, local infiltration, and an orthosis yielded only mild improvement.

Comments. The negative laboratory findings, the images obtained over a period of years, and the MRI scans all support the diagnosis of advanced degenerative changes in segment L4/L5. There is no hard indication for a fusion procedure, as there are no radicular findings, and the intervertebral space can be expected to solidify over time.

4. L4/L5 Protrusion (**Fig. 11.114**)

Clinical presentation. This 50-year-old man complained of chronic, recurrent low back pain occasionally

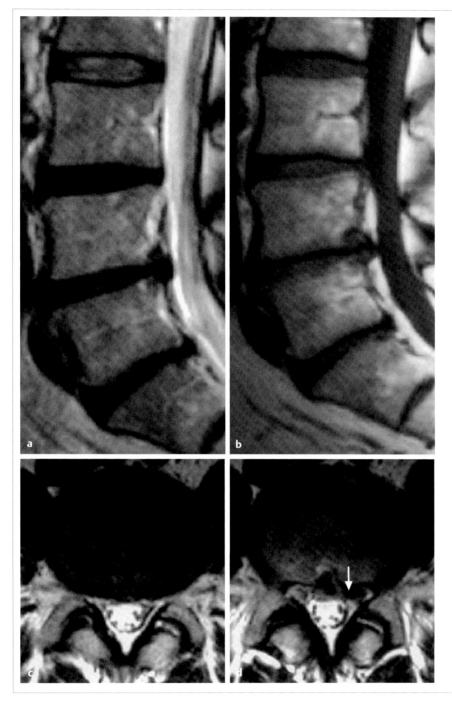

Fig. 11.114 a–d Study sequences (from Krämer and Köster 2001).
a T2 TSE, sagittal, median.
b T1 SE, sagittal, median.
c, d T2 TSE, axial, L4–L5 (**c**) and superior end plate of vertebra L5 (**d**).

11

radiating into the left buttock and lateral thigh. These symptoms had been present for several years and increased in intensity over the course of the day. Examination revealed lumbar spasm limiting the range of motion of the lumbar spine in every direction. No sensory or motor deficit was found, the deep tendon reflexes were normal, and the Lasègue sign was negative on both sides.

MRI. The study sequences are shown in **Fig. 11.114.**

Findings. The lower three intervertebral disks are markedly diminished in height and signal intensity, indicating degenerative disk disease (**a**). Mild disk protrusions, without significant compression of the dural sac, are present at multiple levels, most pronounced at L4/L5 (**a–c**). A circumscribed area of hypointensity (→, **d**) is seen medial to the left L5 nerve root. Whether this represents a calcification, an osteophyte, or a small sequestrated fragment cannot be determined.

Diagnosis. Mild protrusions of the intervertebral disks of the lower three segments, grade II dislocation, most pronounced at L4/L5.

Treatment. Conservative treatment was provided, with facet joint infiltration and epidural infiltration because of persisting left L5 radicular symptoms, in addition to physiotherapy, positioning to flatten the lumbar lordosis, and stabilizing exercises.

Comments. Segments L3/L4, L4/L5, and L5/S1 showed obvious degenerative changes in the form of "black intervertebral disks," in addition to other signs of degenerative disk disease. The collapse of the L4/L5 and L5/S1 intervertebral spaces, in particular, gave rise to a facet joint syndrome. The circumscribed area of hypointensity medial to the left L5 nerve root (**d**, →), whether it represents an osteophyte or a calcified sequestrated fragment, may be responsible for the radicular symptoms. Surgical correction was not recommended, as postoperative scarring would probably have worsened the patient's symptoms. Spinal fusion at L4–L5 was also contraindicated, for the following reasons:

- The symptoms were only moderately severe.
- The adjacent L3/L4 and L5/S1 intervertebral disks were markedly degenerated and might have become increasingly symptomatic after fusion at L4/L5.
- Spontaneous solidification can be expected in the near future.

5. L4/L5 Protrusion and Anular Tear (**Fig. 11.115**)

Clinical presentation. This 36-year-old woman felt a sudden, stabbing pain in the sacral area upon making a rotational movement, in the course of her housework. She was temporarily rooted to the spot, "as if paralyzed." The pain and impaired movement necessitated hospital admission. Examination revealed marked lumbar spasm limiting the range of motion of the lumbar spine in every direction. The patient could not bend forward, but passive and active motion of her hips, knees, and ankles were unimpaired. There was no neurologic impairment or sphincter dysfunction.

MRI. The study sequences are shown in **Fig. 11.115.**

Findings. The contrast-enhanced T2 images reveal diminished signal intensity in the L4/L5 intervertebral disk, with a circumscribed area of increased signal intensity in the posterior peripheral portion of the anulus fibrosus. Disk displacement is slight at most (**a, b, e, f,** →). The nonenhanced T1 image (**c, d**) reveals no significant signal change.

Diagnosis. Lumbago due to a peripheral annular tear in the L4/L5 intervertebral disk, with mild protrusion and degenerative disk disease.

Note. These are the typical MRI findings of an anular tear.

Clinical course. The laboratory findings were normal and acute lumbago was diagnosed. Conservative treatment was provided (step positioning, local heat application, diclofenac). Three days later the patient had improved sufficiently for discharge.

Comments. Acute low back pain due to intradiscal tissue displacement and an anular tear (without perforation) occurs suddenly and can be very painful. Laboratory tests and diagnostic imaging studies must be done to rule out infectious or inflammatory processes and pathologic fractures. The sudden pain is typically felt, not in the affected segment (in this case L4/L5), but lower in the sacral area. Low back pain due to an anular tear usually resolves with conservative treatment. Back school is recommended to prevent recurrent anular tearing upon the resumption of activities such as housework.

6. L4/L5 Prolapse with Infradiscal Extension (**Fig. 11.116**)

Clinical presentation. This 40-year-old man had suffered from severe low back pain, without radiation into the legs, for 8 weeks. Neurologic examination revealed no evidence of radiculopathy and, specifically, no evidence of cauda equina syndrome.

MRI. The study sequences are shown in **Fig. 11.116.**

Findings. The second-to-last intervertebral disk is of diminished signal intensity, but only slightly diminished height. At this level, there is a medial posterior displacement of disk tissue of relatively high T2 signal intensity (**a, c,** →). Elevation of the posterior longitudinal ligament and/or the anuloligamentous complex (**a, b, d,** ▶) is evident. The disk prolapse extends approximately 1.5 cm below the intervertebral space (**a, b,** →).

Diagnosis. Medial infradiscal subligamentous prolapse at L4/L5 (grade V dislocation).

Treatment. Surgery was not recommended because of the normal neurologic findings, and further conservative treatment was provided.

Clinical course. The sacral pain gradually resolved. Six months later, the patient was largely asymptomatic but still could not completely straighten his lumbar spine.

Comments. Located entirely in the medial zone and covered by the anterior epidural membrane, this infradiscal extrusion did not represent an indication for

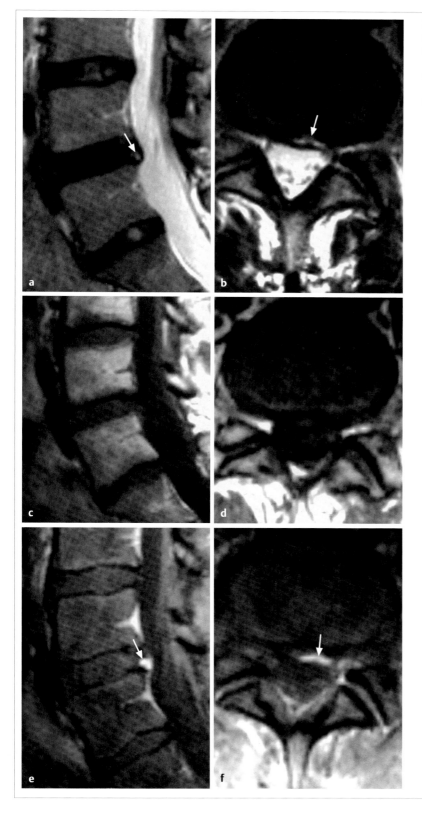

Fig. 11.115 a–f Study sequences (from Krämer and Köster 2001).
a, b T2 TSE, sagittal, left parame-dian (**a**) and axial, L4/L5 (**b**).
c, d T1 SE, sagittal, left parame-dian (**c**) and axial, L4/L5 (**d**).
e, f T1 SE, sagittal, left parame-dian (**e**) and axial, L4/L5 (**f**), fat-saturated with IV injection of gadolinium.

11

surgery. Surgical exposure would have required extreme medial retraction of the dural sac and the nerve roots.

This in itself could have caused leg pain, from which the patient had not suffered previously.

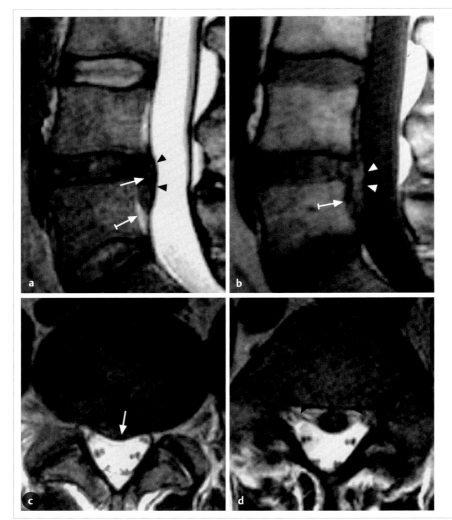

Fig. 11.116 a–d Study sequences (from Krämer and Köster 2001).
a T2 TSE, sagittal, median.
b T1 SE, sagittal, median.
c, d T2 TSE, axial, L4/L5 (**c**) and at the level of the cranial third of the L5 vertebral body (**d**).

Summary: Conservative Treatment

The initial treatment of lumbar syndromes usually consists of heat application, step positioning, and analgesia with over-the-counter medications. Additionally, patients are given "back school" advice of the type that is universally available, along with the instruction to keep active rather than stay in bed. The effectiveness of these measures is supported by scientific evidence, and they have no adverse side effects (**Table 11.23**). If the symptoms should fail to improve, a physician will usually prescribe stronger medications, which, however, have more side effects. Over the further course of the illness, other treatments can be given whose success is partly due to the fact that they are personally administered by a physician or other therapist, e. g., acupuncture, physiotherapy, manual therapy, and massage. Local injections, manual therapy, orthoses, and traction are not universally held to be effective in the current literature: only specially trained therapists should attempt these treatments. Lumbar syndromes are managed conservatively in different ways depending on the severity of the patient's symptoms and on the particular training and skills of the therapist. Multimodal treatment programs centered on physiotherapy, movement, and behavioral training offer the greatest chance of success.

Patients with neck and back pain are likely to improve with any treatment because of:
- the natural history of neck and back pain
- the physician's intention
- the physician's expectations of treatment effects (Nachemson 2000).

Conclusion

An optimally designed multimodal treatment programme, initiated in timely fashion, can help prevent a lumbar syndrome from becoming chronic and make further invasive measures unnecessary.

Table 11.23 Conservative treatment of lumbar syndromes (evidence-based)

Treatment	Effectiveness	Side effects	Level of evidence
Staying active	+++	–	A
Heat application	+++	–	C
Step positioning	+++	–	C
Physiotherapy	+++	–	A
Back school	+++	–	A
Acupuncture	+++	–	A
Medications	+++	++	A
Local injections	++	+	C
Manual therapy	++	+	A
Massage	++	–	C
Orthoses	++	+	C
Electrotherapy	+	–	B
TENS	+	–	B
Traction	+	–	B
Bed rest	–	+	A

A: many randomized controlled studies
B: few randomized controlled studies
C: expert opinion, nonrandomized studies
Strength of evidence: +++, strong; ++, intermediate; +, weak; –, no evidence.

Minimally Invasive Therapy of Lumbar Syndromes

Definition: In the context of the treatment of lumbar syndromes, minimally invasive therapy consists of the percutaneous introduction of needles, catheters, or endoscopic instruments to treat the changes in the lumbar motion segment that are producing symptoms. It occupies an intermediate position between conservative and open surgical treatment.

It is important to distinguish between "true" minimally invasive procedures for diagnostic and therapeutic purposes and minimally invasive approaches for curative surgical procedures. Typical examples for minimally invasive diagnostic and therapeutic procedures include different kinds of infiltrations including epidural catheters, root blocks, facet joint block, discography, intradiscal electrothermal therapy, and others (Mayer 2004).

Classification of Minimally Invasive Therapy

Procedures can be classified by their different **purposes:**
- periradicular therapy (PRT) to treat inflamed nerve roots
- intradiscal therapy to threat displaced disk tissue
- facet therapy to treat activated facet joint arthrosis.

They can also be classified by the **instruments** used:
- infiltrating needles
- catheters
- endoscopic instruments, including optical devices and tissue extractors
- laser probes
- thermal probes
- electrocoagulation probes.

The following **categories** arise from a joint classification by purpose and instrumentarium:
- periradicular therapy as a single infiltration or with a catheter
- intradiscal therapy by injection (e. g., chemonucleolysis) or by extraction or direct treatment of the disk tissue in a percutaneous nucleotomy, laser ablation, or thermal treatment (IDET)
- facet treatment by infiltration or electrocoagulation
- intradiscal or epidural endoscopic techniques for the removal of disk tissue.

Lumbar Spinal Nerve Analgesia as a form of Periradicular Therapy

Synonyms: Posterolateral perineural injection, paravertebral injection (old technique), nerve root block.

Principle. Posterolateral injection of local anesthetic into the foramino-articular region of the motion segment.

Purpose of treatment. Analgesia and desensitization of the spinal nerve root through repeated periradicular infiltration of local anesthetic, at low concentration, to achieve permanent reduction of pain. Lumbar spine nerve analgesia (LSPA) cannot be used to produce total analgesia, e. g., in preparation for surgery (**Fig. 11.117**).

History. Reischauer (1953) originated an immediately paravertebral injection aimed at the ventral branch of the spinal nerve. McNab (1971), too, described a strictly sagittal orientation of the needle for nerve root block. In the LSPA technique developed at the Düsseldorf University Orthopedic Clinic (Krämer 1978), the needle is introduced obliquely through an insertion site 8–10 cm lateral to the midline and advanced at an angle of approximately 60° toward the intervertebral foramen, next to the intervertebral joint (foramino-articular region).

Indication. The main indication for LSPA is an acute or chronic lumbar root syndrome of any type. Irritative conditions in the lumbar motion segment that are produced by osteroporotic collapse, spondylosis, pain of neoplastic origin, spinal canal stenosis, and inflammatory changes, mainly in the intervertebral joints, also respond well to this form of treatment.

11

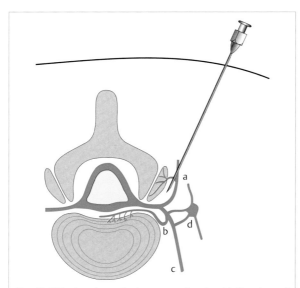

Fig. 11.117 Lumbar spinal nerve analgesia with flooding of the spinal nerve in the foramino-articular region. The following structures are infiltrated: (**a**) dorsal branch (intervertebral joint, back muscles), (**b**) meningeal branch (posterior longitudinal ligament, dorsal portion of anulus fibrosus), (**c**) ventral branch (dermatome in lower limb), (**d**) ramus communicans to the sympathetic chain.

The aid of imaging techniques is not normally required for LSPA, as it can be effectively guided by the palpation of anatomical landmarks. The use of imaging techniques employing ionizing radiation (fluoroscopy, CT) is excluded because LSPA is carried out repeatedly to desensitize the painful nerve root.

When the instructions for injection are precisely followed, an adequate infiltration of the neural structures named in **Fig. 11.117** can be achieved with the injection of 5–10 mL of a dilute solution of local anesthetic. The LSPA procedure can be learned in special workshops or from an instruction manual (Theodoridis and Krämer 2006)*.

Side effects and complications. Like any type of local infection, LSPA can be complicated by orthostatic circulatory reactions, infections, and intolerance to medication. There are also side effects and complications that are specific to LSPA itself. Numbness of a leg accompanied by a transient motor disturbance (buckling of the knee) may arise as a transient side effect (not a complication) if the infiltrated local anesthetic spreads by diffusion to involve the neighboring nerve roots. The anesthetic can also diffuse through the intervertebral foramen into the epidural space. Patients must be monitored for at least 30 min after each injection for the possible development of paresis. Rarely (in less than 0.3% of our clinical cases), the injection of local anes-

* The English translation of this book is due to be published in 2009.

thetic into a nerve root sleeve produces partial or total spinal anesthesia, which then lasts 3–4 h. A single application of 10 mL or less of a dilute solution of local anesthetic should not cause severe circulatory reactions (e. g., cardiac arrest); in more than 100 000 lumbar spinal nerve analgesia procedures over the last 15 years, we have never experienced such a complication. The effects of lumbar spinal nerve analgesia on the cardiovascular system have been studied by a group of cardiologists (Hanefeld et al. 2005), who concluded that specific cardiovascular monitoring is not necessary during LSPA. Patients at risk for vasovagal circulatory reactions have a typical profile: age, a prior history of syncope, and LSPA for the first time. In such cases, intravenous volume administration during LSPA may be useful to lessen the severity of the vasovagal reaction. We recommend pulse oximetry as a simple means of monitoring the cardiovascular system during these procedures, but there should always be a medical emergency kit on hand whenever spinal injections are used for pain therapy or for any other purpose. The emergency kit should contain intubation apparatus, the corresponding medications, and an EKG machine. The staff of the medical office or unit where the injections are administered should be trained in emergency procedures.

In our clinical series there were two serious complications: one case of a paravertebral abscess that required incision and drainage, and another of a renal capsular hematoma after obviously faulty placement of the needle (no contact with bone). In both cases the complication was treated surgically and there was no further harm.

Results. The English-language literature contains retrospective reports on nerve root blocks by Kikuchi and Hasue (1984), Xavier et al. (1988), Bonica and Buckley (1990), Stanley et al. (1990), Derby et al. (1992), van Akkerveeken (1993), Riew et al. (2000), and others. The results were mostly positive. The procedure was also judged positively in the reviews of Borenstein et al. (2004) and Herkowicz (2004).

In terms of obtaining a satisfactory of nerve root block, there is no difference between 1% lidocaine and 2% lidocaine. In view of the risk of complications, 1% lidocaine may be preferred (Yabuki 2006).

Experimental studies on the diminution of pain and desensitization of compressed nerve roots with lidocaine and other local anesthetics were carried out by Yabuki et al. (1998), Rydevik et al. (1989), and Onda et al. (2001). Experimental results suggest that the acid-sensing ion channel ASIC3 in dorsal root ganglia (DRG) neurons may play an important role in nerve root pain caused by lumbar disk herniation. Lidocaine decreased ASIC3 expression in DRG neurons and pain associated with the disk herniation model (Ohtori 2006).

The effects and side effects of LSPA as a component of minimally invasive, in-patient spinal therapy were described by Haaker et al. (1995), Schmidt (2000), Wiese et al. (2001), and Siebertz (2002). A randomized controlled double-blind study showed that mepivacaine and bupivacaine are significantly more effective than normal saline (Krämer et al. 1997). Grifka et al. (1995) studied the effectiveness of acupuncture compared to LSPA and placebo, and found that LSPA was more effective than placebo.

Lumbar Facet Infiltration

Principle. Inactivation of nociceptors in the lumbar intervertebral joint capsules by temporary blockade with a local anesthetic, possibly in combination with steroids. Facet blocks remain at the posterior surface of the facet joint (Farfan 1996).

Indication. Symptoms arising in the intervertebral joints, e. g., facet syndrome, hyperlordosis-related low back pain, pseudoradicular syndromes, spinal stenosis by facetitis.

Technique. Once the clinician has gained sufficient practice with this procedure, fluoroscopic or CT guidance is not necessary for intervertebral joint injections. Facet infiltration under ultrasonographic guidance is recommended so that the dorsal intervertebral joint complex can be reliably reached and so that this can be documented (Grifka 1992). Further details can be found in Theodoridis and Krämer 2006.

Results. Many retrospective studies and case reports have been published, but there have been no randomized controlled studies to date. Good results from facet infiltration were reported by Carrera (1980), Farbank et al. (1981), Destouet et al. (1982), Lynch and Taylor (1986), and Jerosch et al. (1998/2000). The effectiveness of lumbar facet infiltration has not yet been proved, however, and this method is viewed with skepticism in the review articles of some well-known authors (Nachemson and Jonsson 2000, Bogduk 2005, Boswell et al. 2007, Tribrewal et al. 2007). Their opinion is that facet infiltrations are not indicated even if carried out under fluoroscopic or CT guidance.

Facet infiltrations for intervertebral joint capsule analgesia are perhaps indicated as a supplementary treatment for combined radicular and pseudoradicular lumbar syndromes. The same can be said of thermo- and cryotherapy of the intervertebral joint capsule.

Percutaneous Facet Coagulation

Principle. Electrothermo- or cryotherapy and coagulation of small branches of the dorsal branch of the spinal nerve that supply the intervertebral joint capsule. Various techniques are used for cryo-, thermo-, or electrodenervation of the intervertebral joints (Jerosch and Steinleitner 2005).

Indication. Symptoms arising from the intervertebral joints, i. e., facet syndromes, hyperlordosis-related low back pain, and pseudoradicular syndromes. Schultiz and Lenz (1984) always carried out facet coagulation in patients who met the following criteria:

- typical pain pattern extending to the knee
- minimal or no radicular signs
- nerve root compression ruled out
- postoperative scarring after disk surgery ruled out
- aggravation of symptoms by physical activity and relief with bed rest
- unequivocal effectiveness of facet infiltration with local anesthetics, at least for a short time.

Results. Retrospective studies on percutaneous lumbar facet coagulation have been reported by Burton (1977), Schultiz and Lentz (1984), Anderson et al. (1987), Jerosch et al. (1993), North et al. (1994), Götze et al. (2000), Hall (2004), Steinleitner (2004), and others. No randomized controlled studies are available. Jerosch (2005) reported that just over 40% of his patients still had a satisfactory result (or better) after 6 years of follow-up, even under the most favorable initial conditions. In general, recurrences occurred most frequently in the first 6 months after treatment, but about 50% of the patients who had initially had a good or very good result went on to suffer a recurrence at some point during 6 years of follow-up, regardless of other patient characteristics. In view of the variably reported results, it remains unclear how much of the effect of percutaneous lumbar facet coagulation is actually a placebo effect.

Epidural Periradicular Therapy

Synonyms: Peridural therapy, lumbar epidural injections and catheters, epidural corticosteroids, epidural steroids, epidural injections.

> **Definition:** Strictly speaking, "epidural" means *outside* the dura mater, and "peridural" means *in the vicinity of* the dura mater. We use the term "epidural periradicular therapy" for these treatments because they involve injection of medication into the epidural space in order to surround the spinal nerve root with medication (in the periradicular region).

Principle. The application of local anesthetics and/or anti-inflammatories in the vicinity of the nerve roots in the epidural space, even at low doses, exerts a clinically useful effect on the site of origin of pain in lumbar root syndrome. The nerve root is surrounded by the injected medication precisely at the point where it is mechanically irritated by disk tissue, bone, or postoperative scarring and is therefore swollen and entrapped in the surrounding tissues. Perineurally applied local anesthetics and steroids travel directly to the spinal nerve roots through microvascular transport mechanisms (Ol-

11

marker 1993). Lumbar epidural and perineural injections are thus among the more effective methods of treating lumbar root syndromes. They work symptomatically to relieve or eliminate pain, as well as etiologically by reducing nerve root swelling and thereby providing the equivalent of an enlargement of the spinal canal at the affected level.

Approaches. There are several ways to reach the lumbar epidural space with a needle or catheter:

- The **interlaminar approach** is used by anesthestists for lumbar spinal and peridural anesthesia to eliminate the pain of surgery and delivery. Sometimes the catheter remains in place for several days for perioperative pain therapy. Aside from the risks and complications of prolonged catheter treatment, its major disadvantage for the treatment of pain due to nerve root compression is the patient's inability to participate in other measures that are part of the usual multimodal treatment program. Therefore, for the treatment of nerve root compression syndromes, a single epidural injection—the so-called single-shot technique—is preferred to the use of an indwelling catheter. The interlaminar approach is used for conventional epidural injections with the loss-of-resistance technique and also for epidural–peridural injections through an oblique approach into the anterolateral epidural space, employing the two-needle technique.
- An approach to the spinal canal through the **sacral hiatus** is also quite popular and is usually used to treat lower lumbar nerve root syndromes. Aside from injections, one can also use this approach to introduce a catheter into the lower portion of the spinal canal (Racz technique).
- An approach through the **intervertebral foramen** is also possible. When lumbar spinal nerve analgesia is carried out in the foramino-articular region, part of the injected medication reaches the lateral epidural space and surrounds the exiting nerve roots at this level. If the operator wishes to advance the needle into the epidural space by way of the intervertebral foramen, image guidance with fluoroscopy or CT is necessary. The transforaminal approach to the spinal canal or into the intervertebral disk (for intradiscal therapy) is also used for endoscopic procedures of various types.
- Finally, one can approach the lumbar epidural space indirectly **through the intervertebral disk** when the anulus fibrosus is dorsally perforated. We exploit this possibility when discography reveals outflow of contrast medium into the epidural space and the originally intended intradiscal therapy, e. g., chemonucleolysis, cannot be done. The anti-inflammatory agent that is injected into the disk in such cases flows out of the disk and directly into the ventral epidural space and to the site of nerve root compression.

Agents for Injection

Steroids are the principal type of medication injected into the epidural space for the treatment of lumbar nerve root syndromes, either in normal saline or in combination with local anesthetic. We have successfully used a crystalline suspension of triamcinolone hexacetonite for many years without any major complications. The dose depends on the type of injection: 20–40 mg for epidural–sacral and dorsal injections, and 5–10 mg for epidural–perineural injections. The crystals gradually dissolve over several days to weeks and exert their anti-inflammatory effect on the spinal nerve roots; it manifests itself mainly as a reduction of root edema (Olmarker 1993). We have repeatedly been able to observe concretions of these crystals in the epidural fat under the operating microscope while carrying out disk surgery on patients who did not respond to injection therapy. The surrounding area was both grossly and microscopically unremarkable, and histological examination revealed no significant pathological reaction of the epidural fat (Krämer, Herdmann, and Krämer 2005). The hypothesis that steroids might inhibit the spontaneous resorption of prolapses in the spinal canal was not borne out by the observations of Karppinen et al. (2003).

Local anesthetics temporarily interrupt impulse conduction at their target site (nerve). Lidocaine and mepivacaine are characterized by an effect of intermediate duration, favorable properties regarding spread, and relatively little toxicity. Bupivacaine is a lipophilic local anesthetic that produces long-lasting analgesia, with preservation of motor function, when given in concentrations up to 0.25 %. In our own controlled study, we found that pure normal saline also has an analgesic effect, probably because it dilutes the inflammatory mediators in the neighborhood of the nerve root or washes them away. Therefore, when steroids are contraindicated, an epidural injection of normal saline or of pure local anesthetic is a reasonable alternative.

Anti-interleukin-1. In view of the well-known side effects of repeated steroid application, alternative anti-inflammatories have long been sought. Clinical neurophysiological and histological methods have been used to address the question whether anti-interleukin-1 (anti-IL-1, also called interleukin receptor antagonist protein [IRAP], and available under the trade name Orthokine) might improve nerve regeneration in compressed nerve roots. The experimental results showed that anti-IL-1 brought about a significant improvement in neurophysiological parameters and clinical functional values, including the overall number of myelinated axons distal to the compression (Wehling et al. 1993, 1998).

In a pilot study, we found that epidurally applied anti-IL-1 derived from the patient's own blood serum had a similar effect to steroids. The ensuing prospective, randomized study comparing anti-IL-1 and triamcinolone hexacetonite revealed that the former worked comparably to the latter and tended to have a longer-lasting effect (Becker et al. 2007). Since then, we have regularly used anti-IL-1 for epidural injection therapy, particularly when repeated epidural injections are needed, as in chronic, recurrent postoperative nerve root compression syndrome (post-discotomy syndrome) and lumbar spinal canal stenosis. As the injection volume in epidural perineural injections is of the order of 2 mL, anti-IL-1 treatment by this method has a further advantage, because the amount of anti-IL-1-containing serum obtained through processing of the patient's own blood is also about 2 mL.

Epidural–Sacral Injections

Principle. Injection into the lumbar epidural space via the sacral hiatus (**Fig. 11.118**). When epidural injections are mentioned in the literature, the epidural–sacral injection technique is usually meant.

Indication. Since other techniques, particularly epidural–perineural injections, are available, we tend to use epidural–sacral injections only to treat coccygodynia or S1 sciatica and postoperative symptoms in post-discotomy syndrome. They can also be used when the interlaminar approach is rendered difficult by prior fusion surgery.

Technique. The injecting needle is passed through the connective-tissue terminal plate of the sacral canal with the patient in a squatting or lateral decubitus position. The approach is found by the palpation of anatomical landmarks, including the sacral horns. An imaging study is not necessary. Details of the technique and certain accompanying phenomena of sacral injections can be found in Theodoridis and Krämer (2006).

Epidural–Dorsal Injections

Principle. Injection through the interlaminar window into the dorsal epidural space of the affected lumbar motion segment with the aid of the loss-of-resistance technique (**Fig. 11.119**).

The interlaminar approach to the dorsal epidural space of the lumbar spinal canal with an injecting needle is regularly used both for peridural anesthesia and in pain therapy (for the treatment of lumbar nerve root compression syndromes). Peridural anesthesia aims at the complete abolition of pain by flooding of primarily healthy nerve roots with a high concentration of local anesthetic. In orthopedic pain therapy, on the other hand, repeated single injections are carried out to flood compressed nerve roots with an anti-inflammatory agent, and sometimes also with a dilute local anesthetic to lessen sensitivity to pain.

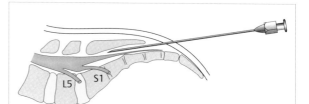

Fig. 11.118 Epidural sacral injection. The needle is introduced into the peridural space of the sacral canal through the sacral hiatus. The injected agent exerts its effect throughout the peridural space, predominantly on the lower lumbar motion segments. In order for the affected nerve roots to obtain the necessary dose, at least 20–40 mg of triamcinolone should be injected in at least 10–20 mL of fluid.

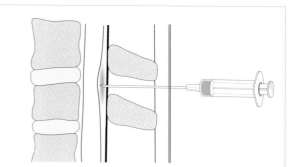

Fig. 11.119 Epidural-dorsal injection through the interlaminar approach. The needle tip lies between the ligamentum flavum and the dura mater.

Indication. Multiple nerve roots can be reached by the dorsal–interlaminar injection technique, on both sides if desired. Thus, their main indications are multisegmental spinal canal stenosis and multiradicular syndromes.

Technique. Depending on the affected root, the interlaminar approach is carried out at L5/S1, L4/L5, or higher levels. For the treatment of spinal canal stenosis, we usually use L3/L4 or L4/L5. The AP plain radiograph of the lumbosacral spine should be visible on a viewing screen in front of the clinician doing the injection, to provide a visual impression of the width of the interlaminar window to be used.

More details on this injection technique can be found in textbooks of regional anesthesia and in our manual on spinal injection techniques (Theodoridis and Krämer 2006)*. The disadvantage of dorsal epidural injections is that large amounts of fluid must be injected to flood the affected nerve roots with the desired concentration of medication, as is also true for epidural–sacral injections. Image guidance or control is not necessary for the interlaminar approach because it is found by palpation of anatomical landmarks (as is ordinarily done by anesthesiologists).

---

* The English translation of this book is due to be published in 2009.

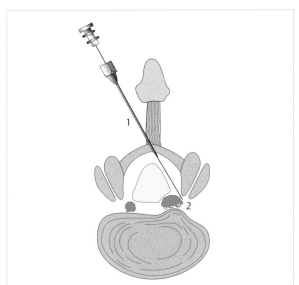

Fig. 11.120 Epidural perineural injection for flooding of the nerve root in the anterolateral epidural space. (**1**) The introducer is inserted from the opposite side, through the skin, subcutaneous fat, and interspinous ligament, at an angle of 15–20°. (**2**) A 12 cm 29-gauge cannula is inserted through the introducer until it makes contact with the bone or intervertebral disk in the anterolateral epidural space.

Epidural–Perineural Injections

Principle. Injection of local anesthetics and anti-inflammatories into the ventrolateral epidural space through an oblique interlaminar approach with the double-needle technique (**Fig. 11.120**).

This method of injection was developed at the Orthopedic University Clinic in Bochum, Germany (Krämer et al. 1997), and has proved its usefulness in several thousand cases. Its special advantage is that a very fine (29-gauge) needle can be introduced into the anterolateral epidural space, where the actual pathoanatomical process is to be found: the site of application is precisely the location in the spinal canal where the nerve root is compressed and inflamed. The main site of application is the anterolateral epidural space between the exiting L5 root and the traversing S1 root. This site is reached by an interlaminar approach between the lower edge of the L5 lamina and the upper edge of the sacrum. Even in the presence of anatomical anomalies, scoliosis, or spinal canal stenosis, the L5/S1 interlaminar window is usually wide enough for a needle to be introduced through it without image guidance. As our experimental studies (Theodoridis et al 2008) have shown, a reliable way of reaching the target is by an oblique approach to the anterolateral epidural space through a needle puncture on the opposite side, with an average injection angle of 16°. When the needle is introduced at this angle and 1 cm below the tip of the spinous process, the trajectory reaches the point where the lateral edge of the

dural sac and the nerve root are at a maximum distance from the medial edge of the articular facet. If a straight (sagittal) approach is used for the injection, the trajectory is shorter. The anterolateral epidural space between the lower edge of the L5 root, the upper edge of the S1 root, and the lateral edge of the articular facet has an average volume of 1.2 mL (Theodoridis and Nottenkämper 2008); thus, volumes of 1–2 mL of local anesthetic, 5–10 mg of steroid, and 2 mL of anti-IL-1 are generally sufficient.

Indication. Monoradicular lumbar root irritation by displaced disk tissue and/or bony compression in spinal canal stenosis, preferentially involving the L5 and S1 nerve roots. The technique can also be used for targeted periradicular infiltration when irritated nerve roots are enclosed by postoperative scar tissue (post-discotomy syndrome).

Technique. In order to advance the fine 29-gauge needle to the site of injection, one needs a double-needle system with an introducer, as is commonly used by anesthesiologists. The 29-gauge needle should be at least 12 cm long. The distance from the skin surface to the posterior edge of the vertebral body (or anulus fibrosus) is 7 cm on average, but may be as much as 10–11 cm if the soft tissues are thick. Further details on the technique of epidural–perineural injection without image guidance can be found in Theodoridis and Krämer (2006)[*].

Results. Epidural steroid therapy for lumbar nerve root compression syndromes has a long tradition. There are many reports on it in the literature, including those of Dilke et al. (1973), Snoek et al. (1977), Barry et al. (1982), Bernau (1984), Cuckler (1986), Ridley et al. (1988), Bush and Hillier (1991), Krämer et al. (1996, 1997), Livesey et al. (1998), Koes et al. (1999), Cannon and Aprill (2000), Nelemans et al. (2001), Dvořák and Grob (2004), Ng et al. (2005), Sell et al. (2005), Mendoza-Lattes (2006), Parke Oldenburg (2006), and Becker et al. (2007).

Corticosteroids do not provide any additional benefit at 3 months. At 1 year there is a trend towards an increased need for further root blocks and surgery in the group of patients who have received bupivacaine alone (Tafazal 2006). Lumbar epidural steroid injections (LESI) are effective in relieving pain and limiting need for operative decompression (Parke Oldenburg 2006). Spinal injections with steroids play an important role in nonoperative care. The transforaminal epidural steroid injection (TESI) theoretically has a higher success rate based on targeted delivery to the symptomatic nerve root (Mendoza-Lattes 2006). Ng et al. (2005) found in their randomized controlled trial that periradicular infiltration provides a sustained reduction in radicular pain and improvement in back-related disability at

* The English translation of this book is due to be published in 2009.

Table 11.24 Randomized controlled studies on the treatment of lumbar nerve root compression syndrome with epidural injections

Author	Year	Approach	Dose	Result
Snoek	1977	Dorsal interlaminar	80 mg triam/NaCl	–
Mathews	1987	Sacral	80 mg triam/lidocaine	(+)
Breivick	1971	Sacral	80 mg triam/bupivacaine	+
Cuckler	1985	Dorsal interlaminar	80 mg triam/procaine	–
Bush	1991	Sacral	80 mg triam/NaCl	+
Klenemann	1984	Dorsal interlaminar	80 mg prednisolone	–
Yates	1998	Sacral/dorsal interlaminar	60 mg triam	+
Krämer et al.	1996	Interlaminar epidural-perineural	10 mg triam/NaCl	+
Krämer et al.	1997	Interlaminar epidural-perineural and epidorsal vs. muscle infiltration	10 mg triam	+
Ng Leslie	2005	Interlaminar dorsal	40 mg triam vs. bupivacaine	+
Becker et al.	2007	Interlaminar, epidural-perineural	17/5 mg triam vs. orthokine	+

3 month follow-up. Corticosteroids did not produce additional benefit in the periradicular infiltration of local anesthetic agents.

The mostly positive results of randomized controlled studies of epidural injections in lumbar nerve root compression and the meta-analyses of Watts and Silagy (1995) and of McQuay and Moore (1998) show that this method of treatment is effective (**Table 11.24**).

The European Guidelines for the Management of Low Back Pain (2006) and the Pharmaceuticals Committee of the German Medical Society (2007) also take a positive view of epidural injection therapy in its guidelines on the treatment of lumbar radicular syndromes. Positive conclusions on the subject were also reached by Nachemson and Jonsson (2000), Nachemson (2004), Borenstein et al. (2004), Herkowitz (2004), and Armon et al. (2007) in their reviews. The European Guidelines (2006) point out that the corticoid should be injected close to the target (nerve root).

There have been only a few reports of serious **complications** and side effects. The main reported complication is post-puncture headache, which arises especially frequently if large-bore injecting needles are used. It is extremely rare when a 29-gauge needle is used for epidural–perineural injections, and, when it does occur in such cases, it is only mild. The overall complications of epidural injections are documented for a very large number of procedures in the anesthesiological literature, which was last reviewed by Hering et al. (2005).

In conclusion, it can be said that epidural injections stand out among minimally invasive treatments of lumbar spinal conditions for their documented effectiveness and their low complication rate.

Periradicular Therapy: with or without the Aid of Imaging Techniques?

Carrying out lumbar spinal nerve analgesia procedures and perineural injections under the guidance of imaging techniques that employ ionizing radiation is problematic. It is in the nature of nerve root compression syndromes to relapse and to take a chronic, recurrent course. Thus, middle-aged patients often require multiple minimally invasive treatment sessions of spinal nerve analgesia and periradicular therapy. If ionizing imaging techniques are used at each treatment, the cumulative radiation dose over the years may be high enough to have serious adverse consequences (Amis et al. 2007). Physicians providing these treatments should, therefore, make it their objective to do so with minimal use of fluoroscopy or CT. Anesthesiologists generally find the peridural space or nerves for regional anesthesia without the aid of imaging techniques. Physicians trained in manual medicine can also normally do paravertebral injections without imaging; there are special training courses and texts that provide a theoretical basis. Nonetheless, imaging techniques are still sometimes needed in special cases.

During the **learning curve** inevitably associated with these procedures, every physician will find it necessary to check that the needle tip is actually in the correct place. This check is particularly important when the injection is ineffective despite apparently normal anatomical relationships and an unequivocal indication for the procedure. The immediate use of fluoroscopic or CT guidance is also indicated if there are special anatomical relationships that make it difficult to find the desired site of injection by the palpation of anatomical landmarks alone, e. g., in patients with **scoliosis** or **transitional vertebrae** and in very **obese patients**. Fluoroscopy or CT may also be needed if a nerve root is to be defined by injection of contrast medium before it is anesthe-

11

Table 11.25 Indications for fluoroscopic or CT guidance for paravertebral injections

- Physician on the learning curve
- Lack of effect after injection without imaging guidance
- Scoliosis
- Transitional vertebra
- Obesity
- Selective nerve root infiltration for diagnostic purposes

Table 11.26 Catheter or single-shot injection for lumbar periradicular therapy?

Catheter	Single-shot
Single introduction of catheter	Multiple injections
With imaging guidance (sacral catheter)	Without imaging guidance
Short-term, intense treatment for very severe pain	Longer-lasting treatment possible
High risk of infection (sacral catheter, antibiotics are required)	Low risk of infection (antibiotics not required)
Limited possibilities for parallel multimodal therapy	No restriction of opportunities for parallel multimodal therapy

tized to abolish pain, e. g., as a preoperative diagnostic test before nerve root decompression surgery. Radiculography, described by van Akkerveeken (1990), is used for this purpose (**Table 11.25**).

Extensive descriptions of the technique of CT-guided perineural injections can be found in Krämer and Köster (2001) and Schmidt and Jergas (2005).

Peridural Catheters

Peridural analgesia through a catheter introduced into the peridural or epidural space is a standard technique in anesthesiology and obstetrics. The main effect of the medication is produced by diffusion of the local anesthetic through the dura mater into the spinal nerve roots. **Peridural anesthesia** is indicated not just to abolish pain and to achieve relaxation in surgical procedures on the lower limbs, but also for pain therapy. Techniques such as the insertion of a peridural catheter for repeated drug instillation or for the attachment of a "pain pump" have opened up a wide range of therapeutic options (Zenz and Jurna 2001). Paravertebral analgesia for the relief of labor pain is considered the gold standard of pain relief in a joint position statement of the American College of Obstetricians and the American Society of Anesthesiologists (Hering et al. 2005). These methods have

also found extensive application in pain therapy. Their advantages and disadvantages are briefly summarized in **Table 11.26.** Their main advantage is the ability to treat very severe pain intensively over the short term without the need for repeated punctures.

The **Racz catheter** is a special type of catheter, incorporating a spring, that is introduced through a guide tube through the sacral hiatus and into the spinal epidural space, and then advanced to the nerve root that is thought to be affected, under fluoroscopic guidance. Once the catheter is in place, contrast medium, local anesthetics, hyaluronidase (a proteolytic enzyme), and/or 10% saline and corticosteroids can be injected through it. An anti-inflammatory effect can be achieved with corticosteroids, an analgesic effect with local anesthetics, or an antifibrotic effect with hyaluronidase. The effectiveness of such treatments has not yet been demonstrated by prospective randomized studies; in particular, it is unclear whether there is really a so-called neurolytic effect against adhesions. Retrospective reports have been published by Lewandowski (1997), Heavner (1999), and Manchikanti and Bakhit (2000). Gerdesmeier et al. (2003) carried out a prospective controlled pilot study documenting efficacy in 25 patients.

Case Illustrations of Periradicular Therapy (from Krämer and Köster 2001)

1. L5/S1 Protrusion (**Fig. 11.121**)

Clinical presentation. This 32-year-old woman complained of sacral pain variably radiating into her left and right legs, of 3 months' duration. The pain radiated from the buttocks across the posterior aspect of both thighs to the popliteal fossa. The mobility of the lumbar spine was limited, especially on forward bending. Neurological examination revealed no deficit. The Lasègue sign was positive on the left at 70° and on the right at the end of the range of motion.

MRI. The study sequences are shown in **Fig. 11.121.**

Findings. There is a circumscribed medial posterior protrusion of the L5/S1 disk, which is of markedly diminished signal intensity and mildly diminished height. The dural sac is compressed, without displacement or compression of the nerve roots (**a–c**).

Diagnosis. Medial protrusion (grade III dislocation) with osteochondrosis at L5–S1.

Note. The relatively thick, dark demarcation (→) represents what is known as the "anuloligamentous complex." Its individual component structures, which cannot be reliably distinguished from one another, include the peripheral portions of the anulus fibrosus, the posterior longitudinal ligament, the epidural membrane,

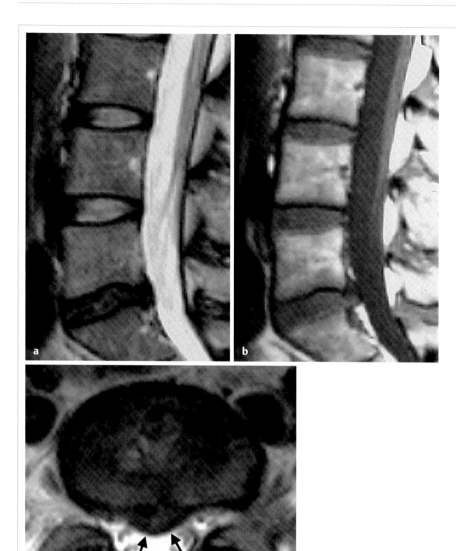

Fig. 11.121 a–c Study sequences (from Krämer and Köster 2001).
a T2 TSE, sagittal, median.
b T1 SE, sagittal, median.
c T2 TSE, axial, L5/S1.

and the dura mater. The definition of a disk prolapse requires perforation of the anulus fibrosus. As the anulus fibrosus cannot be reliably distinguished from the other structures listed, it is difficult to distinguish a subligamentous prolapse from a circumscribed protrusion in cases like this. In a circumscribed disk displacement, thickening of the anuloligamentous complex most likely represents portions of the anulus fibrosus and would therefore suggest a protrusion rather than a prolapse.

Treatment. Conservative therapy was provided, as no clear radicular syndrome was present.

Clinical course. There was marked and lasting improvement after the patient was treated with step positioning, application of a flexion orthosis, and local injections, especially epidural–perineural injections and spinal nerve analgesia.

Comments. There was no evidence of direct nerve root compression, so conservative therapy for several months was recommended. No surgery should be done in cases like this, because exposure of the medial protrusion would require strong retraction of the dural sac and nerve roots. Aside from this, the disk in question is

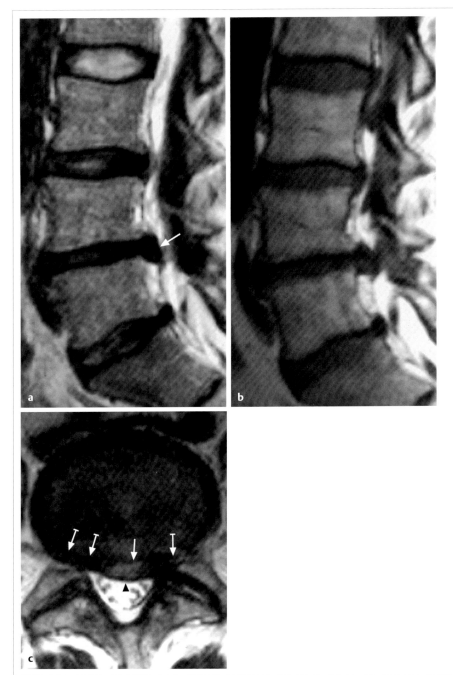

Fig. 11.122 a–c   Study sequences (from Krämer and Köster 2001).
a T2 TSE, sagittal, left para-medial.
b T1 SE, sagittal, left parame-dial.
c T2 TSE, axial, L4/L5.

intact. If the disk pathology should recur and leg symptoms reappear, intradiscal therapy, such as chemonucleolysis with chymopapain, might be considered.

2. L4/L5 Protrusion (**Fig. 11.122**)

Clinical presentation. This 34-year-old man had suffered for 3 years from progressively severe low back pain radiating into the left leg in an L5 dermatomal pattern. Examination revealed a positive Lasègue sign on the left at the end of the range of motion. There was no motor or sensory impairment, and the reflexes were normal.

MRI. The study sequences are shown in **Fig. 11.122**.

Findings. The lowest three intervertebral disks are of diminished height and signal intensity. The L3/L4 and L4/L5 intervertebral disks show slight posterior protrusions (**a, b**). In segment L4/L5, the disk tissue is markedly posteriorly displaced along its entire width, with a circumscribed area of relatively high signal intensity (**a**, **c**, →), which is demarcated posteriorly by a thin, dark line (**c**, ▶). The mediolateral and lateral peripheral portions of the anulus fibrosus are intact (**c**, →). There is secondary stenosis of the intervertebral foramina and lateral recesses at this level (**c**).

Diagnosis. Marked intervertebral disk protrusion (grade III dislocation) with circumscribed subligamentous sequestrum or large anular tear at L4/L5; mild protrusions at L3/L4 and L5/S1.

Note. MRI cannot reliably distinguish peripheral portions of the anulus fibrosus from the posterior longitudinal ligament and the dura mater, as these structures all possess the same, low signal intensity. It can thus be difficult to differentiate between a protrusion and a subligamentous prolapse involving a rupture of the anulus fibrosus. In this particular case, the tissue of high signal intensity (nucleus pulposus and inner portions of the anulus fibrosus) is demarcated posteriorly only by a thin line of low signal intensity (posterior longitudinal ligament and dura mater), which implies that the protrusion is accompanied either by a subligamentous prolapse or by a major anular tear. The contrast study that would have been needed to differentiate these lesions was not carried out, as it would not have had any therapeutic consequences.

Treatment. Conservative treatment was provided, as the disk protrusion was contained.

Clinical course. The patient was treated with epidural–perineural injections, spinal nerve analgesia, and physiotherapy. The treatment centered on traction in the step position and the application of a flexion orthosis. After 10 days of intensive treatment, there was marked improvement, which persisted until the follow-up examination 3 months later. There was only occasional radiation of pain into the left leg.

Comments. Intradiscal tissue migration with an intact anulus fibrosus is not an indication for surgery. Local analgesia reduces the lumbar spasm and interrupts the vicious circle of spasm, disk displacement, and pain, thus allowing the displaced disk tissue to retract back into the intervertebral space. Should the symptoms prove refractory to this form of treatment, intradiscal therapy can be considered.

3. L3/L4 Prolapse with Supradiscal Extension
(**Fig. 11.123**)

Clinical presentation. This 60-year-old man complained of the sudden onset of moderately severe pain in the anterior aspect of his right thigh, radiating to the patellar region. Examination revealed mild right quadriceps weakness and a diminished right patellar reflex. Nonetheless, the patient was able to climb stairs and stand up from a squatting position. He was in only moderate distress.

MRI. The study sequences are shown in **Fig. 11.123**.

Findings. The L3/L4 disk is of diminished height and signal intensity (**a**, **b**). Prolapsed tissue originating from this disk is seen at the supradiscal level (**a**, **b**, →) and is of high signal intensity in the T2 image (**a**, **c**). The dural sac is compressed, and the right L3/L4 intervertebral foramen is narrowed (**c**, →).

Diagnosis. L3–L4 disk prolapse with supradiscal extension (grade V dislocation), causing stenosis of the intervertebral foramen. The prolapse consists largely of nucleus pulposus material.

Treatment. Conservative therapy was provided because of the moderate pain and tolerable weakness, especially in light of the MRI finding of high water content in the prolapsed tissue.

Clinical course. The symptoms abated under conservative therapy consisting of epidural injections, step positioning, heat application, and intensive quadriceps training. The patient reported a daily increase in strength in the thigh. On follow-up examination 6 months later, he was entirely asymptomatic. The knee extensors were of symmetrical strength, although the right quadriceps reflex was still diminished.

Comments. The patient's moderate level of distress and the apparent high water content of the prolapsed disk tissue justified conservative management. The retrovertebral position of the prolapsed tissue favors its enzymatic breakdown.

4. L1/L2 Prolapse with Supradiscal Extension
(**Fig. 11.124**)

Clinical presentation. This 59-year-old woman complained of back pain radiating into the anterior aspect of the right thigh, which had arisen suddenly 2 weeks before presentation. The pain was worse on coughing or straining. Examination revealed limitation of right lateral bending, mild right quadriceps weakness (grade IV), a diminished right patellar reflex, and a negative Lasègue sign.

MRI. The study sequences are shown in **Fig. 11.124**.

Findings. There is posterior displacement of intervertebral disk tissue at L1/L2, a large part of which extends to the supradiscal level (**a**, **b**, →) and into the right lateral recess of vertebra L1 (**c**, arrow), elevating the posterior

11

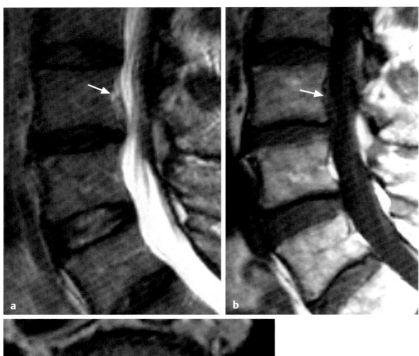

Fig. 11.123 a–c   Study sequences (from Krämer and Köster 2001).
a T2 TSE, sagittal, right para-median.
b T1 SE, sagittal, right para-median.
c T2 TSE, axial, inferior end plate of the L3 vertebral body.

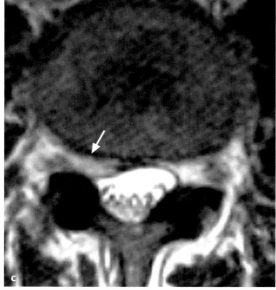

11

longitudinal ligament (**a, ▶**). The T2 image reveals an interface between the intervertebral disk and the supradiscal portion of the extrusion (**a, →**). Stenosis of the right intervertebral foramen at L1/L2 is also seen (**d, →**).

Diagnosis. Right L1/L2 intervertebral disk prolapse with a free fragment extending supradiscally (grade B dislocation).

Treatment. Conservative management was provided because of the brief history and only moderately severe neurologic findings.

Clinical course. The symptoms resolved within a few days under conservative treatment consisting of spinal nerve analgesia, step positioning, heat application, a Discoflex orthosis, and ibuprofen. On follow-up 3 months later, strength had returned in the right quadriceps.

Comments. The prolapsed fragment, originating from the L1/L2 intervertebral space, lay in the concavity of the posterior aspect of the L1 vertebral body and caused only mild compression of the dural sac. The right L1 nerve root and the intrathecal portions of the L2 and L3

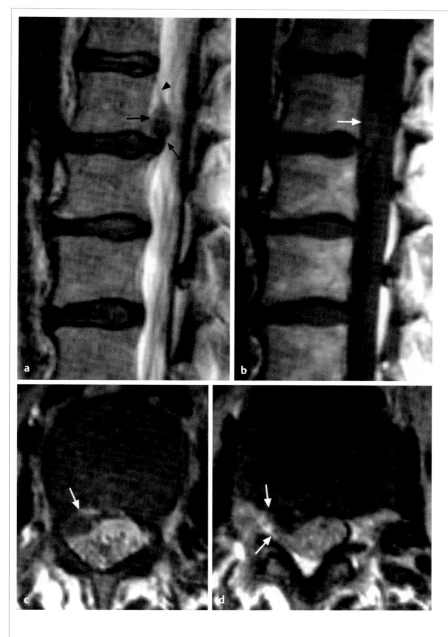

Fig. 11.124 a–d Study sequences (from Krämer and Köster 2001).
a T2 TSE, sagittal, right paramedial.
b T1 SE, sagittal, right paramedial.
c, d T2 TSE, axial, inferior margin of the L1 pedicle (c) and inferior end plate of the L1 vertebral body (d).

nerve roots were temporarily affected. Spontaneous resorption of the fragment can be expected.

5. L1/L2 Prolapse with Supra- and Infradiscal Extension (Fig. 11.125)

Clinical presentation. This 66-year-old woman had suffered from chronic back pain for many years. In the 3 weeks leading up to presentation, the pain had acutely begun to radiate across the lateral aspect of the left thigh into the anterior aspect of the calf and the dorsum of the foot, in an L5 dermatomal pattern. Examination

revealed a mild, chronic left L5 radiculopathy, with no florid evidence of denervation.

MRI. The study sequences are shown in **Fig. 11.125**.

Findings. A soft-tissue mass is seen posterior to, and in tenuous contact with, the L1/L2 intervertebral disk (a–c). The extruded fragment extends to both the infradiscal (→) and supradiscal levels (▶) and exhibits marked peripheral contrast enhancement (c). A signal of intermediate intensity, not typical of liquid, is seen in the T2 and FLASH images (d, e, →). The dural sac is

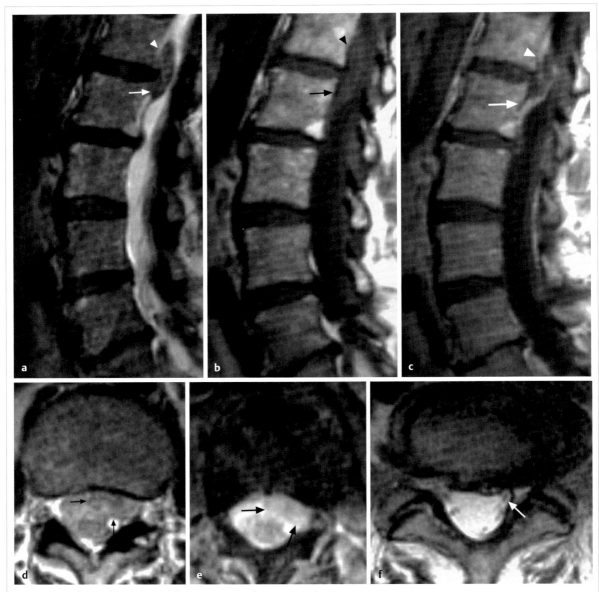

Fig. 11.125 a–f　Study sequences (from Krämer and Köster 2001).
a　T2 TSE, sagittal, left paramedial.
b　T1 SE, sagittal, left paramedial.
c　T1 SE, sagittal, left paramedial, with IV injection of ga-
　　dolinium.
d　T2 TSE, axial, inferior end plate of vertebra L1.
e　FLASH, axial, inferior end plate of vertebra L1.
f　T2 TSE, axial, L5/S1.

severely compressed, with mild compression of the conus medullaris (**a–e**). There is also a broad-based displacement of the markedly degenerated L5/S1 intervertebral disk, causing mild compression of the dural sac immediately medial to the traversing left S1 nerve root (**f**, →).

Diagnosis. Left paramedial L1/L2 intervertebral disk prolapse with a small infradiscal and a larger supradiscal sequestrum. Protrusion at L5/S1.

Note. The T1 images raise the possibility of an epidural abscess, which is, however, ruled out by the findings of the T2 and FLASH images.

Treatment. In light of the discrepancy between the mild left L5 radiculopathy and the disk prolapse at L1/L2, conservative treatment was initially recommended.

Clinical course. The patient's symptoms improved markedly within a week with conservative treatment

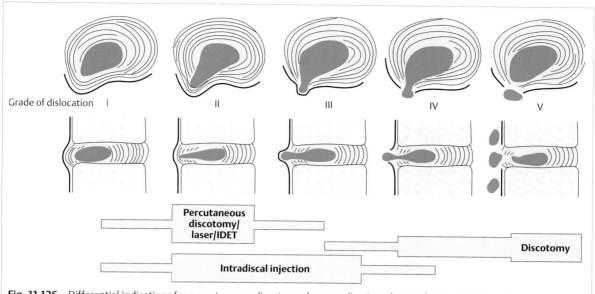

Fig. 11.126 Differential indications for percutaneous discotomy, laser application, thermotherapy (IDET), and open discotomy (when the corresponding clinical manifestations are present).

consisting of left L5 nerve root blocks. Outpatient treatment was continued. On follow-up examination, back pain was still present, but the left L5 symptoms had largely resolved.

Comments. Although a sequestrum was present supradiscally at L1/L2, surgery was not carried out, because this did not correlate with the clinical findings. Fragments that are not in contact with the nerve root and do not cause cauda equina syndrome tend to be spontaneously resorbed by enzymatic action.

Percutaneous Lumbar Intradiscal Therapy

Principle. The percutaneous introduction of needles or instruments via a guide tube into a lumbar disk through a posterolateral approach.

Surgery on an intervertebral disk may use an open approach through the spinal canal, or, alternatively, a percutaneous posterolateral approach. The posterolateral approach had been used by orthopedists for many years for percutaneous biopsies of the vertebral bodies and intervertebral disks for the diagnosis of neoplasia or infection, so it was clear that this approach could also be exploited for therapeutic purposes.

Classification. There are four varieties of percutaneous lumbar intradiscal therapy:
- lumbar intradiscal injection of medications, e. g., chymopapain, collagenase, aprotinin, or anti-IL-1
- mechanical intradiscal therapy (percutaneous nucleotomy),
- intradiscal laser therapy
- intradiscal thermotherapy (IDET).

The common feature of all of these techniques is that they require no skin incision other than a small stab wound through which the instruments are introduced. They are all done under image guidance, usually with fluoroscopy. The position of the tip of the instrument must be verified and documented before the actual treatment is applied. Percutaneous lumbar intradiscal therapy is done under local anesthesia in order to
- reproduce the patient's typical pain (memory pain) during discography
- avoid injuring the spinal nerve root in the foramino-articular region.

Indication. Puncturing the intervertebral disk for the purpose of destroying or altering disk tissue enzymatically, mechanically, thermally, or with a laser is a (minimally) invasive procedure carrying the same risks as open surgery, though they are possibly less frequent. It also disturbs the integrity of the disk as an osmotic system. This form of treatment should therefore be considered only when all conservative treatments, including periradicular therapy, have been exhausted and the patient nevertheless remains in distress because of the pain. Once the clinical indication is present, the choice of operative procedure is largely determined by the pathoanatomical situation in the motion segment. Noninvasive diagnostic techniques such as CT and MRI provide important guidance for the further diagnostic work-up and treatment. A final decision is reached after discography, which is carried out immediately before percutaneous intradiscal therapy. Intradiscal therapy is an option only if the disk remains closed (**Fig. 11.126**, **Table 11.27**).

11

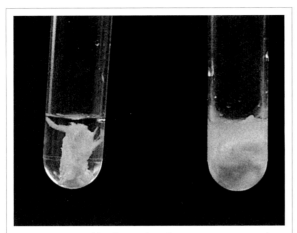

Fig. 11.127 Freshly obtained prolapse tissue in normal saline (left): the solution remains clear. In chymopapain solution, the fluid immediately becomes turbid through dissolution of the disk tissue (right).

Table 11.27 Indications for percutaneous lumbar intradiscal therapy

- Sciatica for > 6 weeks
- Radicular signs
- Positive Lasègue test at < 60°
- Severe pain
- Positive CT/MRI
- Reproduction of pain by discography
- Discography reveals closed disk

Even when the disk is still closed, it still makes a difference whether the displaced disk tissue lies within the intervertebral space (grade I or II dislocation, see **Fig. 11.26**) or protrudes into the epidural space, enveloped by a thin membrane or the outer layers of the anulus fibrosus (grade III dislocation). The ventral epidural space cannot be reached be percutaneous mechanical techniques, nor is it accessible to laser therapy or thermotherapy (IDET). Furthermore, the adjacent neural structures would be at risk. The only intradiscal procedures that are possible in such cases involve the instillation of medications in liquid form, e. g., chymopapain or anti-IL-1. These medications, like intradiscally injected contrast medium, surround the displaced disk tissue but do not flow out of the disk into the epidural space.

Lumbar Intradiscal Injection

Principle. The injection of chondrolytic or turgor-reducing agents into the disk alters the consistency and volume of a disk protrusion. Volume reduction and sof-

tening of the displaced disk material lessens pressure on the nerve root.

The lower intervertebral disks are relatively easy to reach with a long needle inserted posterolaterally under radiologic guidance. The experience previously gained with lumbar discography provided important information on the optimal technique for lumbar disk puncture and thus prepared the way for intradiscal injection therapy. The earliest speculation about the therapeutic possibilities of this form of treatment is found in a report by Witt (1951), who observed marked symptomatic improvement after discography in a number of patients. He hypothesized that an altered tissue turgor due to the introduction of contrast medium might have led to shrinking of the disk prolapse.

Injected agents. Chymopapain is the most frequently used substance for intradiscal injection therapy; others that have been used include cortisone (Feffer 1956, Chapchal 1957), aprotinin (Laturnus et al. 1977, Braun 1979, Krämer and Laturnus 1982, Dubuc 1984, Lesoin et al. 1984), and collagenase (Hedtmann et al. 1987, Steffen et al. 1991, Steffen 1993). Anti-IL-1 is also suitable for intradiscal injection.

Chemonucleolysis with chymopapain. Chymopapain is a proteolytic enzyme derived from the papaya plant (*Carica papaya*). Thomas (1956) discovered its chondrolytic effect in animal experiments: the intravenous administration of chymopapain to rabbits led to transient drooping of the ears. L. Smith (1962) experimentally demonstrated the lytic effect of chymopapain on disk tissue and then, in 1963, carried out the first intradiscal injection of this substance in a man. It was Smith who coined the term *chemonucleolysis* (cf. **Fig. 11.127**).

Results. Chemonucleolysis rapidly became very popular and was reported on in many publications (Branemark et al. 1969, Brown 1969b, Day 1969, 1974, Ford 1969, Gesler 1969, Stern 1969, Schoedinger and Ford 1971, Sussman 1971, 1973, 1975, Beatty 1973, Parkinson and Shields 1973, Nordby and Lucas 1973, Schneider 1975, Watts 1975, Wiltse et al. 1975, Finneson 1980). Intradiscal chymopapain injection is the only minimally invasive method of treating lumbar disk-related symptoms whose effectiveness has been documented in multiple double-blind studies (Fraser 1982, Javid and Nordby 1983, Agre 1984, Dabezies et al. 1988).

Despite the evident effectiveness of chemonucleolysis, there has been a downward trend both in the use of this technique and in the number of publications about it. The reason for this is presumably to be sought in the complications that chemonucleolysis can cause.

Side effects and complications. The most serious complication is a neurological one, namely **transverse myeli-**

tis, which can occur after unintentional intrathecal injection (Agre 1984, Daniel 1985).

Chymopapain chemonucleolysis can also induce allergic reactions, as chymopapain is a protein that is foreign to the body. The frequency of allergic reactions to chymopapain is given in the literature, on average, as 0.2% (Nietzschke et al. 1986, Sutton 1986, Bouillet 1987). This number included both purely immunological (anaphylactic) and pseudo-allergic (anaphylactoid) reactions. Anaphylactoid reactions cannot be reliably predicted by prior testing. Prophylactic pre-treatment with H_1- and H_2-receptor blockers and cortisone can be given to keep allergic reactions in check.

The main reason for the current reluctance to recommend intradiscal injection therapy with chymopapain is **post-injection low back pain.** After chymopapain is injected into the disk, though sciatica disappears, a new low back pain can arise that persists for weeks or even months. The frequency of this side effect is estimated in the literature at 20–40% (Hedtmann et al. 1986, Bouillet 1987). If another substance is used and the dose is lowered, the frequency and intensity of post-injection low back pain can be reduced, but the problem is still not eliminated. The cause of post-injection low back pain after chymopapain application is probably the relatively sudden instability and loss of height of the affected disk due to loss of matrix and water. The osmotic system of the disk responds to the loss of proteoglycan with a rapid reduction of tissue turgor.

As explained in Chapter 8, rapidly occurring topographical changes in the motion segment are associated with pain, mainly because of the telescoping together of the intervertebral joints and the resulting tension on the joint capsules. The loss of stability and height has been demonstrated both in animal experiments and in our own in-vitro tests (Steffen 1993). All post-injection low back pain is reversible and is best initially treated with anti-inflammatories, local injections, step positioning, flexion orthoses, and stabilizing patient exercises. If residual symptoms of root irritation persist, epidural steroid injections can be considered. Post-injection low back pain after chymopapain application can be reduced still further if it is possible to let the enzyme act briefly on the disk protrusion only, without extending its action to the entire disk. This is achieved with a highly targeted application of a low dose of chymopopain, followed by post-injectional neutralization or elimination of the enzyme after it has performed its lytic function within the protrusion.

Percutaneous Lumbar Discectomy

Principle. A small stab incision is made through which a guide-tube system is advanced for the introduction of endoscopes, rongeurs, or motorized instruments into the intervertebral disk. When a defect in the disk is created ventral to the protrusion, the dorsolaterally dis-

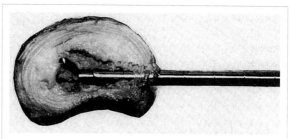

Fig. 11.128 The principle of percutaneous discotomy: central disk tissue and protruding material is removed with percutaneously introduced rongeurs and drilling instruments.

placed disk tissue shifts back toward the center of the disk. It is sometimes possible to remove part of the protrusion with special curved rongeurs and suction cutters (**Fig. 11.128**).

Indication. The clinical criteria underlying the indication for percutaneous lumbar discotomy are the same as those for chemonucleolysis. Only grade I and II dislocations can be treated successfully with percutaneous lumbar discotomy. Disk protrusions that extend far beyond the edge of the vertebral body cannot be reached with percutaneously introduced suction cutters. It would be too dangerous to advance these instruments into the subligamentous portion of a grade III dislocation.

Complications. The most important complication is discitis, which has been reported in up to 8% of cases. Frequent changes of instruments and long duration of the procedure, e. g., when it is carried out at the l5–S1 level, are presumed to be contributing factors. Furthermore, there is a danger of bowel perforation or injury of the great vessels that lie anterior to the disk if the fluoroscopic guidance for the procedure is inadequate, e. g., in very obese patients.

Results. The results of percutaneous lumbar discotomy have been reported in many publications, most of which, however, concern noncontrolled retrospective studies (Kambin and Gellmann 1983, Onik et al. 1985, Schreiver and Suezawa 1986, Caspi et al. 1987, Jentea et al. 1989, Kahanovitz et al. 1989b, Kaps and Cotta 1989, Mayer and Brock 1989, Stern 1989). The randomized multicenter study of Revel et al. (1995) yielded a success rate of 37% at 1 year for automated percutaneous lumbar discotomy, compared to 66% after chemonucleolysis. Chatterjee et al. (1995), in their prospective randomized study, likewise found a success rate of 29% for percutaneous lumbar discotomy. In the treatment of lumbar disk disease, a success rate of 29% or 37% is no better than a placebo effect.

11

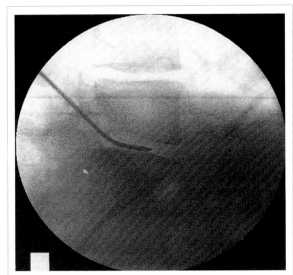

Fig. 11.129   Laser applicator in the intervertebral space.

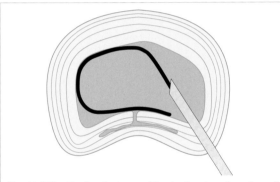

Fig. 11.130   Final catheter position in the dorsal portion of an intervertebral disk in intradiscal electrothermal therapy (IDET).

Percutaneous Lumbar Laser Therapy

Principle. Removal of disk tissue from the intervertebral space by laser vaporization (**Fig. 11.129**). Just as in percutaneous mechanical discotomy, a defect is created in the disk ventral to the protrusion. The dorsally displaced disk material shifts centrally, so that the pressure on the nerve root is reduced.

Indication. The indication is the same as for percutaneous lumbar discotomy or chemonucleolysis, i. e., a grade I or II dislocation. If the disk tissue is displaced any further than this, extending beyond the edge of the vertebra, it can no longer be reached by laser therapy as currently practiced without creating an unacceptably high risk of injury to the dura mater and the nerve root.

Results. Good results of laser therapy have been reported, with success rates between 70% and 80% (Mayer 1993b, Siebert and Behrendson 1993, Steffen et al. 1993), but only in retrospective studies. These good results were not confirmed by the randomized controlled studies of Sherk (1993) and of Steffen et al. (1996) in our clinic. The success rate that was found in the latter study, 31%, was similar to that of placebo treatment.

Intradiscal Electrothermal Therapy (IDET)

Principle. A navigable catheter is advanced into the disk through a guide tube under fluoroscopic guidance and placed so that its active end is in the desired position at the transition from the nucleus pulposus to the anulus fibrosus (**Fig. 11.130**). The tip of the catheter is then electrically heated.

Indication. The intradiscal electrothermal therapy (IDET) method is mainly used to treat discogenic pain due to intradiscal tissue displacement. It is thus recommended for use in patients with chronic, intense back pain that has been refractory to all forms of conservative treatment for at least 6 months. Neurologic deficits or impingement on neural structures, as revealed by an MRI scan, are contraindications to this form of treatment.

Results. There have been retrospective studies (Saal and Saal 2000), case-control studies (Karasek and Bogduk 2000), and randomized controlled studies with variable results: Pautzer et al. (2004) found a significant improvement of symptoms in patients treated with IDET compared to a control group, but the studies of Barendse et al. (2001) and Freeman et al. (2005) revealed no difference between the two groups. Further studies, some with positive results and some with negative results, have been reported by Kleinstueck et al. (2001), Wetzel et al. (2002), Spruit and Jacobs (2002), Andersson (2004), Singh et al. (2005), and Bass et al. (2006).

This method is an option only for a small group of carefully selected patients. The unequivocal diagnosis of discogenic pain is an essential prerequisite. A further important consideration is the very high dose of ionizing radiation required for the correct placement of the heatable catheter under image guidance, because most of the physicians using this technique are still on the steep portion of their learning curve. A central catheter position renders the procedure ineffective, and an extradiscal or peripheral position carries the danger of heat-induced injury to the neural structures in the spinal canal.

Endoscopic Disk Surgery

It is possible, in principle, to remove a disk prolapse from the spinal canal by a percutaneous endoscopic technique rather than by open surgery. This form of treatment is technically demanding, and complications during the learning phase are frequent. The approach is either interlaminar or transforaminal (Rütten et al. 2005).

Summary: Minimally Invasive Treatment

The minimally invasive treatment of lumbar disk disease occupies an intermediate position between conservative treatment and open surgery. When all conservative measures have been properly and consistently applied, but the symptoms have still not been relieved, open surgery should not be the immediate consequence; rather, one should consider whether one of the minimally invasive techniques can be used instead. The indication for these techniques is an intractable local (especially radicular) lumbar syndrome with a clear correlation between the clinical and radiological findings. The choice of procedure is determined by the demonstrated effectiveness of the various procedures in relation to their possible complications and side effects. The side effects to be considered include the possible damage resulting from the employment of multiple minimally invasive procedures under image guidance using ionizing radiation. From this point of view, the optimal form of minimally invasive treatment is a single-shot epidural injection, which requires no radiation exposure whatsoever.

Among the intradiscal techniques, chemonucleolysis has the highest degree of effectiveness, as demonstrated by numerous randomized and controlled studies, but it is also fraught with significant side effects (**Table 11.28**). The other intradiscal techniques have either not been shown to be effective (laser therapy, percutaneous nucleotomy) or have not yet been adequately tested (IDET). The same holds for facet infiltration and facet coagulation. The Cochrane Review (Gibson and Waddell 2007) concludes that the evidence for minimally invasive techniques remains unclear except for chemonucleolysis using chymopapain, which is no longer widely available. For the procedures whose efficacy has not been demonstrated, one should always bear in mind the real damage that can be caused by exposure to ionizing radiation when procedures are carried out repeatedly under image guidance.

Conclusion

If open surgery is not urgently indicated, a lumbar syndrome that has not responded to conservative therapy can be treated with a minimally invasive procedure. Periradicular therapy is the best of the available options.

Table 11.28 Minimally invasive treatment of lumbar syndromes (evidence-based)

Treatment	Effectiveness	Side effects	Level of evidence
Epidural single-shot	+++	+	A
LSPA	+++	+	B
Facet infiltration	+	+	C
Epidural catheter	++	++	C
Chemonucleolysis	+++	+++	A
Percutaneous laser	–	++	B
Percutaneous nucleotomy	–	++	B
IDET	+	++	B
Facet coagulation	+	++	C

A: many randomized controlled studies
B: few randomized controlled studies
C: expert opinion, nonrandomized studies
Strength of evidence: +++, strong; ++, intermediate; +, weak; –, no evidence.

Surgical Treatment

Definition. When a lumbar syndrome is treated with open surgery, as opposed to minimally invasive treatment, the involved area of the spine is operatively exposed.

The number of patients who finally need surgery is very small compared to the vast numbers whose lumbar syndrome can be treated conservatively; according to Frymoyer (1990), surgically treated patients make up 0.25 % of the total. Surgery is reserved for severe conditions that cannot be controlled with conservative or minimally invasive treatment. There are a number of possibilities for the surgical treatment of lumbar disk disease. In this section, we present only the types of operation that are in common use at the present day, which nonsurgical specialists also need to know about—above all, with regard to their indications and postoperative management. The most important types of surgical intervention (like the most important types of minimally invasive intervention) are **those that are carried out on**

the disk itself (discotomy), aiming to remove the displaced disk tissue to relieve pressure on the nerve root. **Fusions, decompressive operations, radiculolysis, and disk replacement operations** are done much less commonly and usually as reoperative procedures.

Open Surgery of Lumbar Disk Prolapses—Discotomy

Synonyms: Nucleotomy (even though this type of operation involves removal not only of the nucleus pulposus, but of the anulus fibrosus as well); prolapse operation; lumbar disk herniation surgery; lumbar discectomy (even though the entire disk is not removed). Kirkaldy-Willis (1988) proposed using the term "discotomy," rather than "discectomy."

> **Definition.** Surgical removal of a lumbar disk herniation through a dorsal interlaminar approach, with opening of the spinal canal.

Micro- or Macrosurgery?

> **Definition.** Microsurgery on the lumbar spine is a surgical approach to the site of the lesion through a narrow incision with lighting and magnification of the operative field as well as the use of special angled instruments.

Whether the dorsal approach is used for the surgical treatment of a lumbar disk herniation or of degenerative spinal canal stenosis, the initial procedure in the depths of the incision is the same: exposure of the lateral edge of the dura mater and nerve root by removal of the overlying portions of the ligamentum flavum, lamina, and intervertebral joint facet. This is all that is necessary to decompress the nerve root when surgery is being carried out for degenerative spinal canal stenosis. If a disk herniation is to be removed, the dural sac and the nerve root must now be mobilized medially ("medialized") to give access to the herniation. The initial procedure for exposure of the root is done in an area measuring roughly 2 × 2 cm. The advantages and disadvantages of a microsurgical approach, as well as its indications and contraindications, are also the same whether the procedure is for a lumbar disk herniation or for degenerative spinal canal stenosis.

The **main advantage** of the microsurgical approach in lumbar disk herniation surgery is the reduced operative trauma, resulting in less postoperative morbidity and enabling earlier mobilization and aggressive rehabilitation of the patient (Mayer 2004). Muscular and neural tissue is spared to a greater extent. There is also less internal scarring, with a correspondingly lower risk of developing post-discotomy syndrome. When microsurgery is routinely used, blood loss is markedly reduced. Direct visibility of the ventral epidural space

under magnification allows easier visual differentiation of the lateral edge of the dural sac and nerve root from disk tissue, which is of practically the same color, and thus injuries to the dura mater and nerve roots are less frequent. The main advantage of microsurgical technique for nerve root decompression in cases of spinal stenosis is the preservation of stability, which renders a fusion procedure unnecessary. Yet another advantage of microsurgical technique in general is that the two-headed operative microscope gives both operating surgeons an equally good view of the operative field and is thus a valuable aid to the training and supervision of residents.

Preoperative surgical planning and the modification of surgical strategies as newer instruments and implants become available are key factors in ensuring the safety and success of minimally invasive spinal surgery (Mayer 2004). The main advantages of minimal access surgery are the reduction in perioperative morbidity and the possibility of early and aggressive mobilization and rehabilitation of the patient. (Mayer 2004)

The main **disadvantage** of microsurgical nerve root decompression is the smaller exposure of the operative field, which requires some getting used to by surgeons accustomed to macrosurgery, and the indirect view of the surgical site through the microscope. Surgeons can no longer orient thmselves by structures lying outside the microscope's field of view.

Indications for Surgery

Among the many clinical manifestations of lumbar disk herniation, only a few are highly relevant to the indication for surgery. These include:
- symptoms and signs of cauda equina compression
- pain
- signs of nerve stretching
- motor deficits.

Cauda equina manifestations, severe and acute loss of strength in important muscles, and persistent, unbearable pain constitute an indication for surgery in themselves, regardless of the time factor, as long as the CT or MRI reveals a disk herniation as the lesion responsible. Clear-cut signs of nerve stretching strongly predict the need for surgery (Dvořák 1988, McCulloch 1990, Postaccini 1998). Less relevant factors with respect to surgical indications include imaging studies, laboratory tests, electrodiagnostic studies, and aspects of the history and physical examination such as the following:
- paresthesiae
- autonomic disturbances
- restriction of movement
- reflex deficits
- muscle cramps
- abnormal posture
- lumbar muscle spasm.

Paresthesiae, abnormal posture, and reflex deficits can admittedly be quite disturbing to the patient as well as to the physician, but they are not decisive factors indicating surgery. Numbness or a sensation of cold or warmth in a leg may persist for a long time even after successful nerve root decompression. Permanent residual findings after the surgical treatment of sciatica due to S1 nerve root compression, for example, can include cramping in the calf, an absent ankle-jerk reflex, and areas of hypesthesia in the S1 dermatome. Younger patients in particular may continue to have an abnormal posture with diminished ability to flex the trunk for months after the pain is relieved by successful treatment, whether conservative or operative.

Conus Medullaris/Cauda Equina Syndrome

The classic complex of manifestations, including
- bladder and bowel disturbances
- saddle anesthesia
- motor deficits

is only rarely encountered as a full-fledged clinical triad in patients with disk herniation. Even massive prolapses are generally more pronounced on one side or the other and cause only partial cauda equina manifestations. The postoperative prognosis of cauda equina syndrome depends critically on the timing of surgery (see p. 270).

Pain and Pain Grades

The pain produced by a lumbar disk herniation compressing a nerve root is highly variable in intensity. When disk tissue presses on the root, there is mechanically induced pain, produced by stimulation of nociceptors and of the nervi nervorum; in addition, freshly extruded disk tissue causes biochemical irritation. The pain of a disk prolapse is initially very severe or unbearable.

   As there is not yet any objective way to measure pain in routine clinical practice, the physician must rely on the patient's statements. The intensity of the pain can be judged from the patient's description of it (in comparison with those of other patients with similar symptoms) and from their analgesic consumption. Numeric rating scales such as the visual analog scale (**Table 11.29**) have proved useful for quantitative pain rating during the course of follow-up.
- **Grade I pain.** When the symptoms of root irritation are only mild, there is occasional, moderately severe pain that radiates in a radicular or pseudoradicular distribution and is bearable enough that the patient consumes no analgesics at all, or only from time to time. Patients generally rate the intensity of the pain in the lowest third of the visual analog scale, but with occasional pain peaks in the middle third after mechanical stress, e. g., after prolonged standing or sitting.

Table 11.29 The visual analog scale (VAS) for pain

No pain	Moderate	Interme-diate	Severe	Unbearable pain
0		5		10

Table 11.30 The assignment of pain grades (1–3) to VAS scores

Pain grade	1	2	3
Pain intensity	Moderate	Intermediate	Severe
VAS	0–4	3–7	6–10

- **Grade II pain.** Pain of intermediate severity more frequently needs treatment with analgesics, particularly when the patient sits or stands for long periods. Patients rate the intensity of the pain in the middle third of the visual analog scale, with fluctuations above and below it corresponding to greater or lesser mechanical stress.
- **Grade III pain.** The pain is severe even when the spine is not under mechanical stress and unbearable with additional loading. The patient can obtain some degree of relief only with powerful analgesics. The intensity of the pain is rated in the upper third of the visual analog scale, with fluctuations downward into the middle third only after prolonged rest or the intake of strong, long-acting analgesics.

Over the course of days and weeks, the pain grade can vary from I to III, mainly as a function of changing body posture (sitting, standing, lying, walking). Patients should be asked to keep a "pain diary" in which they write down the predominant pain intensity for each day (**Table 11.30**).

Signs of Nerve Stretch

A Lasègue test that is positive when the leg is raised only a few degrees strongly implies that a lumbar disk herniation needs to be surgically decompressed. Lifting the extended leg displaces and stretches the spinal nerves L4, L5, and S1. If the nerve root is irritated and swollen with edema, it has correspondingly less room to move around in comfortably. Thus, the Lasègue sign indicates not just the size of the prolapse, but also the state of irritation of the nerve root. The contralateral (crossed) Lasègue test is positive when the prolapse lies medially. If a positive Lasègue sign is found, confirmation with the sitting-up and reclination tests is recommended (see Chapter 13).

   In radicular syndromes of the higher lumbar roots (L1–L3), the sciatic nerve stretch tests are negative, but a positive femoral nerve stretch test may be obtained with the patient prone.

11

Motor Disturbances

Most of the lower limb muscles are innervated by two or more nerve roots, but for each nerve root there is at least one muscle that is predominantly supplied by that root alone. The degree of dominance is variable: the quadriceps, for example, is supplied by the L3 and L4 roots and, to some extent, by the L5 root, but the extensor hallucis longus is almost exclusively supplied by the L5 root. This is why L5 root compression leads to a complete loss of function of the extensor of the great toe, whereas complete compression of the L3 or L4 root causes only partial weakness of the quadriceps. Certain indications of muscle dysfunction can be detected simply by observing the patient attempting to stand and walk on tiptoe, and then on the heels. The observed weakness may be so slight that the patient has not noticed it. Fibrillation of the affected muscle groups is occasionally seen. From the patient's point of view, the most prominent manifestation of a quadriceps palsy is difficulty climbing stairs, and that of a peroneus palsy is tripping over the dropped foot. Even when these deficits are severe, patients often cannot say exactly when they arose.

Longer-lasting compression of motor fibers in the spinal nerve leads first to muscle weakness and then to loss of muscle bulk, ranging to irreversible atrophy. Loss of bulk due to lumbar nerve root compression is easiest to observe in large, superficially lying muscles such as
- the glutei (S1)
- the quadriceps (L3, L4)
- the tibialis anterior (L4) and peronei (L5)
- the triceps surae (= gastrocnemius and soleus) (S1).

Marked visible and measurable atrophy of a muscle predominantly innervated by a single root still does not constitute an indication for surgical nerve root decompression unless there are further reasons, such as severe pain correlating with the anatomical finding. If, as is usually the case, the patient has almost no pain (any more), surgical decompression cannot achieve anything further if muscle atrophy has already set in, and indeed may cause worse postoperative pain because of scarring and segmental destabilization. Surgery is likewise not indicated for quadriceps and peroneus palsies of other causes, such as diabetic polyneuropathy, which can be severe though they are usually not associated with any marked degree of pain.

Because of their multisegmental innervation, the quadriceps and triceps surae muscles often show a surprisingly good functional recovery after intensive strength training, electrotherapy, and gait training.

Important and Less Important Muscle Palsies

The physician must be able to identify and grade pareses of individual lower limb muscles due to nerve root compression, not only to arrive at the correct diagnosis but also to determine whether surgery is indicated. Some muscles, such as the extensor hallucis longus, the adductors, and the glutei, are very useful for diagnostic purposes but of lesser relevance to the decision whether to operate.

Weakness of the quadriceps or of the foot dorsiflexors produces a marked functional deficit. In younger individuals, a complete loss of plantar flexion also produces a disturbing gait impairment and makes it difficult to participate in sports.

Quadriceps. Acute loss of function of a sizable portion of the quadriceps muscle causes difficulty walking, standing, and above all climbing stairs. Weight-bearing on the slightly flexed leg leads to buckling of the knee, so that patients will fall if they do not check the fall quickly enough with their arms.

> **!** Quadriceps weakness of acute onset, with marked difficulty standing, walking, and climbing stairs, accompanied by the corresponding pain and a correlated neuroradiological finding, constitutes an indication for surgical decompression.

Surgical treatment is not indicated, however, if weakness has been present for a longer time, only a moderate degree of pain is present, and/or the patient is suffering from other conditions such as diabetes or polyneuropathy. The best test for quadriceps weakness is the one-legged squatting and standing test. If the patient can still do this, surgery can be deferred and the need for it can be reassessed later, as long as there is no other urgent reason to operate (such as unbearable pain).

Foot dorsiflexors. Marked dorsiflexor weakness causes marked gait impairment (steppage gait). Because the forefoot cannot be raised, the patient must lift the leg higher than normal so that the toes clear the ground during the forward stride. Once the foot drop has become permanent, it can only be treated with a peroneal splint that passively holds the forefoot in dorsiflexion. The relevant practical tests for a foot drop are heel-standing and heel-walking. These tests must be carried out with precision in all positions, particularly if the patient is in severe pain, because pain often restricts the patient's ability or willingness to dorsiflex the foot, as this maneuver also stretches the sciatic nerve. In such cases, dorsiflexor strength should also be tested with the patient in the supine position with the knee flexed, or in the sitting position.

⚠ Dorsiflexor dysfunction of acute onset with marked impairment of heel-walking and heel-standing, if it is accompanied by the appropriate additional manifestations and explicable by the radiological findings, is an indication for operative decompression.

Plantar flexors of the foot. Patients often do not notice weakness of the plantar flexors, e. g., due to compression of the S1 nerve root, until they are asked to stand on the tips of the toes on one foot or to walk on tiptoe, whereupon the affected foot sinks back onto the heel. Bilateral tiptoe standing often remains possible. Commonly, though not invariably, this finding is accompanied by a band of pain in the S1 distribution as well as weakness or absence of the Achilles reflex. Although the strength of the triceps surae muscle can also be tested in the supine position by having the patient plantar flex the foot against resistance, the examiner may fail to detect any weakness by testing in this way, even if the S1 nerve root is severely compressed: the calf musculature may still be able to generate a very intense force even though some of its component muscle groups are partially dysfunctional. Often, weakness of the plantar flexors due to an S1 lesion does not cause any significant functional impairment because of intact mechanisms of muscular compensation and reactivation; thus, the indication for surgery should primarily be based on other features, such as the intensity of the pain and the size of the radiologically demonstrated prolapse.

⚠ Moderately severe acute weakness of the plantar flexors is not an indication for surgical decompression in patients with moderate or no pain.

The threshold degree of plantar flexor weakness for which surgical treatment should be offered is lower for patients who are, and wish to remain, highly physically active in their professional and leisure-time activities, including sports. Even in such patients with a milder degree of weakness, however, a complete recovery of plantar flexor strength cannot be expected with any confidence if the weakness has already been present for a longer period. An alternative treatment would be intensive exercise of the calf muscles to increase their strength, along with corresponding instruction in proper gait.

Dorsiflexor of the great toe (extensor hallucis longus). Isolated weakness of the extensor hallucis longus results from compression of the L5 nerve root. Paresis or paralysis of this muscle is generally not noticed by the patient and causes no significant functional impairment.

⚠ Isolated weakness of dorsiflexion of the great toe is not an indication for surgical decompression even when it arises acutely, unless there are other reasons to operate, such as severe pain and a corresponding finding in the imaging studies.

Table 11.31 Grades of strength (modified, after Hoppenfeld)

5	Fully mobile against gravity and maximal resistance	Normal
4	Fully mobile against gravity and submaximal resistance	Good
3	Fully mobile against gravity, but not against resistance	Moderate
2	Fully mobile, but not against gravity or resistance	Poor
1	Immobile; only slight muscle contractions or fibrillations visible	Very poor
0	No movement, no contractions	Plegia

Adductors. A lesion of the L3 nerve root can cause adductor weakness on the affected side. The adductor muscles are also innervated by the L2 and L4 roots. Their function is tested with the patient in the supine position with the leg bent at the knee and hip. Because of their multisegmental innervation, adductor weakness is not an indication for surgery unless there are other reasons to operate, such as severe pain and a corresponding finding in the imaging studies.

Gluteal muscles. Lesions of the S1 nerve root can affect the gluteus maximus, and lesions of the L5 nerve root can affect the gluteus medius. Weakness of these muscles can be detected by having the prone patient attempt to extend the leg at the hip against resistance; it has no significance with respect to the indication for surgery.

Grading of Strength

To avoid excessive subjectivity in the assessment and nomenclature of degrees of muscle weakness that are found at physical examination, a semi-objective scale ranging from total paralysis (0) to normal strength (5) is normally used (**Table 11.31**). This is commonly called the "MRC scale," because it was introduced many years ago by the United Kingdom Medical Research Council (Medical Research Council [United Kingdom] 1976).

Because of multisegmental innervation, the degrees of weakness found in lumbar nerve root compression are generally between 2 and 4, with 4 being the most common. Here, too, there is room for subjectivity in the examiner's judgment of the degree of resistance exerted by the patient.

Assessment of Motor Impairment

The assessment of motor impairment is based not only on the degree of weakness as such, but also on the functional importance of the affected muscle and on the duration of the paresis. This assessment is, in turn, the most impor-

Table 11.32 Grades of paresis

1	Insignificant	Paresis of insignificant muscles; longstanding paresis
2	Significant	Acute paresis of important muscles, strength grade 4
3	Severe	Acute paresis of important muscles (1–3 days old), strength grade 0–3

Table 11.33 Absolute indications for surgery when the MRI/CT findings are unequivocal

- Cauda equina manifestations
- Acute paresis (strength grade 0–3) of important muscles
- Continuous, unbearable pain

Table 11.34 Relative indications for decompressive surgery in discogenic nerve root compression when the MRI/CT findings are unequivocal

- Moderate to severe intractable pain
- Acute, mild paresis (strength grade 4) of important muscles

Table 11.35 Indications for decompressive surgery in discogenic nerve root compression: overview

No indication for surgery		Relative indication		Absolute indication
S1	S1	S2	S2	S3
P1	P2	P1	P2	P3, cauda equina syndrome

tant factor in the decision whether to proceed to surgical nerve root decompression (**Table 11.32**).

Grade 1 paresis: insignificant. This category includes pareses of unimportant muscles and muscle groups, regardless of their severity. It is functionally irrelevant, for example, if an extensor hallucis longus muscle is completely paralyzed (MRC grade 0–3) on one side, as long as the patient is not in any great degree of pain. The multisegmentally innervated muscles, on the other hand, rarely develop significant weakness from a lesion of a single nerve root. Furthermore, if the paresis has already been present for weeks or months, surgery should be used sparingly, particularly in older patients, because the paresis is unlikely to resolve completely after decompression.

Grade 2 paresis: significant. Acute weakness of important muscles such as the foot dorsiflexors or the quadriceps, leading to a significant loss of strength against re-

sistance (MRC grade 4), can be an indication for immediate nerve root decompression. Important accompanying factors in the decision whether to operate include the degree of pain, the age of the patient, and the size of the finding in the imaging studies.

Grade 3 paresis: severe. Acute weakness of important muscles with a total loss of functional strength (MRC grade 2–3), e. g., acute, total loss of dorsiflexor or quadriceps function—or, in some cases, of plantar flexion—in a younger patient, is a major determinant of the need for surgery. "Acute," in this context, means "having arisen within the past 1–3 days." If the total loss of functional strength has been present for a longer time, it is no longer an indication for surgical decompression.

Summary of the Indications for Surgical Decompression in Cases of Discogenic Nerve Root Compression

Surgery absolutely indicated (Table 11.33): Cauda equina syndrome, acute paresis of important muscles with MRC grade 0–3 (grade 3 paresis) and very severe continuous pain (grade 3 pain), accompanied by a corresponding finding on MRI or CT, are all in themselves absolute indications for surgical decompression. That is to say, cauda equina syndrome and acute grade 3 paresis call for surgical treatment even in the absence of pain. Conversely, very severe continuous pain is an indication for surgery in the absence of any significant weakness. When a decompressive lumbar operation is absolutely indicated, the physician's determination that this is so plays a decisive role. Physicians must use all their powers of persuasion to make it clear to the patient that an operation is necessary.

Surgery relatively indicated (Table 11.34): Moderately severe pain (grade 2 pain) and acute weakness of important muscles that is only moderate in degree when tested against the examiner's resistance (grade 2 paresis) are relative indications for surgery. In such situations, other parameters besides pain and weakness can be taken as evidence of the degree of nerve root compression, e. g., signs of nerve stretch, impairment of the quality of life, and the site and extent of the prolapse in the MRI or CT image. Surgery is also relatively indicated for patients with continuous, moderate or severe pain (grade 2 pain) accompanied by insignificant (grade 1) paresis or none at all, as well as for younger patients suffering from intermediate degrees of functional impairment of important muscle groups (grade 2 paresis) but only mild pain (grade 1 pain). In cases such as these, the patient's attitude and readiness to be operated on play an important role in establishing the indication. Patients must state that they can no longer tolerate the pain and functional impairment and are suffering from a severely impaired quality of life (**Table 11.35**).

11

Surgery not indicated or contraindicated. The lack of an indication for decompressive surgery in nerve root compression is not the same thing as a contraindication. Surgery can still be done without harm, in some circumstances, even if it is not indicated, but it must not be done at all if it is contraindicated. Contraindications include local infection in the area of the surgical approach, life-threatening systemic illnesses, or the patient's refusal to undergo surgery. On the other hand, situations where surgery is not indicated include moderate and tolerable pain (grade 1 pain), weakness of insignificant muscles, and longstanding weakness. Paresthesiae, asymmetry or loss of reflexes, postural abnormalities, and lumbar spasm play no role in the indication for surgery. The same is true of radiological findings, even if they are quite impressive, when the pain is not very intense (grade 1 pain) or when the weakness affects only insignificant muscles or is longstanding (grade 1 paresis). The presence of a mild or moderate sensorimotor deficit does not contraindicate conservative therapy, as the likelihood of resolution is comparable with either conservative therapy or surgery (Postacchini 1999). These criteria are valid for discogenic nerve root compression, i. e., compression by protruding and prolapsed disks. The indications for decompressive surgery in lumbar spinal stenosis are subject to different considerations; here, gait impairment (spinal intermittent claudication) and accompanying illnesses play an important role.

Informed Consent for Decompressive Surgery

Provision of adequate information to the patient before surgery and the patient's explicit declaration of consent assume additional importance in open lumbar disk surgery because of the risk of complications in operations of this type, and also because of their generally unfavorable public reputation. In most malpractice cases arising from disk surgery that has gone awry, the complaint has less to do with the complication itself than with the alleged lack of adequate information about it before surgery. Preprinted information sheets are available that include sketches of the operative technique and lists of possible complications. Generally speaking, when such information sheets are used, the pictures and explanations given should be supplemented, either orally or in writing, by the surgeon personally. Patient education regarding the diagnosis, the course of the illness and its treatment, and the risks of the proposed intervention should refer to the pictures that are provided, as far as is possible.

In principle, all possible complications need to be explained before surgery. The commoner ones—e. g., postoperative leg pain and epidural adhesions—should be explained at length. Rare but serious complications, such as intraoperative injury to abdominal vessels and viscera, should also be mentioned, though with a reference to their rarity: the surgeon may say, for example,

"For legal reasons, I am also required to inform you that there is a very small risk of ..."

Positive reinforcement. The informational discussion before surgery should not take on excessively negative overtones because of the many potential complications that have to be mentioned for medicolegal reasons. The surgeon should also take care to emphasize the positive aspects of the proposed operation, with statements such as these:

- "You can't go on having so much pain and nerve dysfunction, and we have already tried all of the conservative treatment options."
- "All of the tests that you've had so far show that you are otherwise in good health and ought to get over the operation without any difficulty."
- "This type of surgery is part of our department's daily routine and will be carried out by a specialized professional team."
- "This is an operation in the lowest part of the spine, below the level where the spinal cord ends."

At the end of the discussion, the patient should understand that the proposed operation is reasonable and necessary. To reinforce the point, the surgeon can tell the patient, "I would want this operation for myself if I were in your situation." A surgeon who is not of this opinion should not be proposing surgery in the first place.

Planning the Operation and Confirming the Level of the Lesion

Open microsurgical nerve root decompression requires precise preoperative determination of the proper site for the skin incision. Mere palpation of the iliac crests and lumbar spinous processes without any radiological studies, as was the practice many years ago, is definitively no longer adequate. Plain lateral radiographs with a needle at the proposed level of operation can be obtained the day before surgery, or else with a fluoroscopic image intensifier immediately before surgery, with the patient already intubated and in position on the operating table. The latter method has the advantage of being carried out by the surgeon him/herself, so that reliance on the radiologist is not necessary. The needle tip should be centered on the level of the disk. A second check of the level of operation is done intraoperatively once the ligamentum flavum has been exposed. A fine dissector is placed in the upper interlaminar corner at the lower edge of the upper lamina at the exposed level, and a radiograph is taken before the spinal canal is opened (**Figs. 11.131, 11.132**).

Lighting. If an operating microscope is not used, the surgeon can illuminate the field with a head lamp or a cold light source built into the discectomy retractor; these methods provide adequate lighting for the sur-

11

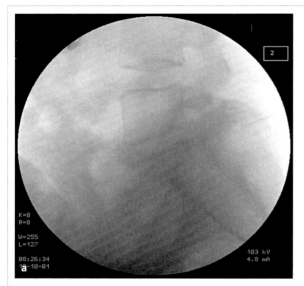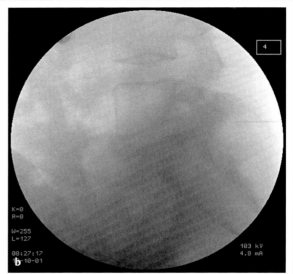

Fig. 11.131 a, b Preoperative radiographs with a needle at L5/S1.

a Improper (oblique) needle position.
b Proper (straight) needle position.

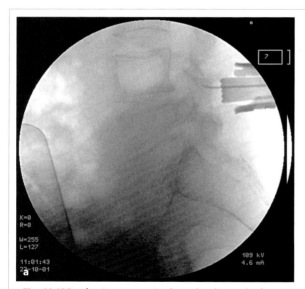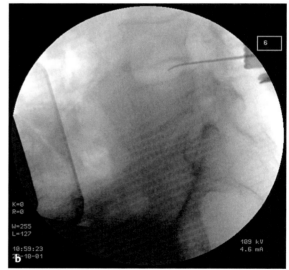

Fig. 11.132 a, b Intraoperative lateral radiographs for segment confirmation (in this case, L4/5) (from Krämer, Herdmann, and Krämer 2005).

a Before opening the spinal canal, at the edge of the lamina.
b Intradiscal (for final documentation).

geon, though not for the assistant. The **operating microscope** enables optimal illumination of the operative field along with the opportunity to magnify the view at will, and it also improves the surgeon's teaching ability, as it gives the assistant an equally good view of the field. Open surgery with an operating microscope affords a better three-dimensional view of the operative field than any closed endoscopic technique.

In case technical difficulties arise with the microscope, or in case of serious intraoperative complications, the surgeon should always be in a position to dispense with the microscope and continue the operation with illumination from a head lamp or a cold light source.

Operative Technique

The operation is carried out in four phases, from the skin incision to the decompression of the nerve root in the ventral epidural space. Each phase has its own characteristic intraoperative appearance at each level of dissection and in each segment of the lumbar spine. The four phases are as follows:

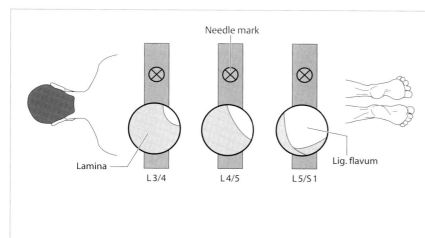

Needle mark

Lamina

L 3/4   L 4/5   L 5/S 1

Lig. flavum

Fig. 11.133 Phase 2 of the operation, with exposure of the lamina/ligamentum flavum layer at the discal level. In the approach to the L5/S1 disk, one palpates and visualizes the lower edge of the next lamina above (L5) in the cranial portion of the operative field. At the L4/5 level, the lower edge of the next lamina above is found in the upper third or the middle of the operative field; at L3/4 and higher levels, it is found in the caudal portion of the operative field. In elderly patients, and when the disk space is narrowed, the lamina overlaps the disk space even more (from Krämer, Herdmann, and Krämer 2005).

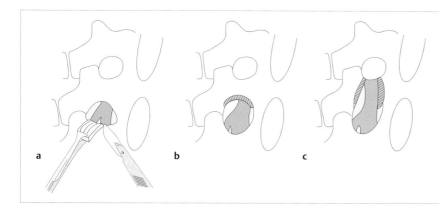

a   b   c

Fig. 11.134a–c Exposure of a lumbar disk herniation by (**a**) fenestration, with removal of the ligamentum flavum (flavectomy, fenestrotomy), (**b**) removal of part of the lamina (laminotomy), and (**c**) removal of half of the lamina (hemilaminectomy).

11

- phase i: skin incision
- phase ii: lamina and ligamentum flavum (**Fig. 11.133**)
- phase iii: posterior epidural space
- phase iv: anterior epidural space (see **Fig. 11.136**).

The actual disk surgery, in the narrow sense of the term, takes place in the anterior (ventral) epidural space. After resection of the ligamentum flavum alone (at the L5/S1 level) or the ligamentum flavum and part of the lamina (at L4/5 and higher levels; **Fig. 11.134**), the dural sac and the nerve roots exiting from it are gently retracted medially ("medialized") to afford a direct view into the anterior epidural space. The free intraspinal disk fragment is removed, and further mobile fragments within the intervertebral space are extracted with a special rongeur fitted with a stop to keep its tip from penetrating the anulus fibrosus ventrally and potentially injuring the abdominal vessels (**Fig. 11.135**). Only free fragments are removed; comprehensive emptying of the in-

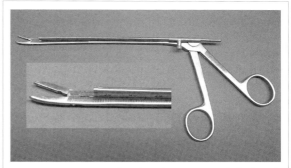

Fig. 11.135 Rongeur fitted with a stop: shaft length 180 mm, width at tip 2 mm, stop with resettable depth preventing insertion of the tip beyond the anterior longitudinal ligament (from Krämer, Herdmann, and Krämer 2005).

tervertebral space brings no further advantage (Fountas et al. 2004, Krämer, Herdmann, and Krämer 2005).

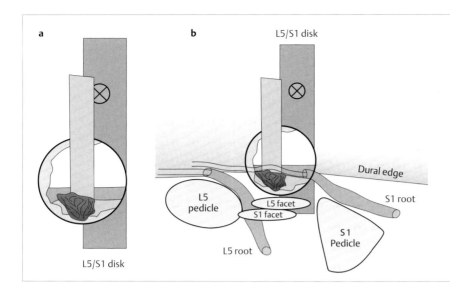

Fig. 11.136 a, b L5/S1 disk herniation at the supradiscal level, phase IV, in the anterior epidural space (from Krämer, Herdmann, and Krämer 2005).
a The operative field as seen by the surgeon. The lower edge of the L5 lamina has been removed. The prolapse is seen immediately superior to the disk (gray zone) after medialization with a nerve root hook.
b Illustration of structures in the vicinity: the L5 nerve root above, the facets laterally, and the L5 and S1 pedicles.

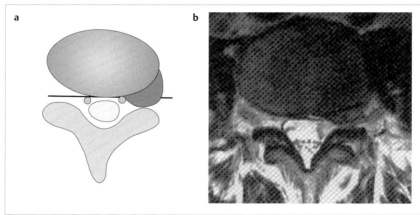

Fig. 11.137 a, b Lateral prolapse at the discal level. Disk tissue at the discal level is seen next to the prolapse. The prolapse impinges on the root outside the foramen (from Krämer, Herdmann, and Krämer 2005).
a Diagram.
b MRI scan.

Once the dislodged disk tissue has been extracted, the quantity of material that has been removed should be compared to the size of the prolapse seen in the pre-operative MRI or CT scan. If there is a discrepancy, the level of surgery should be checked once again with an intraoperative lateral radiograph, with a dissector lying inside the disk space that has been evacuated (third check of the level of surgery if necessary, **Fig. 11.132 b**).

Lateral Disk Herniation

Synonyms: Lateral prolapse, intraforaminal prolapse, extracanalicular prolapse.

Definition: Lateral disk herniations lie outside the spinal canal, lateral to the border defined by the medial edge of the pedicle. They compress the exiting nerve root of the segment above. Often, the dorsal root ganglion is compressed at this site. At the discal level, the prolapse may still be invested by a thin membrane corresponding to the outermost layer of the anulus fibrosus. Supradiscal lateral disk herniations are usually free sequestra (**Figs. 11.137, 11.138**).

Clinical Features and Indications

The frequency of lateral disk herniations as reported in the literature ranges from 2.2% to 11.7% (Crock 1993, Melville 1994, Epstein 1995, Frankhauser 1998, McCulloch 1998, Krämer, Herdmann, and Krämer 2005). Lateral herniations are usually found in older patients, with a mean age of 60 years; men are more commonly affected than women. In comparison, the peak age for lumbar disk herniations that are operated on by the interlaminar approach is 40. Lateral herniations are usually found at the L4/5, L3/4, or L5/S1 level, from most to least frequent (**Figs. 11.139, 11.140**). Neurological examination reveals evidence of nerve root dysfunction with pain and band-like hypesthesia in the appropriate segmental distribution, i.e., usually L4, less commonly L3 or L5.

The best type of imaging study for the demonstration of a lateral disk herniation is MRI, as it depicts all of the lumbosacral segments simultaneously and enables easier identification of the displaced disk tissue in the in-

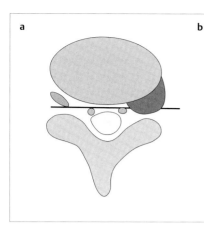 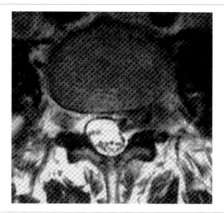

Fig. 11.138 a, b Lateral disk herniation at the supradiscal level. The upper portion of the vertebral body is seen next to the disk herniation. The prolapse lies in the foramen and compresses the exiting nerve root intraforaminally (from Krämer, Herdmann, and Krämer 2005).
a Diagram.
b MRI scan.

tervertebral foramen. If the symptoms and signs are unclear, and particularly when imaging does not yield an unequivocal diagnosis, radiculography and nerve root block can be carried out. Depiction of the exiting root in the intervertebral foramen with contrast medium, followed by local anesthesia of the root, is a clinically important means of demonstrating a symptomatic lateral disk prolapse and simultaneously a potential option for conservative treatment. Patients with lateral herniations are free of pain at once when this is done, so it is certainly worthwhile to inject some cortisone locally immediately afterward and then continue to manage the patient conservatively.

Indications for Surgical Treatment of Lateral Disk Herniations

Three factors determine the indication for surgery on lateral disk herniations:

- Continuous, unbearable pain and the lack of a pain-free position, if correlated with an unambiguous MRI scan, constitute an indication for surgery.
- Acute quadriceps weakness with marked gait impairment and spontaneous buckling of the knee is an indication for surgery even if the patient is free of pain. The indication is not as strong if quadriceps weakness has been present for longer periods of time or if there is an accompanying polyneuropathy (e. g., of diabetic origin).

A precondition to surgery for these two indications is the unequivocal identification of the lateral prolapse in the imaging studies (**Figs. 11.137–11.139**).

The operative technique consists of four phases, just like the technique of the interlaminar approach. The transverse approach to the lateral lumbar area requires special attention to topographical anatomical orientation, because these procedures are done less commonly and in an area containing many blood vessels. Disorientation in the lateral lumbar area is the main cause of errors and complications. The intertransverse area is usu-

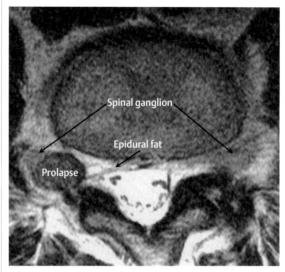

Fig. 11.139 MRI scan of lateral prolapse at L3/4, right (from Krämer, Herdmann, and Krämer 2005).

ally exposed too far laterally, so that further dissection into the depths between the transverse processes can endanger the retroperitoneal soft tissues. The lateral approach has the advantages of less danger of injuring the dura mater and the absence of postoperative epidural fibrosis.

Complications of Lumbar Discotomy

Microsurgery has, in principle, the same potential complications as conventional disk surgery. Injuries of the dura mater and spinal nerves are less likely because of the better view of the operative field, though problems with orientation are more common, particularly among surgeons who are just getting used to the operating microscope. There is a high prevalence of **surgery at the wrong level** among spine surgeons (Mody et al 2008).

11

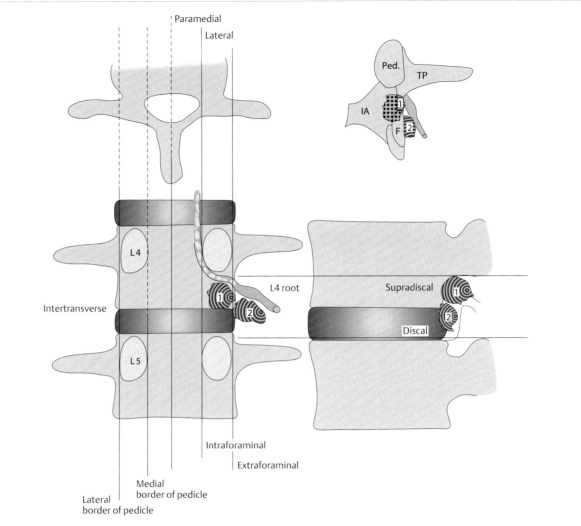

Fig. 11.140 Classification of lateral disk herniations. The lateral zone is defined as lying lateral to the medial border of the pedicle. The foraminal zone extends to the lateral border of the pedicle. The intervertebral foramen extends from the lower edge of the pedicle to the upper edge of the next pedicle below. A supradiscal lateral disk herniation (**1**) lies within the foramen and displaces the root cranially. A lateral disk herniation at the discal level (**2**) lies extraforaminally and displaces the root further outward, cranially and dorsally. The small diagram shows the pars interarticularis (IA), the facet joint (F), and the transverse process (TP). Prolapses **1** and **2** are completely covered by the pars interarticularis and the facets. They can be reached through a medial approach only by resection of large portions of the pars interarticularis and facets (from Krämer, Herdmann, and Krämer 2005).

Even if the operation is precisely planned with a preoperative radiograph of a needle in the appropriate intervertebral space, it is still possible for the operation to be done at the wrong level, e. g., in an adipose or scoliotic patient. This is why we recommend checking the level three times (see **Figs. 11.131, 11.132**).

Bleeding from epidural veins is not a complication in the strict sense. Epidural venous plexuses, particularly just behind the vertebral body, can be torn when a disk prolapse is extracted. Bleeding disrupts the operation when it occurs in a very small operative field and should therefore be controlled as well as possible with bipolar electrocoagulation forceps. Epidural venous bleeding will generally not compress the dural sac, because the venous pressure is relatively low (Bell 1996, Hanley 1996, McCulloch 1998, Findlay 2000, Kraemer et al. 2003). On the other hand, arterial bleeding from the paravertebral musculature and the joint capsule can dangerously compress the dural sac postoperatively if not adequately controlled.

Intraoperative opening of the dura mater (durotomy) occurs in 1–5 % of all lumbar disk operations (Bell 1996,

Getty 1996, McCulloch 1998). In our series of 1281 operations, durotomy occurred in 4.3% of cases involving surgeons who were still on their learning curves and in 0.8% of cases operated by surgeons who had at least 100 such operations behind them (Wiese et al. 2004). Tears up to 3 mm in size can be covered with a piece of muscle or fat, but all larger tears should be sutured together, or patched if there is a punched-out dural defect. Suturing under the operating microscope can be difficult and may require extension of the operative field to expose the full length of the tear.

The most serious complication of lumbar disk surgery, whether done under the operating microscope or by the conventional technique, is injury to the large abdominal vessels through a ventral perforation of the anulus fibrosus. In the large series of De Saussure (1959), Reulen (1991), and Grumme and Kolodziejczyk (1994), this type of complication was found to be very rare. It should not happen when a rongeur fitted with a stop is used, as shown in **Fig. 11.135**.

Wound infection, spondylodiscitis. The literature distinguishes superficial from deep wound infections. Superficial epifascial infections of the skin and subcutaneous fat down to the fascia are reported to have a frequency of 2–3% (Bell 1996, McCulloch 1998, Postacchini 1998). Deep subfascial infections can be of the following types:

- infection limited to the epidural space (epidural abscess)
- infection involving the intervertebral space (discitis) with a greater or lesser degree of involvement of the adjacent vertebral bodies (spondylodiscitis)
- infection penetrating the dura mater (meningitis).

Table 11.36 Epidemiology of spondylodiscitis after lumbar disk surgery

Author	Year	Number of operations	Spondylodiscitis (%)	
Marchetti	1980	6374	0.9	
Lindholm	1982	3576	0.8	
Rawlings	1983	4500	0.2	
Puranen	1984	1100	0.7	
Frank	1988	6632	0.2	
Young	1988	1500	0.13	
			Micro-surgery	**Macro-surgery**
Dauch	1986		0.4	2.8
Stolke	1988		0.5	1.4
Caspar	1991		0.6	3.0
Sollmann	1988	**Operations for recurrence**	1.5	

Microsurgical lumbar disk surgery is widely reputed to have a higher risk of infection, but this notion is not supported by any statistics in the literature (**Table 11.36**).

Postoperative Care

Postoperative rehabilitation programs are generally recommended (McCullach 1998, Postacchini 1998, Borenstein, Wiesel, and Boden 2004). Physiotherapy-based rehabilitation following a first-time disk herniation operation is effective in the short term when compared in a randomized controlled trial with no therapy (Erdogmus et al. 2007).

Table 11.37 Postoperative care after lumbar disk surgery

Phase	1	2	3	4	5
Time	First 24 h	First week	First 3 months	3rd–12th month	After 1 year
Pathoanatomical processes taking place	Clotting	Inflammation	Granulation	Soft scar formation	Solid scar formation
Orthosis	Flexion orthosis	Flexion orthosis	Flexion orthosis	Flexion orthosis (sometimes)	No orthosis
Back school	Body hygiene, mobilization (**Fig. 11.141**)	Sitting, standing, walking	General back school	General back school	General back school
Physiotherapy	Breathing exercises	First aid exercises	First aid exercises, training therapy	training therapy	Sports and gymnastics
Work			Light work, lifting and carrying loads < 15 kg	Moderately heavy work, lifting and carrying loads < 25 kg	Heavy work, lifting and carrying loads > 25 kg
Sports		Walking, stationary bicycle, wading pool	Running, swimming, cycling	Ball sport training	Ball sports, competitive sports

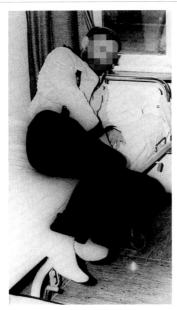

Fig. 11.141 A patient who has undergone disk surgery rolling out of bed while keeping the lumbar spine stiff. The pelvis serves as the fulcrum for this maneuver.

Postoperative care begins when the patient comes round from the anesthetic, and has five phases (**Table 11.37**):

- the first 24 hours
- the first week
- the first 3 months
- the first year
- after the first year.

Postoperative care is adapted to suit the degree of wound healing that is present during each phase, as well as the biomechanical changes that occur in the motion segment after the prolapse is surgically removed. The surgical wound heals in the same phases as wounds from other types of surgery and trauma: coagulation, inflammation, granulation, scar formation, and scar retraction. The smaller the operative site, the less extensive the inflammation, granulation, and scarring that arise after surgery. The exposed neural elements in the spinal canal, which communicate directly with the dorsal wound canal in the interlaminar approach, stand to benefit most from a small operative exposure.

The decisive factor affecting the postoperative management is the **biomechanical alteration of the motion segment** after disk tissue has been removed. The spontaneous extrusion (disk herniation) or operative removal of disk tissue from the intervertebral space fundamentally alters motion segment biomechanics in several ways. The disk loses its mechanical buffer function because of **loss of height and elasticity.** Relatively rapid loss of height increases the transmission of force to the intervertebral joints, which become telescoped into each other, particularly under conditions of axial stress and hyperlordosis. When this process occurs gradually and asymptomatically over many years, in the physiological degenerative loss of disk height accompanying normal aging, the intervertebral joints and nerve roots have the opportunity to adapt. In contrast, when height is rapidly lost in the posterior portion of the disk, the adjoining structures are acutely placed under increased mechanical stress and cannot compensate for it adequately, giving rise to pain. **In the first 3 months after surgery, reduction of stress on the intervertebral joints and gradual adaptation to the new biomechanical demands placed on them can be promoted by keeping the back in mild flexion with flattening of the lumbar lordosis.** This is the essential principle underlying flexion physiotherapy in the step position with exercises out of the stress-reducing posture; it is also the essential principle underlying the use of flexion orthoses. In order to ensure a gradual transition from a flattened lordosis back to a normal lordosis, it is best to use modularly constructed orthoses that can be gradually adjusted to go from a flexing effect to a normal lordotic effect.

Likewise, the physiotherapy exercises that should be done in parallel are first done in the step position, and then, later on in the first 3 months after surgery, with extended hip and knee joints.

Results. The reported data on the results of surgery are variable. Varying indications among surgeons and a high degree of subjectivity in follow-up assessment are two reasons for this (Korres et al. 1992). In our clinic, the results improved markedly after the introduction of microsurgical technique. Statistics on large patient popula-

Table 11.38 Results of lumbar disk surgery

Author	Year	Number of operations	Satisfactory (%)	Moderate (%)	Unsatisfactory (%)
Oppel and Schramm	1976	3238	88	10	2
Finneson	1980	1000	93	–	7
Rothman and Simeone	1982	1500	77	20	3
Söllner et al.	1988	2020	90	–	10
Krämer, Herdmann, and Krämer	2005	1280	90	8	2

tions are the most informative (**Table 11.38**). The success of treatment is judged by the degree of relief of the radicular syndrome by surgery. The proportion of very good and satisfactory results is generally 80–90%, even in large series, and that of moderately good and unsatisfactory results is generally around 10%.

It makes no difference to the results whether a sequestrectomy is done alone or the disk space is evacuated as completely as possible after sequestrectomy (McCulloch 1998, Postacchini 1999, Kaast et al. 2005). The overall outcome after aggressive removal of disk tissue is less satisfactory, especially during the first year after surgery (Carragee et al. 2006). A prospective randomized study in our clinic (Bernsmann et al. 2001) revealed that the results in postoperative follow-up were no better if a free piece of fat was placed on the nerve root at the primary operation to prevent the formation of adhesions. There are fewer complications, and the results in postoperative follow-up are better, if the operation is done by more experienced surgeons rather than less experienced ones (Wiese et al. 2004). The pre- and postoperative symptoms depend on the histological composition and pathological anatomical classification of the disk herniation (McCulloch 1998, Carragee et al. 2003). This observation is confirmed by a study from our clinic showing that, even before surgery, more severe symptoms are present if the disk herniation consists mainly of hard fragments of the anulus fibrosus and cartilaginous end plates (Willburger et al. 2004).

The degree to which the patient still has radicular manifestations after surgery depends mainly on two factors:

- The preoperative duration of symptoms: patients who have suffered from radicular symptoms for a short time do better than those who have suffered from them for years.
- The findings at surgery: the removal of massive herniations and free intraspinal fragments of disk tissue yields better results than the removal of protrusions whose features on CT and/or MRI are not clearly correlated with the clinical manifestations.

! Symptoms attributable to the underlying condition, i.e., disk degeneration and slackening rather than disk herniation per se, cannot be relieved by discotomy.

Most patients continue to have intermittent low back pain even after successful disk surgery and can still have pain on certain maneuvers such as lifting, carrying, and bending. Both Thomalske et al. (1977) and Hasenbring (1992) followed up patients who had undergone disk surgery and concluded that there is an emotional component to negative judgments about the operative result. They found that patients often attributed residual back pain to the operation, even if it was no more severe than the back pain occasionally felt by normal individuals who have not had surgery. The surgeons, on the other hand, uniformly stated that the operation had been a success. Patients who had already received disability compensation judged their operations successful, whereas those who had applied for it but not yet received it were more likely to judge them unsuccessful.

In a meta-analysis involving a total of 2504 patients who had undergone disk surgery, Spangfort (1972) found that the success of the operation depended primarily on the intraoperative findings. Patients who had only a disk protrusion as the cause of their sciatica had success rates between 40% and 65%. The moderate success rates in such cases justifies the use of all possible conservative treatments, with surgery as a last resort.

Recent reports on the results of disk surgery appear to be consistent with the earlier literature (Vaccaro and Fehlings 2007). The two SPORT (Spine Patient Outcomes Research Trial) studies of Weinstein et al. (2006a, 2006b) parallel the outcomes in the study by Weber (1983) and the Maine lumbar spine studies (Atlas et al. 1996, 2005), which demonstrated that most patients will improve with nonoperative or operative management, but that the surgical group improves much more quickly even for back pain (Pearson et al. 2008). The Cochrane Review of the effects of surgical intervention for the treatment of lumbar disk prolapse (Gibson and Waddel 2007) comes to the conclusion that surgical discectomy for carefully selected patients with sciatica due to lumbar disk prolapse provides faster relief from the acute attack than conservative management, although any positive or negative effects on the lifetime natural history of the underlying disk disease are still unclear.

Postoperative symptoms. It is rare for patients to be fully asymptomatic immediately after disk surgery (**Table 11.39**). In addition to the expected incisional pain, there is usually some residual pain from the radicular syndrome. The persistence of radicular irritative phenomena of the same kinds that were present before surgery is evidence of a post-compressive partial **conduction block** in the nerve root: *hypesthesia, diminished reflexes,* and *weakness* may resolve only over the course of several months, if at all (Kobayashi et al. 2007).

Autonomic phenomena, including relative *coolness and hypoperfusion of the affected leg,* are also a part of the post-sciatic symptom complex that is seen after either surgical or conservative treatment. There is also a

Table 11.39 Causes of persistence or recurrence of severe sciatica after lumbar disk surgery

- Inadequate nerve root decompression
- Recurrent prolapse in the same segment
- Prolapse or protrusion in another segment
- Adhesions (PDS)
- Deep wound infection (discitis)

11

transient tendency to have *calf cramps* after an S1 syndrome. These post-sciatic symptoms usually resolve spontaneously and respond well to interference current therapy or lumbar sympathetic chain blocks.

Severe **radicular pain and postural abnormalities** that persist without change or recur a short time after discotomy are attributable to a number of factors. Symptoms persisting at the same level of intensity after surgery indicate inadequate decompression of the nerve root; reasons for this may include an operation at the wrong level, or failure to notice a second disk herniation compressing the same root at an adjacent level. Deep wound infections such as **discitis** are generally suspected because of a persistent fever and then confirmed radiologically.

Recurrent disk prolapse at the operated level through the extrusion of a further disk fragment can also occur after a longer period of time. Reoperative discotomy in such cases is made more difficult by extensive epidural adhesions. Disk protrusions or prolapses that appear later in a different segment cannot be blamed on the primary operation and should not be labeled as "recurrences."

The literature contains many articles on recurrences after disk surgery: see, for example, De Palma and Rothman (1970), Thomalske and Schäfer (1973), Schneider and Rosenkranz (1974), Oppel and Schramm (1976), Thomalske et al. (1977), Krämer and Klein (1980), Wilkinson (1992), McCulloch (1998), and Krämer, Herdmann, and Krämer (2005).

Case Illustrations (from Krämer and Koster 2001)

1. L5/S1, Prolapse at the Disk Level (**Fig. 11.142**)

Clinical presentation. This 55-year-old man complained of very painful sciatica in the left S1 distribution, of 6 weeks' duration, refractory to orthopedic outpatient treatment with spinal analgesics. There was an ipsilateral postural deformity on forward bending. A band of pain and hypesthesia with formication was present on the lateral margin of the foot. The Achilles tendon reflex was absent on the left side, and the Lasègue sign was positive on the left at 40° and negative on the right.

MRI. See the study sequences in **Fig. 11.142.**

Findings. Left paramedial posterior displacement of disk tissue is seen. The dural sac is not compressed, because the vertebral canal is wide, but there is marked displacement of the left S1 nerve root, which is difficult to distinguish in the T1 and T2 images (→, **c, d**). The L5/S1 intervertebral disk makes broad-based contact with the nerve root (**a, b**).

Diagnosis. Large left paramedial intervertebral disk prolapse at L5/S1 without sequestration and with compression of the left S1 nerve root.

Treatment. The severe pain (the patient constantly required powerful analgesics, both day and night) and MRI findings demonstrating disk prolapse constituted an indication for surgery, which was scheduled for the next day during normal hours.

Operative findings. An interlaminar approach at L5/S1 was used. The ligamentum flavum lay in the middle of the surgical exposure, and the severely thickened S1 nerve root was immediately beneath it. The extruded disk tissue lay directly under the nerve root, part of it projecting into the root axilla. Part of the extruded disk was still located within the posterior confines of the disk space (grade IV dislocation). A fragment of the superior end plate was visible within the intraspinal portion of the prolapse. This fragment was in direct medial contact with the nerve root.

Histologic findings. Fragmented disk structures were found, consisting of 50% nucleus pulposus, 40% anulus fibrosus, and 10% superior end plate fragment.

Postoperative course. The patient was free of pain immediately postoperatively. Some residual formication was present on the lateral margin of the foot. There was hardly any need for postoperative analgesics.

Follow-up examination. Three months postoperatively, the patient remained free of symptoms except for formication on the lateral margin of the foot.

Comment. Severe pain due to nerve root compression by hard extruded fragments provided the surgical indication. Because of this compression by hard fragments, the patient still had paresthesia in the distal S1 dermatome postoperatively. In view of the clear clinical situation and MRI correlation, surgery could have been done earlier.

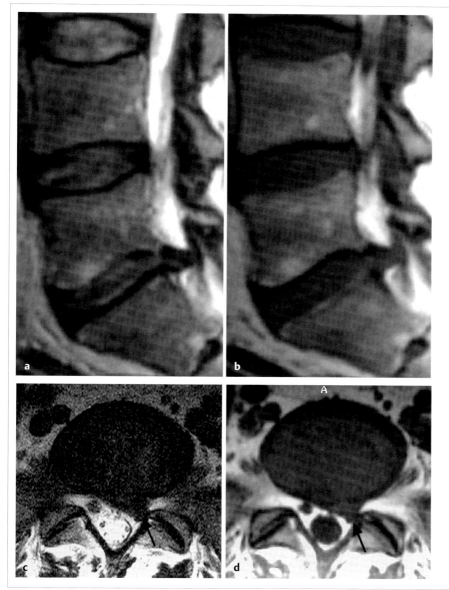

Fig. 11.142 a–d Study
sequences (from Krämer and
Köster 2001).
a T2 TSE, sagittal, left paramedial.
b T1 SE, sagittal, left paramedial.
c T2 TSE, axial, L5/S1.
d T1 TSE, axial, L5/S1.

11

2. L5/S1, Prolapse with Supradiscal Extension
(Fig. 11.143)

Clinical presentation. This 48-year-old woman had undergone surgery for an acute right-sided disk prolapse at L5/S1 (at disk level) 3 years previously. She presented a second time with acute pain radiating into her left leg, of 1 week's duration. The pain radiated across the buttocks to the posterolateral aspect of the left high. Examination revealed marked weakness in the left dorsiflexors, such that the patient was unable to walk on her heels (grade 3 weakness). There was an area of hypesthesia and hypalgesia corresponding to the left L5 dermatome. The Achilles tendon reflexes were symmetrically strong.

Electromyography. Abnormal spontaneous activity was found in the left L5 index muscles (tibialis anterior and extensor hallucis longus), with high potentials and no more than mild evidence of reinnervation, indicative of acute injury to the left L5 nerve root.

MRI. See the study sequences in **Fig. 11.143**.

Findings. Left cranial displacement of disk tissue originating from the L5/S1 disk is seen, with stenosis of the left L5/S1 intervertebral foramen (**a–d**). Demarcation is much less distinct in the T2 image (**a**, →) than in the T1 image (**b**, →), but the T2 image exhibits considerable motion artifact. The extruded tissue (→) is in contact with the left L5 spinal ganglion (>), which appears slightly swollen (**c, d**). No significant scarring is present from the prior disk surgery on the right side at L5/S1.

Diagnosis. Supradiscal, intraforaminal left L5/S1 disk prolapse.

Treatment. It was decided that immediate surgery was indicated because of the position of the herniated tissue with weakness of the dorsiflexors and signs of acute nerve root injury at electromyography.

Operative findings. The inferior margin of the L5 vertebral arch was removed to expose the supradiscal space. Findings superior to the last intervertebral disk included a supradiscal, lateral prolapse projecting into the intervertebral foramen, directly adjacent and inferior to the exiting left L5 nerve root.

Postoperative course. The patient was free of symptoms immediately postoperatively. The dorsiflexor weakness regressed during the first few days after surgery and was absent 3 months later.

Comment. Surgery was clearly indicated by the relatively acute dorsiflexor weakness, with evidence of acute denervation. The disk operation that had been done under the operating microscope 3 years earlier had evidently left no more than a few, barely visible contralateral changes. This effectively rendered the current operation equivalent to an initial intervention.

11

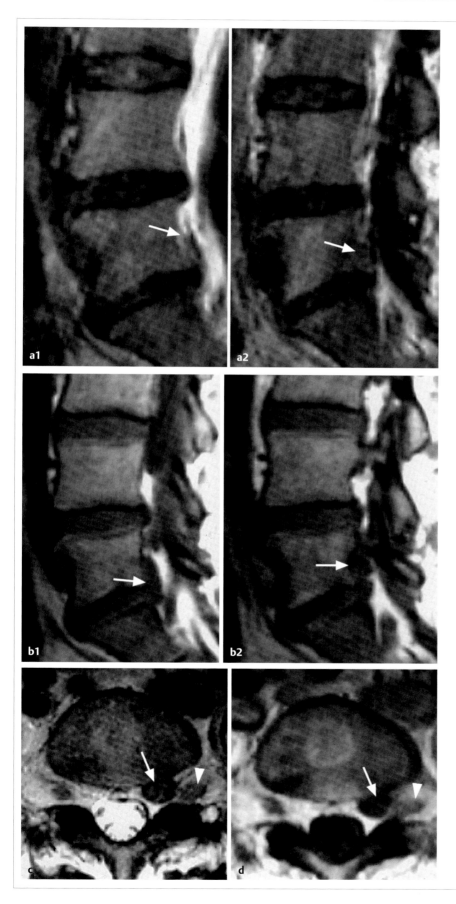

Fig. 11.143 a–d Study sequences (from Krämer and Köster 2001).
a T2 TSE, sagittal, left para-median (**a1**) and left lateral (**a2**).
b T1 SE, sagittal, left parame-dian (**b1**) and left lateral (**b2**).
c T2 TSE, axial, L5/S1.
d T1 SE, axial, L5/S1 after IV injection of gadolinium.

11

3. L5/S1, Prolapse with Infradiscal Extension
(**Fig. 11.144**)

Clinical presentation. This 55-year-old man had suffered for several years from low back pain and sciatica, occurring alternately on both sides, which had never been accompanied by weakness and had always been treated conservatively. He now complained of a new pain in the right posterior calf in an S1 dermatomal distribution, and weakness of plantar flexion on the right, of about 3 weeks' duration. On examination, he could not walk on tiptoe with the right foot, and the right Achilles tendon reflex was absent. There was hypesthesia on the lateral margin of the patient's right foot and the posterolateral aspect of the calf. The Lasègue sign was positive on the right at the end of the range of motion.

MRI. See the study sequences in **Fig. 11.144.**

Findings. Posterior to the first sacral vertebra, there is a soft tissue mass of inhomogeneous signal intensity that does not communicate with the L5/S1 intervertebral disk (**a, b,** →). There is marked compression of the dural sac and the right S1 nerve root, which is poorly visualized (**c, d,** →). All of the lumbar disks are of diminished height, and some of them exhibit marked protrusion. Disk degeneration and Modic type II bone marrow changes are present in the L4/5 segment. (P = prolapse.)

Diagnosis. A right paramedial infradiscal fragment is present at the S1 level; the parent intervertebral space cannot be identified with certainty. Several segments exhibit disk degeneration, with posterior and anterior protrusion and Modic type II bone marrow changes.

Treatment. The severe pain, paralysis of plantar flexion, and relatively large fragment in the sacral canal, with severe compression of the dural sac and a high risk of cauda equina syndrome, constituted an urgent indication for surgery, which was scheduled for the next day during normal hours.

Operative findings. The skin incision was centered 2 cm inferior to the marked disk level. A lateral flavectomy was carried out in the inferior portion of the interlaminar window. The superior margin of the sacrum was removed. Sequestrated disk tissue was found anterior to the ligamentum flavum and sacrum, and lateral and posterior to the S1 nerve root. The opening of the sacral canal on the right side was carried well inferior to the point of exit of the S1 nerve root. The S1 nerve root was found to be edematous, with bluish-red discoloration, over a length of more than 2 cm. The fragment lay well inferior to the L5/S1 intervertebral space. It was decided to remove the fragment without a discectomy at L5/S1 or at higher levels.

Histologic findings. The specimen consisted of fibrous cartilage with focal degenerative changes of intermediate severity. Focal areas of myxoid necrosis were present. The percentages of the various components were not analyzed.

Postoperative course. Leg pain was markedly diminished, but formication in the right S1 dermatome remained and was still present 3 months later. The sacral pain was unchanged.

Comment. This patient had suffered from disk-related symptoms in the lumbar spine for years, with sacral pain and sciatica occurring alternately on both sides. The symptoms became acutely severe when a large fragment was extruded into the vertebral canal on the right side at level L5/S1. This produced neurologic deficits relating to the right S1 nerve root. Surgery was indicated only for relief of the symptoms due to the fragment in the sacral canal. The MRI findings correlated with the clinical neurologic findings. The associated changes at levels L4/5 and L3/4 were not clinically relevant. The medial compression of the dural sac at level L4/5 demonstrated by MRI did not correlate with the patient's symptoms. Therefore, the decision was made not to undertake any surgical correction of levels L3/4 or L4/5, and the operation was limited to the removal of the fragment. Further correction would have produced epidural scarring, which, in combination with the protrusions at L3/4 and L4/5, might well have caused a worsening of symptoms postoperatively. The changes at levels L3/4 and L4/5 were managed conservatively, as before.

11

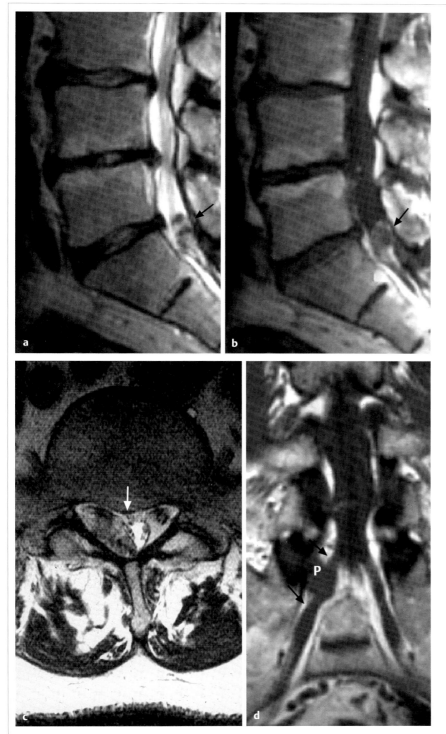

Fig. 11.144 a–d Study sequences (from Krämer and Köster 2001).

a T2 TSE, sagittal, right paramedian.

b T1 SE, sagittal, right paramedian.

c T2 TSE, axial, S1.

d T1 SE, coronal.

11

4. L5/S1, Prolapse with Infradiscal Extension and Cauda Equina Syndrome (**Fig. 11.145**)

Clinical presentation. This 37-year-old patient complained of severe pain in the left leg and less severe pain in the right leg, radiating across the posterolateral aspect of the leg to the heel. There was weakness of the urinary sphincter as well as "saddle" hypesthesia, more pronounced on the left side.

MRI. See the study sequences in **Fig. 11.145**.

Findings. Posteriorly displaced disk tissue is seen (**a, b, c1, d1**) which communicates with the parent disk (→). There is also sequestrated disk material (**a, b, c2, d2**) in the vertebral canal (>), extending inferiorly as far as the rudimentary S1–S2 intervertebral disk. The left S1 nerve root is markedly displaced and, in some images, poorly visualized (**c, d**). In **d2** the arrow (→) indicates the left S1 nerve root.

Diagnosis. Massive prolapse with sequestration at the infradiscal level of segment L5/S1, about 2 cm inferior to the disk space.

Note. The relatively high signal intensity in the T2 image suggests that the displaced material consists of nucleus pulposus tissue, or of inner portions of an anulus fibrosus that has not yet undergone marked degeneration.

Treatment. The presence of cauda equina syndrome constituted a surgical emergency, and the patient underwent immediate surgery.

Operative findings. A massive fragment was found in the sacral canal, medially displacing the dural sac. Portions of the fragment were situated directly beneath the ligamentum flavum.

Postoperative course. The cauda equina findings and leg pain subsided immediately postoperatively.

Comment. Emergency surgery was clearly indicated by the clinical findings. The MRI revealed the size of the fragment and thereby enabled this intervention to be done as a microsurgical procedure through a narrow exposure. The preoperative images clearly showed absence of disk-related pathology cranial to the L5/S1 disk level and thus obviated the need for exploration above this level.

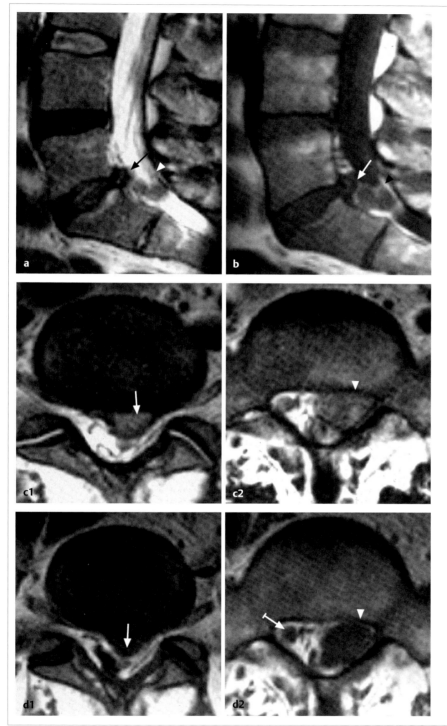

Fig. 11.145 a–d Study sequences (from Krämer and Köster 2001).
a T2 TSE, sagittal, paramedian.
b T1 SE, sagittal, paramedian.
c T2 TSE, axial, L5/S1 (**c1**) and at S1 superior end plate (**c2**).
d T1 SE, axial, L5/S1 (**d1**) and at S1 superior end plate (**d2**).

11

5. L4/5, Lateral Prolapse (Fig. 11.146)

Clinical presentation. This 66-year-old man complained of extremely severe pain in the lateral and anterior aspect of the right thigh, occasionally radiating into the shin. There was marked weakness of the right quadriceps, and the right patellar reflex was absent. A band of hypesthesia covered part of the right L4 and L5 dermatomes and corresponded to the area of the pain.

MRI. See the study sequences in **Fig. 11.146.**

Findings. The images demonstrate displacement of soft tissue from the intervertebral disk at L4/5 into the right lateral recess and intervertebral foramen at that level (**a–d**, →). The nerve root cannot be clearly identified (**a, b, d**), and the spinal ganglion (**c**, →) is displaced. There is lack of continuity of the displaced tissue with the L4/5 parent disk. The numbers 3, 4, and 5 indicate the corresponding lumbar nerve roots on the left side.

Diagnosis. Right L4/5 intervertebral disk prolapse with a foraminal, lateral, supradiscal fragment.

Treatment. Because of the severe pain and subacute quadriceps weakness, the patient was admitted for surgery, which was scheduled for the next day during normal hours.

Operative findings. Exposure was gained through a lateral intertransverse approach. A relatively solid extruded fragment was found at the supradiscal level, in the foramen, at the lateral inferior margin of the L4 vertebral body. The fragment had displaced the nerve root superiorly. After removal of the fragment, a marked indentation was seen in the nerve at the site of its previous compression. This indentation also involved the dorsal root ganglion.

Clinical course. The symptoms improved markedly immediately after surgery. A slight ache on the anterior aspect of the thigh persisted for several weeks. The quadriceps weakness resolved over time.

Comment. Surgery was recommended because of the severe pain and marked quadriceps weakness. As the weakness was several days old by the time of presentation, emergency intervention was not warranted, and the patient underwent surgery as a priority case the next day during normal hours.

11

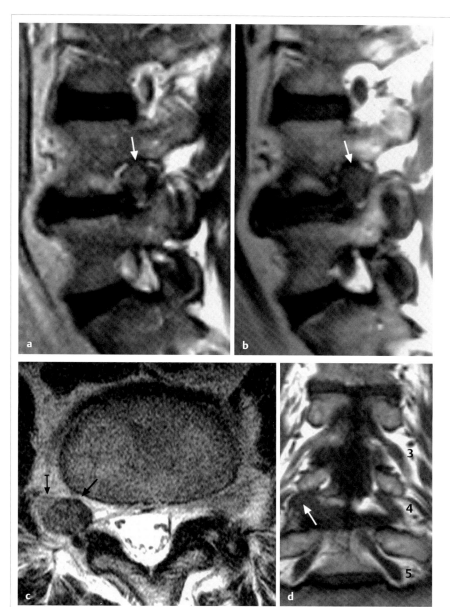

Fig. 11.146 a–d Study sequences (from Krämer and Köster 2001).
a T2 TSE, sagittal, right lateral.
b T1 SE, sagittal, right lateral.
c T2 TSE, axial, L4/5.
d T1 SE, coronal.

11

6. L3/4, Prolapse with Supradiscal Extension
(**Fig. 11.147**)

Clinical presentation. This 42-year-old woman complained of severe pain in the anterior aspect of her left thigh, radiating to the knee, which had arisen suddenly 4 days earlier and then persisted. She had no back pain. Examination revealed moderately limited mobility of the lumbar spine. There was a band of hypesthesia corresponding to the area of the pain, the left quadriceps was markedly paretic (grade 3 weakness), and the left patellar reflex was diminished.

MRI. See the study sequences in **Fig. 11.147.**

Findings. Degeneration of the lowest three intervertebral disks (**a**) is seen, with marked protrusion of the L4/5 disk and mild protrusion of the L5/S1 disk. A soft tissue mass of high signal intensity (>), located posterior to the L3 vertebral body, appears to maintain contact with the L3/4 intervertebral disk (**a, →**). The left L3/4 intervertebral foramen is completely occluded (**b, c, →**), and the dural sac is severely compressed. Marked peripheral enhancement of the soft tissue mass is seen after IV injection of gadolinium (**c**).

Diagnosis. Left L3/4 paramedial intervertebral disk prolapse with foraminal and supradiscal extension.

Treatment. Surgery was undertaken because of the quadriceps paresis, severe pain, and unequivocal, correlative MRI findings.

Operative findings. An interlaminar approach was used to expose a large fragment at the supradiscal level of segment L3/4 that severely compressed the dural sac and extended laterally into the L3/4 intervertebral foramen. The entire fragment was removed through the interlaminar approach.

Clinical course. The symptoms improved markedly after surgery. On discharge from the hospital, the patient still had formication in the anterior aspect of the thigh. The strength in the quadriceps had improved, but was still noticeably impaired. The left patellar reflex was absent.

Comment. Surgery was undertaken on the basis of the unequivocal MRI findings corresponding to the clinical symptoms and signs. Although the prolapse extended into the intervertebral foramen, an initial interlaminar approach was chosen, because the main mass of the prolapse was located within the vertebral canal. A second, intertransverse approach should be considered in such cases if a satisfactory removal of the foraminal portion of the fragment appears not to be feasible.

11

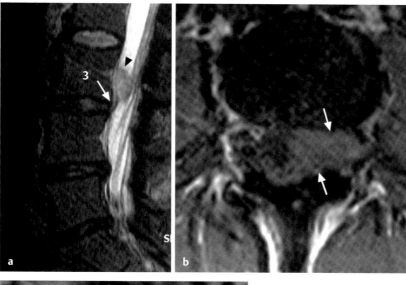

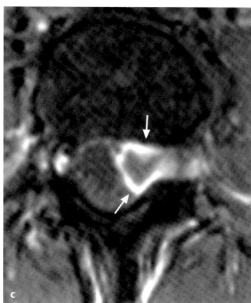

Fig. 11.147 a–c Study sequences (from Krämer and Köster 2001).
a T2 TSE, sagittal, left paramedian.
b FLASH, axial, inferior end plate of vertebra L3.
c FLASH, axial, inferior end plate of vertebra L3, fat-saturated, with IV injection of gadolinium.

11

Summary: Open Disk Surgery

Of all operations carried on the spine, open decompression of a lumbar nerve root after a disk herniation is currently the most important and the most commonly undertaken. Despite all the advances in conservative and minimally invasive treatment of spinal disorders, there are still absolute and relative indications for the removal of a herniated disk from the spinal canal through a posterior approach.

The indication for open surgery depends on clinical criteria. The symptoms and signs are rated with special scores for the degree of pain and paresis, and these scores must be well correlated with the radiological findings. Psychological factors (yellow flags) must be given due consideration. Proper patient selection for open lumbar disk surgery is the decisive factor for the success of the operation.

There is a clear trend toward the use of the microsurgical technique, even though it has not been shown unequivocally that this yields better results than the previously conventional technique—understandably, there are no prospective randomized studies. Microsurgery places high demands on the operating team both in the planning of the procedure and in its execution.

Opening the spinal canal to decompress nerve roots can lead to complications and cannot be considered minor surgery. Intra- and postoperative complications, when they occur, require special management.

In disk surgery, large amounts of disk tissue are removed and the osmotic system of the disk is disrupted. This has implications for postoperative management, which must therefore be carried out under the supervision of an experienced physician and according to the specific paradigm discussed in this chapter.

Conclusion

The open surgical treatment of lumbar intervertebral disk herniations can be expected to yield satisfactory results if it is undertaken for correct indications and the pre-, intra- and postoperative care is delivered according to the appropriate professional standards.

Post-discotomy Syndrome

! **Definition:** The term "post-discotomy syndrome (PDS)" designates all persistent and severe symptoms in the aftermath of open lumbar disk surgery (discotomy) that are attributable to segmental instability and adhesions in the spinal canal.

The alternative designations "post-nucleotomy syndrome" and "post-laminectomy syndrome" are not quite accurate, as it is not always just the nucleus pulposus that is removed at the initial operation, nor is a laminectomy necessarily carrie dout. The English-language literature generally uses the term "failed back surgery syndrome" (Burton et al. 1981) or "failed spine" (Boden and Bohlman 2003, Szpalski and Gunzburg 2005). Wilkinson (1992) made a case for the designation "failed back syndrome," arguing that this complex of symptoms need not always be produced by a prior operation that went awry; it can also develop after an operation that went well. Nonetheless, PDS can be expected to be more frequent after procedures that are complicated by bleeding and injuries to the dura mater and nerve roots.

Both retrospective and prospective studies show that 3–14% of all patients undergoing disk surgery later develop such severe symptoms that a further operation is necessary (Spangford 1972, Cauchoix 1978, Shaw et al. 1978, Wilkinson and Schuman 1979, Lewis et al. 1987, Waddell and Reilly 1988, Cooper et al. 1991, McCulloch 1998, Herkowicz 2004, Krämer, Herdmann, and Krämer 2005, Martin et al. 2007).

Etiology and pathogenesis. Whenever disk tissue is surgically removed, two major changes occur in the motion segment (**Fig. 11.148**):
- slackening and loss of height of the intervertebral space through loss of disk tissue
- the development of adhesions (scarring) in the area of surgery.

The extent of postoperative scarring (e. g., epidural and intrathecal) largely depends on the patient's intrinsic tendency toward scar formation. Exogenous factors such as traumatic surgery and suboptimal postoperative care can also promote scarring.

PDS arises only when the factors depicted in **Fig. 11.148** are all simultaneously present and operate in synergy. *A symptom complex such as that seen in PDS has so far never been observed after conservative treatment or the use of minimally invasive techniques.* Nor is scarring

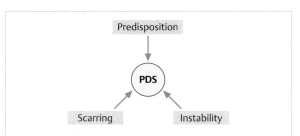

Fig. 11.148   The pathogenesis of post-discotic syndrome.

alone sufficient to cause PDS when the patient is not intrinsically disposed to it and when there is no instability. There are still patients who remain asymptomatic after extensive, multisegmental laminectomy and correspondingly extensive scar formation.

Postoperative instability. Perforation of the anulus fibrosus and removal of disk tissue from the intervertebral space, either spontaneously by herniation or through surgical extraction, disrupts the integrity of the disk as an osmotic system. Loss of height and elasticity adversely affect its biomechanical properties. Relatively rapid loss of height increases the transmission of force to the intervertebral joints, which become telescoped into each other. At the same time, the lateral recess of the spinal canal narrows at the site where the nerve roots run vertically and then exit from the canal horizontally. Lateral recess stenosis arises or becomes worse if it is already present. Instability, in turn, leads to the formation of bony appositions on the edges of the vertebral bodies and the intervertebral joint facets; these bony appositions also narrow the residual space available for the neural elements in the spinal canal, causing **spinal canal stenosis.**

This step-by-step process of loss of disk height, formation of bony appositions, and narrowing of the spinal canal is part of the normal, age-related ("degenerative") development of the lumbar spine and as such generally causes no symptoms. Our studies of the aging spine with plain radiographs and CT in individuals with and without symptoms have confirmed this fact. After the surgical removal of a large part of a disk, however, analogous changes occur very rapidly, so that the joint capsules and neural structures lack the time to adapt.

Scarring. All of these pathoanatomical changes in the motion segment after disk degeneration and postoperative deformation would be of less clinical significance were it not for the additional contribution of adhesions (scarring) to the narrowing of the spinal canal. Scar forms after surgery of any type, including disk surgery.

! Depending on the extent of the surgical intervention, a
• greater or lesser degree of scarring develops in the operative field through connective-tissue organization of the residual blood and serous fluid in the wound. This scarring involves the dura mater and the nerve roots as well.

We have seen by endoscopic inspection that patients with PDS have postoperative adhesions and connective tissue strands in the subarachnoid space as well (Krämer and Klein 1980). The pathoanatomical development of these changes begins with local aseptic arachnoiditis and radiculitis and then progresses to adhesive arachnoiditis and perineural fibrosis surrounding the nerve root, constricting the nerve fibers and leaving them very little residual space.

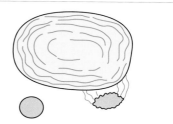

Fig. 11.149 The postoperative adhesion fastening the nerve root to the disk makes the nerve root sensitive to even the least change of disk volume or consistency.

Epidural scarring can take the form of broad adhesions between the nerve root and the adjacent bone in the lateral recess, but it can also appear as connective tissue strands looping around the nerve roots in a type of harness that strangulates them when certain types of movement are performed. In addition to the dura mater and spinal nerves, the epidural venous plexuses are also affected by scarring and develop varicose enlargements. Postoperatively, epidural fat is also lacking in the wound. The epidural fat normally serves as a friction-reducing layer that permits easy movement.

Rigid scar tissue fastening the nerve roots to the surrounding tissues fundamentally alters the state of the motion segments. The L5 and S1 roots, which are normally able to slide over the dorsal portion of the corresponding disks during movement, may now be stuck to the disks instead. This anchoring by scar tissue transmits every alteration of the shape and consistency of the disk to the already irritated nerve root (**Fig. 11.149**).

! Even small intradiscal tissue displacements that would
• have caused no more than transient lumbago in the patient's previous, nonoperated condition can now induce very severe radicular symptoms and neurological deficits.

Perineural fibrosis in the dorsal portion of the spinal canal is also problematic. Adhesions between the nerve roots and their bony surroundings in the lateral recess and the intervertebral foramen hinder the normal sliding of the roots with each movement. Any already existing asymptomatic spinal stenosis, on either a congenital or a degenerative basis, can become symptomatic through the additional factor of scarring.

Why does PDS not develop after every discotomy?
The occurrence of PDS depends not only on the factors mentioned above, both endogenous (predisposition) and exogenous (the trauma of surgery), but also on the configuration of scarring and on the overall condition of the motion segment. Scar tissue forms after all operations, without exception, but usually leaves enough

11

Table 11.40 Manifestations of post-discotic syndrome

- Bilateral mixed radicular and pseudoradicular signs
- Bilaterally positive Lasègue sign
- Inability to incline the trunk or to sit with legs extended
- Myelography: nerve root sleeve cutoff and narrowing of the dural sac
- CT/MRI: epidural scarring

room for the neural structures in the spinal canal. The excursions of movement in the postoperative motion segment are not large enough to induce pulling on the nerve roots by scar tissue. Wilkinson (1992) pointed out that some patients with "failed back syndrome" already had arachnoiditis simulating the symptoms of a disk prolapse long before they underwent disk surgery. In our experience, however, such patients are rare and are presumably suffering from another condition that must be considered in the differential diagnosis of PDS.

Clinical features. After operations that have been carried out without complication, the typical symptoms of PDS tend to arise after an asymptomatic interval of several months. The scars must first solidify before they can cause symptoms. Moreover, the patient becomes more and more mobile over the course of normal recovery from the operation, so that postoperative instability does not make itself felt until a certain period of time has elapsed. On the other hand, after operations that have been complicated by extensive bleeding and injuries of the dura mater and nerve roots, symptoms may arise immediately after surgery and immediately develop into the symptom complex of PDS.

PDS is characterized by bilateral, mixed radicular and pseudoradicular manifestations (**Table 11.40**). Often, multiple nerve roots are involved. Neurologic deficits, if present, are attributable to the operation itself and cannot necessarily be considered a part of the PDS. Severe neurological problems are rare. The nerve roots are strangulated by strands of connective tissue, but nonetheless they are not fully cut off. In our follow-up studies of PDS patients, we did not find any cases of cauda equina syndrome due to scarring, even though the dural sac was often considerably narrowed.

The pseudoradicular component results from segmental instability with ensuing irritation of the intervertebral joint capsules and from irritation of the meningeal and dorsal branches of the spinal nerve. The nerve roots are fastened to the adjoining tissues and do not allow the patient much room to move without pain.

! The strands of connective tissue around the dura mater and nerve roots can be compared to bell-ropes that are activated whenever the patient makes an unthinking movement.

Any larger movement considerably distorts the nerve and induces inflammatory root swelling, which then further narrows the residual space available within the spinal canal. A vicious circle is set up that mainly limits the sliding of the sciatic nerve roots when the patient bends forward; the limitation can also be observed when the patient raises the extended leg or sits up with the legs extended. In severe cases of PDS, the Lasègue sign is present with the leg elevated as little as 10–20°. The dura mater and nerve roots often have so little ability to slide within the spinal canal that the typical symptoms can even be elicited by inclination of the head. Patients with severe PDS after multiple disk operations are markedly impaired in their ability to function in everyday life. They cannot sit, stand, or lie normally. Because they usually do not have a severe neurologic deficit, they are often wrongly held to be malingering or exaggerating their symptoms because of psychological overlay. In our study, we found that patients with PDS were no more likely than other individuals to suffer from underlying mental illness.

It is often difficult to distinguish a possible recurrent disk herniation from scar tissue in the operated area by **CT scan,** even with the most modern apparatus. Both involve tissue of the same radiodensity. The injection of contrast medium enables the distinction to be made, but only when the recurrent herniation is fresh (enhancement): the well-perfused scar tissue takes up more contrast medium than the nonperfused disk tissue. With time, the prolapse undergoes connective-tissue organization, and this distinction is lost. An **MRI** scan with the injection of gadolinium-containing contrast medium is the best technique for distinguishing scarring from recurrent or residual disk herniation. Capillaries in the scar tissue take up more contrast medium than the nonperfused prolapsed disk tissue (**Fig. 11.150**).

When CT and MRI scans are done a long time after surgery, a conglomerate with the grayish signal intensity of disk tissue is usually seen on the operated side, extending without interruption from the disk to the dural sac. There is no epidural fat at these levels. Displacement of the dural sac and nerve roots at adjacent levels may be an indication of pulling by scar.

The following general rule applies especially to postoperative CT and MRI scans:

! The decisive factors for diagnosis and for treatment planning are the severity of the patient's symptoms and the clinical manifestations, rather than the radiological findings (in PDS).

Extensive scarring that causes marked changes in the myelographic, CT, or MR image may be associated with only mild symptoms, e. g., when the second pathogenetic component—instability—is absent because the segment has become immobile. This is the state that regularly arises in normal aging; thus, all patients with PDS can be told that improvement is expected with time (Willburger 2004).

Conversely, even a few strands of scar tissue that are barely visible in the myelographic, CT, or MR image can be associated with severe symptoms if they pull the nerve roots in an unfavorable direction.

Degrees of severity. The severity of PDS is judged above all by the subjective impairment that it causes. Objective criteria, such as neurologic deficits and the degree of scarring and/or instability, are not necessarily the primary considerations for medicolegal assessment or for determining the indications for a fusion procedure. Patients must therefore be seen multiple times and carefully observed by more than one examiner so that the actual degree of severity of their symptoms can be accurately defined. The straight-leg raising test in the lying and sitting positions is relatively reliable, as is observation of the patient while sitting with the legs extended, while taking shoes and socks off, and while bending forward to perform other tasks (**Table 11.41**).

Treatment. The initial mainstays of treatment are simple methods of pain relief such as analgesics, anti-inflammatories, and heat application. Massage and traction should be used sparingly, because movement causes repetitive irritation of strangulated nerve roots. Local injection treatment is better than systemic anti-inflammatory therapy because it can exert a direct local influence on the aseptic inflammatory pathogenetic process. As long as there is no medical contraindication, we recommend epidural and intrathecal cortisone applications with a depot preparation (triamcinolone crystalline suspension or anti-IL). The epidural injection must be one or two segments higher or through the sacral canal, because the epidural space at the level of surgery may well be occluded by scar. A direct effect on the constricted, edematous nerve root can be gained by

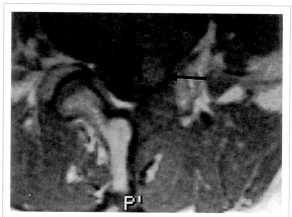

Fig. 11.150 Recurrent disk prolapse (→) within scar tissue at the discal level of a previously operated segment.

epidural, perineural injection of steroids or anti-IL by an interlaminar approach. Intradiscal injections can be considered if the postoperative CT or MRI still shows broad-based indentations in the dural sac caused by disk protrusions.

In cases of persistent pain arising mainly from the dorsal and meningeal branches of the spinal nerve, a trial of transcutaneous electrical nerve stimulation (TENS) or epidural spinal electrostimulation (ESES) is justified.

In order to address the second pathogenetic component of PDS, i. e., instability, treatment with a truncal orthosis can be tried. The flexion orthoses depicted on page 226, which reduce the mechanical stress on the dorsal portion of the motion segment, appear to be suitable for this purpose. In parallel, we recommend isometric stabilizing exercises proceeding from the stress-reducing position.

There has been no lack of attempts to help patients with PDS by undertaking additional surgery. The break-

Table 11.41 Post-discotic syndrome: degrees of severity

Grade	Pain	Lasègue	Medications	Functional impairment	Medicolegal assessment	Degree of disability
1	None at rest, mild on exertion	-	Sometimes	Limited ability to do hard physical labor and high-performance sports	Capable of working but not of hard physical labor	< 20 %
2	Mild at rest, severe on exertion	+	Generally mild medications, sometimes stronger ones	Cannot do any work that places a load on the spine, cannot participate in sports	Often unable to work; cannot work in a given occupation if it involves loading of the spine	30–80 %
3	Severe, continuous pain	+ at < 30°	Continuous need for strong medication	Cannot walk except with an accessory device or another individual to help	Unable to work	100 %

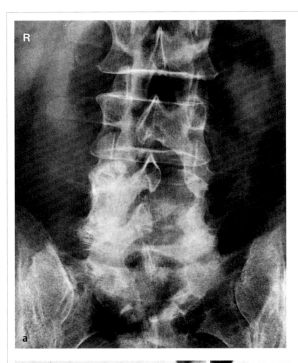

Fig. 11.151 a–d   Clinical findings: 46-year-old man with PDS after three disk operations because of scar-related pain; left L4 and L5 hemilaminectomy with fat-pad graft, persistent symptoms afterward. Treatment plan: test application of a truncal cast, spondylodesis if this brings about mild improvement.
a Anteroposterior plain radiograph of the lumbar spine: status post left L4 and L5 hemilaminectomy with removal of medial portions of the facets.
b–d CT: Status post left L4 and L5 hemilaminectomy with fat-pad graft. Fatty tissue (black) is seen dorsally within the postoperative scar. The dural sac, left S1 root, and bony wall of the spinal canal are still adherent to one another in the left lateral recess.

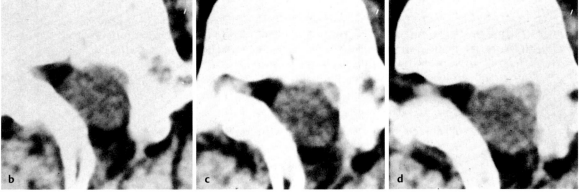

ing-up of scar tissue adhesions and the painstaking dissection of nerve roots free of the surrounding scar, known as radiculolysis, brings only transient improvement, if any. New scar tissue arises that is usually even more extensive than before. The patient's condition worsens after each new operation.

If reoperation is truly necessary, e. g., because of a recurrent disk herniation, we recommend taking a pad of subcutaneous fat and laying it on the exposed dura mater and nerve roots just before closing the wound. The purpose of this is to prevent adhesions (Kirkcaldy-Willis 1988). Experimental and CT follow-up studies have shown that most of the transplanted fatty tissue remains vital and leaves behind a mobile scar (Krämer and Klein 1980, Schroeder 1983, van Akkerveeken 1984,

Burton 1984, Gill 1984, Krempen 1984, Langenskiöld and Valle 1985, Krämer, Herdmann, and Krämer 2005). Despite the impressive CT images showing preserved fatty tissue (**Fig. 11.151**), however, the clinical results are not as good as might be expected, and this is especially true in PDS. The patient's symptoms often persist. The attempt to make all of the scar-tissue adhesions, particularly those between the disk and the nerve roots, adequately and permanently mobile evidently cannot succeed.

Although the attempt to eliminate one pathogenetic component of PDS—recurrent scar formation—often seems to be a vain enterprise, a fusion procedure (spondylodesis) to eliminate the second component—instability—promises greater success.

! Bony fusion of the lower lumbar motion segments reduces the degree of relative motion between the spinal canal and the adherent nerve roots.

Nonetheless, the displacement of the nerve roots in the Lasègue test and by straight-leg raising is not changed after a lumbar fusion (Smith et al. 1993) (**Table 11.42**).

Furthermore, when fusion is combined with distraction of the dorsal portions of the motion segments, it yields an additional widening of the spinal canal and the intervertebral foramina, making more room available for the nerve roots. Most patients with PDS can expect their symptoms to improve after a lumbosacral distraction spondylodesis. About 10%, however, have unchanged symptoms afterward. With all of the available treatment methods taken together, including surgery, patients can only be offered a chance of improvement, rather than cure; most patients are ready to accept this, in view of the degree of pain they are already suffering. This underscores the importance of prevention of PDS.

Prophylaxis and course. The number of patients who remain unsatisfied after surgery is so large that many attempts have been made over the years to reduce the degree of postoperative scarring in the spinal canal. Early or late mobilization of the patient and the routine application of truncal casts or orthoses were found to make no difference. Membranes of synthetic material (Gelfoam) and the systemic or local application of cortisone were also found to have no effect on perineural adhesions. Our prospective randomized trial revealed no benefit from the intraoperative application of a crystalline suspension of cortisone in the epidural space and the affected nerve root sleeves (Vent et al. 1977).

! One reliable way of keeping the formation of scar after surgery to a minimum is to keep the operation itself as small and atraumatic as possible.

For discotomy, this means using a microsurgical technique after unequivocal preoperative determination of the segment to be operated on. Surgical trauma to the tissues dorsal to the dura mater and nerve roots that must be traversed as part of the operative approach should be kept to an absolute minimum. Epidural veins should be preserved and retracted to one side like nerve roots, so that both hemorrhage and electrocoagulation can be avoided. Epidural fat, too, should be spared as far as possible. If a second decompressive operation should nevertheless become necessary, e. g., to free the nerve root after lateral recess stenosis has developed, we recommend the insertion of an epidural fat pad, as in the radiculolysis procedure.

The most important means of preventing PDS remains the correct determination of the indications for the initial disk operation. The studies by Spangfort (1972), McCulloch (1998), and Krämer, Herdmann, and

Table 11.42 Treatment of post-discotic syndrome

Conservative	*Operative*
▪ Physiotherapeutic exercises ▪ Back school ▪ Flexion orthosis ▪ Local injections	▪ Neurolysis with fat-pad graft ▪ Fusion surgery with or without spinal nerve decompression

Krämer (2005) unequivocally showed that postoperative symptoms are much more likely to arise when no more than a disk protrusion, or no disk abnormality whatsoever, is found at the initial operation. An unsatisfactory intraoperative finding necessitates widening the operative field to include the neighboring levels; this, in turn, leads to more extensive scarring than after a simple, monosegmental removal of sequestrated disk tissue.

The natural course of disk prolapse disease is characterized by spontaneous shrinking of the displaced disk tissue and adaptation of the affected nerve root; significant improvement, sometimes even cure, are the universal result if enough time and patience are brought to bear. When conservative measures, are used, the symptom complex of PDS cannot arise.

Conclusion

If no severe, acute neurologic deficit is present, and doubt remains about the indication for surgery, then the patient should not be operated on. Patients who do not undergo discotomy cannot develop PDS.

Fusion Procedures

! **Definition:** A fusion, or stabilization, procedure on the spine is also termed "spondylodesis" and can be done dorsally, ventrally, or both in a combined procedure (so-called 360° spondylodesis). These procedures can be undertaken with and without the implantation of stabilizing material (see **Fig. 11.152**).

Indications and Contraindications

The endeavor to stabilize degeneratively slackened motion segments with a fusion procedure is as old as the recognition of the pathoanatomical processes involved in disk degeneration itself. Thus, for as long as the surgical treatment of lumbar syndrome has been an issue, various types of stabilizing procedure have been considered alongside surgery on the disk itself (discotomy). A prolapse operation—the most common type of surgical intervention in the lumbar spine—removes the cause of nerve root compression; it does not, however, address

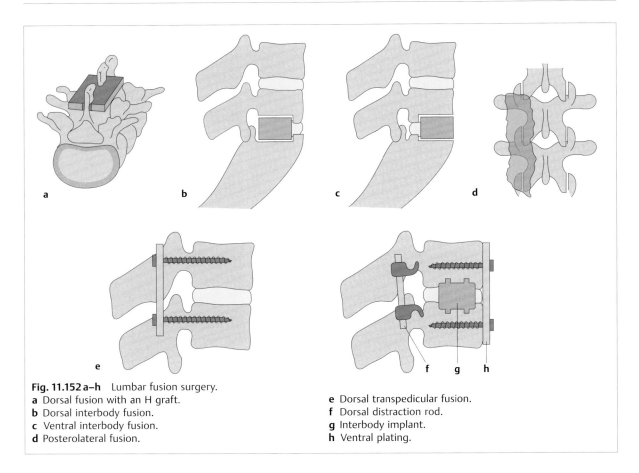

Fig. 11.152 a–h   Lumbar fusion surgery.
a Dorsal fusion with an H graft.
b Dorsal interbody fusion.
c Ventral interbody fusion.
d Posterolateral fusion.
e Dorsal transpedicular fusion.
f Dorsal distraction rod.
g Interbody implant.
h Ventral plating.

the other component of the disease process, namely, the instability of the motion segment due to loss of elasticity, which is actually worsened by partial removal of the disk. Local radicular and pseudoradicular symptoms arise that may not be controllable by conservative means but can be improved by a fusion procedure. Alternatively, an artificial lumbar disk (mobile prosthesis) can be implanted to preserve the mobility of the motion segment.

A lumbar fusion operation is clearly indicated (see **Table 11.43**) in certain kinds of spinal condition not affecting the intervertebral disks, e. g., symptomatic spondylolisthesis that does not respond to conservative treatment, unstable fractures, and neoplasia affecting the spine (where fusion is carried out palliatively). As far as disk disease is concerned, a diagnosis of lumbar instability is insufficient by itself to justify doing a spinal fusion, which is a very demanding procedure. The severity of symptoms and the clinical and radiological findings must be taken into account, and alternative means of treatment must be considered, including intensive physiotherapy for the truncal musculature, temporary wearing of a corset, and the exhaustion of all conservative therapeutic modalities. Psychosocial factors (yellow flags) should be taken into account; we consider them contraindications for fusion. The indication for a lumbar fusion in a patient with disk disease can only be established after the patient has been extensively interviewed and examined—in the best case, after several days of observation in the hospital before surgery. During this time, preoperative procedures can be carried out, including for example the determination of the proper segment for surgery by means of discography and radiculography. The segments adjacent to the area of the intended fusion should be studied by MRI and, when indicated, by discography. Finally, the patient should temporarily wear a truncal cast that also prevents movement of the thigh on the side of the predominant radiating pain, in order to determine whether trial

Table 11.43 Indications for lumbar fusion surgery in disk disease

- Severe pain
- No psychosocial abnormality
- Identifiable unstable segment
- Neighboring segments normal
- Symptoms improved by wearing a cast that immobilizes the leg and pelvis
- Stabilizing portions of the lamina were removed in a prior decompressive operation

immobilization (or partial immobilization) of the lumbar spine yields any benefit. Testing with external fixation is more informative, but also much more demanding.

The contraindications (**Table 11.44**) can be inferred from the above discussion of the indications. Symptoms that are only moderately severe do not justify an invasive fusion procedure and should instead be treated conservatively. Psychosocial factors (yellow flags, see p. 198 and **Table 11.8**) should be absent; their presence guarantees the persistence of symptoms postoperatively. In particular, patients for whom the medicolegal issue of compensation has not yet been resolved should not undergo a fusion procedure. The integrity of the adjacent segments is often difficult to assess, and the surgeon can thus be tempted to fuse more segments than necessary; this is known to yield poorer results. It is hoped that mobile disk prostheses will not have any adverse mechanical effect on the adjacent segments, but this has not yet been demonstrated. Further criteria of exclusion are a negative cast test (see above) and osteoporosis in an elderly patient.

Fusion Techniques

Implant-free Techniques

Ventral interbody spondylodesis (**Fig. 11.152c**) has not gained general acceptance as a single procedure because of a high rate of pseudarthrosis leading to a poor clinical outcome. Posterolateral fusion with pieces of autologous cancellous bone (**Fig. 11.152d**) is in wide use; this operation is also, in fact, the actual "fusion" component of dorsal fusion procedures with instrumentation. In posterolateral fusion, autologous cancellous bone is taken from the iliac crest and inserted in a prepared site between the transverse processes and joint processes, including the intervertebral joints. Instrumented components of fusion procedures are intended only as temporarily stabilizing measures until the bone graft solidifies in place. The use of osteoinductive substances such as bone morphogenetic proteins has helped implant-free posterolateral fusion to acquire a new popularity.

In lumbosacral distraction spondylodesis (LSDS, **Figs. 11.153, 11.154**), a posterolateral fusion is combined with of an interspinous H-shaped bone graft (**Fig. 11.152a**) (Krämer et al. 1984, Wittenberg et al. 1990, 1993).

Fusion Techniques with Implants (Instrumentation)

- **Dorsal** instrumented fusion usually involves the implantation of internal fixator rods bearing transpedicular screws.
- **Interbody fusion.** Two vertebral bodies can be fused to each other through a variety of approaches and techniques.

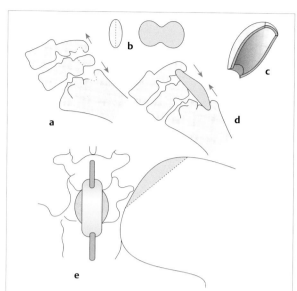

Fig. 11.153 a–e Lumbosacral distraction spondylodesis with cortical-cancellous bone graft from the posterior iliac crest. The L4 and S1 spinous processes are grooved to create an acceptor site for the bone graft (**a**). The L5 spinous process is split down to its base; its two halves are turned down to either side to form a bed for the bone graft (**b**). The graft is notched with a Luer rongeur at its upper and lower ends (**c**) and then solidly inserted between L4 and S1 (**d**). Additionally, a bilateral posterolateral fusion is carried out (**e**).

Table 11.44 Contraindications to lumbar fusion in disk disease

- Only moderate symptoms
- Yellow flags
- Symptomatic segment cannot be precisely identified
- Negative cast test
- Osteoporosis, advanced age

The ventral portion of the lumbar spine is reached through a ventral transperitoneal (or, better, retroperitoneal) approach. This is considered the standard approach, offering the widest possible exploration. This type of procedure is commonly known as anterior lumbar interbody fusion (ALIF). The intervertebral space is bridged with bi- or tricortical bone grafts, which can be either autologous or homologous. Alternatively, metallic interposed elements of various types can be used (see **Fig. 11.152g**).

In posterior lumbar interbody fusion (PLIF), the intervertebral space is entered by a posterior approach after laminectomy and facetectomy. Here, too, either autologous bone grafts or metallic interposed elements, so-called "cages," can be used (**Figs. 11.155, 11.156**).

11

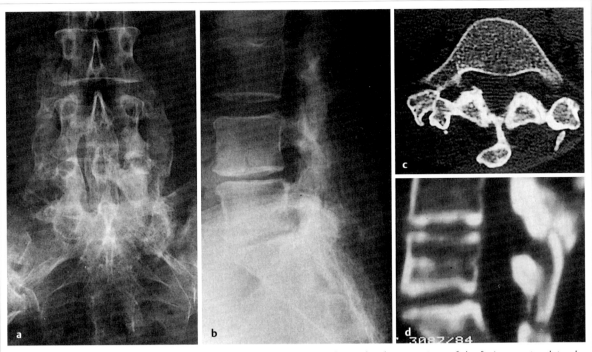

Fig. 11.154 a–d Lumbosacral distraction spondylodesis with autologous bone graft and posterolateral fusion.

   a, b A triple fusion is seen: posterolateral, intertransverse, and the bone graft from L4 to S1.

c CT shows the three portions of the fusion, posterolateral and dorsal–interspinous.

d Lateral reconstruction.

Complications

After the customary initial euphoria, the difficulties of fusion procedures on the lumbar spine involving implants were soon recognized (Haaker 2004). There are the expected general complications of relatively demanding and invasive surgery, including wound-healing disturbances, transfusion-related complications, and thromboembolism; there are also complications of the fusion itself, which are listed in **Table 11.45**. The implanted fusion material can break because of primary excessive stress on the implant or because of secondary excessive stress developing because of the failure of a bony fusion to solidify ("take"). The implant-associated risks of faulty pedicle screw placement, leading to fusion of the segment in an improper position and/or neurological complications, are among the causes of early failures of this type of surgery. The rate of pseudarthrosis is lower than that of the implant-free techniques, but it is not zero, and extensive reoperations or reinforcing ventral fusion procedures are sometimes necessary.

Soon after the introduction of these techniques with implants, the first studies were published demonstrating the increased likelihood of the development of disease in the segments immediately above and below a monosegmental fusion (Schlegel et al. 1996, Haaker 2004). The important findings included the development of instability ranging to spondylolisthesis, spinal canal stenosis, and so-called stress shielding in the adjacent segments.

Table 11.45 Causes of symptoms after lumbar fusion surgery
▪ Residual symptoms after prior disk surgery (PDS)
▪ Infection
▪ Pseudarthrosis
▪ Segment fused in improper position
▪ Implantation error
▪ Neurologic deficit
▪ Implant fracture
▪ Implant intolerance
▪ Post-fusion syndrome

Table 11.46 Post-fusion syndrome in the lumbar spine

- Instability of segment(s) adjacent to fusion
- Sacroiliac joint symptoms
- Scar problems

Post-fusion syndrome

! **Definition:** The term "post-fusion syndrome" refers to fusion-specific symptoms that can arise even after a successful fusion procedure (**Table 11.46**).

Altered spinal statics and dynamics after fusion. The L4/5 and L5/S1 segments are exposed to considerable static and dynamic stress even in their normal state. This is why, for example, these two segments manifest signs of wear and tear earlier than other segments. After a surgical procedure in which these two segments are anatomically and functionally fused with the sacrum, their biomechanical tasks must be assumed by the neighboring segments and by the sacroiliac joints. Visible and symptomatic degenerative changes in the segment just above the intended fusion are a contraindication to lumbar spondylodesis unless the fusion is extended to include that segment as well. Imaging techniques including dynamic plain radiographs in flexion and extension ("function studies") and discography usually enable visualization of these degenerative changes. Sometimes, however, incipient degenerative changes are not visible; much more commonly, they

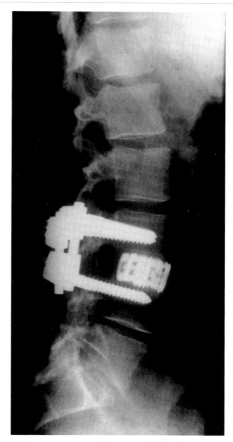

Fig. 11.155 Dorsoventral fusion with dorsal internal fixator rod and ventral titanium cage.

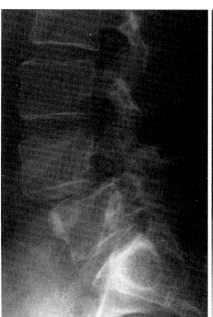
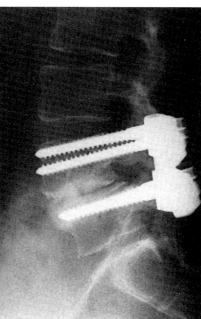

Fig. 11.156 Degenerative spondylolisthesis at L4/5 in a 55-year-old man with increasing neurological manifestations relating to the L4 and L5 nerve roots bilaterally. Instrumented dorsal fusion and additional ventral fusion with autologous bone span.

11

develop only in response to the greater biomechanical demands occasioned by fusion surgery. If, for example, one or more segments above L5/S1 are fused, then the L5/S1 segment is placed under greater than normal biomechanical stress. This situation is called a **floating fusion** (i.e., a fusion with mobile segments above and below).

Segmental instability adjacent to a fusion manifests itself as a facet syndrome with band-like pain at the level of surgery. Function studies in maximal flexion and extension may reveal hypermobility; MRI shows rolling out of the anulus fibrosus. The diagnosis is finally established with test infiltrations of the facets and—if the discogenic component is most prominent—with discography, in which the patient's typical symptoms can be reproduced ("memory pain").

Degenerative changes after fusion surgery are about as common as in normal, asymptomatic individuals who have not undergone any surgery. Furthermore, most degenerative changes after fusion surgery are found at multiple levels, or at levels not adjacent to the fusion; thus, these changes are more likely due to constitutional factors than to increased stress arising from the fusion (Wai et al. 2006).

The many types of artificial disk prosthesis that have been developed represent an attempt to circumvent the problem of segmental pathology adjacent to a fusion.

Sacroiliac joints. Uni- or bilateral sacroiliac joint pain can arise after fusion of the lower lumbar motion seg-ments and is usually felt especially severely upon axial loading of the spine. Local test injections point the way to the appropriate treatment.

Scars. Unlike microsurgical lumbar disk surgery, lumbar fusion inevitably results in extensive scarring. Conventional dorsal fusion with or without instrumentation leaves a large bilateral scar; if the fusion is carried out after a previous disk operation, as is commonly the case, this scar extends all the way from the epidural space to the skin. The scar tissue encases not just the surgically traumatized musculature, but also divided or compressed portions of the dorsal branch of the spinal nerve. After a pain-free interval, the nociceptors and the traumatized nerves and nerve stumps resume their signal-transmitting activity. The resulting deep back pain and cutaneous hypersensitivity are often difficult to treat.

Scarring or surgical trauma involving the sympathetic chain on the ventral side of the spine may lead to sexual dysfunction, among other problems.

Outcomes after fusion procedures (Table 11.47). Most reports of outcomes after lumbar fusion procedures are derived from retrospective case series involving a mixed patient population (Wai et al. 2006), in which the operations were undertaken for diverse indications, including spondylolisthesis, other types of deformities, and neoplasia. Lumbar fusion procedures that are undertaken to treat post-traumatic instability arising from fractures, or

Table 11.47 Results of retrospective and prospective studies of fusion surgery for degenerative spinal disorders and spondylolisthesis with and without instrumentation (rates of pseudarthrosis and rates of good outcome) (after Schultz 1996, Haaker in Wirth and Zichner 2004)

Authors	Condition treated/ surgical technique		Results (%) With instrumentation	Without instrumentation
Bernhardt et al. 1992 (retro)	PDS VSP, lumbosacral	Pseudarthrosis Good results	22 67	26[**] 70[**]
Grubb and Lipscomb 1992 (retro)	PDS U-rod, lumbosacral	Pseudarthrosis VAS score	6 4	35[++] 2.5[**]
Zucherman et al. 1992 (retro)	PDS VSP, L3/4-S1	Pseudarthrosis Good/excellent results	10 74	17[**] 80
Lorenz et al. 1991 (prosp)	PDS VSP, monosegmental	Pseudarthrosis VAS score (improved)	None 77	58[++] 41
Bridwell et al. 1993 (prosp)	PDS VSP, L3/4, L4/5	Pseudarthrosis Functional improvement	13 83	30[++] 30[++]
Wittenberg et al. 1992 (prosp)	Socon L4-S1 Spondylolisthesis	Pseudarthrosis Analgesic medication	6 25	3[**] 45
McGuire and Amundson 1993 (prosp)	VSP, L4-S1 Spondylolisthesis	Pseudarthrosis	22	28
Zdeblick 1993 (prosp)	PDS TSRH	Pseudarthrosis Good/excellent results	5 95	35[++] 71[**]

Significant[++], insignificant[**].

various types of deformities, especially spondylolisthesis, result in far better outcomes then those intended to treat degenerative disk disease, particularly when a foregoing disk operation has led to an unsatisfactory result (PDS) (Wittenberg et al. 1993, Nachemson and Jonsson 2000, Haaker 2004, Willburger 2004, Martin et al. 2007).

Fusion procedures without instrumentation have a higher rate of pseudarthrosis than those with instrumentation (**Table 11.47**), but the use of cages or any form of instrumentation is associated with increased risk of complications compared with bone-only fusions (Maghout-Juratli 2006).

The Cochrane Review does not permit any firm conclusion to be drawn about the relative merits of dorsal, ventral, and dorsoventral fusion (Gibson and Waddell 2005), nor are there any convincing data indicating the superiority of fusion surgery over conservative treatment (Fritzell et al. 2001, Kwon et al. 2006, Mirza and Deyo 2007). However, there has been a marked increase in rates of fusion in recent years and a parallel increase in costs (Weinstein et al. 2006).

Summary: Fusion

Fusion procedures on the lumbar spine have not proved their worth in the treatment of intervertebral disk disease to the extent that they have in the treatment of spondylolisthesis, fractures, or neoplasia. In the case of degenerative disk disease, the list of indications for fusion is short, but the list of contraindications is long. Appropriate patient selection is important. In particular, psychosocial contraindications must be ruled out before surgery.

The operative technique of fusion procedures has undergone an evolution from implant-free to instrumented surgery. This has enabled a decline in the rate of pseudarthrosis as well as more rapid postoperative mobilization.

Conclusion

The only moderate success of fusion surgery and its peri- and postoperative complications, potentially including severe fusion-specific symptoms (post-fusion syndrome), imply a need to establish the indication for this type of surgery very firmly. It should always be borne in mind that the natural course of disk disease is favorable, as a stabilization of the motion segments tends to occur spontaneously.

Intervertebral Disk Prostheses

 Definition: Intervertebral disk prostheses are implants that are inserted into the disk space to preserve segmental mobility.

Synonyms. Artificial disks, disk replacements, disk prostheses, disk endoprostheses (corresponding to endoprostheses of the hip and knee joints).

Classification. Partial prostheses are distinguished from total disk endoprostheses. Partial prostheses are intended to replace the nucleus puloposus; they usually consist of one piece only. Examples include Fernstroem's steel ball (1950) and the PDN prosthesis, which is made of a hydrophilic gel. Total disk endoprostheses usually consist of three pieces. The SB-Charité and Pro-Disc prostheses, for example, are made of two metal plates that are fixed in the end plates of the vertebrae above and below, and a polyethylene component in between (**Fig. 11.157 a, b**).

Many other types of disk prosthesis have been devised that have not yet come into widespread use (see **Table 11.48**).

History. Since the first implantation of metal balls in the lumbar intervertebral spaces by Fernstroem (1950), more than 100 different types of motion-preserving intervertebral implants have been described in the literature (Spalski 2002). Only a few of them have seen extensive clinical use. Despite the marked functional differences among the various types of prosthesis, a broad classification into partial and total prostheses remains useful.

The first prosthesis to be widely used was the three-component **SB-Charité** prosthesis, a metal–polyethylene–metal construct devised by Schellnack and Büttner-Janz in 1984. Like hip and knee endoprostheses, it is designed to function with a low degree of friction at the two interfaces between metal and low-molecular-

11

Table 11.48 Classification of disk prostheses

Replacement for	Designation	Examples
Nucleus pulposus	One-component partial prosthesis	Steel ball (Fernstroem)
Disk	Three-component total prosthesis	SB-Charité Pro-Disc

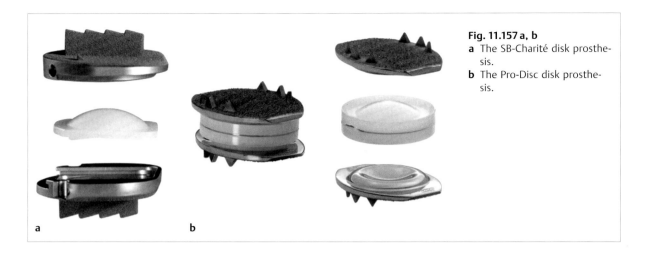

Fig. 11.157 a, b
a The SB-Charité disk prosthesis.
b The Pro-Disc disk prosthesis.

Table 11.49 History of lumbar disk prostheses

Year	Author	Classification	Principle	Product name
1950	Fernstroem	Artificial nucleus pulposus	Steel ball	
1984	Schellnack and Büttner-Janz	Artificial disk	Metal/polyethylene/metal	SB-Charité
1988	Steffee	Artificial disk	Metal/polyethylene/metal	Arcoflex
1990	Marnay	Artificial disk	Metal/polyethylene/metal	Pro-Disc
2002	Mathews	Artificial disk	Metal/metal	Maverick
2002	Schömmyer and Ray	Artificial nucleus pulposus	Hydrophilic gel	PD

Table 11.50 Indications for disk prostheses

- Symptomatic monosegmental lumbar degenerative instability
- Failure to respond to 6 months of conservative treatment
- VAS continuously > 5
- Age 30–50
- Distension pain on discography
- Correlative radiologic findings:
  - only mild loss of height of the intervertebral space
  - MRI: degeneration

weight polyethylene. Three different prototypes of the SB-Charité prosthesis have been developed and implanted in human patients, all of them operating on the same functional principle. Prostheses of the most recent of these three types have been implanted in more than 6000 patients since 1987. Of all the other types of total endoprosthesis, the only one that has seen widespread clinical use to date is the **Pro-Disc prosthesis** of Marnay, which was developed in the 1980s. Its initial version was first implanted in 1990, and it has been used in increasing numbers of patients since then (**Table 11.49**, **Fig. 11.157**).

Indications. The main indication is symptomatic, degenerative, monosegmental instability of the lumbar spine between L2 and S1. The segment most commonly involved is L4/5. A prerequisite for this type of surgery is at least 6 months of persistent pain (of intensity greater than 5 on the visual analog scale), refractory to conservative treatment, in a patient between 30 and 50 years of age (**Table 11.50**).

The clinical findings should be correlated with imaging studies showing mild loss of disk height, monosegmental disk degeneration on MRI, and positive discographic findings without any contrast medium flowing into the spinal canal but with reproduction of the patient's typical pain.

The loss of disk height should be no more than mild because the space-occupying prosthesis must be implanted not in the cancellous bone, but in the end plates. Functional radiography is not required (Büttner-Janz 2004, Fraser 2004), because it does not prove the presence of instability. Disk prostheses can also be implanted in selected patients with PDS who otherwise meet all of the criteria for a good indication (Büttner-Janz et al. 2002).

Contraindications. The indications listed in **Table 11.50** also imply the contraindications, including age below 30 or above 50. Multisegmental degeneration, instability of nondegenerative origin, and pain that mostly fails to reach an intensity of 5 on the visual analog scale are further contraindications (**Table 11.51**).

The more important contraindications of medicolegal significance include conditions in which anchoring of the implant is likely to be disturbed, e. g., osteoporosis, infection, deformity, status post fracture, tumors, and malformations. The lamina must be entirely intact; thus, spondylolysis or status post facetectomy is a contraindication. The intervertebral joints may not be totally or even partially lacking (status post facetectomy), nor should there be any degree of arthrosis or spinal canal stenosis. Axial deviations in the frontal and/or sagittal planes (scoliosis, kyphosis, hyperlordosis) make the implantation of an endoprosthesis problematic.

As in any other type of spinal surgery, psychosocial disorders (yellow flags) are a contraindication to the implantation of disk prostheses.

Technique of implantation. Disk prostheses are implanted through an anterior approach, with different techniques for the deeper part of the procedure depending on the target segment (L5/S1 vs. L4/L5 or L3/L4). Orthopedic surgeons without extensive experience in abdominal surgery work in collaboration with a visceral surgeon ("access surgeon") until the intervertebral disk is reached. Particular caution must be exercised in the mobilization of the great vessels and in the dissection and tying-off of the ascending lumbar vein. The full breadth of the affected disk must be exposed to enable implantation of the prosthesis. An optimal selection of the prosthesis components to be implanted and optimal positioning of the prosthesis in the intervertebral space are decisive factors for the success of treatment. The Pro-Disc and SB-Charité prostheses are implanted in essentially similar ways.

Complications. Alongside the general intra- and postoperative complications that can arise in any disk operation carried out through a ventral approach, including injuries to major blood vessels, the ureter, and the bowel, hemorrhage, sexual dysfunction, spondylitis, and adhesions, **prosthesis-specific complications** can also arise. These include fractures at the implantation site, faulty positioning of the prosthesis and its components, and, above all, **migration of the prosthesis** (Schnake et al. 2007). The prosthesis can migrate intraoperatively, immediately postoperatively, or later, through a gradual sinking of its relatively hard components into the vertebral cancellous bone when the latter is affected by **senile osteoporosis** (Kraemer et al. 2005). The prosthesis can also become ventrally or dorsally dislocated. The great vessels lie ventrally, the spinal canal dorsally. Material allergies are a potential problem with any type of prosthesis as well as wear debris and the potential for osteolysis with total disk replacement (van Ooij et al. 2007).

Table 11.51 Contraindications to the implantation of a disk prosthesis

- Conditions likely to cause problematic implantation:
  - osteoporosis
  - infection
  - deformities
- Multisegmental degeneration
- Axis deviation (e. g., scoliosis)
- Abnormal posterior elements:
  - spondylolysis
  - status post facetectomy
  - spondylarthrosis, spinal stenosis
- Lack of correlative radiologic findings
- VAS < 5
- Age < 20 or > 50 years
- Negative distension test in discography
- Psychosocial disturbances (yellow flag)

Table 11.52 Prosthesis-specific complications

- Faulty implantation
- Vertebral body fracture
- Migration of prosthesis
- Material allergy/wear debris
- Facet-related symptoms
- Spinal canal stenosis
- Heterotopic ossification
- Spontaneous fusion

Facet-related symptoms and spondylarthrosis are the expected results of faulty implantation causing excessive mechanical loading of the intervertebral joints. Hypertrophy of the joint edges may lead to **spinal canal stenosis.** Heterotopic ossification with formation of bone around the disk prosthesis, ultimately leading to fusion of the motion segment, might be regarded as a positive end result of disk prosthesis surgery, as a benign autostabilization of the spine occurs in old age in any case. The currently available data on prosthesis-specific complications are highly variable, with complication rates ranging from 0 % (usually in small series) to 26 % implantation errors (**Table 11.52**).

Results. Beyond a merely historical summary of who first implanted which prosthesis and when (**Table 11.49**), numerous retrospective studies and reviews have addressed the question of outcomes (Zöllner et al. 2000, Hopf et al. 2002, Anderson et al. 2004, German et al. 2005, Goel et al. 2005, Martinoetzel 2005, Mayer 2005, Schulte et al. 2005, Serhan et al. 2006, Siepe et al. 2006, 2007, Shim et al. 2007, Zigler et al. 2007). Wai and Fraser (2003) collected the results of disk prosthesis surgery reported in peer-reviewed publications (**Table**

11

Table 11.53 Results of disk endoprosthesis surgery as reported in peer-reviewed publications and summarized by Fraser (2004)

Author	Year	Number	Type	Follow-up (months)	Results	Prosthesis-specific complications
David	1993	29	SB-Charité	19	15 good 6 moderate 2 poor	1 periprosthetic ossification 1 fusion
Griffith	1994	139	SB-Charité	12	65%	4.3%
Cinotti	1996	56	SB-Charité	38	63%	26%
Lemoere	1997	105	SB-Charité	51	79%	2.9%
Büttner-Janz	1998	91	SB-Charité	72	85%	< 10% (11 reoperations)
Bertagnoli	2002	108	Pro-Disc	3–48	90.8%	None
David	2002	92	SB-Charité	96	77%	12 reoperations (fusion)

11.53), as revealed by a search of the PubMed and Ovied-Medline databases up to October 2002. They assessed the reported results in terms of the restoration of segmental mobility, preservation of the adjacent segments, and, finally, the overall outcome, including complications. They found that the definition of a "good clinical result" was highly variable, and success rates varied accordingly from 63% to 90%. So far, no randomized controlled studies have been carried out. Overall, the results of disk prosthesis surgery seem to be comparable with those of fusion procedures.

The use of artificial disks must await long-term scientifically reliable studies. The preliminary trials suggest equivalent results to spinal fusion, which generally is not effective (Nachemson 2005).

Pros and cons. The merits of disk prosthesis surgery have been hotly debated since its inception. Its proponents (**Table 11.53**) and detractors (Weinstein 2003, Boden et al. 2004, Bono et al. 2004, Dejo et al. 2004, Nachemson 2005) make the following arguments:

- **Pros:**
  - Only a single surgical approach is needed.
  - There is no pain at the bone-graft removal site (because there is no bone graft).
  - The operation is less extensive than fusion, and the patient can be mobilized immediately afterward.
  - The mobile implant preserves the biomechanical function of the adjacent segments.
  - Good results have been obtained in long-term studies (Büttner-Janz 1998, David 2002, 2007).

- **Cons:**
  - The long-term outcome of prostheses in patients who are young at the time of implantation is unknown.
  - Operative revision is problematic.
  - There are no controlled studies.
  - The indications are questionable (imprecise diagnosis).

- Pressure from the companies manufacturing the prostheses seems to be a factor promoting their implantation.

Furthermore, when a large lumbar interbody device needs to be removed through an anterior approach, the proximity of the great vessels and other vital organs, scarring from earlier surgery, and the pathology associated with implant failure all combine to make the revision procedure extremely difficult and potentially disastrous (Fraser 2004, Nguyen et al. 2006). Ureteral or vascular stents should be used in late revisions or in cases with significant extrusion of the device (Leary et al. 2007).

There are no prospective randomized studies with long-term data, which would be especially desirable in comparison to the long-term outcome of conservative treatment. Such studies are difficult to do, however, because patients who were adequately informed about both the surgical and the conservative options would be unlikely to allow themselves to be randomized, and also because, if such a study were proposed, it might not be permitted by an ethics committee.

Minimum requirements for disk prosthesis surgery include the following:

- Ongoing scientific assessment, with careful review of the indications in every case (obtain a second opinion).
- Implantation by an experienced team in a specialist spinal surgery center.
- Revision surgery only with the participation of a visceral surgeon and a vascular surgeon.
- Central documentation and regular follow-up.

Disk replacement remains experimental and controversial, and well-designed randomized controlled trials are needed to show safety and efficacy before it can be widely applied (Gravius et al. 2007).

Disk Prostheses

Mobility-preserving intervertebral disk implants are classified as nucleus pulposus replacements and total disk replacements. After a long phase of historical development, the two types of disk prosthesis that have come into wide clinical use and whose merits can be scientifically assessed are the SB-Charité model and, more recently, the Pro-Disc prosthesis. Nucleus pulposus and total disk replacements for the cervical spine are still in an experimental phase.

Lumbar disk prosthesis surgery has a short and not unproblematic list of indications and a long list of contraindications. The ventral surgical approach requires very precise technique if implantation errors that have a major detrimental impact on the outcome are to be avoided. Among the various prosthesis-specific complications, prosthesis migration and reactive facet arthrosis leading to spinal canal stenosis are the most important.

Heterotopic ossification leading to spontaneous fusion is a type of complication that can be considered positive in the long run. Reports on the outcome of disk prosthesis surgery mainly concern the SB-Charité model; some of these include several years of follow-up. Controlled studies are entirely lacking, to date.

Arguments in favor of disk prostheses include the relatively good short-term results, the use of a mobile prosthesis that can be implanted by a single surgical approach, and the resulting functional preservation of the adjacent motion segments. Arguments against them include the relatively young age of the patients undergoing this type of surgery, who will carry their prostheses for many years with an uncertain long-term result, and the difficulty and probable high rate of complications of revision surgery, should it be necessary. Thus, reasonable requirements for this type of surgery include a very precise indication, implantation and revision in experienced, professional hands in specialized centers, and central documentation with regular follow-up.

Conclusion

Caution is advisable for the time being because of the uncertain long-term results of disk endoprosthesis surgery. Are today's disk prosthesis carriers the problem patients of tomorrow?

Treatment Planning—Integrated Care

Certain uniform clinical syndromes, such as acute lumbago or S1 sciatica, can be appropriately managed with a uniform therapeutic approach. The treatment of lumbar disk disease, like that of cervical syndrome, follows a certain stepwise plan that is fitted to developments over time in the course of the disease and in which certain steps can be omitted depending on the circumstances. The treatment can be more or less invasive depending on the intensity and duration of the pain, which is usually the most prominent symptom.

Physicians should work out their own algorithms for the conservative treatment of lumbar syndrome together with physical therapists. Our poll of orthopedists in private practice and university clinics showed that most of them had the same treatment algorithm with regard to the most important questions (**Fig. 11.158**).

Outpatient treatment. The initial treatment usually consists of nonspecific, general measures including local heat application, analgesic and anti-inflammatory medication, and step positioning (*not* bed rest).

When the symptoms are mild, one can also try to manage the patient without medication (**Table 11.54**). Waddell (2004) recommends the following to outpatients dealing with an attack of back pain:
- Use something to control the pain.
- Modify your activities for a time, if necessary.
- Stay active, and get on with your life!

 In most cases of acute lumbar syndrome, improvement ensues within a few days, not least because of the tendency of disk-related symptoms to resolve spontaneously.

If the symptoms do not improve within 1–2 weeks, patients should be referred to a specialist if their care has not been in specialized hands from the beginning.

In the second stage of treatment, special therapeutic techniques such as manual therapy, electrotherapy, and local injections can be applied. The treating physician can decide, on the basis of individual experience, whether to use these techniques sequentially or in parallel.

In-patient treatment. Ambulatory treatment is of limited usefulness in persistent radicular syndromes. Patients should be admitted to hospital at once if paresis of major muscles or cauda equina syndrome develops; these problems usually require immediate surgical treatment. Patients whose radicular syndromes fail to respond to several weeks of conservative out-patient treatment should, at first, undergo new imaging studies, either MRI or CT. It can then be decided, on the basis of the clinical neurological findings as well as all other circumstances bearing on the decision, whether to proceed to surgery right away or to attempt further conservative management in hospital with minimally invasive therapeutic methods. Multimodal ambulatory and

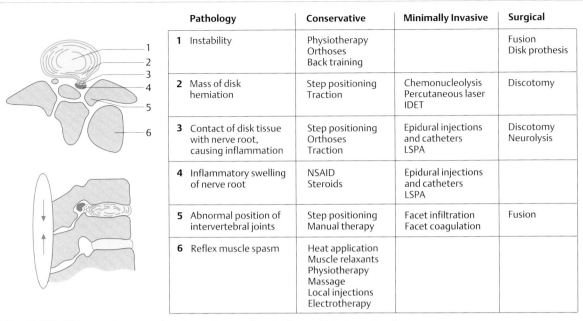

	Pathology	Conservative	Minimally Invasive	Surgical
1	Instability	Physiotherapy Orthoses Back training		Fusion Disk prothesis
2	Mass of disk hemiation	Step positioning Traction	Chemonucleolysis Percutaneous laser IDET	Discotomy
3	Contact of disk tissue with nerve root, causing inflammation	Step positioning Orthoses Traction	Epidural injections and catheters LSPA	Discotomy Neurolysis
4	Inflammatory swelling of nerve root	NSAID Steroids	Epidural injections and catheters LSPA	
5	Abnormal position of intervertebral joints	Step positioning Manual therapy	Facet infiltration Facet coagulation	Fusion
6	Reflex muscle spasm	Heat application Muscle relaxants Physiotherapy Massage Local injections Electrotherapy		

Fig. 11.158   Therapeutic approaches depending on the site from which the pain arises.

Table 11.54 Treatment plan for lumbar syndrome

Outpatient treatment (for all types of lumbar syndrome)
1 Symptoms arising for the first time
  - heat (cold) application
  - stress-reducing positioning
  - analgesic medications
2 Chronic, recurrent symptoms
  - heat application
  - electrotherapy
  - local injections

If the symptoms of a root syndrome persist → CT/MRI and referral to hospital. Immediate referral in case of motor deficit or cauda equina syndrome.

In-patient treatment (for cauda equina syndrome or intractable nerve root syndrome)
1 Conservative management
  - strict step positioning
  - peridural intradiscal therapy
2 Surgical treatment
  - discotomy
  - decompressive surgery
  - fusion surgery/disk prosthesis
  - postoperative rehabilitation: back school

in-patient treatment, comparable to that delivered in the "nonsurgical spine clinics" described by Rasmussen et al. (2005), has proved its worth in our institution and has significantly reduced the number of operations that are ultimately necessary (Theodoridis and Krämer 2006)[*].

There is no good alternative to surgery if the symptoms fail to improve in response to in-patient conservative management. Fusion operations are generally undertaken only as second procedures and only as a last resort.

Regardless of the extent and invasiveness of treatment that is required before the patient's lumbar syndrome ultimately improves, the treatment should be followed by a program of rehabilitation and recurrence prevention, involving both physiotherapy and instruction in disk-sparing behavior. These are best provided in the setting of a formal back school.

[*] The English translation of this book is due to be published in 2009.

Summary: The Treatment of Lumbar Syndrome

The spectrum of treatment of lumbar disk disease ranges all the way from fango packs to dorsoventral fusion surgery. The large variety of treatments can be classified as conservative, minimally invasive, and open operative.

A number of **conservative treatments** have proved their worth over time and are used successfully despite the lack of controlled studies. These include heat application, step positioning, and special exercises. In the few studies of conservative treatment that are available, the patients who received personal attention from their therapists have always been found to do better. This accounts for the reported success of acupuncture, local injections, manual therapy, and physiotherapy.

Minimally invasive treatments include all procedures in which percutaneous cannulae, catheters, or probes are introduced into the intervertebral or epidural space or the foramino-articular region, sometimes under endoscopic guidance. No controlled studies have been done on any of these techniques except for chemonucleolysis, epidural injections, and lumbar spinal nerve analgesia. New minimally invasive techniques for the treatment of lumbar disk disease tend to become popular very soon after their introduction, before they have been subjected to adequate scientific study. This fact testifies both to the high placebo rate of treatment for this condition and to the widespread fear of open disk surgery.

Among **open surgical procedures**, nerve root decompression by removal of the disk herniation is the most commonly undertaken and most important spinal operation. It is increasingly carried out using microsurgical technique. The results of this type of surgery are much better than its (undeservedly) poor reputation if it is carried out for the proper indications and in judicious, experienced hands.

Fusion operations for lumbar disk diseases should be viewed with caution because their results are poor. It remains to be seen whether the results of disk endoprosthesis surgery will be any better.

In view of the fact that intervertebral disk disease is a self-limiting illness, the various types of iatrogenic injury that can be caused in the course of its treatment should be avoided. These include:

- gastrointestinal diseases caused by long-term administration of NSAIDs
- slackening of the motion segments through inappropriate manual therapy
- radiation injury after repeated radiologically guided local injections
- postoperative syndromes (post-discotomy and post-fusion syndromes)
- implants whose long-term outcome is unknown
- treatment-related emotional disturbances.

An integrated treatment plan, agreed upon and carried out in collaboration by the general practitioner, medical specialist, and in-patient clinic, will both promote the patient's best interest and limit unnecessary costs. "Evidence-informed management" of chronic low back pain (Haldeman and Degenais 2008) is necessary to avoid surgery as far as possible.

Conclusion

All treatments for lumbar disk disease must be measured against its benign spontaneous course. It is better to lose a patient to another physician than to lose one's reputation by doing unnecessary back surgery (Wiltse 1977).

11

12 Natural Course and Prognosis of Intervertebral Disk Diseases

The pathoanatomical changes of the intervertebral disk and the disease states that may result from them take a characteristic course. In particular, there are three processes with their own typical time curves:

- degenerative changes of the intervertebral disk with advancing age
- disk disease over the course of life
- natural course of an acute episode of disk disease.

■ Pathoanatomical Changes of the Intervertebral Disk

The natural course of degenerative changes in the intervertebral disk is to increase steadily from about age 20 until age 50–60, by which time disk degeneration has progressed to almost its final extent (**Fig. 12.1**). Plain radiographs reveal loss of disk height and spondylotic osteophyte formation (osteochondrosis, spondylosis), changes that are not considered pathological in themselves. Degenerative changes of the intervertebral disk are normally found at autopsy as well, particularly in the lower cervical and lower lumbar segments. Findings of this type from the older studies of Schmorl (1932), Coventry (1945), Hirsch and Schajowicz (1952), and Schmorl and Junghanns (1968), have been confirmed more recently by Kirkaldy-Willis (1988), Anderson (2002), Benoist (2002), Ito (2002), Greenough (2004), and Singer and Farzy (2004). These degenerative changes, like graying of the hair and wrinkling of the skin, are normal accompaniments of aging. They ultimately lead to spontaneous solidification, i. e., fibrous ankylosis of the intervertebral disks.

Discosis is normally more severe in some motion segments than in others. Impressive degenerative changes, with bridging spondylotic processes, are mainly found at C4–C7 and L4–S1. The lower segments of the thoracic spine are also more severely affected than its upper segments.

Degenerative changes of the intervertebral disk often remain asymptomatic. Boden et al. (1990) found asymptomatic disk protrusions in the MRI scans of 20 % of normal individuals under 60 years of age, and 36 % of individuals over 60. These findings were replicated by Jensen et al. (1994) and Boos et al. (1995).

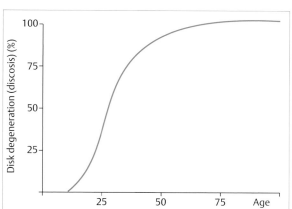

Fig. 12.1 This graph of the prevalence of discosis (degenerative disk disease) as a function of age reveals that 100 % of individuals have it by age 70–80.

■ Disk Disease over the Course of Life

The disease curve is not parallel to the degeneration curve. Disk diseases such as lumbago, sciatica, stiff neck, and shoulder–arm syndrome occur most commonly in midlife and become steadily less frequent and less intense after the fifth decade. This frequency distribution is found both in statistical studies of conservatively managed patients (Krämer 1973, Krämer and Nentwig 1999) and in surgical statistics (McCulloch 1998, Postacchini 1999, Krämer et al. 2004). It has also been confirmed by more recent epidemiological studies (Stephens and Bell 1993, Leboeuf 1998, Bendix 2004, Kuhlmann 2004, Jarvik 2005) (**Fig. 12.2**).

Different clinical manifestations are produced by disk degeneration at different times of life (**Table 12.1**):

- In **younger patients,** intradiscal tissue displacement leading to disk protrusion can produce clinical symptoms: the typical clinical picture is extension stiffness

of the hip and thigh (cf. Chapter 11). The MRI may reveal protrusion of the posterior edge of the disk. The "board sign" is the most notable finding on physical examination, and radicular signs are usually absent. Pain usually radiates into the leg no further down than the proximal portion of the affected dermatome. Because younger patients' disks remain closed even when they protrude, conservative management is recommended, including traction, physiotherapy exercises, and stress-reducing positioning. The course of disk disease in young individuals is slow but generally favorable, i. e., disk prolapse usually does not ensue as long as patients modify their behavior appropriately and correct treatment is provided.

- In **midlife,** the frequency and intensity of disk disease rise. Protrusions and prolapses, with outward displacement of the central, mobile disk tissue, exert pressure on the nerve root. The basic pathogenetic mechanism consists of two factors: a still high turgor pressure in the disk, combined with an already somewhat torn and less durable anulus fibrosus (see Chapter 4). Disk disease can be present in middle age in either the cervical or the lumbar spine.

- **Comfortable rigidity of the aging spine** (Kraemer 1995). In the third phase of the spontaneous pathoanatomical process of disk degeneration, the intervertebral disks develop fibrotic ankylosis. The disks show marked degenerative changes, with signs of wear and tear, but the disk tissue has dried out to such an extent that it has little tendency to become displaced.

! The intervertebral disks wither with age.

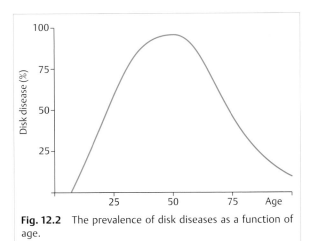

Fig. 12.2 The prevalence of disk diseases as a function of age.

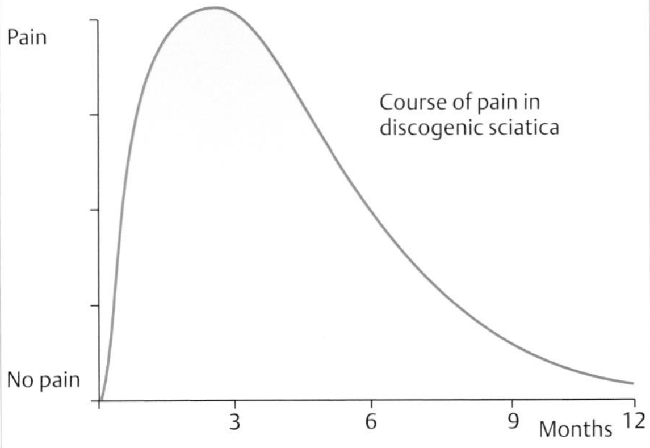

There may be an osteophytic reaction, with narrowing of the spinal canal potentially leading to the so-called spinal stenosis syndrome, but disk degeneration itself is usually asymptomatic in old age. The main feature of the structural–biomechanical constellation of asymptomatic disk degeneration in old age is dehydration of the disks with fibrotic ankylosis of the motion segments. In addition, elderly individuals are generally less physically active than they were when younger. Recent studies confirm that the spontaneous course of disk disease in old age is benign (Cinotti et al. 1998, Kirkaldy-Willis 1988, Martikainen 1998, Ferguson 1999, Anderon 2002, Greenough 2004, Nakagawa 2004). The comfortable rigidity of the aging spine in old age can still be disrupted, however, by accidental trauma or inappropriate behavior (e. g., vigorous gardening) as well as by misguided treatments such as chiropractic manipulation or mobilizing physiotherapy exercises.

Fig. 12.3 The temporal course of pain of acute sciatica.

Course of pain in discogenic sciatica

Table 12.1 Intervertebral disk diseases over the course of life

Stage	Age	Pathological anatomy	Clinical manifestations	
			Cervical spine	Lumbar spine
1	10		Torticollis	
	20	Intradiscal tissue displacement		Extension stiffness of the hip and thigh
	30	Protrusion	Acute local cervical syndrome	Acute lumbago
2	40	Prolapse	Acute radicular irritation syndrome	Sciatica
	50	Intervertebral narrowing	Chronic cervical syndrome	Chronic lumbar syndrome
	60			
	70	Bony reactive changes	Chronic radicular irritation syndrome	Spinal canal stenosis syndrome
3	80	Fibrous ankylosis		

■ The Spontaneous Course of Acute Intervertebral Disk Disease

In addition to the spontaneous course of disk degeneration and disk disease over the course of life, there is also a characteristic spontaneous temporal pattern of each acute episode of disk disease. Discogenic sciatica reaches its peak within a few days and then gradually subsides (**Fig. 12.3**). The acute symptoms are caused not just by mechanical compression, but also by biochemical reactions induced by the liberation of inflammatory mediators as a response to irritation of neural tissue (Rydevik 1990, Saal and Herzog 1990, Willburger et al. 1998). This implies a potential therapeutic role for the epidural injection of anti-inflammatories and local anesthetics, or even of saline solution, to neutralize or dilute the inflammatory mediators.

Severe pain due to mechanical compression and biochemical processes is brief: 90% of all patients feel much better in 2 months, and 99% in 1 year (Krämer and Nentwig 1999). The displaced disk tissue is resorbed through a combination of enzymatic digestion, phagocytosis, and vascularization. Many studies have described this process (Rydevik 1990, Kobajaschi 1998, Haro et al. 2000, Nakai et al. 2000, Deyo and Weinstein 2001, Kato 2003, Karppinen et al. 2004). Plentiful clinical evidence indicates that conservative treatment relieves pain in most patients after a few days to several months. The symptoms can resolve regardless of the type or size of the herniation The presence of motor or sensory deficits of mild or moderate severity is not a contraindication for conservative therapy, since the chances that these will be resolved are comparable to those following surgical treatment (Postaccini 1999).

The spontaneous subsidence of pain is also associated with changes in its character and temporal distribution. McKenzie (1981) described what he called the **centralization phenomenon:** the pain, which at first radiates into the leg, slowly retracts proximally until, as often happens, only back pain remains. Our own studies (Krämer and Nentwig 1999) and other reports in the literature have confirmed this experience (Donelson et al. 1997, Martikainen 1998, Trasimeni 1998, Fergusson 1999, Albert 2004, Nakagawa 2004).

The likelihood that the symptoms of a disk herniation will resolve spontaneously depends on whether the disk fragment consists primarily of nucleus pulposus material or of anulus fibrosus or cartilaginous end plate. Nucleus pulposus material is more readily resorbed. If the spinal canal is still of normal width, the chance of spontaneous recovery is good. A final decisive consideration is the site of the fragment: fragments lying behind the vertebral body are more likely to be spontaneously resorbed, because perfusion in this area is better than in or near the disk. Extradiscal sequestra that have broken loose from the rest of the disk are also more readily resorbed than subligamentous pieces of disk material that remain connected to the disk's still functioning osmotic system.

These observations on spontaneous improvement apply not just to lumbar disk disease, but also to cervical disk herniations. The likelihood of spontaneous resolution of symptoms in the cervical spine is even higher than in the lumbar spine. This is particularly true of cervicobrachial syndromes (McNab 1989, Aoshida 1991, Saal et al. 1996, Mochida 1998, Rubenthaler and Senge 2004, Garvey 2005).

Cervicomedullary syndromes are the main indication for surgery at present (Mochida 1998, Garvey 2005) (see also Chapter 9).

12

L5/S1 Case Illustration: Prolapse with Infradiscal Extension and Spontaneous Resorption

Clinical presentation. This 29-year-old woman complained of acute back pain radiating into the left leg in an S1 dermatomal pattern. Severe lumbar spasm was present. Examination revealed mild weakness of the left plantar flexors and a diminished Achilles reflex on the left.

MRI. The study sequences are shown in **Fig. 12.4**.

Findings. There is a prolapse originating from the L5/S1 disk and extending to the infradiscal level with compression of the dural sac and displacement of the left S1 nerve root (**a,** →). Three years later, only a small amount of soft tissue is seen at the same site, without compression of the dural sac (**b2, c,** →). The L5/S1 intervertebral disk is of diminished signal intensity. The disks of the upper segments of the lumbar spine appear normal. Lumbarization of S1 is seen, with a hypoplastic intervertebral disk (**d,** →).

Diagnosis. (a) A large infradiscal medial and left paramedial disk prolapse is present at L5/S1. (**b–d**) Subtotal "regression" of the prolapse has occurred, with residual disk tissue or scar tissue anterior to the dural sac, and without any compression of the dural sac or nerve root. The L5/S1 intervertebral disk is degenerated.

Clinical course. The patient underwent conservative treatment consisting of step positioning, analgesic medication, and local injections (spinal nerve analgesia). There was subjective improvement within a few days, so that surgery was deemed unnecessary.

The patient returned for examination 3 years later. She still had mild back pain, occasionally radiating into the left leg, especially with weather changes. There was no motor deficit or other positive neurologic findings other than a diminished left Achilles reflex.

Comment. The L5/S1 disk prolapse was largely resorbed by enzymatic action. Remnants persist in the form of fibrous tissue in the anterior epidural space, without compression of the root or dural sac.

Even a large disk prolapse does not require immediate surgery if there is no major neurologic deficit and if the pain is only moderately severe. In young patients, the prolapse consists primarily of nucleus pulposus tissue and will be more readily broken down by enzymatic action than a comparable amount of extruded tissue in older patients.

12

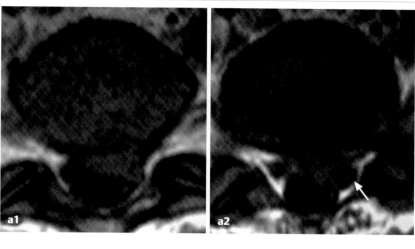

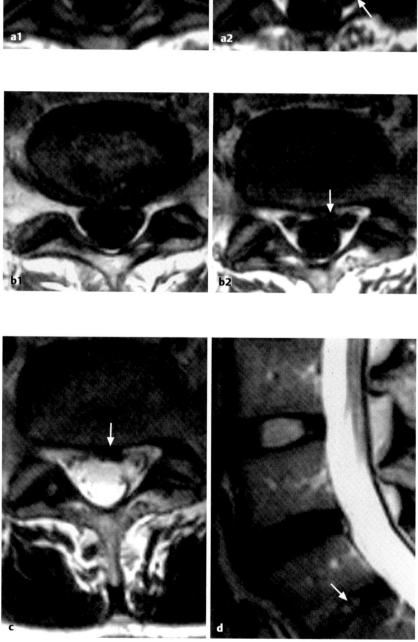

Fig. 12.4 a–d   Study sequences (from Krämer and Köster 2001).
a T2 SE, axial, L5/S1 (**a1**) and L5 inferior end plate (**a2**).
b T1 SE, axial, L5/S1 (**b1**) and L5 inferior end plate (**b2**).
c T2 TSE, axial, L5/S1 at L5 inferior end plate.
d T2 TSE, sagittal, median.
b–d were obtained 3 years later than **a**.

12

L4/5 Case Illustration: Spontaneous Resorption of an Infradiscal L4/5 Disk Prolapse

Clinical presentation. This 24-year-old woman complained of pain alternating between the right and left legs, but mainly on the left side. A band of pain was present in the L5 dermatome and part of the S1 dermatome, on both sides, but more pronounced on the left. There was no motor deficit. The Lasègue sign was positive on the left at 30°, and the crossed Lasègue sign was positive on the right at 40°.

MRI. The study sequences are shown in **Fig. 12.5.**

Findings. The L3/4 and L4/5 intervertebral disks are of diminished height and signal intensity. Hypoplasia of the L5/S1 disk is seen, with sacralization of the L5 vertebra (**a, b**). At the L3/4 level, there is mild posterior displacement of disk tissue, with a circumscribed area of high signal intensity in the T2-weighted image (**a**, →). At L4/5, there is marked posterior displacement of disk tissue, which remains in continuity with the parent disk. The prolapse extends to the infradiscal level (**a–c**) and raises the posterior longitudinal ligament (**a**, >). There is a moderate degree of compression of the dural sac, and the extruded tissue makes contact with the traversing L5 nerve root (**c**, →), as well as with the intrathe-cal portion of the S1 nerve root (**c**, >). The arrows (→) indicate the corresponding nerve roots on the right side.

Diagnosis. Subligamentous, left paramedial prolapse of the L4/5 intervertebral disk, with infradiscal extension. Mild protrusion of the L3/4 disk, with a posterior anular tear.

Treatment. Because of the patient's only moderate degree of pain and her disinclination to undergo invasive treatment, conservative treatment was provided, including local injections, spinal nerve analgesia, epidural injections, step positioning, and physiotherapy.

Clinical course. The patient's leg pain improved markedly within 2 weeks. Practically the only residual symptom was lumbar spasm with a positive Lasègue sign on both sides.

Follow-up examination. The patient remained free of leg pain 3 and 6 months later. There was no neurologic deficit, and the mobility of the lumbar spine was essentially normal. The prolapse was no longer visible on an MRI scan obtained 1 year after the acute episode.

Comment. The displaced disk tissue apparently consisted solely of nucleus pulposus material and caused no more than mild, transient nerve root compression.

12

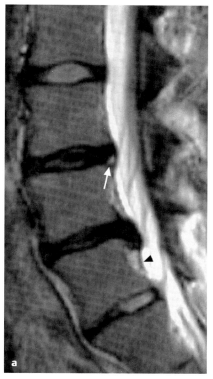

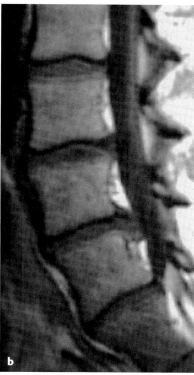

Fig. 12.5 a–c   Study sequences (from Krämer and Köster 2001).
a T2 TSE, sagittal, left para-medial.
b T1 SE, sagittal, left para-medial.
c T2 TSE, axial, L5 superior end plate.

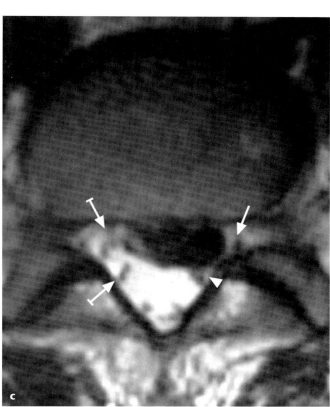

Published information regarding the spontaneous course of disk disease. The literature contains many reports of the spontaneous resorption of dislocated intervertebral disk tissue as well as a few noteworthy studies documenting the benign spontaneous course of disk disease. The best known of these is Weber's (1983) prospective randomized study of patients with lumbar disk herniation. A group of patients who underwent surgery and a control group of patients who did not had identical outcomes at 4 and 10 years after randomization. In another study of patients with at least 6 weeks of symptoms from a disk herniation (Weinstein 2006), those treated surgically improved more rapidly and had better relief of symptoms and better function at 1 year than those treated conservatively. The advantage of surgery diminished somewhat over the second year of follow-up. Moreover, placebo-controlled double-blind studies provide a good insight into the likelihood of spontaneous cure in many different types of disease; a large number of such studies were done when intradiscal therapy with chymopapain was introduced as a treatment for lumbar disk protrusions (Fraser 1982, Agre 1984, Dabezies 1988, Deburge 1993). The studies

showed chymopapain to be very effective, but they also showed that 50% of the patients in the control group, who had only been given a placebo, did just as well. The rate of spontaneous cure, or of cure after placebo treatment, in lumbar disk syndrome is among the highest in all of evidence-based medicine. The response rate of neck and back pain to placebo treatment is variable, but typically around 50% (Nachemson 2000). Back pain is a common, benign, and self-limiting symptom (Schöne 2004); in all too many cases, patients with back pain might have been better off if they had never seen a doctor, and especially not a surgeon (Waddell 2004).

We, too, gained personal experience of the spontaneous improvement of the symptoms of lumbar disk herniation around the time that chymopapain was introduced (Krämer 1988). When this method was at the height of its popularity, our waiting list was long. For many patients, by the time it was finally their turn to be admitted some 2–3 months after the initial presentation, their symptoms had subsided to such an extent that they no longer needed invasive treatment. We called this the **"waiting-list phenomenon."**

Summary

Unlike many other diseases, such as arthritis, diabetes mellitus, and Parkinson disease, intervertebral disk disease is self-limiting. It rapidly reaches a peak of intensity, causing severe suffering, and then subsides spontaneously. This observation is true of the lifelong course of disk disease as well as of the course of individual acute episodes of cervical or lumbar syndrome.

Although disk degeneration progresses continually from age 20 onward and regularly reaches its full extent in old age, disk disease has a different temporal profile, peaking in midlife. Symptoms due to slackening and displacement of intervertebral disk tissue tend to increase in frequency and intensity up to the fifth decade of life and to subside thereafter, with some degree of individual variation. This process ends in the benevolent partial solidification of the spine that is seen in old age.

Individual episodes of disk disease tend to resolve spontaneously in a relatively short time. Not only the

common, acute pains in the neck and low back, but also the symptoms of discogenic nerve root compression, generally subside within a few weeks or, at most, a few months. The "waiting-list phenomenon" and the success of unconventional modes of treatment are both attributable to this tendency toward spontaneous cure. Longer-lasting symptoms, which become chronic, are generally due to an iatrogenic component, psychosocial factors, or a combination of both.

Conclusion

The invasiveness, expense, and risks of diagnostic and therapeutic procedures should always be weighed against the mainly benign spontaneous course of intervertebral disk diseases.

13 The Spine and the Mind

> ! As spinal syndromes and behavioral disturbances are both common, it comes as no surprise that they are often seen in the same patient.

pair bodily integrity, painful disk syndromes take their emotional toll; conversely, primary mental disorders can cause symptoms closely resembling those of intervertebral disk disease.

Furthermore, either of these two types of disorder can induce or worsen the other. Like other diseases that im-

Psychosomatic Processes

Psychosomatic interactions in spinal diseases are of interest both to physicians and to psychologists. The literature on the subject is extensive (Waddell and Turk 1992, Katz 2000, Pfingsten et al. 2001, Blumenstiel et al. 2005, Hildebrand et al. 2005, Dersh et al. 2006, Clays et al. 2007, Heneweer et al 2007, Becker et al. 2008). Studies have shown that cortical processing is abnormal in patients with chronic low back pain and illness behavior (Findlay 2006).

The term "psychosomatic," derived from the Greek words *psychē* (soul) and *sōma* (body), refers both to the emotional/cognitive and to the physical aspects of the individual. The psychosomatic approach to the diagnosis and treatment of disease is based on the principle that these two aspects always function in tandem. The contribution of emotional factors to disease processes such as bronchial asthma, duodenal ulcer, migraine, and eczema is well known. Some diseases, such as gastric ulcer,

meet the strict definition of a psychosomatic condition in that they are associated with a specific organic pathoanatomical lesion. In other, so-called functional disorders, there is no evident organic abnormality: these include, for example, cardiac neurosis, headache, and disturbances of gastrointestinal peristalsis. The organic/functional distinction is not always easy to apply to spinal disorders, because the pathological substrate underlying them is often poorly defined (as in chronic low back pain).

Over the last 15 years, interdisciplinary research on the etiology and pathogenesis of chronic pain has increasingly centered on the gradual process of transition from acute to chronic (Pfingsten 2005). Many prospective studies, some of them specifically concerned with back pain, have convincingly shown that psychosocial mechanisms are generally much better predictors of symptoms becoming chronic than are somatic factors (Linton 2000).

Mind–Body Interactions as Described in the Literature

> ! Unlike psychosomatic diseases in other parts of the body, chronic, recurrent spinal syndromes are not associated with any specific personality type.

Beck (1975), writing about the personality type of individuals with psychosomatic pain localized to the musculoskeletal system, emphasized the role of pent-up **aggressive conflicts** causing muscle spasm and chronic pain.

The electromyographic studies of Wolf (1963) showed the influence of emotional states on cervical muscle tone. Patients with chronic musculoskeletal pain tend to have neurotic disturbances including an impaired ability to express emotion, exaggerated self-control, and a tendency to demand too much from themselves. We consider musculoskeletal pain to be an additional indication that the patient's emotional defense mechanisms are inadequate.

Weintraub (1975) viewed **pent-up strong emotions** and **an excessively rigid approach to life** as the causes of static postural abnormalities and painful muscular hypertonia. He considered these painful states to be the neuromuscular equivalents of conflict-evoked behavioral and defense mechanisms. Psychosomatic low back pain, in particular, is in this view an expression of long-standing excessive mental stress and of the subjective inability to cope with the demands of one's family or occupation. These patients typically have difficulty dealing with their internal and external problems.

Sternbach (1974) found that patients with low back pain had significantly elevated values on scales for hysteria, depression, hypochondria, and hypomania. Male patients were significantly more depressed, irritable, passive, and anxious than female patients. We explain these findings as probably resulting from the higher demands placed by society on men in terms of their occupational and social function, which constitute an additional stressor over and above their actual organic illness.

Although there is a great deal of individual variation, it is clear that chronic pain must be viewed as the result of a process that can be influenced by psychological factors (Pfingsten 2005). The patient's behavior is chiefly guided by factors of perception, attention, cognitive interpretation, and general emotional condition. Caldwell and Chase (1977) postulated that patients with abnormal emotional behavior obtain "secondary gain" from chronic low back pain.

Pain expectation anxiety is a condition characterized by the avoidance of potentially pain-producing situations. Thus, a patient's desire for early retirement may be motivated by a desire to avoid the further pain that might result from a resumption of heavy manual labor, including lifting. Beals and Hickman (1972) studied patients who had had disk surgery and found the severity of their emotional disturbance to be correlated with the number of disk operations they had undergone. A control group consisted of patients with limb injuries. We think that, in such cases, a type of neurosis was probably already present before the onset of disk disease and was then exacerbated by surgery and persistent postoperative symptoms.

Blumetti and Modesti (1976) carried out a follow-up study comparing patients with low back pain who did and did not improve 6 months after the initiation of treatment with various medical modalities. The unim-proved group had significantly higher hysteria and hypochondria scores than the improved group.

Personality tests. Wiltse and Rocchio (1975) found that patients with high hysteria and hypochondria scores on the Minnesota Multiphasic Personality Inventory (MMPI) consistently responded less well to chemonucleolysis than patients with normal scores on these two scales whom the treating physicians judged to have no psychosomatic disturbance. These results have since been replicated a number of times (Hasenbring 1992, Hasenbring et al. 1994). Croft et al. (1996) showed, in a prospective population-based study, that individuals suffering from serious emotional problems (depression) were twice as likely to develop back pain over the course of 1 year as individuals with mild or no psychosocial impairment. A currently depressive mood was also found to be a significant risk factor for acute, nonspecific back pain becoming chronic. The cognitive, emotional, and behavioral aspects of pain processing and coping are very important. The processes of classical and operant conditioning play a central role in the maintenance of these factors (Hasenbring and Pfingsten 2005).

Spring and Wörz (1976) studied patients with discogenic low back pain pre- and postoperatively with the MMPI, a symptoms questionnaire, and a scale assessing the overall emotional state. Patients with a neurotic personality type were found to develop new symptoms after surgery significantly more frequently than patients who did not have a neurotic personality type.

The spine and the mind. Stein and Floman (1990) found a correlation between chronic low back pain and depression: 60–100% of patients with chronic low back pain had demonstrable manifestations of depression, often accompanied by neuro-vegetative signs. Antidepressants improved both back pain and depression. Hasenbring (1992), on the basis of extensive studies, defined risk factors for poor recovery from disk disease after surgical or conservative treatment. Beyond depressivity, which had already been identified by other authors as a risk factor, these factors also included impaired cognitive-emotional pain-processing skills as well as certain inappropriate ways of coping with the pain. The latter two factors were found to have a very marked influence on the resulting pain experience. Avoidance behavior, distraction strategies, and the avoidance of social activities play a decisive role. The studies showed that both short-lasting and long-lasting pain can be predicted, to an extent that is both statistically and clinically significant, by a combination of medical, psychological, and social parameters. Early retirement with receipt of a pension within 6 months of discharge from hospital could be predicted in 85% of cases merely on the basis of two psychological factors—a depressive state and the degree of stress generally present in the workplace. No correlation was found between the extent of dislocation of disk tissue (an indication of the severity of nerve root displacement) and the psychological risk factors.

> **!** Psychological factors operate in every patient, regardless of whether a protrusion or a massive disk herniation is present.

Many other authors have discussed the interactions of the spine and the mind, including Waring et al. (1976), Cailliet (1978), Frymoyer and Pope (1980), Pope et al. (1980), Aronoff and Evans (1982), Blumer (1982), Leavitt (1982), von Bayer (1983), Cameron and Shepel (1983), Bradley and van der Heide (1984), Hendler (1984), McCulloch (1984), Weber and Niethard (1984), Feuerstein et al. (1985), Ryden et al. (1985), Adams et al. (1986), Crisson et al. (1986), France et al. (1986), Keefe et al. (1986), Schofferman (1986), Villard et al. (1986), Watkins et al. (1986), Love (1987), Dvořák et al. (1988), Manucher (1988), Waddell and Reilly (1988), Stein and Floman (1990), Greenough and Fraser (1991), Hazard et al. (1991), Hasenbring (1992), Basler (1998), Pfingsten (2004, 2005), Waddell (2004), Kovacs et al. (2006), Clays et al. (2007), Heneweer et al. (2007), and Becker et al. (2008).

Our own comparative study of 93 patients with chronic lumbar syndrome in our institution and in the outpatient offices of our colleagues in private practice showed that their scores on a number of sub-scales of the Freiburg Personality Inventory (FPI-A) differed significantly from those of a control group of patients with gonarthrosis (Bösken 1986).

> **!** Patients with lumbar syndrome have significantly higher scores for nervousness, depressivity, and emotional lability.

Two basic questions emerge from **our review of the literature and our own studies:**

- One question concerns the extent to which psychosomatic processes contribute to spinal symptoms, i.e., the extent to which mental disturbances can be transferred to the spine.
- The other question concerns the somatopsychic aspect, i.e., the extent to which chronic, recurrent disk disease with an overtly organic pathogenesis can affect the patient's mental functioning.

In the following section, we will present and interpret the findings of studies carried out on our own patients regarding these two questions. Further information on the subject is found in Chapters 8 and 11.

■ The Spine as a Projective Field for Mental Disturbances (Psychosomatic Changes)

> **!** The mental state of individuals can be judged from their behavior.

The spine is the central element of the musculoskeletal system and as such plays a leading role in behavior. The various constitutional and psychological types described by Kretschmer, Jung, Adler, and others all have their specific bodily expressions, which manifest themselves not just in body condition and habitus but also in certain types of movement, gait, and sitting posture. An introverted, asthenic individual sits, walks, and stands differently from an extroverted, pyknic individual. Varying degrees of self-observation, predisposition to excessive muscle tension, and sensitivity of pain receptors will determine whether a given mechanical stimulus results in pain that ceases soon after it begins or in a vicious circle of pain, muscle spasm, and more pain. These things will also determine whether reflex inhibition of movement will develop through what Brügger (1979) termed a nociceptive–somatomotor blocking effect.

The mental state of patients with a spinal syndrome can be discerned from their external appearance, posture, and gestures. Some aspects of body language reflecting both the physical and the mental state of an individual are listed in **Table 13.1**.

> **!** An upright vs. a drooping stance and a tensed neck vs. a head held low are two illustrative examples of postures that have a major psychosomatic component.

The combination of psychological and organic factors. On the other hand, one should be wary of designating any disease process as psychosomatic just be-

Table 13.1 Body language and the spine

Cervical spine	Thoracic and lumbar spine
"holding one's head high"	Stiff posture
"heads up"	Erect posture
"keep your head down"	Poor posture
"my head is bloody, but unbowed"	Stooped posture
	Good posture
"stiff-necked"	Bad posture
"rubber-necking"	"take a stand"
"breaking my neck"	"spineless jellyfish"
"a pain in the neck"	"show some backbone"
	"ramrod spine"
	"back-breaking effort"
	"get off my back!"
	"kow-tow"
	"cringe"
	"bowing and scraping"
	"buckling under"

13

Table 13.2 Characteristics of psychosomatic and organic spinal symptoms

Psychosomatic spinal symptoms	Organic spinal symptoms
Not positionally dependent	Positionally dependent
Poorly localized (the whole left side)	Precisely localized
Described as continuous, unbearable, with frequent use of superlatives	Evident causality; fluctuation in response to external factors; becomes bearable with proper positioning, traction, and analgesics
Unresponsive to apparently correct treatment	Only mild improvement with distraction
Disappear when the patient is distracted	
The patient is not awakened by the pain but has it upon awakening	The typical pain awakens the patient if he or she involuntarily gets into the "wrong position" while sleeping

when the painful condition is useful to the patient for combating some type of negative emotional situation.

> **!** For these patients, psychological treatment is just as important as physical treatment.

Psychosomatic spinal symptoms differ from purely organic pain in a number of characteristics, which are listed in **Table 13.2**. Further useful diagnostic information comes from the positional dependence of true spondylogenic pain and its immediate responsiveness to stress-reducing positioning and traction. The fine points of clinical history-taking and physical examination are diagnostically important here. The characteristics listed in **Table 13.2** are merely rough indications and should not be misread by physicians as implying that any patient who fails to respond to treatment has a psychogenic overlay. All other diagnostic and therapeutic possibilities should be exhausted before a psychogenic condition is diagnosed and treated. On the other hand, patients with **purely psychosomatic symptoms** can also get better with physically directed treatment. This may happen either through a placebo effect or because

> **!** Some patients simulate a good response to treatment because they would rather be treated by an orthopedist than by a psychiatrist.

The latter can happen because patients realize that people with organic conditions are generally treated with more sympathy and consideration than those with psychogenic disturbances. One way to reach the correct diagnosis in such cases is to administer a placebo, such as a purportedly strong analgesic tablet or local infiltration with normal saline.

In practice, there is often no easy way to separate psychosomatic and somatopsychic disorders. As was already pointed out at the beginning of this chapter, disk disease is so common that even individuals with pre-existing abnormal behavior can develop genuine cervicobrachialgia or sciatica. Yet, whenever psychosomatic factors are found to be operative, either as the sole cause or (more commonly) as an overlay that worsens the patient's symptoms, these factors must also be addressed by the therapeutic plan.

> **!** Pain that is produced or exacerbated by psychosomatic factors causes just as much suffering as pain that is of purely organic origin.

The treatment of this type of pain, however, differs from the treatment of organically derived pain. Organic pain can be successfully treated by specifically targeting its pathoanatomical substrate, e. g., by appropriate positioning, traction, local injections, or surgery. Psychosomatic spinal symptoms, on the other hand, are treated in one of two ways: either by "discovery," i. e., by an at-

cause it cannot be definitively attributed to organic pathology. Discogenic symptoms are often accompanied by so little in the way of objective findings that one may be tempted to "write off" the entire constellation of symptoms as psychosomatic. Theoretically, one could devise a psychogenic explanation for almost any disease process, as there is hardly a human being anywhere who does not have some type of past or present emotional conflict that might be imagined to be a causative psychosomatic component of disease.

For example, we saw a 19-year-old woman with a painful sciatic postural abnormality as the sole manifestation of an L4/5 disk herniation with a subligamentous, paramedian free fragment. She had no neurological deficit. After extensive psychoanalysis and psychotherapy, she herself believed that her faulty posture was psychogenic, and she presented herself to our outpatient department under this assumption. Once MRI had revealed the true cause, the disk fragment was surgically removed and the "psychogenic" postural abnormality disappeared.

Yet the organic origin of a spinal syndrome is not always as clear as it was in this case. Typically, mental and physical factors are intermingled. One can safely assume that low back pain and sciatica generally have some type of organic substrate. The biomechanical processes in the motion segment that cause positionally dependent pain can hardly be induced by emotional stress, like gastric ulcer or migraine. But when a small degree of low back pain is already present in a patient with a certain psychological make-up, it may develop into severe low back pain through a vicious circle of pain, muscle spasm, and more pain. This can happen, for example, tempted causal treatment with psychotherapy, or by "covering-up," i. e., by symptomatic treatment, with (for example) a targeted physiotherapy program including exercises, traction, and back training. Invasive diagnostic and therapeutic measures should be avoided for these patients, in order not to expose them to unneces-

sary risks, and lest such measures counter-productively reinforce the symptoms that they are meant to improve. The old saying serves as a warning:

> **!** "Do not operate on the spine of a patient who is also being treated by a psychiatrist."

■ The Effect of Disk Disease on the Mind (Somatopsychic Changes)

Disk disease tends to affect middle-aged individuals who have never been seriously ill.

> **!** A disk herniation causing severe pain and marked limitation of movement can be an unpleasant shock to both the body and the soul of a previously well 40-year-old.

The way patients deal with the shock depends in large measure on their psychological make-up. Many patients alter their basic attitude so that, even after the acute episode of pain has subsided, they live in fear that it will recur. This is particularly common among individuals whose work or family situation requires intense physical labor. Formerly robust and active individuals who used to rise to any challenge become frail, fearful, and seemingly averse to work. Often, they go to the doctor for even the most trivial back pains to obtain a sick note. Problems arise at work because of their diminished performance and frequent absences due to illness. Unless they can be retrained or transferred to another line of work for the same employer, they are often asked to take early retirement.

> **!** In many occupations, lumbar syndrome leads to a decline of the sufferer's social status

—and this puts them under additional emotional stress. Once the mechanisms of giving up work and applying for a pension have been initiated, the sufferer enters into a new situation in which the presence of lumbar syndrome repeatedly needs to be demonstrated to colleagues at work, family members, and the physician, even when the low back pain has subsided or disappeared. Treating patients in this phase of their illness is one of the more thankless tasks that physicians face. Successful treatment, leading to full relief of symptoms, would be incompatible with the already established concept of the patient as a permanent sufferer, which needs to be maintained. The patient has every incentive to use low back pain and the resulting limitation of movement as means to satisfy pressing personal needs.

> **!** In this way, an organic disturbance of posture metamorphoses into a psychosomatic disturbance of attitude.

■ Deliberate Simulation or Exaggeration of Disk Disease

Malingering. Sometimes an organic substrate for the manifestations of disk disease is present to only a minor degree, or is entirely lacking, in patients who deliberately simulate or exaggerate their symptoms as a means of advancing their personal interests. There must be some sort of secondary gain: approval of a pension, avoidance of unpleasant work, or an excuse for inadequate performance of any type, including sexual. Such individuals actually have a normal personality type and are deliberately trying to seem ill to others, particularly physicians, in order to gain personal advantage. Some malingerers become so wrapped up in their role that the simulated illness is transformed into a real one.

> **!** Most of the time, however, these are emotionally normal individuals who simulate the manifestations of illness more or less skillfully although they are really not suffering from them at all, or only to a minor extent.

Methods of assessment. Physicians called upon to assess such individuals medicolegally face a difficult situation when the patient simulates illness with nothing more than a complaint of pain, e. g., severe neck pain, low back pain, or sciatica. Such patients are said to be

> **!** Playing pain games with the doctors.

The physician must take a meticulous history, asking about all of the characteristic features of discogenic symptoms (positional dependence, fluctuating course). Uninterrupted, severe pain and stocking-like sensory deficits in the limbs, for example, are not typical components of degenerative spinal syndromes.

The task of the medicolegal assessor is easier when the patient attempts to simulate not only pain, but postural and functional disturbances as well.

13

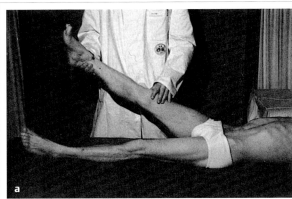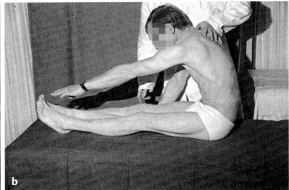

Fig. 13.1 a, b   The Lasègue test (**a**) and the straight-leg-sitting test (**b**).

> ! A sciatic postural abnormality, with its characteristic torsion of the trunk, is difficult to simulate.

Malingerers generally fail to keep up the pretense of a sciatic postural abnormality consistently, particularly while dressing and undressing and while climbing onto the examining table. Individuals truly suffering from sciatica avoid all movements involving forward bending of the trunk with extended hip and knee joints; they use the buttocks as a fulcrum and keep the trunk straight. Any deviation from this antalgic posture causing even minimal contact of the prolapse with the nerve root provokes severe pain radiating into the leg. Sudden, twitching movements due to pain are not a feature of spondylogenic disorders.

The straight-leg-sitting, reclination, and kneeling tests. The Lasègue test (**Fig. 13.1 a**), i. e., the provocation of pain by raising the straightened leg when the patient is supine, is a widely used test that is well known among patients. The sciatic nerve can be stretched for diagnostic purposes just as effectively with the so-called **straight-leg sitting test** (**Fig. 13.1 b**).

If the patient complains of severe pain on straight-leg raising in the Lasègue test and can then sit up with extended knees and touch the dorsa of both feet, for example in response to the examiner's request to demonstrate just how far down the pain radiates, then the Lasègue test certainly was not truly positive. Similarly, the examiner can lift up the leg of the seated patient by the heel, extending the knee, as if to check the pedal pulse. If the patient's upper body then deviates backward, the reclination test is positive, and this makes any other positive sciatic nerve stretch tests more credible. On the other hand, if the patient remains bolt upright during the **reclination test** (negative reclination test), then the cause is not organic. The same holds for the **kneeling test:** a patient who claims to be unable to bend forward either while standing or while kneeling is not to be believed (**Fig. 13.2**).

If a patient complains of pain immediately when the examiner begins raising the straightened leg or as soon as being asked to bend forward from an upright position, then the straight-leg sitting, reclination, and kneeling tests can provide good evidence for either an organic or a nonorganic cause. The suspicion of a nonorganic cause arises if a single test is positive; if two or all three are positive, then our experience (Nentwig et al. 1993) implies that the credibility of the patient's complaints is questionable.

If the patient claims to have used the affected limb to a lesser extent than normal, or not at all, for several months because of allegedly continuous pain—typical statement: "I haven't been able to use my arm for a long time because it's so weak"—then the examiner can assess the veracity of this claim (e. g., for an arm) by measuring and comparing the circumferences of the affected limb and its unaffected counterpart, inspecting the hands for calluses and other evidence of manual labor, and comparing the radiographic bone density on the two sides.

These examining techniques can also be used to some extent in patients who are not malingering but have psychosomatic symptoms. A good deal of clinical experience is necessary in order to be able to distinguish psychosomatic syndromes and simulated disease manifestations from genuinely organic spinal syndromes. An examiner who is not entirely certain how to judge the situation must always treat the patient as if the problem were truly somatic.

> ! The worst thing that can happen to patients with an organic disturbance, such as a compressed nerve root, is to be treated by the physician as if they are malingerers or mentally ill.

The large number of noninvasive diagnostic and therapeutic techniques that are available for degenerative spinal disorders can be used to gain time to reassess the patient in repeated follow-up, and thereby achieve a clearer picture of the underlying problem.

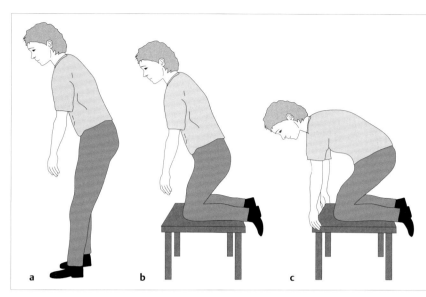

Fig. 13.2 a–c A kneeling test is done if the patient cannot bend forward at all from the standing position with extended knees because of alleged pain in the back and legs (**a**). The patient is asked to kneel on a chair and bend forward. If the patient apparently can bend forward only slightly or not at all (**b**), a nonorganic cause should be suspected. This is because, when the knees are bent, the sciatic nerve and ischiocrural muscles are under so little tension that even a patient with acute lumbar syndrome and nerve root compression should be able to bend forward from the hips (**c**).

■ Psychotherapy and Relaxation Techniques

Psychological diagnostic and therapeutic techniques are used alongside somatic techniques in the care of patients with lumbar disk disease. Emotional disorders and reactive disturbances can be treated, and relaxation techniques such as autogenic training or progressive muscle relaxation can also have a directly beneficial effect on the somatic problem.

Treatment by a psychologist or psychiatrist is indicated in cases of anxiety, and depression (emotional shock due to disk herniation in middle age) and when the pain experience is out of proportion to the physical findings or pain seems about to become chronic (Engle and Ströbel 1990, Basler 1998, Pfingsten 2005). Talk therapy, conflict evaluation, and the guidance of a psychologist in finding new ways of coping with the pain and learning relaxation techniques have all proved useful. The treatment can be considered successful when the patient can deal with the pain and maintain a positive attitude toward life despite all functional impairments and limitations. This is especially true for patients with intractable PDS.

The main relaxation techniques, as listed by Kröner-Herwig and Pfingsten (2005), are the following:
- progressive muscle relaxation (described by Jacobson 1993)
- autogenic training
- biofeedback
- hypnosis
- other methods of imagery and meditation techniques.

The relaxation technique that is by far the most commonly used in the multimodal therapy of disk disease is *progressive muscle relaxation,* as described by Jacobson, which has now largely replaced autogenic training.

Autogenic training, a method derived from hypnosis, was introduced by J. H. Schulz in 1930. It enjoyed wide use in many different variations as an auto-relaxation technique. A relaxed state is actively generated by the repetition of a set of formulae involving visualizations of parts of the body. The resulting diminution of muscle tension breaks the vicious circle of pain, muscle spasm, and more pain. We use autogenic training as an ancillary treatment for disk disease in small groups of patients in both in-patient and outpatient settings. Our goal is to replace these patients' initial "coachman" posture with the more beneficial step posture.

> **!** Generalized relaxation and reduction of tone in the truncal and proximal limb muscles creates appropriate conditions for the disturbed motion segment to return to its original, normal position.

Disk protrusions become flattened, and the position of the intervertebral joints becomes normal again.

Progressive muscle relaxation (PMR) leads even more directly to relaxation in the stress-reducing position. This is a method whose only purpose is relaxation. It is useful both for the correction of abnormal postures of muscular origin and for the relief of pain.

The essence of PMR is that the patient first gains control over the degree of tension of a muscle or muscle group and then consciously relaxes it, gradually, minute

13

by minute, in response to the therapist's instructions. As with autogenic training, these exercises are later continued by the patient working alone.

The main advantages of PMR over other relaxation techniques are that it is easy to learn and that it usually yields rapid results (Kröner-Herwig and Pfingsten 2005).

Summary

Disk disease is often accompanied by psychological changes. These changes, in turn, play a major role in the transition to a chronic disorder. The spine and the mind interact in both directions. Psychosomatic disorders can be projected on to the spine; conversely, long-standing and painful disease of the spine can take an emotional toll.

Both the organic and the psychosocial component have to be taken into account in the diagnosis and treatment of back pain. Physicians in training should be instructed in the psychological aspects, and, conversely, psychologists in training should be instructed in the medical aspects. The examiner should be able to recognize behavioral disturbances and to assess the clinical findings properly, e. g., genuine vs. simulated pain on stretching of the sciatic nerve.

A systematic review within the framework of the Cochrane Collaboration Back Review Group concluded that behavioral treatment seems to be an effective treatment for patients with chronic low back pain, but what type of patients benefit most from what type of behavioral treatment (van Tulder et al. 2000) is still unknown.

If risk factors for a spinal disorder becoming chronic are noted early on in the course of treatment (ideally at the first visit), then the medical treatment of the spinal syndrome per se should be accompanied by an appropriate program of psychological treatment.

Conclusion

The management of disk disease requires attention to the mind as well as the body.

14 Back School

Back school (*ryggskola* in Swedish, *Rückenschule* in German) was introduced in Sweden in 1969 by Marianne Zachrisson-Forsell (1980) and Alf Nachemson. In subsequent years it has become the gold standard for rehabilitation and prevention of low back pain.

! Back school is the training of proper posture and behavior
• for the prevention of injury to the back.

Underlying principle. As part of the rehabilitation and prophylaxis of spinal injuries, particularly disk diseases, patients do muscle-strengthening exercises and learn back-friendly methods of lifting, carrying, bending, sitting, standing, and lying. They also learn and practice the proper movements and bodily postures for a variety of everyday activities such as dressing and undressing, washing, and household chores. The **subject matter to be learned** consists, essentially, of three parts:

- information about the structure and function of the spine
- systematic training in the back school rules for lifting, bending, sitting, standing, lying, etc.
- active protection of the spine through gymnastics and sports.

Information is imparted and demonstrations are given in group sessions, which are then supplemented with practical exercises. The **target population** for back training as a means of secondary prevention consists of patients who have been through an episode of disk disease and wish to avoid a recurrence. The teachings and exercises of back training are also used as primary prevention for individuals who have not yet had a bout of disk disease, but are at risk: children and adolescents with poor posture, adults with an invariant posture at work (sedentary occupation) and in their spare time, and all individuals with weak muscles.

■ The Biomechanical Principles Of Back School

Activating the osmotic system of the disk (**Fig. 14.1**) (see Chapter 5). The pressure-dependent shifting of fluid into and out of the disk as an osmotic system is the basis of

! Back school rule 1 (**Table 14.1**): Thou shalt exercise.

The regular alternation of loading and unloading of the spine, through activities including sports and gymnastics, promotes metabolic exchange in the intervertebral disk.

Avoiding excessive intradiscal pressure (**Fig. 14.2**) (see Chapter 5). As discussed in Chapter 5, experimental studies have shown that certain bodily postures and

Table 14.1 The 10 rules of back school

1 Thou shalt exercise.
2 Keep your back straight.
3 Kneel to bend.
4 Don't lift heavy objects.
5 Spread out loads evenly, and keep them next to your body.
6 When sitting, keep your back straight and support your upper body.
7 Do not stand with straight legs.
8 When lying down, keep your legs bent.
9 Do sports, particularly swimming, running, or cycling.
10 Train your spinal muscles every day.

14

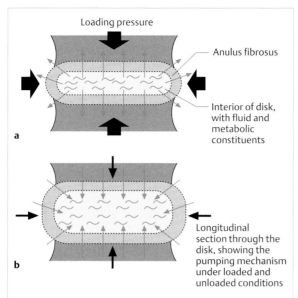

Fig. 14.1 a, b The intervertebral disk as an osmotic system.
a Load > 80 kg: fluid and metabolic waste products are pressed out of the disk.
b Load < 80 kg: fluid and nutrients are taken up into the disk.

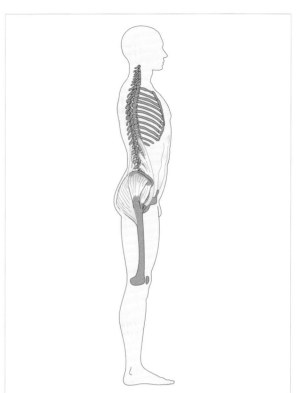

Fig. 14.3 Muscular stabilization of the lumbar motion segments by the muscles of the trunk and hips.

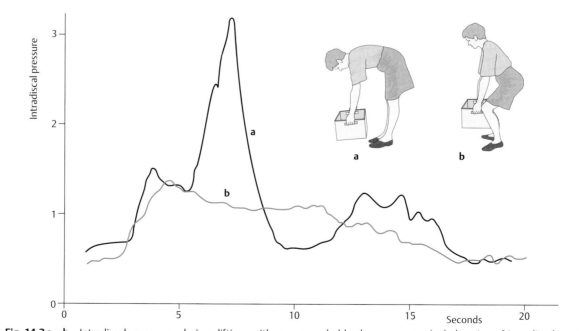

Fig. 14.2 a, b Intradiscal pressure during lifting with a rounded back (**a**) and a straight back (**b**). Lifting with a rounded back causes a marked elevation of intradiscal pressure with a sharp peak (Nachemson 1966, Wilke 2004).

movements markedly elevate the intradiscal pressure. Back school teaches how these postures and movements can be avoided. Experimental studies and clinical observations both show that high intradiscal pressure, combined with asymmetrical loading of the intervertebral disk, leads to displacement of disk tissue and ultimately to disk protrusion and prolapse. Back school rules 2–6 are based on these biomechanical facts. The purpose of back school is to avoid increasing intradiscal pressure (Farfan 1996).

Avoiding telescoping of the intervertebral joints. Axial loading causes the lumbar intervertebral joints to become telescoped into one another. Lordosis and hyperlordosis augment this effect. The joint capsules are overstretched. This unfavorable situation can be counteracted by gently folding the legs (rules 7–8).

Building up the trunk musculature (**Fig. 14.3**) (see Chapter 5). Training of the abdominal, erector spinae, and proximal leg muscles stabilizes degeneratively slackened lumbar motion segments from without.

■ Sitting

The stress-reducing effect of brief sitting. Sitting is wrongly considered to be generally harmful to the intervertebral disk. Many individuals suffering from low back pain are glad to be able to sit down for a short time after prolonged standing and walking, e.g., in a museum or while shopping. The deep and unbearable pain in the low back subsides immediately. The reason for this is that the hyperlordosis that sets into the lower lumbar motion segments after prolonged standing is flattened again when the individual sits, so that the intervertebral foramina become larger and the spinal canal becomes wider. That the lumbar motion segments are under reduced stress in this flattened or kyphotic posture is also demonstrated by the observation that the antalgic posture adopted by individuals with sciatica always includes a mild forward bending of the trunk.

! Sitting with the hips and knees flexed and the lumbar lordosis neutralized restores the spine to the natural curvature that it had early on in ontogenetic development.

The sitting position is also phylogenetically older than the erect posture, in which the hip joints are extended. Sitting abolishes all of the postural elements that were acquired along with the upright stance: lumbar lordosis, hip extension, and knee extension. The sitting position also corresponds to the stress-reducing step position, albeit with a 90° rotation, so that there is additional stress on the spine from gravity. A proper sitting posture is therefore crucial, so that spinal loading can be distributed evenly and held to a minimum.

There are three sitting postures, in which the center of gravity is located in front of, immediately above, or behind the sitting surface.

Sitting Forward

! In the sitting-forward posture (**Fig. 14.4 a**), the intradiscal pressure is almost twice as high as during standing.

Increased loading of the anterior edge of the intervertebral disk, combined with high intradiscal pressure, leads readily to disk tissue displacement in a dorsal direction, i.e., to a protrusion or prolapse. According to the measurements of Andersson et al. (1974), the loading pressure on the disk is much lower when a individual sits upright with a flattened or lordotic lumbar spine than during sitting with a fully rounded back. It is of course possible to sit up actively from the sitting-forward posture, putting the lumbar spine into a lordotic position; this requires much truncal and muscular work, however, and can only be transiently maintained, because the lumbar spine normally assumes a kyphotic position when the hips are flexed to 90° and the pelvis is tilted backward (**Fig. 14.4 a**).

A backrest with a lumbar support was suggested as early as 1889 by **Staffel** as a means of counteracting maximal kyphosis and giving the spine its normal shape when the individual leans back (Staffel 1889). The beneficial effect is only brief, however, and then the lumbar support presses against the flattened or ky-

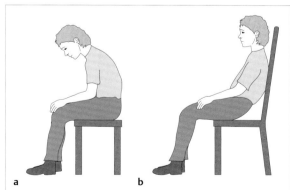

Fig. 14.4 a, b.
a The sitting-forward position: lumbar intradiscal pressure 0.65 MPa.
b The sitting-backward position: lumbar intradiscal pressure 0.3 MPa.

14

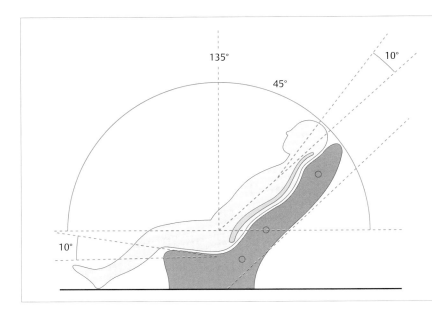

Fig. 14.5 The stress-reducing sitting position: lumbar intra-discal pressure 0.3 MPa.

photic lumbar spine at certain points. As Grandjean and Burandt (1962) observed, the desired correction also fails to occur when the individual, as usually happens, does not lean back properly or when the buttocks slide forward on the seat.

Sitting Back

> ! The appropriate position for sitting is one that puts the least stress on the disks, ligaments, and muscles.

As only lying down brings about a near-total unloading of all of these elements, individuals who must sit for a long period of time should attempt to sit in positions most closely approximating the lying position. Most individuals meet this requirement unconsciously by sliding forward in the seat while reclining the upper body backward, as long as the sitting surface offers enough room to do so. The final result is the extreme sitting-backward position with the pelvis tilted back (**Fig. 14.4 b**). This position is felt as pleasant at first, because the weight of the upper body is partly supported by the backrest. Nonetheless, if the backrest is high and close to the vertical, lack of lumbar support will lead to the development of a maximal kyphosis, not just of the lumbar spine but also of the cervical spine.

The stress-reducing sitting position. If, however, the backrest is shaped to correspond to the physiological curvature of the spine, and the head and neck are supported at a more favorable angle, then reclining to 45° results in a sitting posture that takes stress off the spine, ligaments, and muscles. The posture-maintaining work required of the cervical and truncal muscles is minimal

in this stress-reducing position (**Fig. 14.5**). The loading pressure on the intervertebral disk is reduced in all portions of the spine. In the lumbar spine, it is less than 0.3 MPa and approximately equal to the loading pressure in the horizontal position (Nachemson 1974, 1976). Both Andersson et al. (1974) and Wilke (2001) showed that the loading pressure on the lumbar disks diminishes the more the backrest is reclined backward. A parallel lessening of activity in the trunk muscles was demonstrated electromyographically by Hosea and Simon (1984).

In the stress-reducing sitting position, the backrest should not be too soft, and it must have a mild protrusion at the lumbar and cervical levels corresponding to the somewhat flattened lordosis at these levels. As the ankle between the thigh and the truncal axis increases to 135°, lumbar support lessens the backward tilting of the pelvis. The main points of support are now at the thoracolumbar junction and in the craniocervical region. To give the seated individual a better viewing angle, the head is inclined 10–20° forward in relation to the truncal axis. The depth of the seat is adapted to the length of the thighs and its surface is inclined about 10° downward from front to back in order to keep the individual from sliding forward in the seat; a footrest may help achieve the same purpose.

One can use a 45° chair of this type to make the sitting position as much like the horizontal position as possible, not just during leisure hours but also during some types of occupational activity. This stress-reducing position can be obtained almost instantly with some kinds of adjustable easy chairs or TV loungers. It has also been found practical for driving (Krämer et al. 1979, 2005), as the low height of the seat above the floor of standard cars forces the driver to assume a sitting-back-

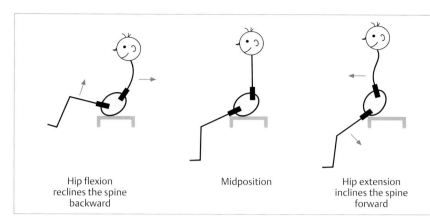

Fig. 14.6 Diagrams from back school showing the effect of hip flexion and extension when the individual is seated. Hip flexion causes kyphosis of the lumbar spine; hip extension causes lordosis of the lumbar spine (from Krämer J. Bandscheibenschäden. Vorbeugen durch Rückenschule. Munich: Heyne; 2005.).

Hip flexion reclines the spine backward

Midposition

Hip extension inclines the spine forward

ward position anyway. Any attempt to bring the spine into an upright position only leads to an even more pronounced lumbar kyphosis.

Guidelines for the **sitting-upright position** with a vertical spine were published by Akerblom (1948), Schoberth (1962), and Berquet (1984). According to these guidelines, the lumbar region should be firmly supported with a suitable backrest that reaches to the border of the pelvis. Chairs must have armrests so that some of the weight of the upper body can be laterally supported on the elbows at least some of the time, reducing the posture-maintaining work demanded of the shoulder and neck muscles. The proper depth of the seat depends on the length of the thighs, and the seat should be inclined downward about 5° from front to back. Writing desks should be of a height that the lower arms can be freely rested on the desktop without any need to raise the shoulders. The workplace, where many individuals spend a large part of their lives, must be adapted to individual body size, and this is best done with direct trials of the sitting position. Bad fitting of the workplace to the worker leads to the indefinite maintenance of harmful postures.

Sitting and the angle of the lumbar spine, pelvis, and leg. The lumbar spine, pelvis, and leg are a biomechanical system connected by ligaments and muscles. Even without muscle activity, the posture of the spine is affected by the position of the leg: hip extension causes lordosis and hip flexion causes kyphosis of the lumbar spine. Changes of leg position have a stronger effect on lumbar spinal posture if the ligaments of the joint capsules and the lumbar muscles are short and inelastic (**Fig. 14.6**). The angle of the lumbar spine, pelvis, and leg has been studied by Nentwig, Krämer, and Ullrich (1997) and Schramm et al. (1997).

In the sitting-forward and sitting-upright positions, therefore, the hip joints should be less flexed; the knees should be below the hips. A seat cushion can be used to help maintain this posture: Schneider and Lippert (1961) suggest the use of a cushion together with a for-

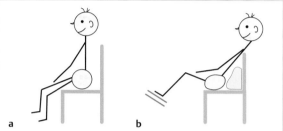

a   **b**

Fig. 14.7 a, b More diagrams from back school.
a The sitting-forward and sitting-upright positions: the knees are lower than the hips.
b The sitting-backward position: the knees must be above the hips to maintain the physiological lumbar lordosis with a normal angle of the lumbar spine, pelvis, and legs.

ward-tilted seat surface. On the other hand, raising the legs (knees above hips) is necessary to maintain physiological angle of the lumbar spine, pelvis, and leg in the sitting-backward position (**Fig. 14.7**).

Dynamic Sitting

The more recent intradiscal pressure measurements of Wilke et al. (1992–2001) have shown a high variability of intradiscal pressure during sitting, depending on position: the values ranged from 0.83 MPa in the sitting-forward position with rounded back to 0.27 MPa in the stress-reducing "relaxed" position. This implies that an alternation of sitting positions can effect an alternation between loading and unloading of the disks, allowing fluid to move in and out of the intervertebral spaces. By temporarily supporting the upper body with armrests (similarly to the parallel bars used in gymnastics), one can even bring the intradiscal pressure down as low as 0.10 MPa. The back school recommendation therefore includes dynamic sitting with alternation of positions and occasional support of the upper body on the armrests.

14

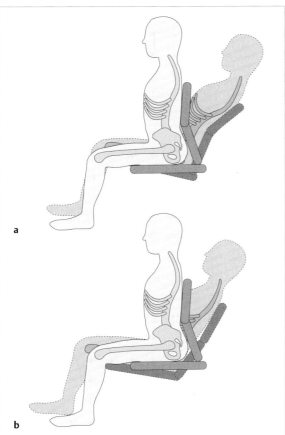

Fig. 14.8 a, b Dynamic sitting with alternation between two positions (Wilke 2004).
a The previous recommendations enabled alternation of loading, but no movement.
b New concept: When the individual leans back, the contour of the backrest changes and the seat surface slides forward. This allows alternation of loading and movement in the lumbar segments. The individual can, for example, work with a desktop computer in either of the two sitting positions.

Some of types of chair that are currently on the market enable dynamic sitting only to a limited extent. A dynamic chair design makes dynamic sitting possible, as required by proper back school. Based on the new understanding of lumbar spine dynamics, Wilke (2004) has proposed a new type of chair design to facilitate dynamic sitting (**Fig. 14.8**). According to this design, the lumbar lordosis is still supported when the individual sits upright, as with previous chair designs. When the individual leans back, the curvature of the backrest continually changes, finally allowing kyphosis once the individual leans all the way back. The seat surface can also slide forward when the individual leans back, so that the spine does not leave the surface of the chair. These two features of this novel chair design enable the spine to be supported over its entire length even in the maximal sitting-backward position. Thus, the intervertebral disks and other participating spinal structures bear a variable load, depending on the sitting position; the changing backrest contour lets the entire spine move, i. e., natural movement occurs even during sitting.

■ Standing

An upright stance with fully extended hips and a lordotic lumbar spine is a newly acquired phylogenetic feature of the human species. Standing places **stress** on the cervical and lumbar disks in a mechanically unfavorable lordotic configuration. Poor posture, with the pelvis tilted forward, further accentuates the lumbar lordosis. Accordingly, many patients with pre-existing damage of the intervertebral disks have back pain after standing for a long time without changing position. The pain arises both from the inadequate postural muscles of the trunk and from the intervertebral joints. In order to prevent such symptoms arising, one should take every opportunity to interrupt long periods of standing with short walks. When an individual walks or runs elasti-

cally, the swinging arm movements and the alternation of each leg between the standing and swinging phases of gait cause a beneficial variation of intradiscal pressure favoring fluid exchange in the intervertebral disk. To reduce intradiscal pressure in the lower spinal segments when standing for longer periods of time, one should try to lean against a wall or support the upper body with the hands on any nearby surface or object.

During standing, the prolonged maintenance of a **half-bowed posture** (e. g., for gardening) has a particularly harmful effect on the disks and back muscles. The intradiscal pressure is higher than in the erect posture. The disks become wedge shaped; if the individual suddenly stands upright, they can protrude posteriorly,

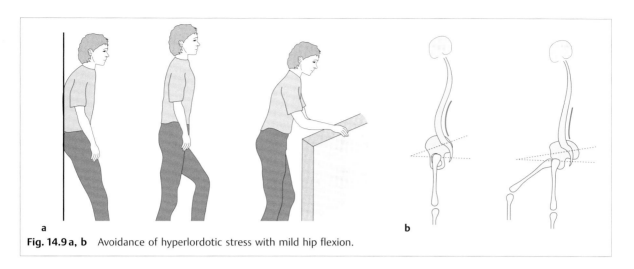

Fig. 14.9 a, b Avoidance of hyperlordotic stress with mild hip flexion.

causing symptoms. Furthermore, the half-bowed position puts excessive demands on the erector spinae muscles, which become painful if they are inadequately conditioned. Therefore, tables and working surfaces should be high enough to allow prolonged activity in an upright, rather than bent, posture. *Tools with long handles* should be used as much as possible for gardening and housework. A *standing desk* is recommended for brief writing tasks.

! Hyperlordosis of the lumbar spine, like extreme kyphosis, • should be avoided.

As discussed in Chapter 11, hyperlordotic low back pain arises from poor posture combined with insufficiency of the back muscles and can also be caused by walking downhill, wearing high-heeled shoes, or working above one's head. This type of low back pain can be prevented by intensive training of the back muscles as well as by certain neutralizing postures for flattening the lumbar lordosis while remaining standing, if there is no opportunity to sit down for a short time. Some degree of relief can even be obtained, for example, by leaning against a wall with the hips mildly flexed and the upper body bent slightly forward, or by supporting oneself temporarily on a railing or banister. One can also flatten the lumbar lordosis by alternately planting first one foot, then the other, on a step or an elevated area of the floor (**Fig. 14.9**) (back school rule 7).

The prevention of hyperlordotic low back pain with a flexion orthosis is discussed in Chapter 11.

■ Lying

The stress-reducing step position is an essential component of the *treatment* of disk disease, but proper positioning and the correct choice of a supporting surface also play an important role in its *prophylaxis*. Many individuals go to bed pain-free and wake up in the morning with pain in the low back or neck. Humans spend about one-third of their lives in the horizontal position and two-thirds erect. In order for the spine to be under as little mechanical stress as possible during lying and sleeping, enabling fluid uptake into the disk, the **supporting surface** should be such as to keep the intradiscal pressure as low as possible. As shown by intradiscal pressure measurements, the disk is minimally loaded when the individual lies supine, or in the lateral decubitus position, on a firm mattress with mildly flexed hips and knees. If the mattress is too soft, a longitudinal depression forms, with its deepest point at the body's center of gravity, which is in the upper lumbar region. The result is that the lumbar spine is bent backward in the supine position, and laterally in the lateral decubitus position. A pillow or wedge below the head further accentuates this unfavorable bending of the spine. This position not only elevates the intradiscal pressure but also, as already described, deforms the disk into a wedge shape in the segments of maximal curvature. Under these circumstances, discogenic pain in the lumbar or cervical spine can easily arise when the individual turns during sleep, or shortly after getting out of bed.

A *slatted bed-frame* under the mattress is a simple way of creating a firm sleeping surface. The head and neck are best positioned on a *neck roll,* which can be easily formed, for example, from any loosely filled pillow (**Fig. 14.10**).

14

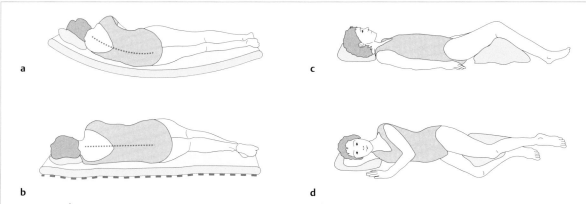

Fig. 14.10 a–d.
a Lateral curvature of the spine caused by an excessively soft mattress.
b With a slatted frame under the mattress, the spine remains straight.

c, d Avoidance of pain due to excessive lordosis (facet syndrome) in the supine and lateral decubitus positions by mild flexion of the hips and knees. Keeping a cushion or folded blanket between the legs in the lateral decubitus position stabilizes the position and prevents torsion of the lumbar spine (back school rule 8).

The **prone position** is beneficial to the intervertebral disks because it promotes lordosis of the cervical and lumbar spine. The cervical spine, however, undergoes not only reclination (lordosis) but also a greater or lesser extent of rotation, which may impair flow in the vertebral artery and/or lessen the space available to the nerve roots in the intervertebral foramina on the concave side. Patients who habitually sleep on their stomachs often complain of a stiff neck or finger paresthesiae in the morning.

Not only the proper choice of sleeping surface, but also the **duration of sleep** is highly relevant to the generation of disk-related symptoms. When the body is horizontal, gravitational loading is removed from the disks, which take up fluid and thereby increase in volume. Unloading for longer periods of time leads to more fluid uptake; pain can then result from stretching of the posterior longitudinal ligament or of the intervertebral joint capsules.

> ! An already existing protrusion can enlarge and cause worse symptoms when the volume of the disk increases through unloading (removal of weight from the spine in the lying position) for longer periods of time.

Thus, simple horizontal positioning for longer periods than are usual in the individual's circadian cycle can cause disk enlargement and pain. Patients typically complain of back pain arising despite a suitably firm mattress and disappearing shortly after they get up. In hospital, too, one often sees patients—usually younger ones—who complain of low back pain after several days of bed rest, despite the obligatory board under the mattress. If the patient's underlying illness does not permit sitting or standing for short periods, it suffices in

such cases to raise the foot or head of the bed and have the patient perform isometric tension exercises for the truncal muscles. These will raise the intradiscal pressure. Prophylactic measures of this type, to prevent abnormal build-up of fluid in the intervertebral disks, are also recommended for astronauts who spend long periods in space under zero-gravity conditions. Height measurements of American astronauts who had spent several months in space showed them to be a few centimeters taller after returning to Earth than they were before their mission.

Results. It is hard to give a succinct, uniformly valid assessment of back school because of the heterogeneity of curricula (and participants), as well as the diversity of evaluative criteria that have been applied (Nentwig 1999, Nentwig and Czolbe-Flothow 2002, Flothow 2003, Ostelo et al. 2004, van Tulder et al. 2004, 2005, Heymans et al. 2005, Airaksinen et al. 2006, Heymans et al. 2006). Schneider and Schiltenwolf (2005) point out that it is precisely those groups of individuals who are at greatest risk of developing disk disease who make significantly less use of preventive measures such as back school. It follows that only randomized controlled studies can yield valid conclusions. The results of 17 such studies are listed in **Table 14.2**: 9 of them support the effectiveness of back school programs, 2 are inconclusive, and 6 do not demonstrate any beneficial effect. These inconsistent results are partly due to a misunderstanding of the concept of back school: a number of institutions, for example, call themselves back schools while offering no more than a program of muscle-strengthening exercises. Information alone, without any practical exercises, is also insufficient. Lastly, the success of a back school program depends not just on the program itself,

Table 14.2 Randomized, controlled studies on the effectiveness of back training (Ullrich et al. 2004)

Authors	Results		
	Positive	Inconclusive	Negative
Berwick (1989)		●	
Berquist-Ullmann and Larsson (1977)	●		
Daltroy et al. (1997)			●
Donchin et al. (1990)			●
Härkäpää et al. (1992)	●		
Hurri (1989)	●		
Keijsers et al. (1990)			●
Lankhorst et al. (1983)			●
Leclaire (1996)		●	
Lindequist (1984)			●
Linton et al. (1992)	●		
Moffett et al. (1986)	●		
Morrison (1988)	●		
Nentwig and Ullrich (1990)	●		
Postacchini et al. (1988)	●		
Stankovic (1995)			●
Walter et al. (2002)	●		
Total	**9**	**2**	**6**

but on the instructors. The concept of back school is one of the more important elements of the management of back pain; it teaches patients to help themselves, under the motto, "Learn to be good to your back, and your back will be good to you" (Kirkaldy-Willis 1988).

Three prospective controlled evaluative studies have been done in Germany to date: two on back school programs for secondary prevention, by Nentwig and Ullrich (1999) and Walter et al. (2002), and one on primary prevention in kindergarten and in the school of Czolbe-Flothow (1994). All three found positive outcomes. Back school is effective for children as well (Geldhof et al. 2006). Czolbe-Flothow (1994) and Nentwig and Ullrich (1999) described a significant improvement of postural and movement behavior among back school participants as compared to an untrained control group. In a controlled prospective study carried out by the health insurance provider AOK in the German state of Lower Saxony (Walter et al. 2002), the participants in a back school program (patients with low back pain of nonspecific origin for less than 6 months) not only had less pain, but also took fewer days off from work than in-

dividuals in the control group. The "return on investment" for back school was calculated to be 3.1:1 overall and 1.3:1 for the insurance company alone, making such programs highly effective from the economic point of view as well. We hope these encouraging findings will lead to further high-quality primary studies, which, as mentioned above, are currently lacking. Back school is a low-cost technology that can be used with great benefit and cost-effectiveness for both primary and secondary prevention (Ullrich et al. 2004). Carefully selected educational materials can change beliefs and attitudes positively, potentially improving clinical outcomes and reducing work absences due to illness (Waddell 2004). The systematic review within the framework of the Cochrane Collaboration Back Review Group (Heymans et al. 2005) concluded that there is moderate evidence suggesting that back schools have better short-term and intermediate-term effects on pain and functional status than other treatments for patients with recurrent and chronic low back pain. In an occupational setting, back school reduces pain and improves function and return-to-work status (Wiese et al. 2008).

14

Summary

Back school is based on four biomechanical principles:
- The intervertebral disks benefit from an alternation between loading and unloading.
- Peaks of intradiscal pressure provoke disk herniation.
- Excessive lordosis strains the intervertebral joints.
- Powerful muscles stabilize the motion segment.

If these principles are disregarded, back pain arises. Lack of exercise, improper lifting and carrying of heavy loads, and weak muscles will sooner or later lead to back pain. Back school is designed to put these principles into practice; the instruction that is provided therefore consists of both information (theoretical education) and practical postural and behavioral training. Back school is a necessary means of diminishing human suffering as well as unnecessary expense. It accords well with the MIRACLE principle stated at the beginning of this book: at a *m*inimum of *i*nvasiveness, *r*isk, *a*nd *c*ost, it has a *l*asting, beneficial *e*ffect.

Conclusion

Observing the rules of back school leads to less back pain.

15 Exercise in a Pain-Free Range of Motion

The concept of exercise in a pain-free range of motion (EPFRM) is based on the observation that exercise reduces pain. The exercise must not be of a type that worsens pain, i. e., parts of the body should be exercised that are not affected by the pain-producing process. In patients with severe, chronic pain at multiple sites, only a few parts of the musculoskeletal system can be activated without pain, and such individuals typically stop doing practically any physical activity, particularly sports and gymnastics. Patients with back pain and arthrosis, too, say things like, "Because of the pain, I've had to give up all types of sports, even my favorites, as they all make the pain worse."

On the other hand, patients with pain commonly state that they have less pain overall when they are more physically active. They find, by experience, which kinds of movement are good for them and do not give rise to further pains that persist even after the activity is over. Thus, the first rule of back school is, "Thou shalt exercise."

Controlled studies have shown that patients with acute low back pain are more likely to become pain-free if they exercise than if they rest in bed (Coomes 1961, Gilbert 1985, Deyo 1986, Postacchini 1998, Szpalski 1992, Malmivaara 1995, Wilkinson 1995). Exercise therapy integrated into a multimodal program is successful in patients with chronic back pain (Hildebrand 1994, Pfingsten 1997).

■ Exercise and Nociception

As long as exercise does not itself produce pain, it has multiple positive effects on the process of nociception in the musculoskeletal region (**Table 15.1**):

- The increased perfusion accompanying all types of exercise promotes the peripheral degradation of inflammatory mediators.
- Muscle activity increases the transport of metabolic waste products out of the muscle tissue.
- Patterns of movement that are beneficial for the spine and joints bring about positive changes in the central nervous pathways for nociceptive impulse conduction and processing.

The latter is implied both by the gate control theory of pain and by the known mechanisms of neural plasticity. Exercise, like antalgic medication, can dampen or even totally interrupt the conduction and processing of nociceptive impulses.

Exercise above a certain level of intensity causes the release of endogenous pain-relieving substances. The activation of endorphinergic neurons leads to the development of pain tolerance, ranging all the way to analgesia (**Fig. 15.1**).

Endogenous opioid peptides activate peripheral opioid receptors and inhibit nociception in damaged tissue. Endorphins travel from their site of production to their target organs in the same way as hormones. They

---

Table 15.1 Exercise in a pain-free range of motion (EPFRM)

- Neutralizes the effect of pain-producing substances by dilution
- Quiets the activity of the nervous system's nociceptive pathways
- Promotes the secretion of endorphins
- Defuses pain-promoting emotional processes and distracts from the pain

"Exercise your pain away!"

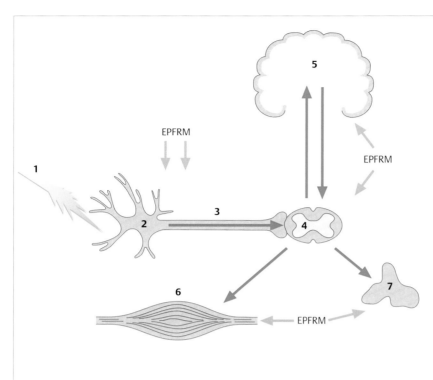

Fig. 15.1 Points along the nociceptive pathway of the musculoskeletal system where the EPFRM program exerts its beneficial effects. Exercise increases perfusion and promotes the removal of inflammatory mediators away from the vicinity of the *noxious stimulus* (**1**), *nociceptors* (**2**) and *afferent fibers* (**3**). New patterns of movement quiet the activity of the pathways for *nociceptive conduction* (**4**) and *nociceptive processing* (**5**) and suppress pain-producing signals. The activation of endorphinergic neurons results in tolerance to pain and diminished pain perception. *The ability to cope with pain* (**5**) and *pain processing* (**5**) are both improved. Metabolic waste products are transported away from the *musculature* (**6**). The concentration of endogenous pain-producing substances is reduced. Better perfusion of the *autonomic nervous system* (**7**) (from Krämer and Nentwig 1999).

inhibit the release of nociceptive neurotransmitter substances, such as substance P, thereby reducing the number of nociceptive action potentials traveling to higher centers. Synaptic activity, with excessive excitation of nociceptive neurons due to a high intracellular calcium concentration, is reduced (Waldvogel 1996).

> ! The most important benefit of exercise in a pain-free range of motion (EPFRM) is psychological. It is highly useful both as a coping mechanism and as a treatment of pain: it distracts the patient from the pain and imparts the feeling of having done something to promote one's own health, including reducing the consumption of medication. The patient's self-esteem improves.

■ Which Exercises are Suitable?

> ! The EPFRM program differs from patient-oriented physiotherapy in three ways: it is not primarily intended to mobilize joints or strengthen muscles, the movements that are used are usually distant from the site of pain, and the purpose is purely that of a dynamic, isotonic exercise program.

The EPFRM program is designed simply to promote exercise as such. It uses only dynamic exercises with isotonic muscle contraction in order to stimulate regional and global blood circulation and metabolism, as manifested by a faster pulse, more frequent respirations, and sweating.

In principle, a particular type of exercise can do no harm to the spine or joints if it is carried out with only minimal or no loading of the moving body part and when the joint is smoothly taken through its comfortable range of motion—i. e., without stretching of the

joint capsule, torsional movements, or asymmetrical forces. The EPFRM program therefore stresses dynamic, "straight-line" types of exercise such as

- swimming
- running
- cycling.

The pattern of movement in these types of exercise is to be contrasted with that of "zig-zag" sports such as tennis, squash, soccer, and volleyball, in which movement is much more often of the stop-and-go variety and puts a greater strain on the joints.

Other types of physical activity besides sports can also be a part of the EPFRM program if they meet the following conditions:

- The activity involves dynamic movement with measurable activation of blood circulation and metabolism.
- Pain is not increased during the activity or afterward.

Gymnastics, aqua-jogging, fitness training, and dancing usually meet these conditions, as do all types of dynamic movement that are involved in gardening, housework, or occupational work.

There is no temporal limit to EPFRM if it is done properly according to these conditions. In other words, a lot of exercise helps a lot.

Exercise Points

Individual types of EPFRM activity have different intensities (**Table 15.2**). Intensity multiplied by duration yields so-called exercise points. The intensities of the typical kinds of spine- and joint-friendly sports and physical activities in the home, the garden, and the workplace were assessed by pulse measurement and by the associated energy use per 10 min period, and were then assigned point scores. Running and its variants rated highest for intensity. Dynamic garden work (raking, lawn-mowing), physical activity at work, dynamic housework (vacuuming, sweeping, etc.), and leisure-time activities such as dancing or walking/hiking were also assigned points that can be added up over the course of each day and logged by the patient in an "EPFRM diary."

Stepwise Program

Patients can engage in different types of exercise and sport over the course of the day, depending on their underlying problem and on how they feel. Those who have severe musculoskeletal pain or are still in the rehabilitation phase after disk surgery, trauma, or acute treatment for spinal disorders must limit themselves to level 1 activities (see **Table 15.2**). As the progress, they can add activities from level 2, after discussion with the treating physician. Before taking up a ball game, for example, the patient can exercise alone with the ball (without an opponent). Tennis begins with long volleys, golf with short games of a few holes.

Table 15.2 Types of sport and exercise and their intensity per unit time when performed with typical power (degree of intensity from 0 [low] to 10 [high]) (from Krämer/Nentwig 1999).

ESFR, level 1	*Intensity points*
Running (jogging)	10
Walking (hiking)	3
Swimming	5
Cycling	6
Aqua-jogging	5
Aerobics	6
Gymnastics	3
Fitness training	3
Arm jogging	4
Dancing	4
Dynamic gardening	3
Dynamic housework	3
Dynamic occupational work	3

ESFR, level 2	*Intensity points*
Soccer	10
Handball	10
Basketball	10
Volleyball	7
Golf	2
Table tennis	5
Tennis	6
Badminton	8
Squash	10
Downhill skiing	4
Cross-country skiing	10
Mountain climbing	5
In-line skating	3
Snowboarding	4
Water polo	10

The intensity of exercise in an EPFRM program normally rises steadily, from a low level just after the acute illness all the way to full capacity. **Patients with chronic pain** generally stop somewhere along this continuum at an individually appropriate point, usually consisting mainly of level 1 activities.

■ EPFRM Units

Running

Endurance running, or jogging, scores the largest number of exercise points per unit time, as it is one of the more intense forms of straight-line exercise. When an individual runs with a slightly bent posture and flexed arms, as most people automatically do, the lumbar motion segments are in their central functional position and subject to a regular, rhythmic alternation of me-chanical loading and unloading. The same holds for the cervical motion segments as long as the head is bent slightly downward and the gaze is directed downward (**Fig. 15.2**). An important prerequisite for the beneficial effect of running on the spine is appropriate footwear with well-cushioned soles. All good running shoes on the market today are of this type.

Running is also the ideal form of exercise for individuals with chronic shoulder pain. The dependent

15

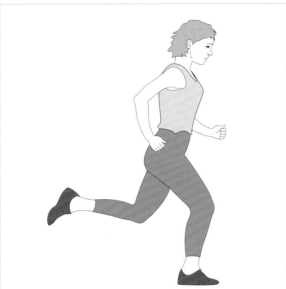

Fig. 15.2 Running, an intense form of straight-line exercise, is a particularly suitable sport for patients with chronic back and shoulder pain. Recommended manner of running: mild inclination of the head and trunk, gaze straight ahead and down, short strides.

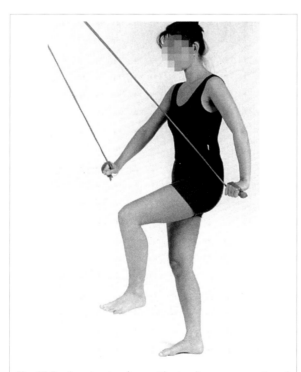

Fig. 15.3 Running in place with simultaneous exercise of the arms using Thera bands. Simultaneous dynamic activation of the upper and lower limbs, to an approximately equal extent (from Krämer and Nentwig 1999).

arms take mechanical stress off of the subacromial space, and their swinging movements promote circulation in this area.

Running is not a suitable form of exercise for individuals with any sort of disease in the lower limbs, particularly hip, knee, or ankle arthrosis. Nor is it useful for individuals with acute spinal syndromes, as each impact with the ground causes pain. In this situation, the basic concept of "exercise in a pain-free range of motion" is not fulfilled.

Running with Simultaneous Activation of the Arms

This is a type of running in place, with activation of the arms, that can be done either on a treadmill or using a special apparatus (e. g., Nordic Trac, Nordic Walking). It corresponds to the traditional style of cross-country skiing. Simultaneous movement of the arms and legs is an intense form of exercise for practically all components of the musculoskeletal system and is particularly suitable for an EPFRM home training program when a limited time is available for exercise (**Fig. 15.3**).

Running with a Reduced Load

While running on a treadmill, individuals can bear part of the weight of the body on the upper limbs by supporting themselves laterally. This reduces the load on the spine and, above all, on the lower limbs. If a treadmill is not available, the individual can do the same while running in place between two chairs (**Fig. 15.4**). This type of exercise is suitable for individuals with painful conditions of the lumbar spine who have pain when running normally. The main indication for it is chronic pain in the hips or knees.

Swimming

Swimming is the ideal type of sport for nearly all chronically painful conditions of the musculoskeletal system. The spinal motion segments and the larger joints can be exercised without excessive loading. Many individuals with chronic pain can exercise without excessive pain in a swimming pool and almost nowhere else.

In water, as elsewhere, the correct posture is important. Chronic pain arising from the intervertebral joints of the cervical and/or lumbar spine worsens when the sufferer does breaststroke. The ideal position in water corresponds to the step position (**Fig. 15.5**), lying on the back. The hip and knee joints are flexed, and the back is straight or lightly reclined backward. The head is bent forward, flattening the cervical lordosis. Rounding (kyphosis) of the back under stress-free conditions is not

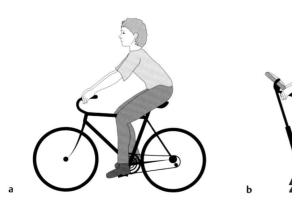

Fig. 15.4 Walking in place between two stationary chairs (from Krämer and Nentwig 1999).

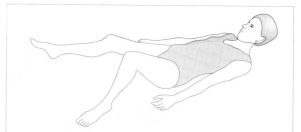

Fig. 15.5 Swimming: backstroke in the stress-reducing position.

Cycling

Cycling is one of the more important activities in the EPFRM program. It can be done by individuals with nearly any type of chronically painful condition of the musculoskeletal system without causing additional pain. Stationary cycling is also an ideal test situation for exercise studies, because it is safe and readily available and because the intensity of performance can easily be measured and quantified.

When an individual rides a bicycle, the weight of the body is not kept above the legs but instead is shifted to the seat and partly to the handlebars. Cycling, therefore, is typically recommended along with swimming to individuals with chronic hip and knee pains that could be worsened by exercise under additional loading. The spine benefits from it, too, even though cycling requires less effort from the truncal musculature than running; the partial support of the upper body on the handlebars takes some of the weight off the spine. Moreover, proper positioning of the handlebars and bicycle seat puts the body in the stress-reducing step position. In their ideal pain-free range of motion (30–40°), the knee and hip joints are mildly flexed and the spine is straight. The hollow of the back (the lumbar lordosis) is largely flattened in this position (**Fig. 15.6**).

harmful, but rather beneficial for the spine. Positive effects are also achieved for patients with chronic shoulder pain, because there are no overhead movements (such as in the breaststroke). This type of swimming is also recommended for those with hip or knee arthrosis. Pedaling movements under water with a 30–40° arc can strengthen the musculature while gently bringing the knee and hip joints through their pain-free range of motion.

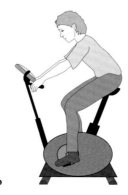

Fig. 15.6 a and b.
a Correct cycling posture: back straight; trunk, thigh, and lower leg in step position.
b Training on a stationary bicycle (ergometer) in the sitting-forward position. The patient sits midway forward with the knees below the hips, the back straight, and the upper body supported in front by the arms on the handlebars. The patient's viewing angle is downward and the display screen is positioned accordingly.

15

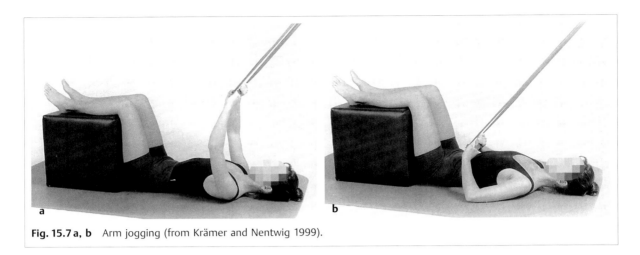

Fig. 15.7 a, b   Arm jogging (from Krämer and Nentwig 1999).

Gymnastics

Any kind of gymnastics that does not increase pain is suitable for the patient with a chronic pain problem. Typically, the suitable EPFRM exercises are those that are carried out with the painful body parts in a position associated with the lowest possible mechanical load, i. e., an intermediate degree of hip and knee flexion and flattening of the lumbar and cervical lordoses. Any exercises that can be done in this position are permissible.

Arm-jogging

Patients with severely painful conditions of the lower lumbar spine (lumbago) or acute irritation of the joint capsules of the hip and knee have pain upon even the slightest movement in these areas. Only the upper limbs can be exercised in such situations; this can be done with the patient in the stress-reducing position (step

positioning). Useful aids include the Bali apparatus (a spring that can be compressed) and the even simpler Thera-Band, an elastic band that can be rhythmically stretched and released (**Fig. 15.7**).

Dynamic Work at Home, in the Garden, and at Work

In addition to all of the types of sports mentioned above, there are many physical activities in everyday life—at home, in the garden, and at work—that can be done without pain and that demand enough exertion from the body to merit the award of exercise points for the patient's EPFRM diary. Such activities include sweeping, vacuuming, raking leaves, etc. As long as patients with chronic back pain obey the rules of back school (see Chapter 14) while carrying out these activities, they should not result in increased pain.

Summary

Patients with chronic back pain (or other painful conditions) can still swim, run, or cycle without having additional pain during or after these activities. The same is true of other level 1 sporting activities (see **Table 15.2**).

Table 15.3 Sporting activities chosen by patients with chronic back pain (n = 300) (from Krämer/Nentwig 1999)

Sport	%
Cycling	35
Swimming	25
Running (jogging)	20
Walking (hiking)	10
Gymnastics	10

In a prospective controlled study, it was found that patients who participated in an exercise program
- had less pain
- used less analgesic medication

than those who did not but were otherwise treated identically (Krämer and Nentwig 1999).

The types of sporting activity that were preferred by pain patients are listed in **Table 15.3**. Women of all ages preferred swimming and cycling, but young men most commonly preferred running. The type of sporting activity that the patient prefers should take a central place in the recommended EPFRM program, to sustain the patient's motivation to participate.

16 Sports

■ Introduction and Literature

Sports play a mixed role in disk disease. On the one hand, suitable types of sporting activity help prevent degenerative changes in the intervertebral disks, according to the motto, "The disk lives by moving." On the other hand, certain harmful types of movement and excessive participation in sports can harm the disks and can, in particular, provoke disk protrusions and prolapses. A review of the relevant literature discloses only a small number of randomized controlled trials on this topic. Most of the available scientific studies on spinal injuries and overuse phenomena in sports are retrospective analyses, theoretical biomechanical papers, and summaries of the authors' personal experience (MacAuley and Best 2002, Schmitt 2004, Göbel et al. 2005, Krämer, Wilcke and Krämer 2005, Lennart and Crabtree 2005).

Just as it has been found difficult to attribute occupation-related spinal changes to a particular pattern of abnormal mechanical stress (Dupuis 1999, Hartmann 1999; see Chapter 17), it has also not been possible to delineate the characteristic features of spinal injury due to any particular sport. There is no "weightlifter's spine," "rower's spine," or "golfer's spine." The literature only contains reports on the frequency and severity of back pain in individual types of sport without indicating any modality-specific patterns of injury (Krämer 1997, Nadler 1998, Day and Giovanni 2001). Fifteen percent of all sporting injuries affect the spine (Day and Giovanni 2001). Female athletes more commonly have low back pain than male athletes (Nadler 1998). Wrestlers

(Granhed and Morelli 1988); triple jumpers, javelin throwers, and gymnasts (Görtzen 1998); power athletes, and weightlifters (Schmitt 2004) have a high lifetime incidence of back pain. Long-distance and marathon runners tend to have less back pain, over the course of their lives, than others. Radiological studies of former high-performance athletes reveal the greatest degree of degenerative change among shot-putters, discus-throwers, and high-jumpers (Schmitt 2004). Despite their marked degenerative changes, however, these former high-performance athletes had fewer symptoms than a control group of individuals who did not have their degree of physical training.

The degree of severity of radiological changes such as spondylosis and osteochondrosis in current or former athletes is much less important than the clinical findings, both with respect to diagnosis and with respect to the medicolegal assessment of any such problems as occupational injuries to the spine. The current state of knowledge on the resilience of the spine to the stresses of sport allows us to make the following statements:

- Trained athletes with well-developed back muscles complain of less back pain than untrained individuals.
- Powerful muscles and taut ligaments are better able to cope with the many mechanical stresses of everyday life than weak muscles and slack ligaments.
- When taken ill, athletes have a strong desire to get well and demonstrate excellent compliance in their aftercare: they are ideal patients.

■ Sports and the Cervical Spine

The special biomechanical properties of the cervical spine owing to the relative heaviness of the head were discussed in Chapter 9. The cervical motion segments

are stabilized by the muscles of the shoulder and the nuchal and anterior cervical muscles. If the physical examination is unremarkable, i. e., in patients without any

16

history of complaints related to the cervical spine and with well-toned shoulder, nuchal, and anterior muscles, there is no reason to advise against any of the usual types of sport. The high acceleration found in motor sports necessitates the use of a cervical support behind the neck. Contact sports such as football, rugby, and wrestling are more likely than other types of sport to cause cervical spine injuries (Watkins and Williams 2004). Whenever a cervical spine injury is suspected, even if it is considered to be unlikely, guidelines for the proper transport of the athlete from the field should be followed. Neck supports extending down to, and resting on, the shoulders should be worn whenever permitted by the rules of the sport.

Individuals with pre-existing spinal injuries and recurrent pain in the shoulder and neck, with or without radiation into the arm, should be especially cautious about combat sports such as judo, karate, and wrestling. They should also be wary of playing soccer (heading the ball) and handball (collision with opponents). Competitive cycling is also problematic because the head is thrust backward during sprinting. In noncompetitive (recreational) cycling, the handlebars can be elevated to bring the upper body into an erect position and avoid the unfavorable configuration of the head and neck. Individuals currently suffering from shoulder and neck pain should not ride a bicycle out of doors, because even mild shocks can exacerbate the pain; in such cases, we recommend a stationary bicycle.

Individuals suffering from chronic, recurrent shoulder and neck pain who nevertheless want to continue participating in a type of sport that is unfavorable for their cervical spine can benefit from compensatory training of the nuchal and shoulder musculature. This should be done with special apparatus under the direction of a physical therapist. Once individuals have become familiar with the apparatus and the exercise program, they can continue the exercises unaided.

■ Sports and the Lumbar Spine

The positive and negative effects of sporting activity on the spine are mainly centered on the lumbar region. Fifteen percent of all sporting injuries affect the spine, and most of these affect the lumbar spine (Day and Giovanni 2001). The most common injuries involve lumbago and sciatica arising either in training or during competition.

The benefit of sport to the lumbar spine is mainly due to the physical exercise associated with most types of sport. Rhythmic loading and unloading of the lumbar spine improves fluid exchange into and out of the intervertebral disks.

> **!** Sports involving exercise improve metabolic exchange in the disks and help prevent disk disease.

Harmful aspects of certain sports with respect to the lumbar spine include the need to maintain an unchanging posture and movements involving forward bending and torsion of the trunk. Mechanical loading of a rounded lumbar spine, particularly when combined with inclination and torsion, causes displacement of slackened disk tissue. The studies of Pope et al. (1980) and Krag et al. (1987), as well as our own (Krämer 1997), have shown that disk protrusions and prolapses can be provoked in the experimental setting by asymmetrical loading of the disk.

> **!** Types of sport involving high intradiscal pressure, asymmetrical loading of the intervertebral disks, and torsion place excessive strain on the disks.

■ Sporting Activities that are Good and Bad for the Intervertebral Disks

A group of orthopedists specializing in sports medicine, with special experience in the treatment of spinal problems in both high-performance and leisure-time athletes, was asked to respond to a questionnaire about which types of sport they considered beneficial and harmful to the intervertebral disks (Warnecke in Krämer et al. 2005), with the main emphasis on leisure-time sport. Experts were asked to make only one assessment per type of sport. All of the experts were approached personally for this study, so the response rate was 100%. The results are shown in **Fig. 16.1**. As expected, **aerobics, running, backstroke swimming, cross-country skiing,** and **dancing** were held to be especially beneficial to the disks. **Horseback riding** also scored high, probably because of the common observation that back pain tends to improve during riding. Contrary to our expectations, however, **cycling** did not score very high, probably because the question about cycling was not specific enough: many experts were apparently thinking mainly of the strongly rounded back, particularly in the sprint posture, which is not a feature of leisure-time cycling. A large group of sporting activities formed a middle category of partly disk-friendly, but also potentially damaging sports, including all types of **team ball games.** Certain very popular types of sport such as **tennis** and **downhill skiing,** as well as **soccer, handball,** and **volley-**

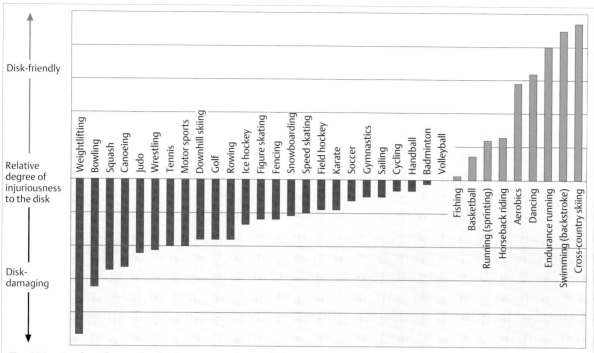

Fig. 16.1 Results of a poll of 18 experts asking which sporting activities they considered beneficial or harmful to the intervertebral disks. The experts were asked for their overall judgment of each sport, with a grade ranging from 1 to 6, in view of the typical movements associated with doing it as a leisure-time activity, rather than competitively (from Krämer, Wilke, and Krämer: Wirbelsäule und Sport, Deutscher Ärzte-Verlag, Cologne 2005).

ball, involve marked axial loading of the spine, with a rounded back and torsional movements.

Weight-lifting, among all sporting activities, was listed as the most damaging to the intervertebral disks. The very heavy weights that must be lifted are, of course, the decisive factor in this judgment. **Golf** and **motor sports** were also largely judged negatively, both because they involve relatively little physical exercise and because they require postures and movements that can be harmful to the intervertebral disks. The relatively neutral assessment of **fishing** and **sailing,** even though both of these activities also require a relatively constant posture, is presumably due to the fact that they can both be done in disk-friendly fashion, in a suitably stress-reducing sitting position, after proper back training. The same is true for other types of sport that were judged as either neutral or harmful, including **downhill skiing, judo, karate, gymnastics, canoeing, bowling, wrestling, rowing,** and **squash:** individuals with spinal problems who want to participate in these demanding sports must undergo compensatory strength and exercise training.

Summary

Any sport that involves exercise has a basically positive effect on the intervertebral disks, but certain types of sport are associated with unfavorable postures and movements that elevate the intradiscal pressure and can thus provoke a disk prolapse. There are no controlled trials on the topic of sports and disk injuries. The available scientific evidence regarding excessive strain on the intervertebral disks and the risk of subsequent disk disease in connection with individual types of sport is confined to retrospective analyses, theoretical biomechanical considerations, and expert opinions. All types of sport involving constantly maintained postures and elevated intradiscal pressures are held to be harmful to the intervertebral disks, while those involving intense physical exercise and little axial loading are held to be beneficial. Anyone who participates in a sport that places excessive stress on the intervertebral disks should also undergo compensatory exercise and strength training and should, for example, regularly run, cycle, or swim in addition.

Conclusion

With a few exceptions, sport is good for the disks.

16

17 Medicolegal Assessment

■ Introduction

Frequency of Medicolegal Assessment of Disk-Related Diseases

Disk-related diseases have a high point prevalence as well as a high annual and lifetime prevalence and are, therefore, frequently the subject of medicolegal assessments by physicians. Indeed, they account for 60 % of all such assessments, followed by disorders affecting the lower limbs (30 %) and upper limbs (10 %). Even when the primary damage is in a limb, e. g. after amputation or after stabilization of a joint, the affected individuals usually claim additional disability because of secondary effects on the spine. Disk disease commonly gives rise to claims of inability to work, inability to pursue one's present occupation, and loss of earning capacity, as well as claims of occupational or accidental injury.

Problems

Pre-existing degenerative disease, the fluctuating nature of the clinical manifestations, and the lack of objective correlates to the pain all complicate the task of medicolegal assessment of disk disease. Because of the diversity of possible interpretations in this area, the judicial process is often protracted, and assessments are often met with counter-assessments and overriding assessments. A further difficulty arises from the fact that, with the exception of small children, all humans have some degree of degenerative disease of the intervertebral disks.

! The spine is much more commonly affected by pre-existing injury than any other part of the musculoskeletal system.

If a disk should be injured still further by a traumatic event, the medicolegal assessor must decide whether to lay more emphasis on the pre-existing injury or on the trauma. In all assessments, the **fluctuating course** of disk disease must be taken into account. The clinical picture varies not only in a circadian rhythm but also over the course of weeks, months, and years, complicating a fair evaluation. Individuals presenting for medicolegal assessment often have no symptoms on the day that they are examined. The physician must then refer to earlier reports in the medical record and to the patient's description of the symptoms at other times. **Imaging studies** yield **only a small amount of information** in the medicolegal assessment of disk disease. On the other hand, an acute cervical or lumbar syndrome that is demonstrably present at the time of examination may subside within a few days or weeks. As discussed in Chapter 12, all types of disk disease tend to improve with age, which implies that all long-term judgments and assessments of diminished working capacity are subject to revision. Follow-up examinations are needed.

As in all other types of medicolegal assessment, attention must be paid to the patient's own attitude to the disease manifestations that they describe. When there is a question of accidental or occupational injury, or indeed of injury while serving in the armed forces or as a consequence of persecution in another country, the most important issue is often that of etiology and pathogenesis. The affected individuals tend to attribute all their symptoms to the event in question. On the other hand, when the assessment concerns the inability to work or loss of earning capacity, causation is relatively unimportant and the main issue is the patient's impaired ability to do their job and the corresponding classification in terms of loss of earning capacity (see **Table 17.7**). In medicolegal assessments concerning an individual's ability to work or to participate in sports, one also finds a certain tendency toward malingering.

> ! Assessing the degree of disability caused by pre-existing spinal damage or trauma is just as difficult as evaluating the ability of individuals with an apparently normal spine to work or take part in sports.

■ Disk Herniations and Accidents

Problems

Everyone who suffers from sudden-onset back pain attributes it to some external event, from a natural tendency to believe that everything must have a cause. Overexertion, faulty posture, or trauma is blamed for the pain. Questions of this type arise in all assessments of possible occupational or accidental injury, and the assessors' opinions are varied. It is sometimes stated that the disks are actually quite robust and that trauma is more likely to fracture a vertebra than to rupture a disk, i.e., that all disk disease is a matter of biological destiny and attributable to degenerative change. Other assessors will attribute the entire disability in disk disease to one or more traumatic events, resulting in the official recognition of the problem as a traumatic injury.

Basic research, above all the studies of Krag (1987), Andersson (1991), Pope (1992), and Waddell (2004), has shown that external factors are part of the multifactorial causation of disk-related diseases and play a role in their etiology and pathogenesis, particularly with respect to the consequences of disk herniation. Individual traumatic events also have a degree of significance as part of this process.

> ! Degenerated disks are highly susceptible to external influences.

In medicolegal assessment, the main issue is in many cases a displacement of disk tissue—intradiscal displacement, protrusion, or prolapse—that may have been provoked or exacerbated by an accident. The assessment is complicated by the possibility that the changes seen in the plain radiographs, CT scans, and MRI scans obtained at the time of the accident might already have been present before the accident without causing any symptoms: 20% of all protrusions and prolapses are asymptomatic.

Pre-existing Damage

Because it can never be assumed that an adult patient had entirely healthy disks before an accident, the demand commonly made by insurance providers for proof of full bodily integrity before the event loses its relevance. No one over 30 years of age has a spine without degenerative changes rendering them more susceptible to external traumatic injury.

There is a particular susceptibility to such injury in midlife, when the biomechanical constellation favors displacement of disk tissue in the intervertebral space (see Chapter 12). Axial forces, particularly when combined with lateral bending and torsion, can bring about a decompensation of the tenuous state of the spine, with intradiscal tissue displacements, protrusions, and prolapses.

Although the structural changes are often impressive, the **clinical findings** are of primary importance for the assessment of pre-existing damage. Protrusions, prolapses, osteochondrosis, and spondylosis can be associated with only mild clinical manifestations, or none at all; on the other hand, there may be relatively marked symptoms when the structural changes are relatively slight. The physician trying to assess pre-existing damage due to degenerative disease must base any conclusions on the history obtained from the patient, and, especially in medicolegal situations, on the information contained in the medical record regarding any previous episodes or low back pain and/or sciatica requiring treatment. When classifying the pre-existing damage, the physician should take account of the fact that so-called simple back pain is a **nearly universal condition** that should **not be designated as a pre-existing illness.** Recurrent low back pain radiating into the leg and requiring medical treatment is of greater significance. Further evidence for the severity of earlier spinal problems can be derived from the very fact that radiological studies were obtained and special treatments such as paravertebral injections, hospitalizations, or surgery were undertaken, if this is the case. Any historical details that the patient cannot remember can be supplemented by information from previously treating physicians and insurance providers.

The Accident

> ! **Definition:** an *accident*, as defined by both private and statutory insurance providers, is a sudden, unpredictable external event that injures the body.

If the accidental event is of a dramatic nature, e.g., a fall, a blow, or a collision, then doubts are generally not expressed as to its having been an accident. Much less dramatic events are usually at issue as the possible cause of disk-related conditions. German law gives a very broad definition of the concept of an accident, particularly in the context of statutory accident insurance, and extends insurance protection not only to the effects of forces originating outside the body but also to a large number of other types of injury that can occur at work. Thus, slipping, twisting one's ankle, stumbling, falling, and catching a heavy weight can all count as accidents. This problem is taken into account in the general conditions for private accident insurance. Insurance protection also extends to strains, sprains, and tears caused by unusually intense exertion on the part of the insured party. The precise course of the traumatic event determines whether it will be legally recognized as the cause of a disk syndrome. It must be determined whether the event described falls under the scope of the insurance policy. Activities that are normally part of the individual's work and are associated with goal-directed movement initiated by the individual him/herself are not considered accidents; activities of this type include lifting and carrying a heavy load, working in a stooped posture, and pushing up a heavy load with the arms. "**Faulty lifting,**" i. e., an attack of pain during the lifting of a heavy object in a stooped posture, is the most common type of event requiring clarification in insurance law. This is a **normal work activity** that cannot be considered a traumatic event and is therefore outside the scope of accident insurance protection. Events of this type are consciously initiated by the individual him/herself. Any disk syndrome or disk herniation that might arise in the course of normal work activities would presumably have arisen at the same time, and with the same degree of intensity, if the individual had been involved in any other activity of everyday life instead.

Normal work activities can, however, be disturbed by external influences. If, in the course of a work activity, the individual must suddenly exert him/herself more than usual, with a sudden, involuntary (reflex) muscle contraction, or when an unusual type of movement is necessitated by an external influence, then this would satisfy the condition of a sudden, unpredictable external event required by the definition of an accident for the purposes of both private and statutory accident insurance.

! The essential feature of an accident is its unpredictability, i. e., being unforeseen and unavoidable.

The effects of such events on the mechanically labile intervertebral disk are much more marked than those of movements that are consciously executed as planned. Such situations arise, for example, when a worker stumbles while lifting and carrying, or when a carrying strap tears and the weight suddenly shifts. A traumatic event is also within the scope of accident insurance protection when, for example, several workers lift up a

Table 17.1 Requirements for a disk herniation or acute disk syndrome to be legally recognized as the result of an accident

- There must be a sufficiently severe trauma, with high intradiscal pressure caused by a violent force originating outside the body and/or an unanticipated exertion that is unforeseen, unpredictable, and unavoidable.
- The typical symptoms must arise immediately.
- The patient must have been free of symptoms immediately before the event.

heavy object simultaneously and then, because the load tilts or one worker drops out, the entire load must suddenly be borne by a single individual. The high intradiscal pressures that come about during such an event, combined with torsion and undue stress on the lateral edge of the intervertebral disk, are produced before the individual has a chance to protect the disk with voluntary contraction of the truncal and proximal appendicular muscles.

Criteria for Recognition

In addition to the presence of a sufficiently intense traumatic event, the state of the individual before and after the accident is of crucial importance in medicolegal assessment. The individual must be asymptomatic just before the event, i. e., the typical post-traumatic symptoms must not have been present immediately beforehand (**Table 17.1**). This question is usually resolved by noting that individuals with low back pain and sciatica generally do not expose themselves to additional mechanical loading of the type involved in the accident. Another important criterion for the recognition of a disk syndrome as being due to an accident is the immediate generation of symptoms. Symptoms that do not arise until hours or days after a given event, but are nonetheless causally attributed to it, should be regarded skeptically. Sudden intradiscal tissue displacements, protrusions, and prolapses cause severe pain immediately. Because the displaced disk tissue can also shift in position after the trauma, it is certainly possible for there to be low back pain immediately after the trauma that then develops into a radicular syndrome over the ensuing days because of further dorsolateral dislocation of the initially displaced tissue. The severe pain and limitation of movement usually cause the affected individual to cease working and present to medical attention within 24 h.

For individuals with the normal degree of pre-existing disk degeneration for their age who sustain a sufficiently intense trauma followed by an acute disk syndrome, the overall compensable injury is apportioned as follows over its further course, in the contexts of legally mandated and private accident insurance, respectively:

Statutory accident insurance. In Germany the principle of contributory causation applies, with all-or-nothing compensation. If the traumatic component predominates, then the overall compensable injury—i. e., the clinical syndrome of post-traumatic low back pain or sciatica—is to be viewed as being entirely the consequence of the accident, for a certain period of time. Only if the disease manifestations caused by the accident subside over time, to be replaced by other manifestations, can the latter be fully ascribed to pre-existing degenerative damage independent of the accident.

Manifestations caused by the accident can be distinguished from manifestations arising independently of it by reference to the spontaneous course of disk disease, as described in Chapter 12.

Private health insurance assumes that the patient's problem, right from the beginning, has both a component that is caused by the accident and an accident-independent, degenerative component. The latter component is referred to as the contribution of events other than the accident. Depending on the extent of the problem that is attributed to accident-independent factors, the accident-related component may initially be assumed to account for up to 100 % of the overall compensable injury and then be gradually scaled back over time. At a future time, the accident-related component might be assessed at, for example, 20 % for 1 year.

Permanent injury. Low back pain and sciatica normally subside over a few weeks to months, even when they are of traumatic origin. All further symptoms arising from the motion segment, particularly any new symptoms that might arise acutely, are a consequence of disk disease rather than of the accident.

If a disk herniation is recognized as being at least partly the result of an accident, then all types of permanent injury that might arise from it will also be the result of the accident, to the same extent as the original herniation. This applies, for example, to residual neuro-logical deficits such as a foot drop after an L5 syndrome, a quadriceps paresis after an L3 or L4 syndrome, or symptoms due to postoperative adhesions (post-discotic syndrome) if the original disk herniation required surgery. Nonetheless, objectifiable permanent injuries, such as adverse sequelae of operations or neurological deficits after a post-traumatic disk syndrome, are encountered only rarely among all cases presenting for medicolegal assessment. In most cases, the expert carrying out the assessment has no evidence for a permanent injury beyond the patient's subjective report of the course of illness. If it is stated that the pain subsided a certain time after the accident and then returned after an asymptomatic interval, then the expert will be able to divide the course of the illness into two periods—one in which the patient suffered from post-traumatic disk syndrome, and another in which the problem was due to degenerative disease.

Such statements by patients are rare. Much more commonly, it is claimed that the pain and impairment resulting from the accident have persisted without interruption from the day of the accident for months and years thereafter. In such cases, the assessment generally involves a stepwise reduction of the percentage of the overall compensable injury that can be attributed to the accident, in accordance with the general medical experience of the spontaneous resolution of disk disease. It can be safely assumed that the entire compensable injury cannot be attributed to the accident alone, because, if there had been no pre-existing damage, a situation of this severity would not have arisen in the first place.

The general medical experience of the spontaneous resolution of lumbar disk herniation (see Chapter 12) implies that the traumatically induced worsening of a disk syndrome undergoes a transition to the normal course of nontraumatic illness within 6 months to 1 year. No precise guidelines can be stated with regard to the percentage distribution of accident-induced and accident-independent factors over time. Any traumatically induced disk herniation that remains symptomatic afterward should be evaluated individually.

Summary

Disk disease is so common (in fact, universal) that the question is often raised whether a particular disk herniation was the result of an accident.

It can be assumed that every human has some degree of pre-existing disk damage (degeneration).

An accident is defined as an unforeseen traumatic event.

The prerequisites for the recognition of an accident as the cause of an intervertebral disk condition are a sufficiently intense trauma, an asymptomatic state before the accident, and typical symptoms immediately after it.

In the German system of statutory accident insurance, all manifestations of disk disease are recognized as being due to the accident, at least for a short period of time, as long as the three prerequisites listed above are satisfied. Private accident insurance, on the other hand, generally assumes a gradually decreasing percentage contribution of the accident to the causation of the overall compensable injury, with an increasing contribution of factors other than the accident.

The medical experience of the spontaneous course of acute disk syndromes implies that permanent damage is not to be expected, unless the disk herniation provoked by the accident has caused a demonstrable, permanent neurologic deficit or has been treated by surgery with consequent adverse sequelae.

Conclusion

Even though disk degeneration is a universal phenomenon in the absence of trauma, a disk herniation can still be legally recognized as the consequence of an accident if certain conditions are fulfilled.

■ Damage to the Intervertebral Disks After the Loss or Permanent Injury of a Limb

! **General considerations:** The partial or total amputation of a limb has an effect on the spine. The motion segments, which normally bear a symmetrical load, are permanently asymmetrically loaded thereafter and develop abnormal signs of wear and tear. The loss or permanent injury of a limb is considered a "pre-discotic" condition, i. e., one that predisposes to the exacerbation of degenerative disk disease.

Cervical Spine

The loss or significant functional impairment of an upper limb induces an asymmetrical posture, particularly in the lower cervical motion segments. The healthy, functional limb is used preferentially; the cervical spine is laterally bent with the convexity on the side of the functional limb (so-called "idemscoliosis"). This abnormal posture, in time, leads to a fixed abnormal curvature of the spine with structural scoliosis. Symptoms arise through the overloading or abnormal loading of the shoulder and neck muscles and through the over-stretching or sprain of the intervertebral joint capsules of the cervical motion segments. On the concave side of the cervical spine, narrowing of the intervertebral foramina can produce signs of nerve root irritation.

Lumbar Spine

When an uncompensated leg-length discrepancy has been present for a long time, as after an amputation or severe knee injury (including fusion of the knee joint), a pelvic tilt develops, with a consequent lateral curve in the spine. The convexity usually points to the shorter, or damaged, side. The lateral curvature can be compensated for at first, but over time a structural scoliosis develops. Leg prostheses for amputees are usually fitted so as to be 1–2 cm shorter than the intact leg, to allow easier swinging of the prosthetic limb during walking, which is particularly useful if the ground is uneven.

Besides this static deviation in the frontal plane, prostheses with a containment socket for the ischial tuberosity also cause a change in the sagittal plane: the pelvis is tilted forward, with consequent hyperlordosis of the lumbar spine. Both of these static abnormalities, lateral curvature and hyperlordosis, are normally well compensated in younger patients, particularly those who actively participate in sports and gymnastics. When these compensatory mechanisms are no longer adequate, because of constitutional or age-related muscle insufficiency, the lumbar motion segments are put under excessive mechanical stress, particularly in the intervertebral joints. Decompensation is illustrated by a fixed lateral curvature of the lumbar spine on an AP plain radiograph, which should be supplemented by functional views in lateral bending to the left and the right. Such changes can also occur after long-standing unilateral functional impairment of a lower limb, resulting, e. g., from fusion of a knee, flexion contractures at the hip and knee joints, or deformities of the foot. The resulting limp places an asymmetrical stress on the spine, particularly the lower lumbar motion segments and the sacroiliac joints. The patient complains of spinal symptoms that arise mainly in the muscles and intervertebral joints. Back pain is most severe when the patient stands or walks. The symptoms are usually those of a local lumbar syndrome. Signs of nerve root irritation resulting from narrowing of the intervertebral foramina are relatively rare.

Medicolegal Assessment

Because of the high prevalence (point prevalence as well as annual and lifetime prevalence) of symptoms in the cervical and lumbar spine (see Chapter 3), amputees and individuals with a damaged limb on one side will often have such symptoms on a degenerative basis alone and then attribute them to their congenital or acquired impairment, simply because of our natural tendency to identify a specific cause for every effect.

There are no statistically valid data on whether amputees or individuals with a damaged limb on one side

17

are more likely to suffer a disk protrusion or prolapse than a comparable control group of healthy individuals. The degree of lateral curvature of the spine, as seen in an AP plain radiograph, is a useful indicator of the severity of the spinal problem caused by a unilateral appendicular injury, and of the likelihood that it will be permanent. Functional radiographs with lateral bending to the right and left will demonstrate whether the curved deformity is "functional" (due to asymmetrical muscle contraction alone) or fixed (i. e., scoliosis, due to structural changes of the spine itself).

Unlike idiopathic constitutional scoliosis, lateral curvatures associated with amputation or severe damage to a limb are free of torsion, i. e., the spinous processes and the oval shadows of the roots of the laminae are projected normally (symmetrically) on plain radiographs. An exception to this rule is seen in permanent unilateral damage to a limb beginning in childhood; in such cases, the scoliosis induced by the injury always has a torsional component as well.

Degenerative changes of the cervical or lumbar spine that would have arisen even without any arm or leg injury must be taken into account as a contributory factor in assessments for private accident insurance and as a contributory cause of symptoms in assessments for statutory accident insurance. The more important changes of this type are loss of disk height in the lower segments of the cervical and lumbar spine and the accompanying local, sometimes radicular manifestations.

Summary

The extent of a unilateral upper or lower limb injury should be assessed. Measurements should be made of any tilting of the pelvis or lateral curvature of the spine, as seen in functional plain radiographs with maximal lateral bending to the right and left. The radiographs should also be inspected for signs of torsion.

If an injury-related lateral curvature of the cervical or lumbar spine is documented, the corresponding injury-related loss of loss of earning capacity should be no more than 10%.

> **Conclusion**
>
> Individuals with a demonstrable scoliosis as the consequence of the loss or permanent injury of a limb are considered to have a loss of earning capacity of up to 10%.

■ Whiplash: Acceleration Injury of the Cervical Spine

> **!** **Definition:** Acceleration injury of the cervical spine ("whiplash") is a painful condition in the nuchal area that results from the forward and backward movement of the head upon abrupt acceleration of the trunk.

Epidemiology

Despite a decline in the frequency of traffic accidents in recent years, there has been a rise in cervical spine injuries after motor vehicle collisions, both in absolute terms and as a percentage of all types of injuries (Kitchel 2004). According to insurance industry data, more than 25 000 claims for whiplash are submitted in Germany each year. The resulting costs, calculated at 1 billion euros annually, are the sum of the costs of judicial proceedings, compensation payments, and, above all, lost income and the costs of treatment (Thomann 2004). The increase in whiplash claims is particularly marked among individuals who were "rear-ended" and were thus not personally responsible for the accident, and who then submit a claim to the other driver's insurance company. The ensuing medicolegal assessments are frequently complicated by a paucity of objective findings combined with a multiplicity of subjective complaints. As a rule, the severity of injury tends to be inversely proportional to the difficulty of the medicolegal assessment.

Terminology

Mechanism of Injury

In a individual sitting or standing upright, the cervical spine is a weak connecting element between the trunk and the relatively heavy head, which is freely mobile in practically any direction. Abrupt accelerations of the trunk causing whip-like movements of the head can occur, for example, when the individual engages in sports, rides a motor-scooter, or—most commonly—is involved in a traffic accident. If there is no headrest, or if the headrest is poorly adjusted, rear-end collisions cause a maximal, undamped backward thrusting of the head followed immediately by a forward rebound (**Fig. 17.1**). If the force of impact comes from the side or obliquely, or—as in some cases—when the individual's head is not oriented straight ahead (in the anatomical position) at the moment of impact, then the cervical spine will be forcibly bent in the frontal plane or in an intermediate plane between the frontal and the sagittal. In addition to these bending forces, there are also forces tending to displace the motion segments forward and backward with respect to one another (translation trauma).

Just as when any other mobile part of the skeleton is subjected to a forcible wrenching (distorsion), a whiplash injury can cause a strain, sprain, or disruption of continuity of the soft-tissue structures of the neck, depending on the intensity of the applied force, together with edema and, in some cases, hemorrhage. The pain of soft-tissue edema may not be felt until a few hours have elapsed (the so-called asymptomatic interval). Severe soft-tissue injuries and fractures, however, are felt immediately.

A traumatizing force applied to the cervical spine, as in whiplash, can also cause dorsal or dorsolateral dislocation of the mobile material in the central portion of a cervical intervertebral disk, as long as there is pre-existing damage of the disk to makes this occurrence more likely. The result may be either a protrusion or a prolapse.

History and Clinical Findings

Individuals who have been injured in rear-end collisions usually state that they did not see the other car and could not have seen it coming. Mild acceleration trauma usually produces no symptoms at first (because of the emotional shock effect, among other reasons). The symptoms tend to arise only after an asymptomatic interval of a few hours, often at night. An important question for medicolegal assessment is whether the patient drove directly home or back to work after taking care of the formalities at the scene of the accident, or instead went to a doctor or was taken to hospital for medical treatment. An asymptomatic interval lasting several days, during which the patient was not seen by a doctor, deserves to be regarded skeptically in medicolegal assessment.

Further important questions regarding the history of the accident include the following:
- Where was the patient seated in the vehicle?
- Was he or she wearing a seatbelt?
- Did the airbag expand?
- What position was the head in at the time of the impact—facing straight ahead, or turned to the right or left?
- Was there any loss of consciousness or amnesia?
- Were there any pre-existing cervical spine symptoms before the accident?

The typical constellation of symptoms largely resembles that of a degenerative cervical spine syndrome: nuchal and occipital pain with painful restriction of the range of

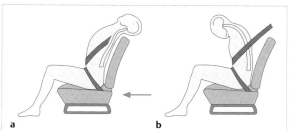

Fig. 17.1 a, b Acceleration injury of the cervical spine in a rear-end collision.
a First phase: sudden forward acceleration of the trunk with retroflexion of the cervical spine.
b Second phase: the head springs back (retroflexion).

motion of the cervical spine. These typical symptoms gradually subside over the course of a few days or weeks. The characteristic symptomatic course of acceleration injuries is thus of the "crescendo–decrescendo" type (Schröter 2004). Depending on the intensity of the applied force and the extent of pre-existing damage, other parts of the motion segment and neighboring structures can also be involved in the injury. The resulting symptom complex can be predominantly cervicobrachial or predominantly cervicocephalic, depending on which structures are affected. Pain in the arm (a post-traumatic cervicobrachial syndrome) can arise in a whiplash injury because of traction on the spinal nerves, which are relatively immobile within the intervertebral foramina. The examiner's report should always mention not only the palpatory findings and range of motion of the cervical spine, but also any neurological abnormalities such as weakness, diminished reflexes, paresthesiae, and sensory deficits.

The clinical examination should include cautious diagnostic assessment of the range of motion with segmental manual testing. If the force of the accident was such that a fracture is a possibility, plain cervical spine radiographs should be obtained before the range of motion is tested. The clinical neurological findings and plain cervical spine radiographs in two planes are part of the primary diagnostic battery for acceleration injuries of the cervical spine. Further optional studies include images specially demonstrating the craniocephalic junction through an open mouth (odontoid views), functional images obtained with inclination and reclination of the head, CT, and MRI.

Degree of Severity

The severity of cervical spine acceleration injuries is assessed as mild, moderate, or severe depending on the degree of tissue injury and the intensity of the post-traumatic symptoms. The Quebec Task Force (Spitzer 1995) proposed the following grading scale:

17

Table 17.2 The distribution of cervical spine accelera-tion injuries according to severity (ACIR, QT force)

Author/date	I	II	III (IV)
▪ Krämer (1997)	77	13.3	9.7
▪ Suissa (1999)	66	28	5
▪ Miettinen (2004)	47.2	10.4	0.7

Table 17.3 Persistent damage after cervical spine ac-celeration injuries

Author/date	Study	Persistent symp-toms 1 year after injury
Obelieniene (1999)	210 cervical spine injuries in traffic accidents, 210 control subjects	4.0% accidents 6.2% controls
Kasch (2003)	141 cervical spine injuries, 40 ankle injuries	7.8% cervical spine 0% ankle
Miettinen (2004)	144 cervical spine injuries	11.8% grades I/II 26.0% grade III

- grade I: neck pain and stiffness, negative physical findings
- grade II: neck pain, positive musculoskeletal findings on examination
- grade III: neck pain, positive musculoskeletal findings on examination, and neurologic signs
- grade IV: fracture or dislocation with corresponding symptoms.

This scale largely corresponds to the modified Erdmann scale customarily used in German-speaking countries (Krämer 1997), which, however, also takes the duration of the asymptomatic interval into account (**Table 17.2**). A grade of severity is assigned on the basis of the findings of the initial examination, most importantly with regard to the presence of any neurological deficits or involve-ment of bony structures. The great majority (91–99%) of all cervical spine acceleration injuries are of grades I and II (Krämer 1997, Suissa 1999, Miettinen 2004, Moorah-rend 2004).

Although it is often hard to judge whether a particu-lar case should be assigned a severity of grade I or grade II because of an inadequate primary examination, posi-tive neurological findings and bony changes are gener-ally evident from the start. Statistics regarding the dura-tion of illness and persistent damage (cf. **Table 17.3**) generally concern grade I and II injuries.

Treatment

The treatment of degenerative cervical spine symptoms and post-traumatic problems of the shoulder and neck has evolved in recent years. Previously, passive methods were preferred, such as heat application, soft cervical collars, and bed rest, sometimes with traction (Glisson traction). Currently, patients are advised to *stay active* and *behave normally,* as long as the cervical spine is not severely injured, which it usually is not (Nachemson and Jonsson 2000, Waddell 2001, Kitchel 2004). In addition, a monitored course of physiotherapy is usually advised, within the patient's range of tolerability. Analgesics, usually NSAIDs, are also given, and sometimes local in-filtrations. Cervical collars are used only transiently, for a few days, if at all.

We prefer this mode of treatment both on the basis of our own experience and because of the findings of ran-domized controlled prospective studies on the subject, which are well summarized in a meta-analysis by Seferidis et al. (2004). These studies compared a very diverse collection of therapeutic paradigms for acute and chronic post-traumatic symptoms (Mealy et al. 1986, McKinney et al. 1989, Pennie et al. 1990, Gennis et al. 1996, Borchgrevink 1998, Bonk et al. 2000, Rosenfeld et al. 2000, 2003, Söderlund et al. 2000).

Course and Prognosis

The organic changes associated with grade I or grade II acceleration injury of the cervical spine heal within a few weeks, or within 3 months at most. Suissa (1999), in an extensive study of 2600 patients with cervical spine acceleration injuries, found that the symptoms per-sisted for an average of 32 days. The prognosis of grade I and grade II acceleration injuries is generally considered good (Waddell 2001, McClune 2002). With appropriate treatment and appropriate behavior on the patient's part (keeping active), rapid recovery can be expected.

A longer time is required for the treatment of grade III injuries with pain and paresthesiae radiating into the upper limb, as well as for the treatment of traumatically induced cervical disk herniations.

Symptoms That Become Chronic

As can be seen from **Table 17.3**, not all individuals with less severe injuries (grades I and II) are asymptomatic 1 year afterward. Even in the well-known controlled study from Lithuania (Obelieniene 1999), a country in which there is no legally enforced basis for the monetary compensation of individuals claiming accel-eration injuries of the cervical spine, 4.0% of patients still had symptoms in the shoulder and neck that they attributed to the traffic accident 1 year after the event.

On the other hand, 6.2 % of the patients in the control group had shoulder and neck symptoms from other causes 1 year after the beginning of the study.

Kasch (2003) compared a group of individuals with cervical spine injuries with another group with ankle injuries. 7.8 % of the former, but 0 % of the latter, still had symptoms 1 year after the initial trauma.

Shoulder and neck symptoms may become chronic after cervical spine acceleration trauma, but apparently not just for somatic reasons (the high density of nociceptors in the cervical spine may predispose to chronic, recurrent symptoms); psychosocial factors also have a role to play. In the cervical spine, just as in the lumbar spine, chronic, recurrent symptoms are more likely to arise when certain psychosocial risk factors (yellow flags) are present, even when the initial findings are not at all severe.

By analogy to the risk factors for chronic back pain, which were discussed in Chapter 11, the risk factors for chronic neck symptoms after acceleration trauma of the cervical spine are listed in **Table 17.4**. The possibility of gain from illness, often considered the most important risk factor, is in fact only one among many. The risk factors listed in **Table 17.4** have not yet been validated and are generally not taken into account at present in the examination and medicolegal assessment of this group of patients. A few of them can already be addressed in primary treatment, e. g., inappropriate conceptions of illness that can be dealt with by adequate explanation and a description of the typical, benign course. Patients with a passive attitude should be told that they have a better chance of a good recovery if they remain as physically active as possible.

Medicolegal Assessment

In recent years, the medicolegal assessment of cervical spine acceleration injuries (whiplash) has tended to pay more attention to the magnitude of the forces responsible for the injury than to the actual medical events themselves. Many studies of whiplash were carried out on healthy volunteers; in some of these studies, the conditions of an accident were simulated (Castro et al. 1997, 1998). In one interdisciplinary study, volunteers were subjected to rear-end collisions with cars and motor-scooters. The primary question to be answered was whether any clinical or radiological (MRI) changes in the cervical spine could be detected after a rear-end automobile collision with a speed reduction of the order of 10–15 km/h. This study revealed, among other things, that none of the volunteers who had undergone collisions with a drop in speed of 11 km/h complained of any symptoms afterward. This result might be taken to imply that whiplash injury is essentially excluded if the reduction in speed during the impact is 10 km/h or less. In consequence, many medicolegal assessments in re-

Table 17.4 Risk factors for symptoms becoming chronic (yellow flags) after acceleration injuries of the cervical spine

- Inability to cope with psychosocial stresses
- Job dissatisfaction
- Low occupational qualifications
- Emotional problems (depression, anxiety)
- Passive attitude
- Inappropriate conception of illness
- Operant factors (gain from illness)
- Other unexplained pains besides neck pain
- Earlier acceleration trauma to the cervical spine for which a claim for compensation was submitted

cent years have been terminated early on, as soon the engineers consulted have been able to determine that the collision was at such a low speed that, for this reason alone, no cervical spine trauma could have occurred. The technical examination, after the fact, of the motor vehicles involved in the collision became the major objective of medicolegal assessment. As a reaction to this, however, many legal complaints and trials ensued, because the medical aspects of the original claims had not been taken into account. A retrospective technical analysis of the change of speed occurring at the moment of collision provides no more than an incomplete representation of the traumatic forces that were applied to the cervical spine during the accident.

The results of experimental rear-end collisions must be interpreted with caution (Di Stefano 1999) and still need to be confirmed by further studies. Even in low-speed collisions, the medicolegal assessment may yet favor the true generation of symptoms by the accident if the cervical spine was not in the anatomical position at the moment of impact (as in all of the experimental studies), but rather in a rotated or laterally inclined position. Pre-existing damage to the cervical spine also needs to be taken account in medicolegal assessment. An experienced assessor can evaluate the patient's description of the accident and the behavior of the physicians who were initially consulted to determine whether the course of subsequent events was truly consistent with a traumatic injury.

Head Position at the Moment of Impact

When the cervical spine is rotated or inclined to one side, it has a lower tolerance for accelerating forces with swinging movements of the head than when it is in its functional middle (anatomical) position. Such a situation arises, for example, when the individual is looking to one side precisely at the moment of collision. Rotation and lateral bending put the soft tissues, particularly the intervertebral joint capsules, under more tension

17

than in the anatomical position, so that an additional impulse is more likely to cause an injury (sprain).

Pre-existing Damage and Injury Resulting from the Accident

When trauma affects a cervical spine that has already undergone degenerative changes, it is generally the most degenerated segments that suffer the most severe injury. Motion segments that have been slackened, and thus rendered partially unstable, by degeneration are exquisitely sensitive to externally applied forces. The pain-sensitive neural elements in the spinal canal, the intervertebral foramina, and the joint capsules are not as well protected in the degeneratively destabilized motion segment as they are in the vicinity of normal disks. Reflex compensatory movements and muscle contractions of the type that can be induced by the sudden, unexpected application of a traumatizing force can lead to neural irritation and pain even when the applied force itself is relatively small. In such cases, the acceleration injury should be regarded as having caused a transient, rather than permanent (i. e., temporally limited), worsening of a process that was already in progress independently of the accident. The overall loss of earning capacity may be the same as in the absence of pre-existing damage but must be divided into accident-related and accident-independent components, the latter of which increases steadily as a percentage of the total over time. In mild or moderately severe acceleration trauma of the cervical spine (grades I and II), the accident-related component reaches a peak shortly after the accident and then gradually diminishes over the course of several weeks (maximum 3 months). Any symptoms that increase in severity after that, such as chronic, recurrent pain in the shoulder and neck that lasts for months or years after the injury, must be attributed to the accident-independent, pre-existing process of degenerative disease.

In the German system of statutory accident insurance, the accident-related component is held to be entirely responsible for the claimant's inability to work for a period of time immediately after the accident (all-or-nothing principle) until the accident-independent component becomes predominant, a maximum of 3 months after the accident. In private accident insurance, the accident-independent component is considered to play a role from the very beginning.

Temporal Course Consistent with a Traumatic Injury

The course of a post-traumatic cervical syndrome resembles that of a purely degenerative cervical syndrome. Its major symptoms are nuchal and occipital pain, painful restriction of movement of the cervical spine, and possibly radiation of the pain into the upper limb or back of the head, depending on the severity of the trauma. The clinical examination involves cautious segment-by-segment manual testing of mobility. The physician called upon to carry out a medicolegal assessment after the fact should bear in mind that the original medical findings immediately after the accident, and the behavior of the patient and the treating physician(s) at the time, can be used to determine whether the temporal course of the problem is consistent with an injury. The notes of the physicians who treated the patient initially are often fragmentary, and often one can only infer that certain symptoms were present from the types of diagnostic and therapeutic measures that were undertaken. These may include, for example, plain radiographs (radiation exposure!), prescriptions for analgesics and anti-inflammatories (with their known side effects), and perhaps local anesthetic infiltrations and manual therapy (also with their known side effects). Generally speaking, physicians would not order these measures unless they seemed to be justified by the findings of the history and physical examination.

The determination of causality requires careful consideration of pre-existing damage (if any), the mechanism and severity of the accident, the patient's subjective complaints, the objective findings of clinical examination, and the subsequent symptoms and measures undertaken by the treating physicians. It is important that the temporal course of the problem should be consistent with a traumatic injury.

Post-traumatic Stress Disorder

Independently of the purely somatic course of the traumatic injury, there may also be an emotional disturbance resulting from the accident, so-called post-traumatic stress disorder (Thomann and Rauschmann 2004). This term has found its way into the international psychiatric diagnostic manuals only in the last two decades. Studies have shown that it does not denote a uniform disease entity but is, rather, a collective designation for a number of different conditions. Emotional responses to accidents are due only in small part to the events of the accident themselves. Such was also the conclusion of the study by Castro et al. (2001), in which 51 subjects were (falsely) led to believe that they had sustained a rear-end collision. 20% of these healthy subjects had pain in the head and neck 3 days later; in 10%, the pain was still present 4 weeks after the initial "trauma." The subjects in this study were volunteers who had no possibility of claiming insurance benefits.

Nevertheless, symptoms that are entirely of emotional origin can be distinguished from the physical consequences of trauma by professional history-taking and clinical examination with the appropriate manual techniques.

Summary

Cervical spine acceleration injuries have a benign course. Typically, the neck pain reaches peak intensity some time after the accident and then gradually subsides over several weeks (maximum 3 months). Severe injuries and permanent damage are rare. The affected individuals should remain active. Recovery is promoted by an early return to normal activities and hindered by rest, passivity, and excessive medicalization of the patient's complaints.

The retrospective analysis of accidents to determine the reduction in speed of the vehicle at the moment of the collision cannot be used as the sole means of medicolegal assessment of cervical spine acceleration injuries. The position of the head at the time of impact, pre-existing degenerative changes, and a temporal course consistent with a traumatic injury are further important criteria.

It remains an open question whether individuals with a persistent emotional disturbance (post-traumatic stress disorder) after an accident should receive compensation even if physical examination reveals no somatic injury.

Conclusion

The medicolegal assessment of acceleration injuries is, at present, still complicated by a lack of clarity in the pertinent terminology, pathogenesis, and symptomatology.

■ Assessment of Loss of Earning Capacity in Lumbar Intervertebral Disk Disease

Definition and Classification of Loss of Earning Capacity

> **!** **Definition: Loss of earning capacity** is the impairment of an individual's ability to earn a living in the general job market, expressed as a percentage of the normal full amount, because of a current impairment of health; in the context of this chapter, because of intervertebral disk disease.

In terms of loss of earning capacity, the degree of disability can be classified depending on the severity of intervertebral disk disease (**Table 17.5**). The **spectrum of disability** due to lumbar intervertebral disk disease extends from no (i. e., no measurable) disability (level 0) in individuals with occasional, simple low back pain, a condition that affects practically everyone, without any significant radiological findings, all the way to very severe disability, e. g., inability to stand or walk combined with permanent sphincter dysfunction after a massive disk prolapse or a disk operation with complications (level 4). When the clinical assessment yields findings of a type that regularly implies significant damage to the spine, it should be possible for the assessor to determine the **loss of earning capacity** on a graded scale. The important criteria to be used for this purpose are the **history, pain, and clinical findings,** only then followed by the **radiological findings.**

Clinical Findings

The clinical criteria to be evaluated include the patient's subjective depiction of the history, the current complaints, information in the medical record concerning the past history of the present illness, and the findings of the assessor's physical examination of the patient. **Pain** is assessed with respect to its localization, whether or not it is dependent on movement, duration, and, above all, intensity. Low back pain that does not radiate into the leg should be assessed as less severe than low back pain associated with radicular or pseudoradicular symptoms; pain of the latter type is generally more severe and longer-lasting.

For the purpose of determining the patient's loss of earning capacity, the **severity of pain** in intervertebral disk disease, as in other painful conditions, can be graded with the aid of a visual analog scale (**Table 17.6**). The patient's statements regarding the intensity of the pain are, however, only of limited use in medicolegal assessment.

Table 17.5 Classification of degrees of disability

Level	Loss of earning capacity (%)	Degree of disability
0	0	None
1	10	Mild
2	10–20	Moderate
3	> 30	Severe
4	> 50	Very severe

Table 17.6 Classification of severity of pain

Pain	Visual analog scale	Loss of earning capacity (%)
Mild	0–3	0–20
Moderate	4–6	20–30
Severe	7–10	> 30

17

The findings of physical examination of the back and leg are incorporated into the assessment. If the patient's symptoms are restricted to the lumbar region, then the patient is suffering from a **local lumbar syndrome** (see Chapter 11). The symptoms of local lumbar syndrome can be alleviated fairly well by the adoption of a correct posture and other correct behaviors, as taught in back school. **Limitations on physical activity** include a limited ability to sit or stand for long periods of time, to work in a stooped position, or to lift and carry weights heavier than 10–20 kg, depending on the intensity of the pain. Walking is beneficial, as is an alternation between walking, standing, and sitting. The therapeutic recommendation is to stay active, rather than rest.

> **!** The loss of earning capacity associated with a local lumbar syndrome is between 10% and 20%, depending on its severity.

In **lumbar radicular syndromes,** the more or less severe symptoms of a local lumbar syndrome are combined with signs of nerve root compression (see Chapter 11). The constellation of clinical manifestations in lumbar radicular syndromes is varied and depends on the severity of the condition and the particular nerve root affected. Serious manifestations that limit the patient's physical activity include severe pain and weakness of functionally important muscles, such as the foot dorsiflexors and knee extensors (quadriceps). Residual reflex abnormalities and sensory disturbances, on the other hand, do not impair the patient's ability to function. Another possible feature that should not be judged as serious is weakness of functionally less important muscles, such as a toe dorsiflexor paresis or a mild weakness of plantar flexion. If only this type of weakness is present and the pain, if any, is mild, no surgical treatment is indicated, even if the imaging studies show an impressive disk herniation.

Nerve root syndromes, unlike local lumbar syndromes, generally do not improve to any great extent when the individual adopts a proper posture and other spine-friendly behaviors. The ability to lift and carry loads, sit, stand, or work in a stooped position for more than a short period of time is impaired. The same therapeutic recommendation applies to lumbar root syndromes as to local lumbar syndromes: avoid bed rest, remain as active as possible, and go about your normal daily activities as far as you can. However, a large part of the employment market is closed to these patients, even for light or moderate physical work.

> **!** The loss of earning capacity for lumbar root syndromes with moderate or severe pain and/or weakness of functionally important muscles is 30% or more.

Persistent, severe cauda equina dysfunction is a special category of lumbar root syndrome and is associated with a loss of earning capacity of more than 50%. The same figure applies to chronic, recurrent lumbar root syndromes corresponding to a grade II or grade III postdiscotic syndrome.

Radiologic Findings

Radiologic findings are assessed for the purpose of rating loss of earning capacity only in conjunction with the clinical findings (history, physical examination). The following may be clinically relevant:
- loss of height in one or more intervertebral disks exceeding the normal age-related loss of height
- intervertebral joint arthrosis (spondylarthrosis)
- dorsal spondylophytes (retrospondylosis)
- disk protrusion
- disk prolapse
- degenerative spondylolisthesis
- retrolisthesis
- postoperative adhesions.

In contrast, sclerosis of the vertebral body end plates, "black disks" in MRI, and spondylosis are clinically irrelevant findings. Osteophyte formation is only of clinical importance, with an impairment of functional ability, in the case of osteophytes that protrude posteriorly into the spinal canal (so-called retrospondylosis) and impinge on a nerve root. Osteophytes growing from the anterior and lateral edges of the vertebral bodies are clinically irrelevant, even if they are very marked and partially or completely bridge one or more intervertebral disks, because they cannot come into contact with any neural structures. They may be of medicolegal importance, however, as a component of the typical stress-related pattern of spinal damage as an occupational illness.

Clinically relevant radiologic findings include marked, rapidly progressive loss of disk height to less than one-third of the original height, causing increased stress on the intervertebral joints and consequent arthrosis (spondylarthrosis), which expresses itself clinically as a so-called lumbar facet syndrome (a particular variety of local lumbar syndrome). The pain and functional impairment that result are not significantly disabling, because they can be alleviated fairly well by the adoption of a correct posture and other correct behaviors, as taught in back school, and by exercise (staying active). The corresponding loss of earning capacity is less than 10%.

On the other hand, more severe disability results from disk tissue displacement, i. e., protrusions and prolapses of the lower lumbar disks with impingement on the nerve roots and the corresponding lumbar radicular syndromes, because inappropriate behavior can easily make the condition worse. The loss of earning capacity in such cases is more than 30%. There is an exception to this rule for disk protrusions (usually solitary ones) that jut out more than 5 mm beyond the line connecting the dorsal edges of the vertebrae above and below but do not (yet) impinge on a nerve root, or do so only to a minimal extent and cause no more than mild symptoms. In such cases, the limitation on the patient's physical ability arises mainly from the possibility of worsening with inappropriate behavior that is suggested by the MRI findings. For similar reasons, any segmental instability that has been documented with functional plain radiographs on inclination and reclination of the spine can also be considered to limit the patient's physical ability to some extent, even if it is associated with little or no pain.

Cessation of Harmful Activity

No matter what type or degree of spinal damage is judged to be present, the medicolegal assessment must state which of the following activities that are demanded of the human body in various occupations can be done only to a limited extent by the patient, as well as the degree of the limitation and the reason for it:

- walking
- standing
- sitting
- working in a stooped posture
- lifting
- carrying loads of various weights
- working above the head.

The **spectrum of loss of earning capacity** due to intervertebral disk disease ranges from low levels, in which a recommendation to continue working is part of the treatment, to higher levels (above 20%), in which the patient is obliged to refrain from harmful activities.

Cessation means entirely desisting from the harmful activity, both because the patient has too much pain and functional impairment to do it and because continuing with it could result in further harm. The obligation to cease the harmful activity should be determined on the basis of objective evidence. There is no such obligation if the level of loss of earning capacity is low. This is because of the current therapeutic attitude toward intervertebral disk disease: the previous idea that bed rest and restricted activity were strongly advisable in cases of low back pain and sciatica has now given way, because of the findings of controlled studies, to a recommendation to stay active and continue going about one's daily activities, including light and moderately heavy physical work (Nachemson and Jonsson 2000, Waddell 2004, Bolm-Audorff et al. 2005, German Back Pain Guidelines 2006, Krämer 2006*).

Levels of Loss of Earning Capacity

Most types of illness are categorized into stages and degrees of severity. The stages of intervertebral disk disease are defined according to the stages of disk degeneration and the corresponding clinical manifestations. Classification systems generally refer to mild, moderate, and severe degrees of illness, but this threefold scheme is too imprecise and not reproducible enough to be used in the rating of loss of earning capacity due to disk disease. A more precise classification, such as that shown in **Table 17.7,** is needed to take proper account of all of the degrees of functional impairment that may be caused by intervertebral disk disease, ranging from insignificant amounts of low back pain to very severe disability due to nerve root compression.

Disk-related Symptoms with 0% Loss of Earning Capacity

Diagnosis. Simple low back pain. This category includes the type of occasional low back pain that affects practically all humans, with a very high point and annual prevalence and a lifetime prevalence of 100% (see Chapter 3).

Clinical features. Every human occasionally suffers from low back pain, e. g., after long periods of free standing or transiently after lifting and carrying heavy objects, but also sometimes without any evident cause. Occasionally, there may also be brief episodes of severe low back pain associated with immobility of the lumbar spine, so-called lumbago.

Radiologic findings. Plain radiographs of the lumbosacral spine reveal the intervertebral disks to be of normal height for age. In individuals doing heavy physical work and high-performance athletes, the greater degree of stress placed on the musculoskeletal system is reflected by sclerosis of the vertebral body end plates, sometimes accompanied by osteophyte formation. These findings are of no clinical importance.

Limitation of physical activity. Such individuals can do any kind of work, including heavy physical labor. An episode of lumbago causes only a transient inability to do heavy physical labor, possibly requiring a doctor's note excusing the patient from work for a limited period of time.

Prevention. Primary preventive measures against intervertebral disk disease are good practice for everyone (see Chapter 14).

---

* The English translation of this book is due to be published in 2009.

17

Table 17.7 Assessment of lumbar disk diseases in terms of loss of earning capacity

Level	0	1	2	3	4
Limitation of physical activity, general	None	Mild	Moderate	Severe	Very severe
Loss of earning capacity	0%	10%	20%	30–40%	50% and above
Diagnosis	Simple low back pain	Local lumbar syndrome with mild low back pain	Local lumbar syndrome with regularly occurring, severe low back pain and occasional manifestations of nerve root irritation	Local lumbar syndrome with severe low back and leg pain, neurological deficits, grade I or II PDS	Lumbar root syndrome, severe motor disturbances, cauda equina syndrome, grade II or III PDS
Clinical features	Occasional low back pain	Regularly occurring, mild low back pain, residual mild manifestations of nerve root irritation	Regularly occurring low back and leg pain without neurological deficits	Local lumbar syndrome, radiation into the leg, severe pain, neurological disturbances	Very severe pain, inability to stand or walk, sphincter disturbances
Radiologic findings	Normal for age	Loss of disk height, spondylarthrosis	Osteochondrosis, spondylarthrosis, protrusion	Protrusion, prolapse, scar tissue	Protrusion, prolapse, scar tissue
Limitation of physical activity, special	No limitation	Frequent work in a stooped posture, manipulation of heavy loads	Work for long periods in a single, maintained posture while sitting and/or standing, more than occasional work in a stooped posture, manipulation of heavy loads	Sitting and standing, work in a stooped posture only for short periods and with frequent breaks, no lifting or carrying	Any type of occupational activity
Prevention	General protective measures	Special protective measures	Special protective measures and, if necessary, refraining from certain activities	Refraining from certain activities	Refraining from certain activities

Level 1: Mild Limitation of Physical Activity (10% Loss Of Earning Capacity)

Diagnosis. Local lumbar syndrome with mild low back pain.

Clinical features. Regularly occurring low back pain, with pain on movement and mechanical loading, muscle spasm, and limited range of motion of the lumbar spine. All of these manifestations persist for longer periods of time. Level 1 also includes residual, mild sensory nerve root phenomena, e. g., in the aftermath of a nerve root compression syndrome or as the patient's final condition after recovery from successful disk surgery.

Radiologic findings. Loss of height of one or more disks, spondylarthrosis.

Limitation of physical activity. Frequent work in a stooped position and the manipulation of heavy loads should be avoided, as these activities can be expected to aggravate the regularly occurring low back pain.

Prevention. The recommendations for individuals with level 1 intervertebral disk disease include ergonomic optimization of the workplace, the use of lifting and carrying aids at work, and participation in sports and gymnastics.

Level 2: Intermediate Limitation of Physical Activity (10–20% Loss of Earning Capacity)

Diagnosis. Local lumbar syndrome with regularly occurring, severe low back pain and occasional nerve root manifestations.

17

Clinical features. Frequently occurring low back pain, with pain on movement and mechanical loading, muscle spasm, and limited range of motion of the lumbar spine. The pain may occasionally radiate into the leg, but there is no neurologic deficit. This category also includes patients with an intermediate degree of functional limitation after surgery.

Radiologic findings. Loss of height of the intervertebral disks, spondylarthrosis, protrusion, postoperative scarring.

Limitation of physical activity. Inability to maintain a single sitting or standing posture for any length of time, to work in a stooped posture on more than an occasional basis, or to manipulate heavy loads.

Prevention. Special protective measures as in level 1; cessation of the harmful activity if it is regularly associated with a stooped posture and/or the manipulation of heavy loads.

Level 3: Severe Limitation of Physical Activity (30–40 % Loss of Earning Capacity)

Diagnosis. Lumbar root compression syndrome with severe low back and leg pain and weakness of functionally important muscles. Grade I or II post-discotic syndrome.

Clinical features. Lumbar syndrome with segmental pain and sensory disturbances that are always present.

Radiologic findings. Protrusion, prolapse, postoperative scarring.

Limitation of physical activity. Sitting, standing, and working in a stooped posture are possible only for short periods of time with breaks in between.

Prevention. The patient should avoid the activities that are harmful to the spine.

Level 4: Very Severe Limitation of Physical Activity (> 50 % Loss of Earning Capacity)

Diagnosis. Lumbar nerve root compression syndrome, severe weakness, cauda equina syndrome, grade II or III post-discotic syndrome.

Clinical features. The patient has very severe pain and must regularly take strong analgesics. There is a marked impairment of stance and gait, and may also be sphincter dysfunction.

Radiologic findings. Protrusion, prolapse, postoperative scarring.

Limitation of physical activity. The patient can no longer pursue a regular job, not just because of the pain, but also because of the regular intake of analgesics, usually opioids, which would make it dangerous for the patient either to drive or to take public transport to work.

Prevention. Cessation of occupational activity.

Problems in Medicolegal Assessment

The requirement that each patient should be assigned a well-grounded percentage loss of earning capacity, after the medicolegal assessment has revealed consistent findings, creates certain difficulties with respect to intervertebral disk disease.

Course and Prognosis

Intervertebral disk diseases take a fluctuating course. Over the human life span, the frequency and intensity of disk diseases reach a peak in middle age (35–45 years) and then decline gradually after age 50. This implies that, when a 40-year-old man presents with a disk prolapse causing a lumbar root syndrome as an occupational illness, is assigned a 30 % loss of earning capacity, and is medicolegally required to cease the harmful activity, his disk disease will normally improve over the next year or two in response to appropriate conservative treatment, gradually developing into a local lumbar syndrome with a loss of earning capacity of less than 10 %. His risk of sustaining a new prolapse is now no greater than in other individuals with level I or II disk disease. It may be difficult, however, to reintegrate him into his original occupational activity after the temporary cessation.

Follow-up examinations and adjustments of the loss of earning capacity are certainly necessary.

Psychosocial Factors

When the patient's complaints of pain and functional impairment do not correspond to the clinical neurological findings or to the radiologic findings, it is difficult to assign an appropriate level of loss of earning capacity. Psychosocial factors (yellow flags) often play a role. In such cases, a psychologist should be consulted.

Variability

The clinical findings and course of disk diseases are highly variable, and the types of findings that are regularly seen may come in different combinations. Some patients with local lumbar syndrome, who by definition have no pain radiating into the lower limb, nonetheless

17

have such severe back pain and functional impairment that their physical activity is severely limited and they must be assigned a loss of earning capacity of 30% or more and required to stop the harmful occupational activity. The cause may be, for example, a rapid loss of disk height causing segmental instability and severe stress on the intervertebral joints (a rare event). A rare occurrence of this type may constitute an indication for a fusion procedure. On the other hand, lumbar root syndromes may be associated with only mild symptoms and cause only a mild limitation of physical activity, with a low level of loss of earning capacity and no requirement to stop the occupational activity in question. All patients must be assessed individually.

Postoperative States

Surgery on a lumbar intervertebral disk (discotomy) or fusion surgery is only rarely followed by a total cure of disk disease without any functional impairment (restoration to the normal state). The motion segment that has been operated upon by discotomy, and also the neighboring segments after fusion surgery, will always remain more than normally vulnerable to externally applied forces. Even a relatively small disk protrusion that would have caused only a transient local lumbar syndrome, or mild symptoms of nerve root irritation, in a patient who had not previously undergone surgery can produce severe and lasting symptoms of nerve root irritation, with marked limitation of physical activity, if it arises in a segment that was previously operated upon, because postoperative adhesions at this site firmly anchor the nerve root to the surrounding structures. A variably severe post-discotic syndrome arises after 10% of all disk operations; if present, this must be taken into account in the assessment of loss of earning capacity. If the surgically treated disk herniation was recognized as an occupational illness by the insurance provider, then all consequences of the operation, potentially including post-discotic syndrome of any degree of severity, must also be recognized as being of occupational origin, and the loss of earning capacity must be determined accordingly. Thus, in view of the relatively high values of loss of earning capacity assigned to patients who must cease occupational activity because of postoperative conditions, insurance providers would do well to pay particular attention to the indications for surgery, and to the manner in which surgery is carried out and postoperative care is delivered, for all patients whose illness might be recognized as being of occupational origin.

The complete list of references can be found online at: http://www.thieme.de/go/kraemer-disks/

17

Subject Index

Notes: Page references in *italics* refer to figures and those in **bold** refer to tables